**Thomas S. Leeson, MD, PhD**
*Professor of Anatomy*
*Department of Anatomy*
*University of Alberta*
*Edmonton, Alberta, Canada*

**C. Roland Leeson, MD, PhD**
*Professor of Anatomical Sciences*
*College of Medicine*
*University of Illinois*
*Urbana, Illinois*

**Anthony A. Paparo, PhD**
*Professor of Anatomy*
*Department of Anatomy*
*School of Medicine*
*Professor of Zoology*
*Department of Zoology*
*College of Science*
*Southern Illinois University*
*Carbondale, Illinois*

# Text /Atlas of
# *HISTOLOGY*

**W.B. SAUNDERS COMPANY**
**Harcourt Brace Jovanovich, Inc.**

*Philadelphia London Toronto Montreal Sydney Tokyo*

**W. B. SAUNDERS COMPANY**
Harcourt Brace Jovanovich, Inc.

The Curtis Center
Independence Square West
Philadelphia, Pennsylvania 19106

**Library of Congress Cataloging-in-Publication Data**

Leeson, Thomas Sydney.
   Text/atlas of histology/Thomas S. Leeson, C. Roland
Leeson, Anthony A. Paparo.
   p.    cm.
Includes index.
ISBN 0–7216–2386–7
   1. Histology. 2. Histology–Atlases.   I. Leeson, C.
Roland (Charles Roland), 1926–        II. Paparo,
Anthony A.   III. Title.
   [DNLM: 1. Histology. 2. Histology—atlases. QS 504
L4872t]
QM551.L425 1988                                    87–26649
611′.018—dc19                                            CIP

To order the accompanying set of 200 color slides (order #0-7216-2824-9),
call 1-800-782-4479 or write HRW/WBS, Attention Order Processing,
6277 Sea Harbor Drive, Orlando, Florida 32821

Listed here is the latest edition of this book together with the language of the translation and the
publisher.

Spanish—1st Edition—Nueva Editorial Interamericana, Mexico City, Mexico

*Editor:*  Martin Wonsiewicz

*Developmental Editor:*  Kathleen McCullough

*Designer:*  W. B. Saunders Staff

*Production Manager:*  Frank Polizzano

*Manuscript Editor:*  Gina Scala

*Illustration Coordinator:*  Walter Verbitski

*Page Layout Artist:*  Dorothy Chattin

*Indexer:*  Susan Thomas

*Illustrators:*  Karen Giacomucci, Glenn Edelmayer, Philip Ashley, Laurence Ward

Text/Atlas of Histology                                    ISBN 0–7216–2386–7

Last digit is the print number:    9    8    7    6    5    4    3

Dedicated to our wives,
Mary, Marjorie, and Kathleen,
and to our respective children

# PREFACE

This edition represents a major change from the format of our previous publications. The fifth edition of our *Textbook of Histology* was published in 1985 simultaneously with the second edition of our *Atlas of Histology*. The textbook and the atlas have been used together in many courses and by numerous students, but, in other courses, only one has proved to be necessary. In some histology courses, the bulk of the material is presented by lectures and demonstrations, with little or no laboratory time allocated. In such situations, the intelligent use by students of an atlas has proved to be of value, although we hasten to add that it never was our intention for the atlas to be regarded as a substitute for the use of the microscope. Student experience with microscopy is invaluable, and, in courses with this as a component, the atlas has been, and we hope will continue to be, useful in the identification and interpretation of tissue sections. It also has proved to be of value in other disciplines, providing, for example, a morphological background for the interpretation of functional activities in physiology and for comparison of normal and diseased states in pathology. In some histology courses, study of a textbook is required and necessary for the acquisition of knowledge, but the use of an atlas is not essential. It is our hope that both textbook and atlas will continue to find acceptance by both students and course coordinators in such situations.

Over the more than 20 years since the first edition of our textbook was published, the suggestion that consideration should be given to the use of more color illustrations has been made on several occasions. The use of color figures obviously has some advantages and, to many readers, is esthetically pleasing. Over the last two decades, the use of color in general has increased, but it does imply an increase in costs and, consequently, an increase in price. Throughout these years, it always has been our aim to keep costs and prices as low as possible, consistent with quality, and we are well aware of the ever-increasing demands upon students in respect to the acquisition of textbooks and other learning materials. It was with these background thoughts that we considered the major change of combining and integrating the material in the textbook and atlas. Didactically, there was little doubt that the concept offered many advantages, and preliminary discussions with our publishers elicited interest, even enthusiasm. While many figures from the current editions of the textbook and the atlas could be, and have been, utilized with a corresponding saving in expenditures, the authors and publishers accepted the need both to replace some figures and to add others. This has been done.

The preparation of this new volume also provided the opportunity to revise and bring up to date the material, and, early in its evolution, we accepted that it was preferable to rewrite entirely. In some chapters, the rewrite also included some reorganization. We decided to maintain the format of the current text and its companion atlas with an Introduction and seventeen chapters divided into two major parts—General Histological Principles and Primary Tissues (Chapters 1 through 7) and Histology of the Organ Systems (Chapters 8 through 17). This is a logical and proven organization of the material and reflects the scheduling of many histology courses designed for science, medical, dental, paramedical, and other students. At the same time, each chapter is a separate entity, and use of this book does not dictate course structure

Histology has a close relationship with other disciplines, particularly cell biology, physiology, and pathology, and, perhaps to a lesser extent, with biochemistry and immunology. These evolving interrelationships have resulted in some change in emphasis and content throughout the book. Careful attention has been given to economy and clarity in the descriptive material. The figure descriptions have been designed to be informative, and, where necessary, they are relatively expansive. This is a response to student suggestions. New also is the provision of an outline at the beginning of each chapter and, at the conclusion, a chapter summary. In many chapters, the summary is in tabular form, highlighting the major components of the tissue, organ, or system, but in other chapters, where deemed appropriate, it provides a functional, rather than a morphological, review. After careful consideration, we have eliminated the list of references at the end of each chapter. It is our experience that few students have the time or interest to pursue further reading in the discipline. If necessary, this can be directed by course coordinators for their courses. Further, the computerization of libraries has facilitated the search for additional material, and such aid now is available to most students.

We hope the new layout of the book and the presentation of the material will prove attractive and inducive to learning. They reflect our desire to coordinate and integrate textual and illustrative material. Within the text, a reference is made to each figure, and an attempt has been made to place each figure in close proximity to the textual material that it illustrates. Where appropriate, several figures have been grouped together. It is hoped that this format will eliminate, or greatly reduce, the necessity of scanning backward and forward in the text or, indeed, of constantly referring from one book to another. We trust that it will prove to be both practical and efficient.

We are especially indebted to Dr. Hai-Nan Tung who allowed us free access to his files of negatives and willingly gave permission to include micrographs, most of which have not been published elsewhere. We would like to express our sincerest appreciation to Drs. Don W.Fawcett, Thomas L. Lentz, Radivoj V. Krstic, Tsuneo Fujita, Keiichi Tanaka, and Junichi Tokunaga, who generously allowed us to use transmission electron micrographs, scanning electron micrographs, and composite fine-structure diagrams from their textbooks. We acknowledge the generosity of their publishers and the courtesy given to us by so many of our colleagues. Above all, we thank our students, who, over the years, have provided the stimulation that has made this professional activity so satisfying. We have become even more enthusiastic about communicating to students by textbook as well as in the classroom, and we hope that this is apparent in our writing and visual explanations.

Our thanks for secretarial assistance go to Ms. Leslie McCormack, Ms. Candida Morris, Ms. Marjorie Gillett, and Ms. Lorie Hatfield. We are particularly indebted to Ms. Leona Allison for her extraordinary artistic talents and for most of the original drawings. We thank Mr. Philip Ashley, Mr. Glen Edelmayer, Mr. Larry Ward, and

Mrs. Karen Giacomucci for some of the colored illustrations and for their personal interest in, and enthusiasm for, this project. In the preparation of this book, we have worked closely with Martin Wonsiewicz, ably assisted by Kitty McCullough, and we thank them and all their associates at the W. B. Saunders Company for their support and encouragement. Our wives and families continue to show forbearance for our continuing, even continuous, abstraction from, and apparent disinterest in, family affairs. We assure them that their support is greatly appreciated.

Anthony A. Paparo<br>
Thomas S. Leeson<br>
C. Roland Leeson

# CONTENTS

# Introduction

## HISTOLOGY: WHAT DOES IT EMBRACE?

Histology, a term derived from the Greek *histos*, meaning tissue, and *logia*, meaning "the study of" or knowledge, literally, then, means the knowledge, or science, of tissues, both plant and animal. This textbook is restricted, in the main, to a consideration of human histology.

What does the term "histology" actually encompass? Anatomy, the science of the structure of the animal body, can be subdivided into that which is visible to the naked eye—*gross anatomy*—and that which can be seen only with the aid of a microscope—*microscopic anatomy*. The latter can be further subdivided into *organology* (the study of organs), *histology* (tissues), and *cytology* (cells). Today the term "histology" is used loosely to include all subdivisions of microscopic anatomy, and it is in this sense that the term is used here.

Although it is often stated that the body is made up of *cells*, it is important to appreciate that the body tissues contain two other important components. If the body were composed of cells alone, it would be too weak to support the mass. To solve this problem, cells of one of the basic tissues, connective tissue, elaborate several kinds of lifeless but not inert *intercellular substances*. Moreover, to maintain their life and functional activity, cells must have a continuous supply both of oxygen and of nutrients, and a method for removal of their toxic byproducts. This is achieved by the *body fluids*, including blood, which circulates within the blood vascular system, and other fluids, which will be considered later. The three components of the body tissues are therefore (1) *cells*, (2) *intercellular substances*, and (3) *body fluids*.

Thus, histology not only involves the study of tissues, composed of cells, intercellular substances, and body fluids, but also embraces a consideration of individual cell types and organ systems. And since histology refers to the study of cells, tissues, and organs, it includes a study of function as well as of structure. Therefore, the study of histology not only complements the study of gross anatomy but also provides a structural basis for the study of physiology. The correlation between structure and function is essential and perhaps provides the reason that histology is such an intriguing and readily understandable subject. Students should find that if they examine the structure of an organ or tissue, they can deduce much about its function. Conversely, if they know its function, they can forecast more easily much of its microscopic structure. It must be emphasized that histology is, in general, a visual discipline. It combines observation with reasoning. Thus, the illustrations in this book must be considered as basic, not supplementary, material.

A knowledge of the normal is a necessary prelude to the study of the abnormal (pathology), which deals with the alterations in structure and function of the body and of its organs, tissues, and cells caused by disease processes. Hence, the study of histology is fundamental to medical and dental curricula. For students of biology who do not intend to pursue degrees in histology, such study provides a reservoir of valuable knowledge. Too often, in many special fields of biological science, the student becomes involved in problems of a functional nature without being exposed to sufficient consideration of the underlying microscopic structure.

## METHODOLOGY

In the study of histology, there are two important considerations with regard to methodology:

1. The type of microscope used.

2. The preparation of the tissue or organ in a manner suitable for viewing with the microscope.

In general, the development of histological techniques has lagged behind the technical achievements made in connection with the various types of microscopes. Perhaps the best example of this applies to the electron microscope. Although the electron microscope was developed in the early 1930s, it was not utilized to any extent in biological work until the late 1940s and early 1950s, when methods of *thin sectioning* were developed. (This technique is described later in this chapter).

Microscopy dates from the 17th century when Hooke and Malpighi employed simple lenses in the study of various structural features. Between 1673 and 1716, Leeuwenhoek developed compound lenses, and by the early 19th century, the compound microscope had become highly sophisticated. In the latter part of the 19th century, the *microtome* (an instrument for preparing sections of tissue for study) was developed commercially, and hand in hand with its appearance came the development of fixing, embedding, and staining techniques. Staining techniques still are in the process of development, particularly with regard to their application to the newer forms of microscopy.

In the study of histology, the student will be introduced to the results obtained from various forms of microscopy and histological technique How these results were obtained should always be borne in mind since it influences their interpretation. Thus, it is important for the student to understand the applications and limitations of the various types of microscopes in use today and the basic principles underlying the different methods of preparation of tissues.

## Microscopy

Several types of microscopes are available for the study of biological material. Basically, they may be classified by the type of light source used. In most general use is the light (or optical) microscope using visible light. Modifications of this type include the polarization, phase-contrast, interference, and dark-field microscopes. Microscopes that utilize a nonvisible light source, the ultraviolet and electron microscopes, are more recent developments.

The usefulness of any type of microscope depends not only upon its ability to magnify but, more important, upon its ability to resolve detail. Beyond certain limits, magnification adds no new detail. The useful magnification of an ordinary light microscope is about 1500 times (1500 ×). The *resolving power* is a measure of the capacity of the microscope to clearly separate two points that lie close together. Beyond the resolving power of any microscope, two points will appear as one. The resolution with lens systems is limited by the wavelength of the light and by the numerical aperture, or light-gathering capacity, of the objective lens. The resolving power of a well-constructed light microscope is about 0.2 micron (μ), or micrometer (μm). (See footnote on units of measurement, p. 5.)

## MICROSCOPES UTILIZING A VISIBLE LIGHT SOURCE

**The Light (or Optical) Microscope.** Basically, the light microscope acts as a two-stage magnifying device (Fig. 1). An objective lens provides the initial magnification, and an ocular (projector) lens is placed so as to magnify the primary image a second time. Total magnification is obtained by multiplying the magnifying power of the objective and ocular lenses. An additional condensing lens normally is employed beneath the stage of the microscope to concentrate the light from its source into a very bright beam illuminating the specimen, thus providing sufficient light for the inspection of

the magnified image. Although the condenser lens does not contribute to the total magnification, it does influence the quality of the image observed.

The path of light rays through the microscope is indicated in Figure 1, on the left. The ocular (projector) lens commonly used has a magnification of × 10, although many microscopes are equipped with alternative eyepieces that provide different magnifications. Generally, the objective lens assembly consists of several detachable lenses mounted on a revolving disc at the lower end of the microscope tube. These lenses can be interchanged as required by rotating the disc through part of a turn. The four objectives routinely used have magnifications of × 10, × 25, × 40, and × 100, respectively. The × 10 objective, called the *low-power objective*, when combined with a × 10 ocular lens, gives a total magnification of × 100. Similarly, the × 25 objective, called the *medium-power objective*,

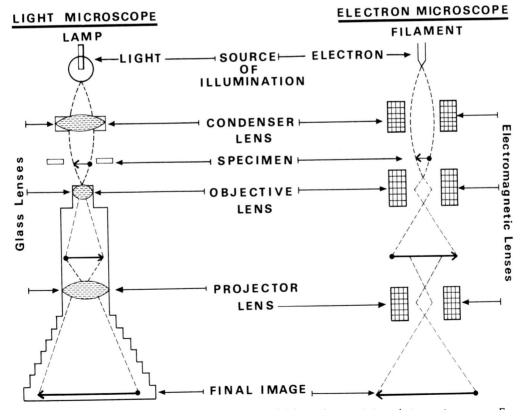

**Figure 1.** *Diagrammatic comparison of the optical systems of light and transmission electron microscopes. For ease of comparison, the system of the light microscope has been inverted and a camera attachment added.*

and the × 40 objective, the *high-power objective*, together with the × 10 ocular lens, provide total magnifications of × 250 and × 400, respectively. The × 100 objective, also known as the *oil-immersion objective*, in combination with the × 10 ocular lens, gives a total magnification of × 1000. When using the oil-immersion lens, it is necessary to replace the air gap between the objective lens and the coverslip of the specimen with an immersion oil of suitable refractive index. This objective must be focused very carefully, since it closely approaches the coverslip. It should be added that the extent of what can be seen in a section decreases in proportion to the magnification being used.

**The Polarizing Microscope.** Many natural objects, including crystals and fibers, exhibit an optical property known as double refraction, or *birefringence*. In histological material, birefringence is caused by asymmetric molecules, too small to be resolved even by the best light microscopic lenses, that are oriented in a nonrandom manner. Thus, an examination of birefringence permits deductions to be made concerning the organization of structure not demonstrable by regular methods of microscopy.

In its simplest form, the polarizing microscope is a conventional microscope in which a Nicol prism (or Polaroid sheet) is interposed in the light path below the condenser lens. This "polarizer" converts all light passing through the microscope into plane polarized light, or light that vibrates in one optical plane only. A similar, second prism, termed the "analyzer," is placed within the barrel of the microscope above the objective lens. When the analyzer is rotated until its axis is perpendicular to that of the polarizer, no light can pass through the ocular lens, resulting in a dark-field effect. The field will remain black if an *isotropic*, or singly refractive, object is placed on the specimen stage. A birefringent object, however, will rotate the axis of the light emerging from the polarizer and will appear as a light structure on a dark background. Birefringence, or *anisotropy*, is exhibited by many biological structures, for example, muscle fibers, certain connective tissue fibers, lipid droplets within the suprarenal cortex, and the rods and cones of the retina.

**The Phase-Contrast Microscope.** Lack of contrast has always presented a problem in biological work because the refractive indices of all parts of a specimen are similar. In normal microscopy, one overcomes this problem by staining differentially, but this is subject to numerous limitations. Phase microscopy provides a method whereby contrast is created by purely optical means.

The *refractive index* is a measure of the optical density of an object, or the speed with which it is traversed by a light wave. Air, for instance, has a refractive index of approximately 1.0, water about 1.3, and glass about 1.5. In other words, light travels fastest in air, more slowly in water, and slower still in glass. Light waves traversing equal distances through air, water, and glass will emerge and be bent out of phase with each other. The phase-contrast microscope contains optical plates placed within the condenser and objective lenses that convert the phase differences into amplitude differences. Briefly, therefore, differences in refractive index are rendered directly visible. Objects ordinarily transparent become visible through contrast differences. The phase-contrast microscope is of no particular assistance in the study of fixed and stained preparations in which transparency differences are not important. The instrument finds its application chiefly in the study of living cells and tissues and of unstained, plastic-embedded thick sections.

**The Interference Microscope.** The interference microscope, like the phase-contrast microscope, depends upon the ability of an object to retard light. However, unlike the phase microscope, which depends upon the specimen diffracting (bending) light, the interference microscope sends two separate beams of light through the specimen. These beams then are combined in the image plane. After recombination, difference in retardation of the light results in interference that can be used to measure the thickness or refractive index of the object under investigation.

**The Dark-Field Microscope.** This microscope utilizes a strong, oblique light that does not enter the objective lens. A special dark-field condenser allows no light to pass through the center of the lens. Light thus reaches the specimen to be viewed at an angle so oblique that none of it can enter the objective lens. The field is therefore dark. However, small particles present in the specimen will reflect some light into the objective lens and will appear as glistening spots. Thus, it is possible to visualize particles far below the limits of bright light resolution. The effect is similar to the phenomenon of dust particles "seen" in a beam of sunlight entering a darkened room. Darkfield examination also is useful in the study of small transparent objects, such as chylomicrons (particles of fat in the blood), which are invisible in the glare of bright-field illumination.

### MICROSCOPES UTILIZING A NONVISIBLE LIGHT SOURCE

All the microscopes that have just been discussed utilize visible light. However, images can be formed by rays other than visible light and, in this instance, since the images cannot be viewed directly, they are made visible by means of a suitably sensitized photographic film. In general, the rays used in these special microscopes all have a shorter wavelength than that of visible light and thus permit higher resolution.

**The Ultraviolet Microscope.** Since ordinary optical lenses are practically opaque to ultraviolet light, quartz lenses are used throughout the lens system. The microscope depends upon the differential absorption of ultraviolet light by molecules within the specimen, and the results are recorded photographically. In principle, this system allows an improvement in resolution about twice that of the light microscope (0.1 micron [$\mu$], or micrometer [$\mu$m]). The system is useful for detecting proteins that contain certain amino acids and in detecting nucleic acids.

Ultraviolet light also is employed in *fluorescence microscopy* (Fig. 2). Many substances have the property of emitting visible light when irradiated by invisible rays. When ultraviolet light is focused upon such a specimen, the specimen glows and can be observed by its emitted fluorescence. Fluorescence may be naturally occurring within the specimen, or it may result from the introduction of fluorescent dyes that bind to specific components of the specimen.

**The Electron Microscope.** In the study of biological material, two types of electron microscopes commonly are used: the transmission electron microscope (TEM) (Fig. 3) and the scanning electron microscope (SEM).

The *transmission electron microscope* (TEM) utilizes a system that, in principle, is analogous to that of the light microscope (see Figure 1). In the electron microscope, the illuminating source is a

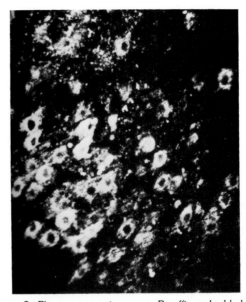

**Figure 2.** *Fluorescence microscopy. Paraffin-embedded sections of the locus ceruleus of an adult rat were exposed to paraformaldehyde vapor prior to examination. A green fluorescence, shown as white in the photograph, is localized in the perinuclear portions of the cells and is considered to be norepinephrine. High power. (Courtesy of Drs. D. Felten and J. Weyhenmeyer.)*

beam of high-velocity electrons accelerated in a vacuum. The beam is passed through the specimen and is focused upon a fluorescent screen or photographic plate by a series of electromagnetic or electrostatic fields. The wavelength of the electrons depends upon the accelerating voltage used. At the voltages used routinely, the wavelengths of the electrons are of the order of 0.05 angstroms (Å).* The electric or magnetic fields used as lenses

---

*Units of measurement. In the past, the terms micron ($\mu$, one thousandth of a millimeter), millimicron (m$\mu$, one thousandth of a micron), and angstrom unit (Å, one tenth of a millimicron) received general acceptance as units of measurement in light and electron microscopy. More recently, it has been recommended that they be replaced by units that relate directly to the metric system.

| Old Terminology | New Terminology (SI units) |
|---|---|
| Micron ($\mu$) | Micrometer ($\mu$m) |
| Millimicron (m$\mu$) | Nanometer (nm) |
| Angstrom unit (Å) | 0.1 nm |

Thus, 0.05 Å (referred to above) becomes 0.005 nm in the new terminology. Since students still will encounter both terminologies in their reading, they should be familiar with both.

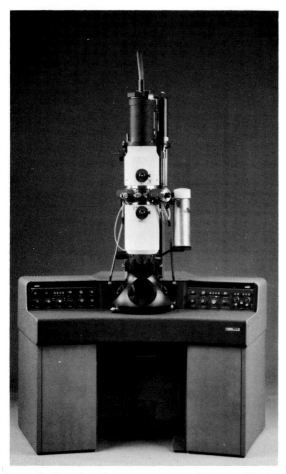

**Figure 3.** A modern electron microscope. (Courtesy of Philips Electronic Instruments.)

are imperfect and do not have the numerical aperture of optical lenses. Thus, the practical limit of resolution of the electron microscope is about 2 Å (0.2 nm), and the usual limit for biological preparations about 3.5 Å (0.35 nm).

More recently, high-voltage (400,000–1,000,000 V) transmission electron microscopes have been utilized in the study of biological specimens. The high speed of acceleration of the electrons in the beam allows the penetration and visualization of relatively thick specimens.

The electron microscope permits the observation of cell and tissue structure beyond that seen with the light microscope. Structures smaller than individual macromolecules now can be visualized.

To describe this particular level of structure requires the use of some special term. The one in most common use is *fine structure*, which refers to those elements of structure that can be visualized only with the electron microscope. The term *ultrastructure*, which is used by many workers in this field, in our opinion is better avoided, since literally it means "beyond structure."

*Scanning electron microscopy* (SEM) is a more recent development, and, unlike transmission electron microscopy, it does not depend upon electrons passing through the specimen under examination. The scanning electron microscope bombards the surface of a specimen with a finely focused beam of electrons. As the beam strikes a point on the specimen, deflected primary and emitted secondary electrons that originate from the surface are collected by a detector. The resulting signals are accumulated from many points to build up an image that is displayed on a television tube. Since the scanning electron microscope is characterized by a great depth of focus, it gives a three-dimensional image of the surface of a bulky specimen.

Just as with light microscopy, TEM and SEM require special techniques for preparing specimens for examination. These will be discussed in the following section.

## The Preparation of Tissues

Cells, tissues, and organs cannot be studied to advantage unless they are suitably prepared for microscopic examination. The methods of preparation fall logically into two groups:

1. Methods involving the direct observation of living cells.
2. Methods employed with dead cells (fixed or preserved).

In the student's personal study of histology, permanent fixed and stained preparations of tissues and organs constitute most of the material used. Living tissues usually are more difficult to handle and are available for a short period only. Nevertheless, it is important that the student be aware of the methods by which living cells may be observed and understand the ways in which they differ from fixed and preserved cells. In the living cell, structure and function may be studied simultaneously. Living cells may be seen to move, to ingest foreign material, occasionally to divide, and to carry on other functions.

## OBSERVATION OF LIVING TISSUES

Unicellular organisms and, occasionally, free cells from a complex organism may be studied directly under the microscope while they still are alive. Free cells are colorless, and structures within them lack contrast. This difficulty can be overcome by using the phase-contrast microscope. Human blood cells are easy to obtain and can be studied in thin films while surrounded by their natural environment, plasma. In this way, ameboid and phagocytic activity may be observed within white blood cells.

Membranes may be thin enough to be viewed directly under the microscope without first sectioning the tissue, for instance, the mesentery, the web of the frog foot, the buccal pouch of the hamster. Thin sections of relatively thick organs such as liver and kidney may be viewed by transillumination with quartz rods, which produce a cold light and avoid heat coagulation of protoplasm. *Glass windows* may be inserted into ears or backs of animals such as the rabbit, thus permitting extended study of processes such as tissue regeneration or vascular activities.

Prolonged preservation of living cells outside the body can be achieved by a technique known as *tissue culture* (Fig. 4). Fragments of tissue are removed aseptically, transferred to a physiological medium, and kept at a temperature normal for the animal from which the tissue was taken. The cultures are placed in thin glass vessels or in hanging drops on a coverglass mounted over a hollow slide. In this way they are available for observation under the microscope. In such cultures, growth, multiplication of cells, and, in some cases, differentiation of cells into other cell types can be observed directly. Tissue culture is a valuable method for the study of cancer and the activity of many viruses.

Microdissection involves the use of an instrument that moves very fine glass needles with precision under the microscope. In this way, small

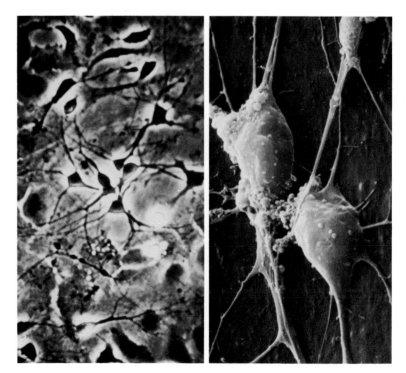

**Figure 4.** *Photomicrographs of tissue culture preparations from the brain of a fetal rat. Left: Primary cultured cells reveal a heterogeneous population of cells that form a background monolayer of flat cells of predominantly glial (supporting) origin, over which individual and clusters of phase bright cells with extensive processes are found. These phase bright cells have been identified as neurons on the basis of fine structural characteristics. Phase contrast. High power. (Courtesy of Dr. J. Weyhenmeyer.) Right: Extensive processes with swellings that appear to be varicosity-like in structure originate from the nerve cell body. Although not evident in this micrograph, synaptic contacts are a prominent feature of the brain cell culture system. Scanning electron microscopy.* × *3000. (Courtesy of Drs. J. Weyhenmeyer and R. Fellows.)*

components of a cell, such as a nucleus, can be removed and the effect observed.

Two staining methods have been applied successfully to living animals or to surviving cells:

1. In *vital staining*, dyes that are not harmful are injected into the living animal. The activity of certain cells will result in the selective absorption of the coloring material by these cells. An example of this procedure is the staining by trypan blue of macrophages on the basis of their ability to phagocytose foreign particles.

2. *Supravital staining* involves the addition of a dyestuff to a medium of cells previously removed from the organism. Examples of this technique are the staining of mitochondria in living cells by Janus green, of lysosomes by neutral red, and of nerve fibers and cells by methylene blue.

Finally, motion picture records aid in the understanding of cellular activities. Lapsed time films made of individual living cells or of tissue cultures help to analyze processes such as mitosis, phagocytosis, and ameboid movement. Slow-motion films of such rapid processes as the beating of cilia permit analysis of the action.

## PREPARATION OF DEAD TISSUES

**Light Microscopy.** The most convenient way to study histology is to use *sections*, each of which is a more or less permanent preparation. A section is prepared by cutting a thin slice from a small piece of fixed tissue, which then is stained, mounted in a medium of suitable refractive index on a slide, and finally covered with a coverslip. The various ways in which sections can be prepared constitute *histological techniques*, about which many books have been written. Detailed information of this kind is not required by students of histology, but they should be aware of the general principles involved in order to use the material intelligently. Since the stained tissue section is the type of material examined most frequently by the student, the method of production is described in some detail. It involves the following stages:

1. *Removal of the Specimen.* For cytological purposes, and for the best histological preparations, the material should be removed from an anesthetized animal or immediately after death of

the animal. In the case of human material, this is scarcely ever possible. Surgical material represents the best source of human tissue, since frequently some normal tissue is removed together with the abnormal or diseased tissue.

2. *Fixation.* The primary objective of fixation is to preserve protoplasm with the least alteration from the living state. Thus, it must be performed promptly to avoid tissue digestion by enzymes present in the tissue (autolysis). Most fixing fluids coagulate protoplasm, thus rendering it insoluble, and harden the tissue so that sectioning is facilitated. They may or may not preserve carbohydrates and lipids. Many fixatives also increase the affinity of protoplasm for certain stains.

The reagents that are employed most commonly as fixing agents are formalin, alcohol, mercuric bichloride, and certain acids (picric, acetic, osmic). No single fixative possesses all the desirable qualities, and this has resulted in the development of several mixtures, such as *Bouin's fluid*, containing picric acid, formalin, and acetic acid, and *Zenker's fluid*, composed of formalin, potassium dichromate, and mercuric bichloride. The choice of a fixative usually is determined by the particular tissue or component that is to be studied and by the staining method to be used.

3. *Embedding.* The purpose of embedding is to provide rigid support to the tissue block so that it may be cut into thin sections. Prior to embedding, the fixed tissue is washed to remove excess fixative and then *dehydrated* by passing it through increasing strengths of ethyl alcohol or some other dehydrating agent. The tissue then is *cleared*. This process involves the removal of the dehydrating agent and its replacement by some fluid that is miscible both with the dehydrating agent and with the embedding agent. *Clearing agents* include xylol, chloroform, benzene, and cedarwood oil. After clearing, the tissue is infiltrated with the embedding agent, usually melted paraffin or celloidin. Following infiltration, the embedding agent is allowed to solidify so that a firm homogeneous mass containing the embedded tissue is obtained.

For special studies, such as rapid study of pathological specimens during surgical procedures or histochemical study of sensitive enzymes, tissue can be embedded in paraffin without subjecting it to preliminary treatment with fixatives, dehydrating solutions, or clearing agents. This is known as the *freeze-drying* method of preparation, in which the fresh tissue is frozen rapidly and dehydrated, while still frozen, in vacuum at a low temperature. The dried tissue then is embedded. In the *freeze-substitution* modification of this method, the ice within the frozen tissue is replaced by alcohol at a very low temperature prior to embedding.

4. *Sectioning.* The hardened paraffin block containing the embedded tissue is trimmed, usually into the form of a block, and is mounted on a microtome. Sections are cut by the steel blade of the microtome to a thickness of between 3 and 10 μm. Each section is transferred to a clean glass microscope slide on which a little egg albumin has been smeared. Water is run under the section, and the slide is placed on a warming stage. The water evaporates, and the section settles down onto the glass surface, to which it becomes attached. The mounted section now is ready for staining.

5. *Staining.* The purpose of staining is to enhance natural contrast and to make more evident various cell and tissue components and extrinsic material. Most stains are employed in aqueous solution, and thus to stain a paraffin section it is necessary to remove the paraffin by placing the mounted section in a paraffin solvent, or *decerating agent*, usually xylol or toluol. This step is omitted in the case of a section which has been embedded in celloidin. The section then is passed through descending strengths of alcohol prior to staining.

6. *Mounting.* After staining, excess dye is removed by washing with water or alcohol, depending upon the solvent of the dye, and the section is dehydrated through ascending grades of alcohol. Following absolute alcohol, the section is transferred to a solution of a clearing agent. After removal of the clearing agent, a drop of mounting medium, for instance, Canada balsam, which has a refractive index similar to that of glass, is placed on the section. The preparation is covered with a coverslip and allowed to dry. After the mounting medium dries, the specimen is available for microscopic examination and storage.

**Electron Microscopy.** In general, the method of preparation of sections for electron microscopy is similar to that employed for light microscopy.

There are some important points of difference about which the student should be aware. Much smaller pieces of tissue are used, since preservation and fixation of cellular fine structure is more critical and requires rapid interaction with the fixative. Blocks are commonly about 1 cu mm or less in size. Tissue must be obtained fresh, since postmortem changes are more obvious at the higher resolution of the electron microscope. Greater care is necessary in fixation in order to maximally preserve structure. A double fixation procedure, using a buffered glutaraldehyde solution first, followed by a second fixation in buffered osmium tetroxide, commonly is employed. The glutaraldehyde retains the protein constituents of the cell, and osmium tetroxide preserves the lipid components, particularly phospholipid. The osmium tetroxide, because it is a heavy metal, additionally plays a major role in electron deflection and image formation when the specimen is viewed in the electron microscope. The procedures of dehydration and embedding, although similar to those employed in light-microscopy preparations, are effected rapidly because of the small pieces of tissue involved. Since paraffin is not suitable for very thin sectioning, it is replaced as an embedding medium by some agent, usually a plastic material such as Epon or Araldite, which produces a firm block. The sections, cut upon a special precision-built microtome with glass or diamond knives, are minute, about 0.25 mm square and about 300 to 500 Å (30 to 50 nm) thick. They are mounted on perforated copper grids and then stained. The stains employed are heavy metal salts, such as lead citrate and uranyl acetate, which possess a high electron-scattering or electron-absorbing capacity. The grid, containing stained sections, is placed in the electron microscope and those portions of the sections that span the holes in the grid may be examined and photographed.

Thick sections, about 0.2 to 1.0 μ (0.2 to 1.0 μm), of such plastic embedded material can be mounted on glass slides, stained, and examined by light microscopy (Fig. 5). Although such sections initially were used to overcome sampling problems encountered in electron microscopic studies, they now are finding increasing usage and acceptance in light microscopy studies and in general histological laboratories. They exhibit

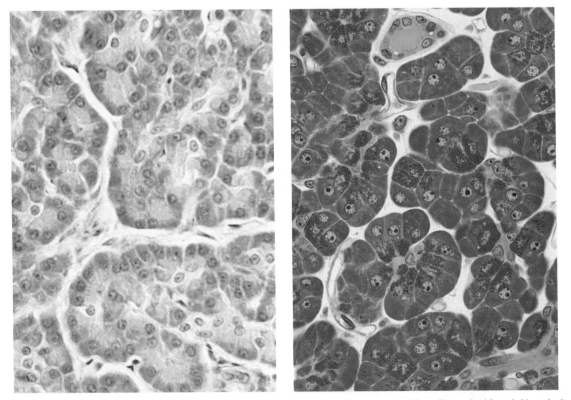

**Figure 5.** *Comparison of the results obtained after routine preparation for light microscopy (paraffin embedding, left) and after preparation for electron microscopy (plastic embedding, right). The clarity of detail generally is better in the latter and is the result of better fixation, less tissue shrinkage during preparation, and thinness of the section. In both sections (pancreas, high power), groups of secretory end-pieces (acini) are present. Darkly staining secretory granules are well preserved in the plastic section. Left: H and E. Right: methylene blue, azure A.*

superior clarity, principally the result of better fixation and plastic embedding. Numerous photomicrographs of this type of preparation are to be found throughout this textbook.

*Freeze fracture* (freeze-etching) is a special method of sample preparation for electron microscopy. A small fragment of tissue is frozen at very low temperatures and then is fractured along a plane approximately that of the plane of the cutting device, a sharp metal blade. The tissue is kept in a high vacuum, briefly warmed to etch the fractured surface by vacuum-sublimation, and a replica of the surface made by heavy metal shadowing. The frozen tissue is removed, and the surface replica can then be placed on a specimen grid and viewed in either a transmission or scanning electron microscope. The method allows examination of the surface of single cells or of such structures as cytoplasmic membrane systems at the macromolecular level.

For *scanning electron microscopy,* the specimen is fixed and dehydrated by special procedures that depend upon the nature of the specimen (Fig. 6). Following drying, the specimen is coated evenly with a layer of metal, for example, gold or platinum, and mounted on a stub, prior to viewing in the microscope. This technique allows the biologist to record accurately in three dimensions the surface features of cells and tissues.

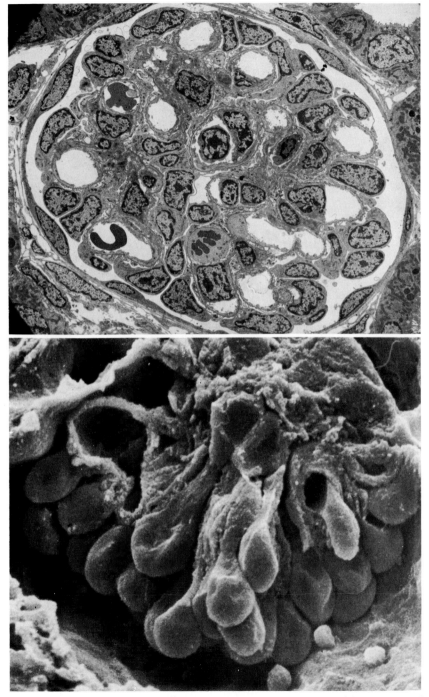

***Figure 6.*** *Comparison of the results obtained from transmission electron microscopy (top) and from scanning electron microscopy (bottom). Both micrographs are of a renal glomerulus. Top: Sectioned capillary loops of the glomerulus appear empty. Bottom: The glomerulus is seen in three dimensions, and a few capillary loops have been cut open. (Courtesy of Professor M. Miyoshi.)*

## AUTORADIOGRAPHY

Autoradiography is a special technique that permits the localization of radioactive substances in cells or tissues (Fig. 7). The technique is coming into increasing prominence in histology as a method of chemical localization. Tracer isotopes introduced into an animal either by feeding or by injection follow the same metabolic pathways as do naturally occurring elements. Their presence in an organ or tissue can be detected by autoradiography. After administration of a tracer isotope, the organ or tissue under investigation is removed and processed for light or electron microscopy in the normal manner. The resulting tissue section then is dipped into a photographic emulsion in a dark room and stored in a light-proof box in a refrigerator. After different exposure times depending upon the radioactive element and the nature of the experiment, the emulsion covering

the section is developed photographically and examined. Black-silver grains indicate the existence of radioactivity in the structures in contact with these granules. The section then may be stained with regular stains and mounted prior to viewing in the microscope. Some excellent results have been achieved by this method—for instance, the localization of radioiodine in the thyroid gland and of phosphorus (using radiostrontium as a substitute) in bone. It is possible to study not only different metabolic pathways but also the speed with which the metabolic processes occur. For example, thymidine is used by the cell in DNA synthesis. It is incorporated into the DNA by cells that are about to divide, since they need to double their DNA content. If radioactive thymidine is injected into an animal and a fixed unit of time is used in the experiment, it is possible to estimate the rate of turnover of specific cell populations.

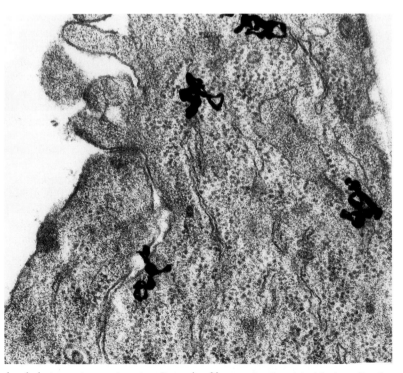

**Figure 7.** *An example of electron microscopic autoradiography. Neurons in dissociated brain cell cultures were exposed to iodinated angiotensin II (ANG II), fixed in aldehyde, sectioned, and stained prior to examination. Radioactive grains, shown as the black label in the photograph, appeared adjacent to the plasma membranes of several infolding nerve fibers and represent the localization of specific ANG II–binding sites. × 14,000. (Courtesy of Dr. J. Weyhenmeyer.)*

## STAINS

Although it is not necessary for the student to be conversant with the details of the various staining techniques used, it is important to understand the general principles, uses, and results of the common staining procedures (Fig. 8).

In general, the dyes in use are complex organic chemicals, and they may be classified in numerous ways. The simplest approach is to base the classification upon use, with regard to tissue and cell components. Dyes may be of general use, staining either the nucleus or the cytoplasm, or they may be more specific with regard to particular components. It must be emphasized that many dyes require special methods of fixation and preparation of the tissue, and the reader is referred to a textbook of histological and histochemical techniques for the details.

Stains in general use are considered to be either acids or bases, but in fact they are neutral salts having both acidic and basic radicals. When the coloring property of the dye is in the basic radical of the neutral salt, the stain is referred to as a basic dye, and the structures that stain with it are termed *basophil*. Basic dyes carry a positive charge. In most instances, the basophil substances that attract the basic dyes are themselves acids, for instance, the nucleic acids of the nucleus and the acidic components of the cytoplasm such as ribonucleic acid (RNA). Similarly, when the staining property is in the acidic radical of the neutral salt, the stain is spoken of as an acid dye, and it carries a negative charge. Structures that stain with acid dyes, for instance, the general cytoplasm, are *acidophil*.

The *basic dye* in most common use is *hematoxylin*, the staining property of which depends upon the presence in solution of its oxidation product, hematein. When stained with such a dye, nuclei appear blue. Iron hematoxylin, which stains nuclei dark blue or black, has a wide application. In most methods employing iron hematoxylin, one overstains with the dye and regressively differentiates in a weak acid or in a ferric salt solution. By careful differentiation, which may be viewed directly under the microscope, such organelles as chromosomes, mitochondria, Golgi apparatus, and the contractile elements of muscle may be visualized.

The basic *aniline dyes* are a group of stains used extensively. This group includes azure A, toluidine blue, and methylene blue, stains that are employed also in the identification of proteoglycans (mucopolysaccharides), which stain *metachromatically* (*meta*, beyond; *chroma*, color). This means that proteoglycans, when stained with one of these dyes, will take on a color different from that of the dye employed. It is thought that substances that demonstrate metachromasia do so because they are capable of concentrating the dye to form aggregates of dye molecules whose absorption properties differ from those of individual dye molecules. Mucin, matrix of cartilage, and granules of mast cells are demonstrated readily by their metachromatic staining. Other basic aniline dyes in common use are brilliant cresyl blue, neutral red, and Janus green, all of which are nontoxic and may be used also as vital or supravital stains in the study of living tissues.

*Acidic dyes*, commonly employed to stain the general cytoplasm, include eosin, picric acid, acid azo dyes such as chromotrope, and the acid diazo dyes, trypan blue and trypan red. The latter two are used also as vital stains.

Most histological sections are stained with both a basic dye and an acidic dye. The most common combination is *hematoxylin and eosin* (H and E), in which nuclear structures are stained blue or dark purple and practically all cytoplasmic structures and intercellular substances are stained pink. Trichrome methods, such as Mallory's connective tissue stain and the Mallory-Azan method, possess the advantage that they differentiate between cytoplasmic structures and intercellular materials. Masson's staining procedure is another trichrome method in general use, in which connective tissue fibers are stained green, cytoplasmic structures red, and nuclei blue or purple. Although there is no truly specific stain for collagen, it is best shown by the acid aniline dyes in a trichrome method. Elastic fibers are brilliantly acidophil and can be stained selectively with orcein or with resorcin fuchsin. Reticular fibers can be demonstrated specifically by precipitation of silver from an alkaline solution. Hence, these fibers are termed *argyrophil*. It must be appreciated that special methods of staining are necessary to demonstrate certain constituents of cells and formed extracellular fibers and that a single staining method will not suffice to demonstrate everything present within a section.

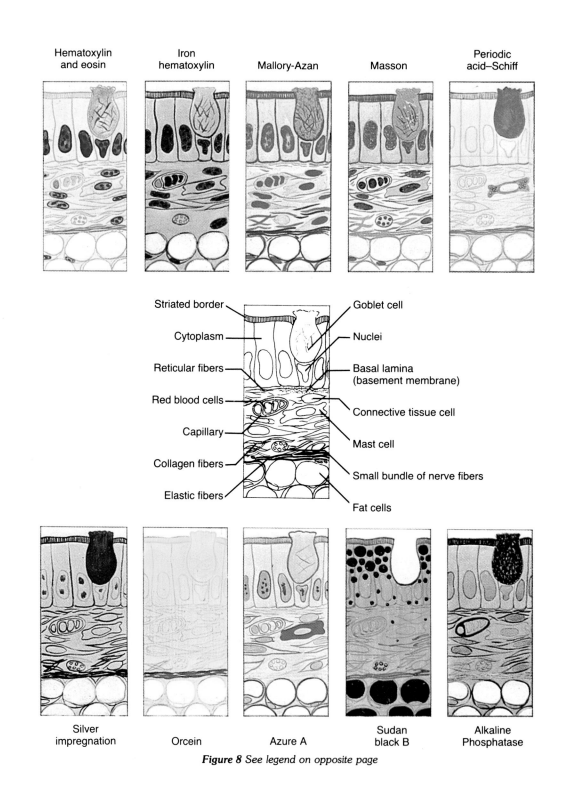

Hematoxylin and eosin    Iron hematoxylin    Mallory-Azan    Masson    Periodic acid–Schiff

Striated border — Goblet cell
Cytoplasm — Nuclei
Reticular fibers — Basal lamina (basement membrane)
Red blood cells — Connective tissue cell
Capillary — Mast cell
Collagen fibers — Small bundle of nerve fibers
Elastic fibers — Fat cells

Silver impregnation    Orcein    Azure A    Sudan black B    Alkaline Phosphatase

*Figure 8 See legend on opposite page*

**Figure 8.** *Diagrammatic representation of a section (partly hypothetical) of a portion of intestine wall as it would appear after different staining procedures.* Hematoxylin and eosin *stains nuclei dark blue, and both cytoplasm and connective tissue fibers pink-red.* Iron hematoxylin *stains nuclei a dark purple-black. It also stains red blood cells. With less differentiation after staining (see text), it would make visible also such cellular components as mitochondria.* Mallory-Azan *and* Masson *are examples of trichrome methods of staining that are useful in differentiating between cytoplasm and connective tissue fibers. In the former method, collagen fibers are stained bright blue; in the latter, they are stained green.* Periodic acid–Schiff *stains positively the brush border, mucus within the goblet cell, the basal lamina, and cytoplasmic granules of the mast cell. All other structures in the section are negative with this stain.* Silver impregnation *and* orcein *are examples of stains used to differentiate between the various types of connective tissue fibers. Impregnation with silver outlines reticular fibers; hence, commonly, they are termed argyrophil. Elastic fibers are stained selectively with* orcein *(and with resorcin fuchsin).* Azure A *is one of the group of basic aniline dyes that stains nuclei blue. It also is employed in the identification of proteoglycans, which stain metachromatically, as do the granules of the mast cell here (see text).* Sudan black B *is a dye that is absorbed by fat and thus stains it selectively. It requires a method of preparation of tissue that avoids the use of fat solvents.* Alkaline phosphatase *is an enzyme that can be localized by a histochemical method (see text). Hence, there is a positive reaction in the brush border and, as often happens, in the cytoplasm of endothelium lining blood vessels. (After Garvin.)*

## HISTOCHEMISTRY

**General Methods.** The fact that deposition of specific stains in certain regions is a result of chemical or physical properties inherent in the tissue forms the basis of histochemistry. This is a field of research that has expanded rapidly and has as its goal the localization within specific areas or cell components of the chemical compounds known already by biochemical analysis to be present. These compounds, both inorganic and organic, can be identified by chemical reactions that produce insoluble colored substances. Some examples of those histochemical methods of histological interest follow.

*Ions.* Sections of tissues or organs containing ferric ions may be identified by an adaptation of the Prussian blue reaction. The sections are incubated in a solution containing potassium ferrocyanide and hydrochloric acid, and the ions form a highly insoluble, dark-blue precipitate of ferric ferrocyanide.

*Nucleic Acids.* The *Feulgen reaction* for the identification of deoxyribonucleic acid (DNA) is an example of a histochemical test that requires preliminary treatment of a section so that the substance under investigation either is liberated or produces a substance for which a specific test exists. Basic fuchsin is a magenta-colored dye that can be bleached by treatment with hydrochloric acid and sodium bisulfite. Reaction with aldehydes produces, in the bleached dye, a new colored compound, also magenta in color. Mild hydrolysis of a section with hydrochloric acid will promote the formation of aldehydes from DNA. If the section then is immersed in the colorless form of basic fuchsin, the aldehydes formed from DNA will react with the dye and exhibit the magenta color. Since both DNA and RNA are basophil, the Feulgen reaction allows a distinction to be made as to which basophil material is DNA.

*Proteoglycans.* Proteoglycans are composed of glycosaminoglycans (formally known as mucopolysaccharides) linked covalently to a protein core. The glycosaminoglycans may be identified by a modification of the Feulgen reaction, known as the *periodic acid–Schiff (PAS) reaction.* Periodic acid is an oxidizing agent that will produce, from glycosaminoglycans, aldehydes that are insoluble. These then react with the Schiff reagent, which is the colorless form of basic fuchsin, to produce a complex compound having a purple or magenta color.

*Lipids.* Not all reactions in histochemistry rely upon chemical affinities. Fat can be detected in sections that have not been exposed to fat solvents by stains such as Sudan III, Sudan IV, and Sudan black B. These stains have a physical affinity for lipid and are absorbed by the fat. Use of such dyes forms the basis for the term *sudanophilia,* the ability to stain substances with this group of dyes.

*Enzymes.* Numerous histochemical methods are available to localize the sites of enzymic activity within cells and tissues. Many enzymes retain a portion of their activity in tissues fixed with aldehyde fixatives such as formalin and glutaraldehyde. In the study of unstable enzymes, however, sections of frozen, unfixed material must be used. The histochemical methods used attempt in principle to localize the site of a specific enzyme by a chemical process similar to that performed by the enzyme *in vivo.* The section under examination is incubated at body temperature in the presence of a suitable substrate, and the product of the resultant chemical reaction with the enzyme is converted into a chemical substance of a definite color. For example, to demonstrate the enzyme alkaline phosphatase, glycerophosphate is used as the substrate in an alkaline medium, and the phosphate liberated by the action of the enzyme is deposited in the presence of calcium ions as calcium phosphate. The deposit of calcium phosphate is converted to an easily visualized black precipitate of cobalt sulfide (or metallic silver) by immersing the section in cobalt acetate (or silver acetate) and then rinsing in ammonium sulfide. Methods are available now for a wide variety of enzymes including phosphatases, lipases, esterases, and oxidases.

*Glycogen.* Glycogen is stained by Best's carmine stain or by the periodic acid–Schiff reagent. In either case, glycogen then can be differentiated from other polysaccharides by the fact that the staining property of the latter substances is resistant to digestion by salivary amylase.

**Immunocytochemistry.** Immunocytochemistry is one branch of histochemistry that has received considerable attention in recent years. At the light microscopic level, the fluorescent antibody technique is a sensitive method for the localization of specific proteins and other macromolecules. The basis of this technique is the fact that the body reacts to foreign protein substances, the *antigens*, by elaborating specific substances, the *antibodies*, which combine with and inactivate the antigens. Fluorescent dye molecules are chemically linked to antibody molecules, and the sites of their reaction with antigens can be visualized in the ultraviolet microscope (Fig. 9). The method has been used to identify the cells of origin of protein hormones, the intracellular localization of various enzymes, and the sites of proteins such as myosin. The method has been adapted for use with the electron microscope by conjugating an antibody with a metalloprotein such as *ferritin*, which naturally possesses a distinct appearance in the electron microscope. This method has localized precisely the site of the antibody-antigen reaction.

To localize an antigen by immunocytochemistry, there are both direct and indirect methods.

1. *Direct method.* Sections suspected of containing an antigen (protein X) are incubated with a specific antibody to X, which has been labeled with a fluorescent dye or other tag. The antibody will combine with X, and the antigen then can be detected by either light or electron microscopy.

2. *Indirect method.* Tissue sections initially are exposed to unlabeled antibody, resulting in the formation of an invisible antigen-antibody complex. The second step involves the production of labeled secondary antibody to the primary antibody by injecting the primary antibody into an-

other species. The secondary antibody is labeled for visibility by a fluorescent dye or other tag. When it is applied to the tissue sections, it combines with unoccupied antigen sites in the primary immune complex and thus makes it visible. This technique increases considerably the sensitivity of the method.

## THE EXAMINATION AND INTERPRETATION OF SECTIONS

Once the student has acquired an understanding of the basic principles underlying microscopy and the preparation of tissues, he or she should be able to move on to an examination of prepared sections of tissue. The ability to interpret a histological section is a skill that must be developed. Initially, it should be recognized that it is most helpful to be able to compare what one sees in a microscope with labeled illustrations of sections of the same tissue. The student, therefore, should refer frequently to relevant illustrations within this text.

However, before proceeding to the examination of a section under the microscope, the student must be advised to hold the section up to the light and to inspect it with the naked eye. As one gains more and more experience, the naked-eye appearance of the stained slice of tissue will

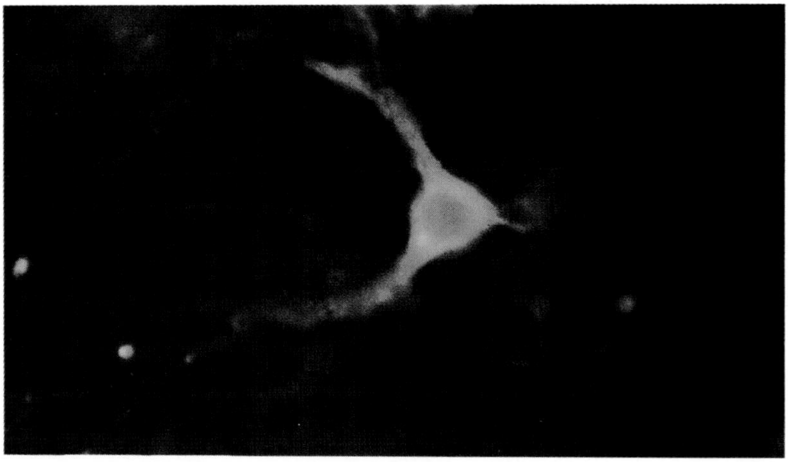

**Figure 9.** An example of the indirect immunofluorescence method for localization of a cellular antigen. Angiotensin II (ANG II) was localized in neurons of dissociated brain cell cultures with a specific antiserum to ANG II followed by a fluorescein-labeled second antibody (anti-IgG). Immunoreactive ANG II is observed in the dendrites (brightly fluorescent large fibrous processes), initial axon segment, and perinuclear portion of the nerve cell body. Oil immersion. (Courtesy of Dr. J. Weyhenmeyer.)

provide helpful hints as to the region or organ from which the section was taken. When the section eventually is placed on the stage of the microscope, the temptation to use the greatest magnification as quickly as possible should be resisted. The low-power objective discloses a much larger area of the section than do the high-power objectives, and, by moving the slide around, it is possible quickly to examine the entire section. Additionally, inspection with the low-power objective enables one to select the best area to center for later inspection with the higher power objectives. The field of view obtained with the low-power objective is about 1500 micrometers (μm), or 1.5 mm, across. It diminishes in direct proportion to the magnification used, and, with the oil-immersion objective, the area of the section under view is only a little more than 100 micrometers wide.

Further, in a study of sections, there is a tendency to think in terms of only two dimensions, since, for all practical purposes, the sections have no depth. *It is important to reconstruct a three-dimensional mental picture of cells, tissues, and organs.* In this respect, the plane of sectioning must be borne in mind. A single section of an organ may give a false impression of its architecture. Thus, it is important to use several sections taken in different planes in order to arrive at an interpretation of the structure of complex organs. As a simple example of this, we can consider the appearance of tubular structures (see Figure 10). Tubes, such as blood vessels, the ducts of glands, and the male genital ducts, are encountered frequently in histological sections. They are most easily recognized when they are cut in cross section. However, if they are cut longitudinally or obliquely or if they are sectioned in areas where they appear tortuous, they must be visualized in three dimensions if they are to be recognized as tubes.

After examination of a histological section, it is not sufficient to arrive at an identification and notation of structures. One must strive to interpret

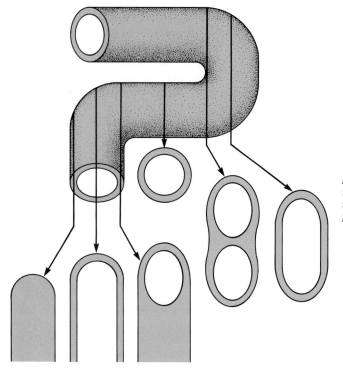

*Figure 10.* Diagrammatic representation of the various appearances, as indicated by the arrows, of a tubular structure when it is sectioned in different planes.

the functional significance of what one observes. Dead structures are examined for the purpose of throwing light upon their condition in life. Conditions that are dynamic in life have been converted to a static form in the permanent histological section. Interpretation further involves an appreciation of the method of preparation and of the staining or histochemical technique used.

## Artifacts

It must be appreciated also that not all sections are perfect. Owing to the techniques used in preparation, sections may not be accurate representations. These alterations, resulting from manipulation, are termed *artifacts*, and they should be recognized as such by the student. Some common forms of artifact are listed below.

**Shrinkage.** The different chemicals with which tissues are treated, principally fixatives, or the heat of the melted paraffin, may cause shrinkage. It tends to be uneven, resulting in the separation of portions of tissue that in life were contiguous and creating a deceptive appearance of empty spaces.

**Precipitates.** If fixative is inadequately buffered or is imperfectly removed from tissues, crystals of it may precipitate and remain behind.

**Folds and Wrinkles.** Sections are so thin that commonly they become folded or wrinkled as they are cut or while they are being attached to slides. Generally, folds and wrinkles appear darkly stained.

**Defects in the Microtome Knife.** If there are any nicks in the cutting edge of the knife, they create defects in the section and appear as pale, straight lines across it.

**Rough Handling.** Rough handling of fresh tissue as it is being removed from an animal, either pinching by forceps or crushing by dull scissors, results in mutilation of the tissue.

**Postmortem Degeneration.** Although not strictly speaking an artifact, postmortem degeneration is an important cause of sections of inferior quality. The importance of rapid fixation already has been emphasized in this chapter. Unless tissues are fixed promptly, they undergo digestion by enzymes present in the tissues, resulting in postmortem degeneration (autolysis).

## SUMMARY

The term histology, although meaning literally the study of tissues, today embraces as well the study of organs (organology) and of cells (cytology). The body itself is composed of cells, intercellular substances, and body fluids. A knowledge or normal histology is a necessary prelude to the study of the abnormal (pathology) and includes a consideration of function as well as of structure.

There are two important deliberations with regard to methodology: the type of microscope used, and the methods of preparation of tissues in a manner suitable for viewing with the microscope. Microscopes may be classified by the type of light source used. Those which use a visible light source include the light- (or optical) microscope and the polarizing, phase-contrast, interference, and dark-field microscopes. Microscopes utilizing a nonvisible light source are the ultraviolet and electron microscopes, both transmission (TEM) and scanning (SEM). The methods of preparation of tissues fall into two groups: those involving the direct observation of living tissues and those employed with dead or fixed tissues.

In the preparation of dead tissue for routine light microscopy, the tissue first is placed in a fixative to preserve protoplasm. Then, it is washed to remove excess fixative and is dehydrated by passing it through increasing strengths of ethyl alcohol. Following dehydration, the tissue is "cleared," a process that involves the removal of the dehydrating agent and its replacement by some fluid that is miscible both with the dehydrating agent and with the embedding medium. After clearing, the tissue is infiltrated with the embedding agent, usually paraffin or celloidin. The embedding agent then is made to solidify so that a firm homogeneous mass containing the tissue is obtained. The embedded tissue is sectioned with a microtome, and each section is transferred to a glass microscope slide prior to staining.

The method of preparation of sections for electron microscopy in general is similar to that employed for light microscopy, although there are some important points of difference. Much smaller pieces of tissue are used, since preservation and fixation are more critical. The common fixatives used are glutaraldehyde, which maximally retains protein constituents of the cell, and osmium tetroxide, which retains the lipid components. Since paraffin is not suitable for very thin sectioning, it is replaced as an embedding medium by some agent, usually a plastic material such as Epon or Araldite. The sections, cut upon a special microtome with glass or diamond knives, are minute and are mounted upon perforated copper grids and stained with heavy metals prior to viewing in the electron microscope.

The purpose of staining for light microscopy is to enhance natural contrast and to make more obvious various cell and tissue components and extrinsic material. Stains in general use are considered to be either acids or bases, but in fact they are neutral salts having both acidic and basic radicals. When the coloring property of the dye is in the basic radical of the neutral salt, the stain is referred to as a basic dye, and structures that stain with it, such as the nucleus, are termed basophil. Similarly, when the staining property is in the acidic radical of the neutral salt, the stain is spoken of as an acid dye and the structures stained, for instance, the general cytoplasm, are acidophil. Most histological sections are stained with both a basic stain and an acidic stain, the most common combination being hematoxylin and eosin (H and E). Trichrome methods, such as Mallory's connective tissue stain and the Mallory-Azan and Masson procedures, possess the advantage that they differentiate between cytoplasmic structures and extracellular materials. Special methods of staining are necessary to demonstrate certain constituents of cells and formed extracellular fibers, and a single staining method does not suffice to demonstrate everything present within a section.

Histochemical methods deposit specific stains in certain regions as a result of chemical or physical properties inherent in the tissue, and they are utilized to visualize ions, nucleic acids, proteoglycans, lipids, enzymes, and glycogen. Specific proteins and other macromolecules may be localized by immunocytochemical methods, a special branch of histochemistry.

Not all sections are perfect, and as a result of manipulation during preparation, artifacts may be introduced, and they must be recognized as such. They include shrinkage, the presence of precipitates, folds and wrinkles, defects resulting from the use of imperfect knives or rough handling, and postmortem degeneration.

# ONE

# GENERAL HISTOLOGICAL PRINCIPLES AND PRIMARY TISSUES

# The Cell

## COMPONENTS OF THE BODY

The body is composed of three different elements: body fluids; intercellular, or extracellular, substances; and the cells.

1. *Body fluids* include blood, confined within the vascular system; tissue or intercellular fluid, found between and around cells; and lymph, draining tissue fluid back to the venous system. There is also a free exchange between blood and the intracellular fluid. These fluid components are usually lost during the preparation of histological sections, with the exception of formed elements (cells) of the blood.

2. *Intercellular, or extracellular, substances* are materials that are found between cells and that support and nourish them. This intercellular material gives a firmness to the tissues and is divided into two main types. The *formed*, or *fibrous*, type includes *collagen* (white fibrous tissue present in meat) and *elastin*, which gives the property of elasticity to tissues. The *amorphous* type forms the ground substance. The latter contains substances called *glycosaminoglycans* and *proteoglycans*. These are carbohydrates that are bound to protein. Glycosaminoglycans (polysaccharides) contain repeating disaccharide units that

1

consist of hexuronic acids and amino sugars. Proteoglycans are formed when these are bound to a protein. Chapter 3 contains a more detailed description of these intercellular substances.

3. *Cells* are the structural units of all living organisms. They are bound by a membrane that "isolates" them from their environment. Cells present the most obvious feature of tissue sections. The cell consists of *protoplasm*, the living substance in the form of a heterogeneous aqueous phase containing biological components whose integrated functions exhibit properties of life. Protoplasm contains protein, nucleic acids, carbohydrates, lipid and inorganic materials that include the chemical machinery for metabolic processes and the hereditary material. It has been recognized that there exist two fundamentally different types of cells. The *prokaryotic* cell is typified by bacteria, in which the metabolic and hereditary components are mixed, since they do not have a nuclear envelope separating the genetic material from other cellular constituents. In contrast, *eukaryotic* cells have a distinct nucleus surrounded by a nuclear envelope lying in the remainder of the cell, or *cytoplasm*. So many biochemical similarities exist between the two types that many investigators have postulated that one group evolved from the other. However, while cells vary in structure and function, most have many features in common.

## PROTOPLASM

Protoplasm, the material of which cells are composed and which has been described as the physical basis for life, exists in a *colloidal state*. It is difficult to define a colloid exactly, but the basic feature of a colloidal solution is that its particles are of such a size that they cannot be filtered through natural membranes, the membrane acting like a sieve and holding back particles. Both the vital, living protoplasm of cells and the nonliving materials between cells exist in the colloidal state. Crystalloids (glucose) can pass through membranes. Proteins show all the characteristics of the colloidal state, and some can exist either as a sol or as a gel. Fluid solutions of colloids

usually are sols but are viscous to some degree. Sol-gel transformations can occur in the protoplasm of cells and are often reversible, as is the case, for example, in the "setting" and "melting" of a solution of gelatin.

## Components of Protoplasm

Protoplasm contains protein, nucleic acid, carbohydrate, lipid, and inorganic material. *Proteins* constitute more than half of the dry weight of the cell and determine the shape and structure of the cell. Protein can exist as pure protein or combine with lipid (lipoprotein) or with carbohydrate to form glycoprotein, proteoglycan, or mucoprotein. Enzymes constitute an important group of proteins. Many hormones, for example, insulin and gonadotropin, also are proteins.

Two classes of *nucleic acids* can be identified. Deoxyribonucleic acid (DNA) forms the genetic material and is found mainly in the nucleus, whereas ribonucleic acid (RNA) is present in both the nucleus and the cytoplasm. RNA carries messages from the nucleus to the cytoplasm and serves as a template for the synthesis of proteins.

*Carbohydrates* provide the chief source of energy of most cells in the form of glucose and glycogen, the storage form of glucose. Complexes of carbohydrates and protein form the constituents of the intercellular material. *Lipids* are major components of the membrane systems of cells. They also serve as an energy source for the cell.

Inorganic materials, particularly potassium and magnesium as cations and phosphate and bicarbonate as anions, account for about 1 per cent of the materials of the body; without them physiological processes are impossible. They are involved in a variety of physiological functions, including maintenance of intracellular and extracellular osmotic pressures, contraction of muscle, transmission of nerve impulses, tissue rigidity (e.g., bone), adhesiveness of cells, and activation of enzymes.

*Water* makes up about 75 per cent of protoplasm: partly free and available as a solvent for metabolic processes and partly bound to protein as a structural component.

## Properties of Protoplasm

Protoplasm is characterized by a number of physiological properties that indicate the functions of cells. All living cells show these properties. The functions of any particular cell type are a direct expression of one or more of these properties of its protoplasm. Accordingly, a high development of a single function in a particular cell type has often been achieved at the expense of the other properties.

*Irritability* designates the ability of protoplasm to respond to a stimulus. It is most pronounced in nerve cells and disappears with cell death.

*Conductivity* is the generation of a wave of excitation (an electrical impulse) throughout the cell from the site of the stimulus. Irritability and conductivity are the most important physiological properties of nerve cells.

*Contractility* is the ability of a cell to change shape, usually in the sense of shortening. It is especially prominent in muscle cells.

*Respiration*, essential for life, is the process whereby cells produce energy by utilizing food substances and absorbed oxygen to produce energy, carbon dioxide, and water.

*Absorption* is the ability of cells to take up substances from the environment.

*Secretion* is the process by which a cell extrudes useful material such as a digestive enzyme or a hormone.

*Excretion* is the elimination from the cell of waste products of metabolism.

*Growth* is the increase in the size of a cell that results from an increase in the amount of protoplasm or from an increase in the number of cells. There are limits to the size a cell can attain. The maximum size of a cell is limited by its surface area (while surface area increases by the square of the diameter, the volume of the protoplasm increases by the cube). Beyond the maximum size, an increase in the amount of protoplasm is accomplished by *cell division*.

## METABOLISM

*Metabolism* of a cell is the total sum of all of the chemical reactions of the cell by which nutri-tion is effected. It may involve the degradation of cell protoplasm or of materials brought to the cell as food supply. This is called *catabolism*. Other reactions are concerned with the build-up or synthesis of materials that either are retained or released by the cell. This process is *anabolism*.

## COMPONENTS OF THE CELL

All cells, whatever their size, shape, or function, are simple units of living matter and exhibit fundamental metabolic activities. The protoplasm of each cell consists of two major components: the nucleus and cytoplasm. In ordinary histological slides, these two components of a cell will be differently stained, that is, the cytoplasm will appear to be a different color from that of the nucleus. The cytoplasm may be small in amount or very lightly stained and, for this reason, difficult to observe.

### Cytoplasm

In many histological preparations, cytoplasm has an even, homogeneous amorphous appearance, but it does in fact contain many small bodies of varying type and function (Fig. 1–1). Cytoplasmic bodies are suspended in a component known as the *cytoplasmic matrix*, or *cytosol*. This portion of the cytoplasm contains many enzymes, various other soluble proteins, nutrients, and constituent building blocks used in the synthesis of macromolecules. Variations in cell function (e.g., an enzyme-secreting cell or a nerve cell) are reflected by different appearances of the cytoplasm, which in turn result in variations in the number and type of these small cytoplasmic bodies. These cytoplasmic bodies may be classified either as *organelles*, which are highly organized, living structural units of cytoplasm that perform specific functions in the cell, or as *inclusions*, which generally represent cell products or metabolites that often are transitory in nature (Figs. 1–2 and 1–3).

Cytoplasmic organelles include the cell (plasma) membrane, the endoplasmic reticulum (ergastoplasm), the Golgi apparatus, the centrioles

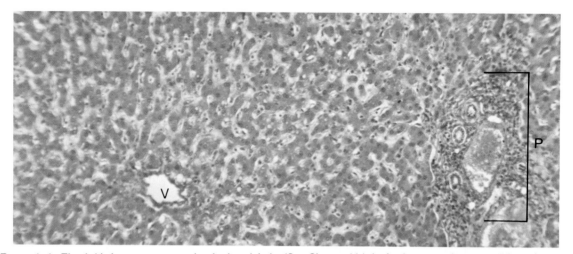

**Figure 1–1.** *This field shows a portion only of a liver lobule. (See Chapter 11.) At this low magnification, cell boundaries are indistinct; however, liver (parenchymal) cells, which are epithelial, are arranged in irregular cords radiating from a central vein (V) and with vascular or sinusoidal spaces between the cords. Other cell types and structures are present. Note that cytoplasm of the parenchymal cells is abundant, eosinophil, and homogeneous. Nuclei of these cells are generally spheroidal and vesicular in type. Smaller, darker-staining (condensed or hyperchromatic) nuclei of cells associated with the sinusoids also are seen. On the right is a portal area (P) containing several tubes (blood vessels and bile ducts) cut in transverse section. This area appears darker owing to the presence of numerous small cells with dark nuclei, packed closely together. Liver. H and E. Low power.*

(or centrosome), mitochondria, annulate lamellae, fibrils and filamentous structures, lysosomes, and microtubules (Fig. 1–4).

Cytoplasm in most cells is regionally specialized. Near the nucleus usually are found the centrosome and the Golgi apparatus. Lysosomes often are seen near the Golgi apparatus. Granular endoplasmic reticulum and mitochondria are found in the basal cytoplasm in a cell that secretes protein. This latter cell also shows the centrosome on the apical side of the nucleus and secretory droplets or granules in apical cytoplasm. Other organelles such as microtubules, microfilaments, and the contractile proteins of muscle cells are arranged in particular arrays. Each cell is bound by a plasma membrane, or plasmalemma, which is one of the organelles (Fig. 1–5).

### CELL (PLASMA) MEMBRANE

A thin plasma membrane, or *plasmalemma*, delimits the cell from the environment (Figs. 1–6 and 1–7). It is only 7.5 nm thick and is invisible by light microscopy. However, it may be visualized if it is sectioned obliquely, thus enhancing its thickness, or if its staining is enhanced by the presence of associated material on its external surface. The cell, or plasma, membrane is defined as the thinnest layer resolved at the cell surface by light microscopy. It is a highly selective filter that maintains the unequal concentration of ions on either side and allows nutrients to enter and waste products to leave the cell.

All biological membranes, including the plasma membrane and the internal membranes of eukaryotic cells, have a common overall structure. They are assemblies of lipid and protein molecules held together by noncovalent interactions with a small amount of carbohydrate. The thickness varies a little from cell type to cell type, and internal membranes usually are somewhat thinner than the plasmalemma. When stained for electron microscopy and observed in cross section under high magnification, this membrane exhibits three

*Text continued on page 32*

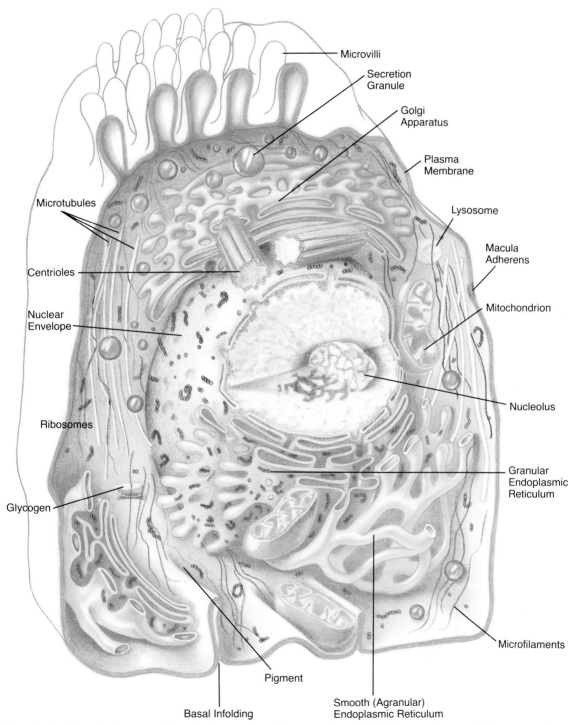

Microvilli

Secretion Granule

Golgi Apparatus

Plasma Membrane

Microtubules

Lysosome

Macula Adherens

Centrioles

Mitochondrion

Nuclear Envelope

Nucleolus

Ribosomes

Granular Endoplasmic Reticulum

Glycogen

Microfilaments

Pigment

Basal Infolding

Smooth (Agranular) Endoplasmic Reticulum

*Figure 1–2.* Schematic diagram of the cell shows many of the organelles and inclusions as they would be seen on electron microscopy.

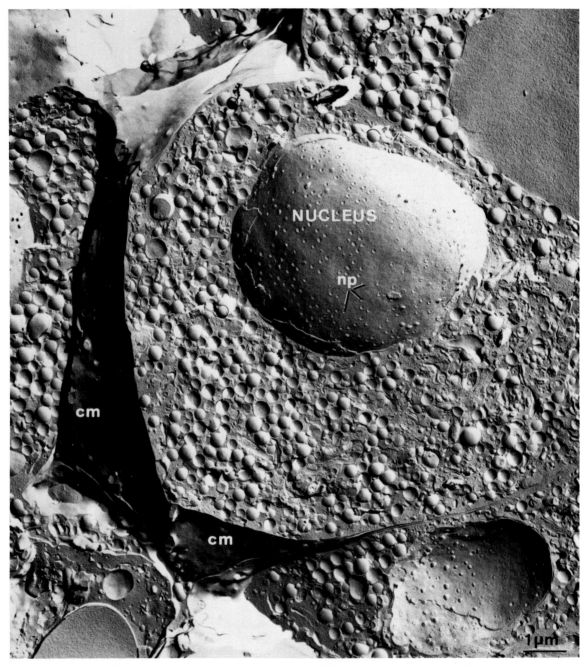

**Figure 1–3.** *Freeze-etch replica from an isolated pancreatic islet. This technique characteristically reveals face views of membranes. The endocrine cells shown here have been cleaved in such a way that a fracturing plane followed cell membranes (cm) for some distance before breaking through into the interior of the cells, revealing the nucleus with numerous nuclear pores (np) or annuli in the nuclear envelope. Most of the globular cytoplasmic profiles represent secretory granules. (With permission from Orci, L.: Morphological characterization of membrane systems in A- and B-cells of the Chinese hamster. Diabetologica 10:529–539, 1974.)*

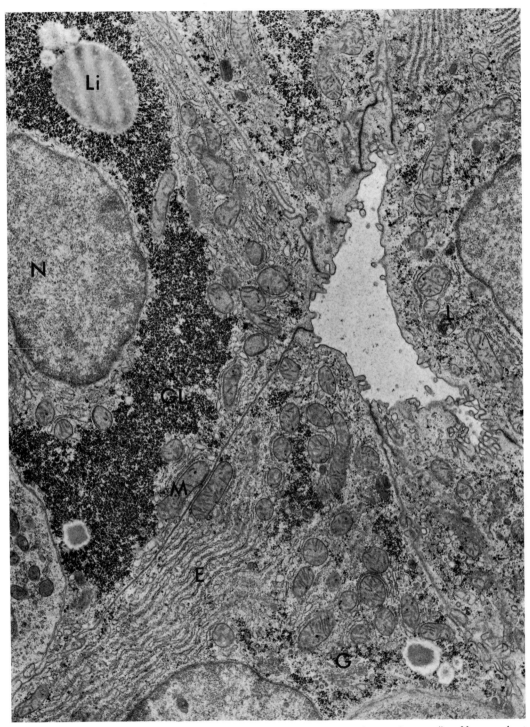

***Figure 1–4.*** *Electron micrograph of rat liver cells illustrating the appearance of several organelles: N = nucleus; M = mitochondrion; G = Golgi apparatus; E = granular endoplasmic reticulum; L = lysosome; GL = glycogen; Li = lipid. The clear space in the center is a bile canaliculus. × 13,000. (Courtesy of J. Steiner.)*

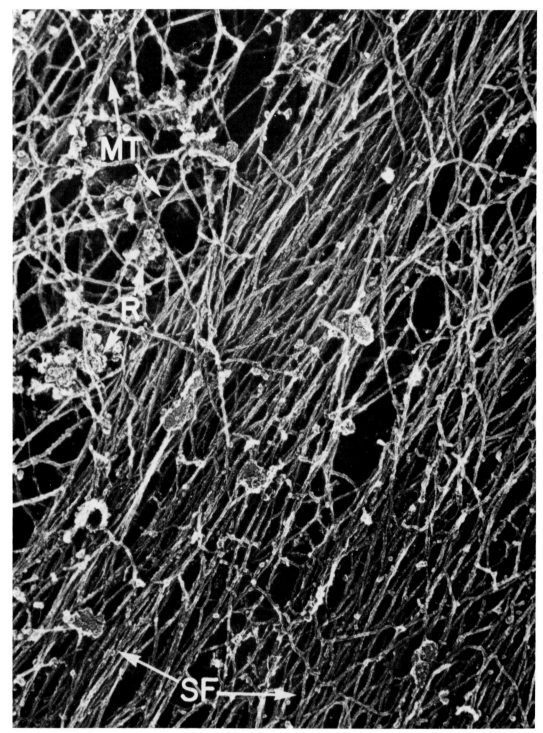

**Figure 1–5.** Platinum replica of freeze-dried cytoskeleton from a fibroblast. Prominent are bundles of filaments called stress fibers (SF). Also visible in upper left-hand corner are two thicker structures thought to be microtubules (MT). Filaments are studded in various places with grape-like clusters that are the size and shape of polyribosomes (R). × 70,000. (From Heuser, J. E., and Kirschner, N. W.: Filament organization revealed in platinum replicas of freeze-dried cytoskeletons. J Cell Biol 86:212–234, 1980; reproduced from The Journal of Cell Biology by copyright permission of The Rockefeller University Press.)

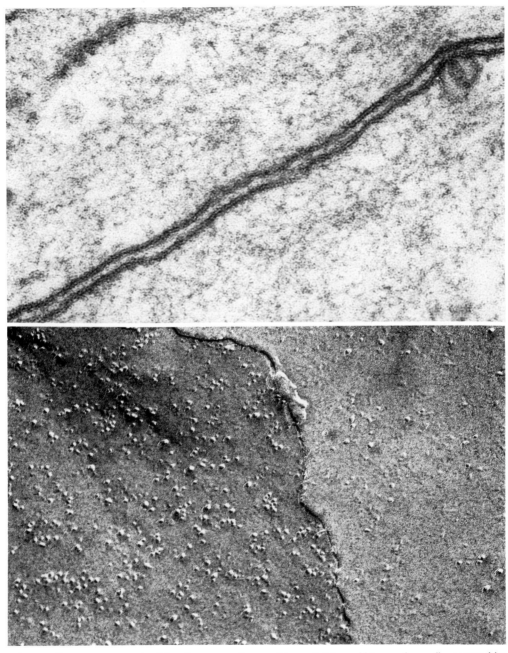

**Figure 1–6.** Top: *Electron micrograph of the plasma membranes of two adjoining rabbit granulosa cells separated by a 15-nm intercellular cleft.* × 240,000. Bottom: *Freeze-fracture replica of a typical plasma membrane from a spermatocyte, showing P-fracture face on the left and E-fracture face on the right.* × 168,000. (Courtesy of Dr. H. N. Tung.)

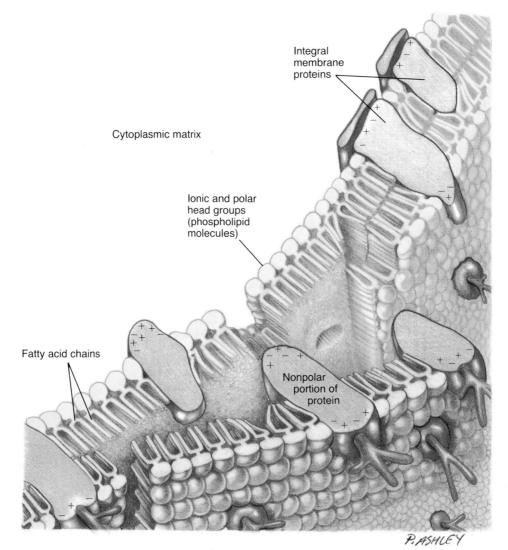

*Figure 1–7. Diagram of the fluid mosaic model of the plasma membrane.*

well-defined layers. The latter arrangement is called the "unit membrane" structure of two dense lines, each about 2.5 nm thick, separated by a lucent intermediate layer of about 3 nm.

Several models have been proposed for the plasma membrane. On the basis of a great amount of experimental data, Danielli and Davson advanced the concept that the membrane consisted of an inner and outer layer of protein, separated by an intermediate bimolecular layer of lipid. Membrane lipids, mostly phospholipids, have a hydrophilic phosphate (polar) end and a hydrophobic, nonpolar end (fatty acid "tail"). In the membrane, the phospholipids are arranged in two monomolecular layers with the hydrophilic phosphate ends on the surface contacting the protein layers and the hydrophobic tails apposed to each other in the center of the membrane.

This configuration is, unfortunately, often referred to with the not too very precise designation of "unit membrane," since its three layers have been considered to correspond to the bimolecular lipid layer with the two surrounding protein layers in the Danielli and Davson model. However, the appearance in recent years of much new information concerning the properties of the cell membrane has led to the proposal of other concepts of the molecular structure of the cell membrane. Of these, the so-called "fluid mosaic model" of Singer and Nicholson is in best accord with present knowledge. This model considers the cell membrane to consist of a bimolecular layer of phospholipids, into which globular protein units are intercalated at varying intervals, forming a mosaic with the lipid layer. These integral membrane proteins have been shown to have hydrophobic and hydrophilic regions, and probably the hydrophobic parts are embedded in the central lipid of the membrane, with the hydrophilic regions exposed at the surface. The phospholipids and proteins in the membrane are believed to be largely independent of each other, since they form true chemical bonds only to a very slight degree.

Although study of electron micrographs and freeze-etch replicas may give the impression that the plasma membrane is a rigid structure, many components, particularly membrane proteins, move freely. During movement, the protein molecules are presumed to maintain their orientation and position in the membrane owing to their polar character.

Substances move selectively through membranes in the living cell. If the cell is killed or the plasma membrane is irreparably damaged, molecules move freely across the membrane, and equilibrium may be attained. Because equilibrium is rarely reached in living systems, the living membrane must serve as a dynamic, regulatory barrier to the entry and exit of molecules and particles. The maintenance of the intracellular environment requires selective membrane transport that is both active and passive, with nutrients passing into the cell and other materials passing out. The rate at which a molecule diffuses across the plasma membrane depends largely on the size of the molecule and on its relative solubility in lipid. The more lipid-soluble it is—that is, the more hydrophobic or nonpolar it is—and the smaller its size, the more rapidly a molecule diffuses across a lipid bilayer. Physiologically, it is believed that there are pores in the membrane, although these have not been demonstrated morphologically. They may be represented by channels in those proteins that traverse the full thickness of the membrane. These transport proteins open only in response to a particular stimulus and are otherwise closed passageways. The stimulus that the plasma membrane receives can come from hormones and neurotransmitters. Hormones, at a "target" cell, either must penetrate the plasma membrane (which occurs with steroid hormones, probably because they are lipid-soluble) or must transmit their message across it without penetrating (which occurs with glycoprotein hormones that ligand-bind to cell-surface receptors).

The plasma membrane differs from other membranes in that its external surface is covered with glycoprotein, the *cell coat* or *glycocalyx*. This coat varies in thickness from 10 to 20 nm according to the functions performed by the particular cells. It can be demonstrated in some cells by the periodic acid–Schiff (PAS) technique, for example, on the luminal surface of intestinal epithelium where it is associated with small, finger-like protrusions of the cell surface called *microvilli*. Intestinal cells possess a thicker glycocalyx because of the variety of substances that come in contact with their surfaces. On electron microscopy, it appears as an internal amorphous substance and external fine filaments called *antennulae microvillares*. The glycocalyx is composed of glycolipids, glycoproteins containing high amounts of sialic acid, and proteoglycans. It is synthesized by coordinated activity of rough endoplasmic reticulum and Golgi apparatus and is transported in vesicles to the cell surface. Aside from the obvious functions of providing a filtration barrier and a suitable microenvironment for materials to enter and leave the cell, the glycocalyx makes it possible to genetically program specific cell recognition at the molecular level. The surfaces of probably all cells show a glycocalyx, although it may be thin, and it is absent only in areas of specialized cell contact (see page 108). This cell coat confers a negative charge on the cell surface that probably is important in cellular contacts and adhesions, most cells being separated by a regular interval of about 20 nm. The variety and amounts of components in the glycocalyx impart to each cell type a special identity. Recognition of cells plays an important role in histocompatibility and helps explain, to some degree, rejection of grafts.

Although the membrane is a bilayer structure, it is not symmetrical. Morphologically, as shown above, glycoproteins, glycopeptides, and glycolipids are situated in the outer layer, and there also are differences in composition of lipids between the two layers.

Solutes, macromolecules, and particles can cross the membrane by processes that involve the formation of membrane-bounded vesicles or the fusion of vesicles with the plasma membrane. In this process, a cell surrounds a part of the environment with a section of its cell membrane. This section then separates from the cell membrane itself and moves into the interior of the cell. The general term for this process is *endocytosis*. If the contents of the vesicle are solid materials, the process is called *phagocytosis*. If the contents are liquid, the process of vesicle formation is *pinocytosis*. Endocytosis is an active process that requires energy, but the exact mechanisms of this process are not clearly understood. Endocytosis does not involve large amounts of materials, but this route of entry does provide a means by which small amounts of even the largest molecules may enter cells. The reverse of this process, that is, extrusion of material, is called *exocytosis*. Here, the membrane bounding an excretory granule or droplet, for example, fuses with the plasmalemma and releases its contents to the exterior. Apart from releasing material from the cell, the process of exocytosis may also generate additional cell membrane when the membranous vesicles fuse with the plasmalemma. Various cell products and secretions (e.g., mucus droplets that are formed in intestinal goblet cells and digestive-enzyme precursors that appear in granule packages from pancreatic cells) may, by exocytosis, leave the cells in which they are produced.

Micropinocytotic vesicles or *caveolae intracellulares* are only about 50 nm in diameter and are involved in transport of proteins and other molecules. They are particularly prominent in endothelial and mesothelial cells (lining vascular spaces and the body cavities) and in smooth muscle cells.

In many cell types, there are modifications in the form of the plasma membrane, the majority of these being visible only on electron microscopy. For example, in cells specialized for absorption, there are at the apical (luminal) surface a series of small, finger-like processes, or *microvilli*. These are simple, tubular evaginations of the plasma membrane with a cytoplasmic core in which there are collections of microfibrils. If the microvilli are regular and closely packed, they collectively form a "brush" or "striated" border, visible on light microscopy, and obviously greatly increase surface area (Figs. 1–8 and 1–9). In addition, the surface area of cells is often increased by numerous infoldings of the basal plasmalemma (Figs. 1–10 and 1–11). Between cells (i.e., at lateral borders), adjacent plasma membranes are separated by a narrow gap of about 20 nm, and, while the interface may be straight and regular with adjacent plasmalemmae parallel, often it is highly irregular with a system of interlocking tongues and grooves. This is termed a "jigsaw" or "zipper" interlocking and is a factor in cell adhesion. Other specializations of the cell surface are discussed later in relation to epithelium. They include *maculae adherentes* or *spot desmosomes* (Fig. 1–12) that appear as small densities scattered along cell interfaces. Occasionally, the intercellular space is widened to form "intercellular canals," usually with microvillus or pseudopodial projections of adjacent cells into the intercellular space.

## ROUGH-SURFACED (GRANULAR) ENDOPLASMIC RETICULUM

By light microscopy, in some cell types, there are areas of the cytoplasm that stain blue with basic stains, such regions being termed the *basophilic component* of the cytoplasm, *chromidial substance*, or *ergastoplasm* (ergastoplasm indicates work, i.e., that component of the cytoplasm involved in synthesis) (Fig. 1–13). All cells contain an ergastoplasm, whose membranes typically constitute more than half of the total membrane in a cell. On electron microscopy, these membranes contain large numbers of small electron-dense particles called *ribosomes*, usually attached to these membranes, which are arranged as a three-dimensional network or reticulum of channels in the form of cisternae or flattened sacs,

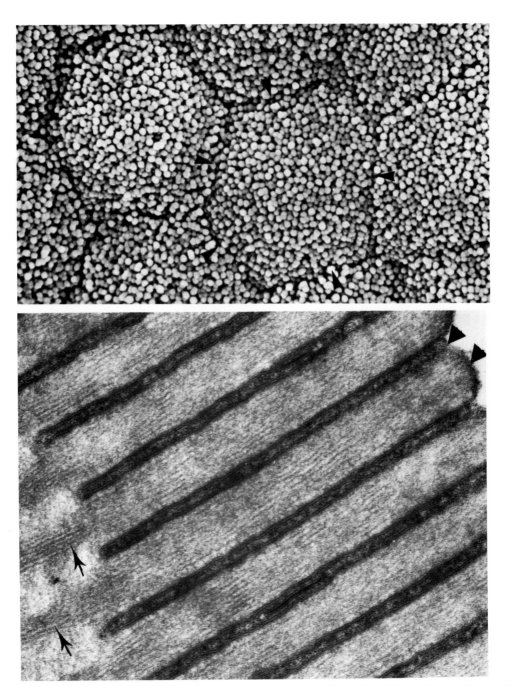

**Figure 1–8.** Microvilli of the brush border. Top: Scanning electron micrograph of cells of the monkey gallbladder. Note cell outlines (arrowheads). × 4000. (Courtesy of Dr. P. Andrews.) Bottom: Microvilli of the lining epithelial cells of the duodenum. Note the trilaminar plasma membrane with associated glycocalyx (arrowheads) and bundles of filaments (arrows) in the cores of the microvilli. × 125,000.

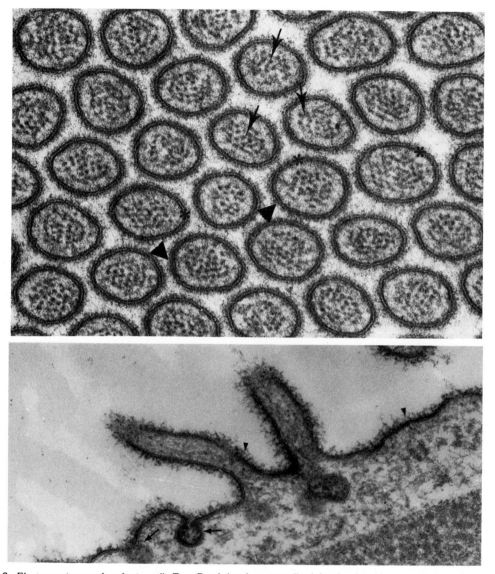

**Figure 1–9.** *Electron micrographs of microvilli. Top: Brush border microvilli of the duodenal lining epithelial cells, in transverse section. Note trilaminar plasma membrane (asterisks) and associated glycocalyx (arrowheads), core of filaments in the microvilli (arrows).* × *125,000. Bottom: Mesothelial cell of pleura showing occasional microvilli, glycocalyx associated with the plasma membrane (arrowheads), and micropinocytotic vesicles, two as invaginations (arrows) of the surface plasma membrane.* × *115,000.*

tubules, and vesicles (Figs. 1–14 and 1–15). This membranous network runs throughout much of the cytoplasm of the cell and is continuous with the cell membrane and the nuclear envelope. The myriad unions of this membranous network to the cell membrane and nuclear membrane lead to the reasoning that the network is derived from an invagination of the cell membrane. The membrane of the reticulum shows a unit membrane or trilaminar structure, usually 6 to 7 nm thick, which encloses a lumen or intracisternal space. This space may contain some flocculent material of moderate electron density that represents newly synthesized protein.

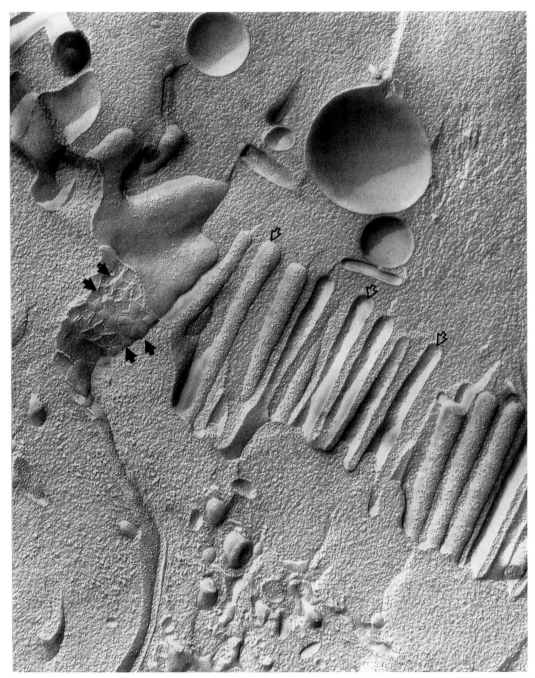

**Figure 1–10.** Electron micrograph of freeze-fracture replica of intestinal absorptive cells depicting microvilli (clear arrows) and a tight junction (solid arrows). × 57,000. (Courtesy of Drs. R. Roberts, H. N. Tung, and R. G. Kessel.)

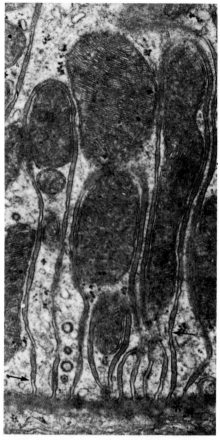

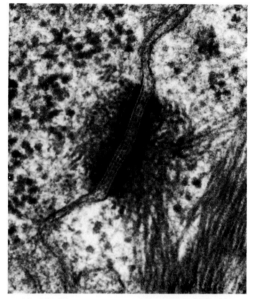

**Figure 1–11.** Electron micrograph of basal infoldings (arrows) of the plasma membrane in an epithelial cell of a kidney tubule. Amorphous basal lamina material is marked with asterisk. × 25,000.

**Figure 1–12.** Electron micrograph of a spot desmosome (macula adherens) on a cellular interface of epithelial cells (epidermis). Note associated cytoplasmic filaments and density of the two plasma membranes. × 64,000.

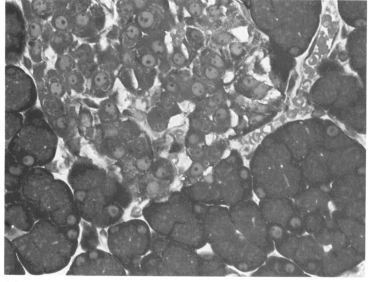

**Figure 1–13.** Photomicrograph to illustrate cytoplasmic basophilia and pink-staining droplets. The zymogen-secreting cells of the pancreas are arranged in groups or acini. The basal cytoplasm of each cell stains intensely basophil (purple) owing to the presence of numerous ribosomes associated with the endoplasmic reticulum. The apical cytoplasm contains pink-staining secretory (zymogen) droplets or granules. Compare the intense basophilia of these cells with the lack of it in endocrine cells of an islet of Langerhans (above). Pancreas. Plastic section. H and E. High power.

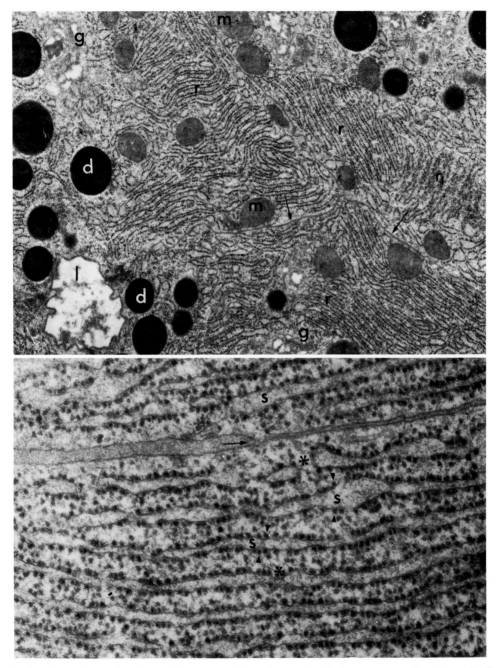

***Figure 1–14.*** *Electron micrographs demonstrate the granular endoplasmic reticulum in pancreatic acinar cells. Top: Large collections of parallel cisternae of granular reticulum are seen (r), also sectioned en face at center right (r). Also seen are mitochondria (m), Golgi apparatus (g), secretory droplets (d), plasma membranes at cell interfaces (arrows), and the lumen (l) of an acinus. × 8000. Bottom: Parts of two cells with a cell interface (arrow), parallel cisternae of granular reticulum with lumina or intracisternal spaces (s) containing some flocculent material and bounded by membranes studded with ribosomes (arrowheads) on their cytoplasmic surfaces. Note pores or fenestrae (asterisks), that is, discontinuities in the cisternae. × 80,000.*

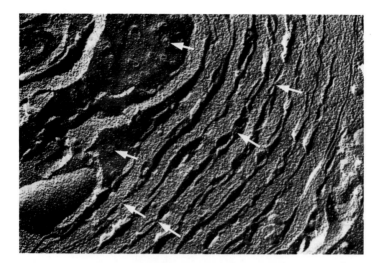

*Figure 1–15.* Freeze-etch preparation of granular endoplasmic reticulum in transverse and longitudinal fracture planes in pancreatic acinar cell of the spiny mouse. Arrows point to fenestrae or pores. × 33,000. (Courtesy of Dr. L. Orci.)

This organelle is particularly well developed in protein-secreting cells, a good example being the enzyme-producing cells of the pancreas. Attached to the outer surfaces of the membranous network are the ribosomes; hence the term rough endoplasmic reticulum. In order to study the functions and biochemistry of the rough endoplasmic reticulum, it is necesary to separate its membranes from other components of the cell. Intuitively, this would seem a staggering task, since this membranous network may connect with the plasmalemma in a few cell types or with nuclear envelope, and in some cells, it shows continuity also with the smooth or agranular endoplasmic reticulum and also communicates via small vesicles to the Golgi apparatus. Fortunately, when tissues or cells are disrupted by homogenization, the endoplasmic reticulum is fragmented into many smaller ($\cong 100$ nm in diameter) closed vesicles called *microsomes*. Microsomes derived from rough endoplasmic reticulum are studded with ribosomes. Ribosomes are always found on the outside surface of such microsomes, with the microsomal lumina containing the secretory product of the reticulum. Because they can be readily purified in functional form, microsomes represent a specially useful preparation for studying the many different processes carried out by this organelle. The vesicles are topologically sealed in the same manner as the rough endoplasmic reticulum, leaving their cytoplasmic surfaces easily accessible to components that can be added *in vitro*. To the biochemist, microsomes represent small authentic versions of the rough endoplasmic reticulum still capable of protein synthesis.

As indicated already, the main function of granular endoplasmic reticulum is synthesis of a secretory protein and its segregation from the remainder of the cytoplasm within the intracisternal space. In some cells (e.g., pancreatic acinar cells), concentration of the product also occurs within the reticulum, although concentration mainly occurs in the Golgi apparatus. The rough endoplasmic reticulum is also involved in the production of lipid components of most of the cell's organelles. Its extensive membranes contain many different biosynthetic enzymes, including those responsible for all of the cell's lipid synthesis.

## RIBOSOMES

Ribosomes are small electron-dense particles measuring about 15 nm in diameter at the widest portion. As indicated earlier, ribosomes are responsible for the cytoplasmic basophilia, and they contain RNA and protein. They are found in all cells except mature erythrocytes and may be attached to, and part of, the granular endoplasmic reticulum, or they may lie free within the general cytoplasm.

In humans and all other mammals, the ribosome has a characteristic sedimentation coefficient of 80S, with the larger, heavier subunit of 60S and the smaller subunit of 40S. Whether they are free or attached, ribosomes are generally found in

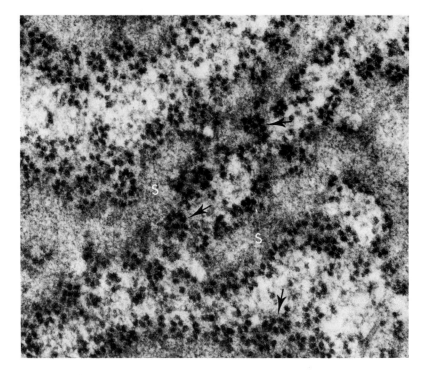

**Figure 1-16.** *Electron micrograph of polyribosomes. Cisternae of granular reticulum cut en face showing intracisternal spaces (s) with polyribosomes (arrows) associated with cisternal membranes. × 61,000.*

clusters called *polysomes* or *polyribosomes* (Fig. 1-16). The clusters represent groups of ribosomes connected by a strand of messenger RNA. Polysomes vary in the number of associated ribosomes, and in general, the larger the strand of messenger RNA, the greater the number of attached ribosomes and the longer the polypeptide chain that is produced. It has been suggested that free ribosomes synthesize the proteins that are used by the cell for its own needs, such as replication, whereas ribosomes attached to membranes synthesize proteins that will be secreted by the cell and used elsewhere in the body.

The role of ribosomes and granular endoplasmic reticulum in protein synthesis is discussed in more detail at the end of this chapter.

### SMOOTH-SURFACED (AGRANULAR) ENDOPLASMIC RETICULUM

In contrast to granular endoplasmic reticulum, agranular, as implied by the term, is devoid of ribosomal granules (Fig. 1-17). Since it does not stain differently from the surrounding cytoplasmic matrix, it was first discovered after the introduction of electron microscopy. This organelle is tubular or vesicular in form and is more likely to appear as a profusion of interconnected channels of variable shape and size than as stacks of flattened cisternae, which characterize rough endoplasmic reticulum. However, the membranes are similar to those of granular reticulum, being 6 to 7 nm thick, with a tubular lumen of about 50 nm. Smooth endoplasmic reticulum membranes arise from rough endoplasmic reticulum and may connect directly with granular reticulum and indirectly with the Golgi apparatus via small vesicles.

Smooth endoplasmic reticulum is not involved in protein synthesis. Although it is plentiful in some specialized cells (see section below), in the great majority of cells, including most secretory cells, smooth endoplasmic reticulum is really nothing more than a small ribosome-free region of rough endoplasmic reticulum. Such regions are called *transitional endoplasmic reticulum*, rather than smooth endoplasmic reticulum. They represent the specialized region of endoplasmic reticulum from which the vesicles bud off for intracellular transport.

Smooth endoplasmic reticulum not only exhibits a diversity of morphological appearances in

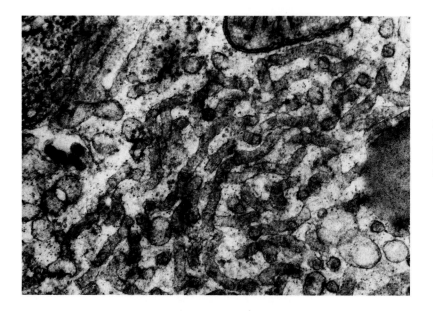

*Figre 1–17.* Electron micrograph of a portion of an interstitial (Leydig's) cell of the rat testis. The cytoplasm largely is occupied by smooth or agranular endoplasmic reticulum. × 34,000.

different cell types but also is associated with a variety of specialized functional capabilities. It may be the most prominent organelle (e.g., in steroid-secreting cells), or it may be represented by a few elements only. In different cell types, it performs different functions. The smooth reticulum functions in the biosynthesis of steroid hormones and is found in abundance in, for example, Leydig's cells of the testis that secrete testosterone, cells of the adrenal cortex that secrete corticosteroids, and progesterone-secreting cells of the corpus luteum of the ovary. In hepatic parenchymal cells, *glucagon*, a hormone produced by the pancreas, induces the formation of new endoplasmic reticulum membranes, which participate in glycogen breakdown to glucose and in lipid synthesis. Glucagon is also concerned with the metabolism of several lipid-soluble drugs such as barbiturates. The hepatic parenchymal cells are the principal site of production of lipoprotein particles for export. The enzymes that synthesize the lipid components of lipoproteins are located in the membranes of the smooth endoplasmic reticulum. This organelle also contains enzymes that catalyze a series of reactions to detoxify both drugs and harmful compounds produced by metabolism. In columnar absorptive cells lining the intestine, it is associated with lipid absorption, resynthesizing triglycerides from monoglycerides and fatty acids that are absorbed into the cells, and passing the

triglycerides into the intestinal lymphatic vessels. In striated and cardiac muscle, a specialized and elaborate smooth endoplasmic reticulum, called the *sarcoplasmic reticulum*, sequesters calcium from the cytosol. The calcium-ATPase that pumps in calcium is the major membrane protein present in this smooth endoplasmic reticulum. The removal of calcium from the cytosol permits the relaxation of the myofibrils following each round of muscle contraction.

The agranular reticulum must be distinguished from other smooth, membranous elements in the cytoplasm such as the Golgi apparatus and vesicles. The fact that it often is connected to cisternae of the rough endoplasmic reticulum suggests that it is derived from the rough reticulum.

### GOLGI APPARATUS

The Golgi apparatus, or Golgi complex, consists of stacks of flattened sacs located in the cytoplasm of many cells (Fig. 1–18). Arrayed around the margins of the flattened sacs are vesicles of various sizes. This organelle may be visible by light microscopy as either a "positive" or "negative" image. After silver impregnation or prolonged exposure to osmium tetroxide, it is seen as a darkly staining network of canals or vacuoles or as an irregular granular mass located near the nucleus and is sometimes multiple. The Golgi

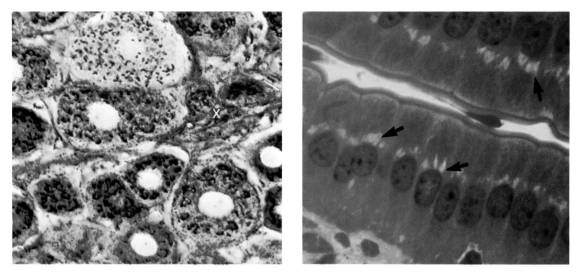

**Figure 1–18.** *Golgi apparatus. Left: The large spheroidal cells are ganglion cells, with large spherical nuclei, of a dorsal root ganglion. In the cytoplasm of these cells is an extensive network of dark (black) small vesicles and tubules. This is the Golgi apparatus as a positive image. In these cells the Golgi apparatus is scattered throughout the cytoplasm and around the nucleus and is extensive. Sensory ganglion. Plastic section. Osmium tetroxide. High power. Right: The mucosal surface of the duodenum shows a negative image of the Golgi apparatus in a supranuclear position (arrows). Duodenal epithelium. Plastic section. H and E. Oil immersion.*

apparatus is frequently disposed about the centriole pair that defines the cell center. The number of Golgi stacks per cell varies enormously, depending on the cell type, from as few as one to hundreds. The Golgi apparatus can even account for a large fraction of the cell volume in some specialized cells. One example is the goblet cell of the intestinal epithelium, which secretes mucus into the gut; the glycoproteins in mucus are glycosylated principally in the Golgi apparatus. Its appearance and location, however, do vary with cell type. In secretory cells, for example, it is supranuclear, but in nerve cells, it usually forms a net around the entire nucleus (Fig. 1–19). After routine H and E staining, in cells with intensely basophil cytoplasm such as osteoblasts and plasma cells, the Golgi apparatus is indicated as a pale, clear area. This is a "negative" image; the "positive" image is seen after special techniques, as indicated earlier. Historically, existence of the Golgi apparatus was questioned as artifact until electron microscopy confirmed not only its presence but also its complex structure and distinctive role in the secretory process of proteins.

With the electron microscope, three membranous components are seen in the Golgi complex: (1) cisternae (flattened plates) or saccules, (2) small vesicles, and (3) larger vacuoles, all lacking ribosomes. The cisternae tend to be bowed, presenting a convex proximal face (toward the nucleus) and a concave distal face (away from the nucleus). The cisternae are relatively compressed at their centers and somewhat dilated peripherally. The Golgi complex, as a whole, looks like a stack of shallow bowls with the concavity directed away from the nucleus. These flattened, curved, smooth-surfaced membranous cisternae are arranged in parallel stacks of 3 to 12, with a regular spacing of 20 to 30 nm between adjacent cisternae. The cisternae may communicate with one another by slender channels at places along their contiguous surfaces. The proximal membranes are thinner than the distal membranes, which are more like those of the plasmalemma (7.5 to 10 nm). The cisternal lumen is about 15 nm wide, but dilation occurs, particularly at the periphery or rim of the saccules. Electron-dense material may be present within cisternae. The term *dictyosome* describes such a stack of cisternae, and this may be the entire Golgi apparatus in a cell, although more usually several dictyosomes are present (Fig. 1–20). The proximal face (that near the nucleus) is relatively free of vesicles and has been termed the convex forming (immature) face.

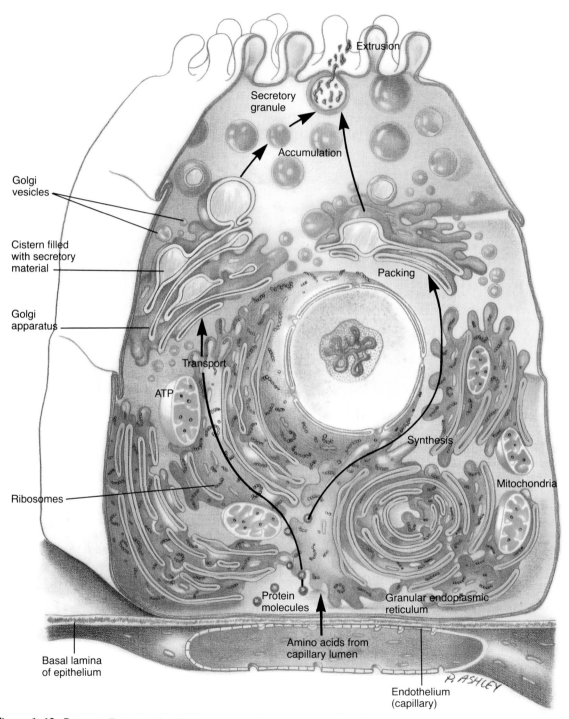

**Figure 1–19.** Diagram illustrating the Golgi apparatus of a secretory cell and its participation in protein and glycoprotein secretion.

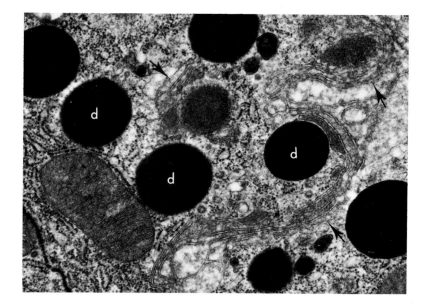

**Figure 1–20.** Electron micrograph of the apical region of a rat exocrine pancreatic cell. Several dictyosomes (arrows) and cisternae containing secretory material with dense secretory droplets (d) are seen. × 19,750.

The distal face (facing out toward the bulk of the cytoplasm), which is typically engaged in granule formation, has been termed the concave (mature) secreting face. Associated with the distal cisternae are vesicles and vacuoles. *Vesicles* are small spheres about 40 nm in diameter, most smooth-surfaced but some with a bristle-like coat of fine filaments radiating from the surface ("coated vesicles"). In addition to mediating a variety of endocytotic processes, coated vesicles appear to be responsible for the transport of membrane proteins between the endoplasmic reticulum and the Golgi apparatus and between the Golgi apparatus and the plasma membrane. Different sorts of coated vesicles would seem to be necessary to account for their diverse array of functions. *Vacuoles* vary in diameter up to 0.5 μm and may contain secretory products of varying density. The larger ones have a dense, homogeneous content and are termed "condensing," or secretory, vacuoles. In the case of the pancreas, secretory vacuoles contain concentrated secretory proteins (zymogen granules). These secretory proteins are discharged from the cell by exocytosis, a process in which the secretory vacuoles fuse with the plasma membrane to release their content to the outside. The location of vesicles and vacuoles in relation to the cisternal stack often is asymmetrical.

The Golgi apparatus is not static but changes continually (Figs. 1–21 and 1–22). Elements of granular reticulum adjacent to the Golgi apparatus lack ribosomes, and from these elements, small "transfer" vesicles "bud" off, enclosing some of the content of the reticulum. The transfer vesicles pass toward and then fuse with a Golgi element, often a cisterna at the forming face, thus releasing the contents into the saccule. Also, secretory vacuoles are formed at the mature face and pass to the cell periphery. The Golgi apparatus, then, appears to accept vesicles from the endoplasmic reticulum, modify their contents and their enclosing membrane, and pass the products in the form of secretory vesicles and lysosomes to other parts of the cell. This involves a movement or "flow" of membrane through the Golgi stack from forming to mature face, the membranes "maturing" from a type similar to endoplasmic reticulum to one similar to the plasmalemma. This process, as secretory vacuoles fuse with the plasmalemma and release their contents by exocytosis, would result in an increase in area of the plasmalemma; it is believed that to balance it some plasmalemma is internalized by endocytosis and then digested by lysosomal action.

In contrast to this concept of "membrane flow" and to recognize the fact that there are differences between the membranes of the endoplasmic reticulum, Golgi apparatus, and plasmalemma, there is the alternative theory of "membrane shuttle." This hypothesis postulates that the membrane types do not mix; however, on the immature face, transfer vesicles release their content into the Golgi saccule and then shuttle back to the reticulum to repeat the process. On the mature face, a similar shuttle mechanism transports secretory material to the surface via secretory vacuoles.

Many types of molecules pass through some portion of the Golgi structure at some stage in their maturation, usually shortly after their synthesis in the endoplasmic reticulum. These include glycoproteins and proteoglycans; glycolipids; plasma membrane glycoproteins: proteins of lysosomes; and secreted proteins. Concentration of secreted proteins occurs by removal of water; although this process starts in the Golgi apparatus, it usually continues after formation of the secre-

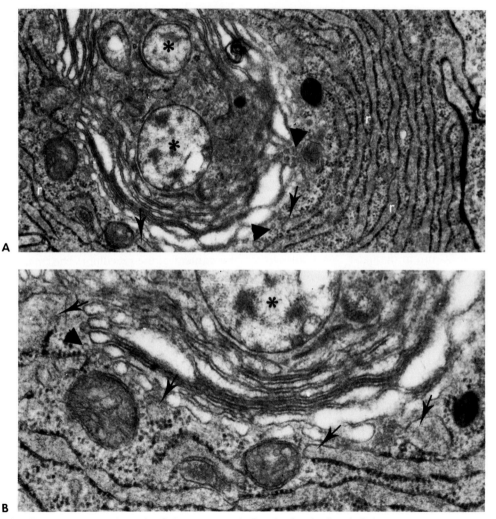

**Figure 1–21.** *Electron micrographs of the Golgi apparatus. A, Rat duodenal cell with Golgi cisternae in a cup or bowl shape, forming face externally and mature face internally with lysosomes (asterisks). The apparatus is surrounded by an extensive granular endoplasmic reticulum (r) with transfer vesicles (arrowheads) and elements of granular reticulum lacking ribosomes (arrows) where it is adjacent to the Golgi apparatus. × 19,750. B, A higher magnification of the top picture. × 34,000. C, A freeze-fracture replica of the Golgi apparatus from rat primary decidual cell. × 61,000. (Courtesy of Drs., H. N. Tung, M. Parr, and E. Parr.)*

*Illustration continued on opposite page*

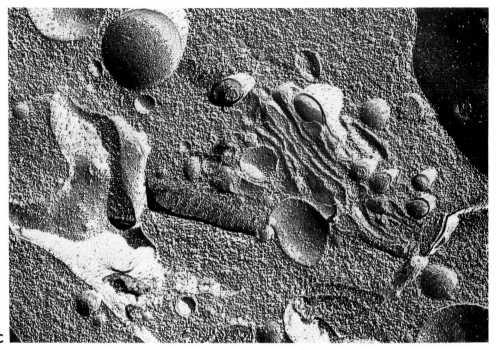

C

*Figure 1–21* Continued

tory granule, which becomes increasingly dense as it matures. In cells in which the secretory product is glycoprotein, some sugars are added to the polypeptide in the endoplasmic reticulum, but synthesis is completed in the Golgi apparatus by the addition of other sugar residues. The Golgi apparatus functions much the same in the secretion of lipids as it does in the secretion of protein. Lipids, however, are synthesized by the smooth endoplasmic reticulum. Some of the lipid is released from the cell surface just as protein secretions are, but some is also released into the cytoplasm of the cell, where it remains in the form of lipid droplets.

The Golgi apparatus is also involved in the synthesis of sulfated mucopolysaccharides (e.g., in goblet cells of the intestinal mucosa). In beta cells of the pancreas, proinsulin synthesized in the endoplasmic reticulum is cleaved into insulin (the active product) and C-peptide within the Golgi apparatus. The carbohydrate components of the plasmalemma are synthesized in the Golgi complex. The Golgi apparatus is responsible for the packaging of hydrolytic enzymes, and the so-called primary lysosomes are pinched off from

the Golgi apparatus. In some cells, a type of smooth reticulum situated near the forming face of the Golgi apparatus is involved in the formation of lysosomes (and possibly also secretory vacuoles), without the involvement of the Golgi apparatus. This reticulum, because of its location, nature, and assumed function, is called *GERL* (Golgi, endoplasmic reticulum, and lysosome).

Thus, the Golgi apparatus is involved in membrane flow; in transport and concentration of secretory materials and their release from the cell; in synthesis of certain secretory products, particularly glycoproteins and mucopolysaccharides; and in primary lysosome formation.

### LYSOSOMES

Lysosomes are membrane-bound cytoplasmic structures that appear granular during inactivity but assume the appearance of vesicles when active (Fig. 1–23). Lysosomes are believed to originate from the Golgi apparatus. However, in certain cells or under certain conditions, they may be derived from portions of the endoplasmic reticulum.

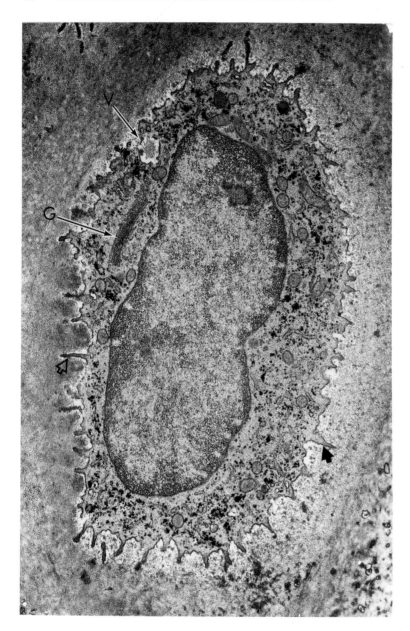

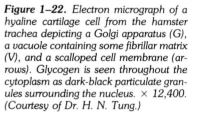

**Figure 1–22.** Electron micrograph of a hyaline cartilage cell from the hamster trachea depicting a Golgi apparatus (G), a vacuole containing some fibrillar matrix (V), and a scalloped cell membrane (arrows). Glycogen is seen throughout the cytoplasm as dark-black particulate granules surrounding the nucleus. × 12,400. (Courtesy of Dr. H. N. Tung.)

Lysosomes constitute an intracellular digestive system capable of breaking down materials originating both outside and within the cell (Fig. 1–24). Owing to their involvement in digestion, their appearance depends upon their functional state, and this results in a great variety of appearances, or pleomorphism. Electron microscopically, they appear as rounded granules that are bound by a trilaminar membrane. Although variable in size, they usually range from 0.2 to 0.4 μm in diameter. Lysosomes are found in all cells except erythrocytes but are numerous particularly in macrophages, neutrophil leukocytes, hepatic cells, and cells of the proximal tubule of the kidney. Some 40 enzymes are known to be contained in lysosomes. They are all hydrolytic

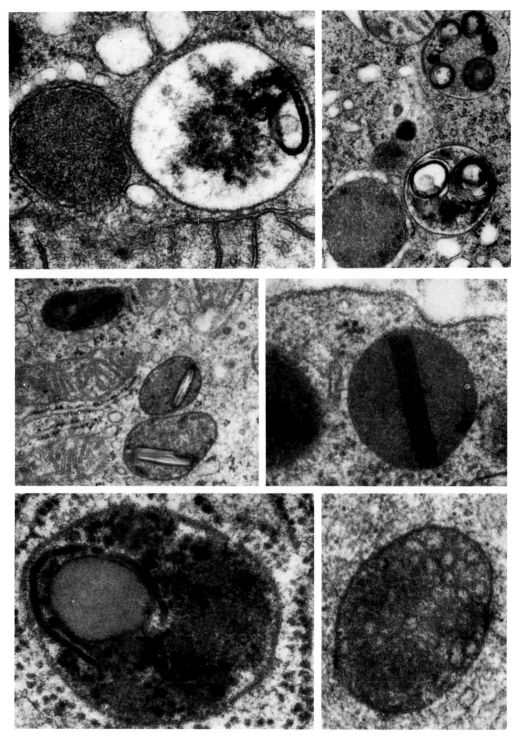

**Figure 1–23.** *Electron micrographs illustrate primary lysosomes (top left and right), secondary lysosomes (center left and bottom left), a lysosome ("specific granule") of an eosinophil leukocyte (center right), and a multivesicular body (bottom right). Top left: kidney tubule cell, × 65,000. Top right: kidney tubule cell, × 31,000. Center left: duodenal epithelial cell, × 21,000. Center right: eosinophil leukocyte, × 28,000. Lower left: pancreatic acinar cell, × 68,000. Lower right: duodenal epithelial cell, × 68,000.*

*49*

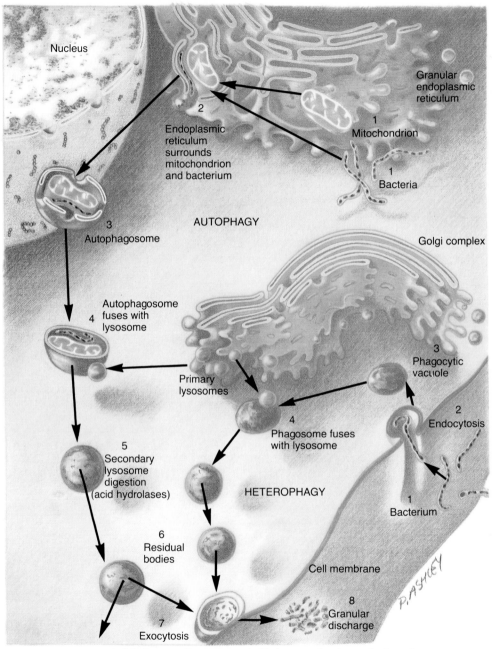

*Figure 1–24. Diagram illustrating probable lysosomal pathways in the cell.*

enzymes, including proteases, nucleases, glycosidases, lipases, phospholipases, phosphatases, and sulfatases. All are acid hydrolases, optimally active near the pH of 5 maintained within this organelle. They can be identified by electron cytochemistry using a modified Gomori technique for acid phosphatase, a commonly used marker, or by reactions for other enzymes they contain. The activity of these enzymes is controlled by the lysosomal bounding membrane. This membrane selectively admits substrates into the lysosome and protects the cells against indiscriminate digestion by its own lysosomal enzymes. Unlike secretory granules, lysosomes are typically not released but remain within the cytoplasm.

Lysosomes can be divided into two main groups. A *primary lysosome* is one that is "resting" and has not entered into the digestive event and, as indicated previously, probably arises in the Golgi complex. A *secondary lysosome* is engaged actively in digestion and occurs after fusion of a primary lysosome with some other membrane-bound body arising from within or outside the cell. The only sure guide to their identification is histological methods to detect the presence of hydrolytic enzymes within these structures. Following digestion of the contents of the secondary lysosome, nutrients diffuse through the lysosomal membrane and enter the cytoplasm. Some material may be indigestible, and the secondary lysosome, now inactive, thus is termed a *residual body*. Morphologically, residual bodies are identified by a content of whorls of membranous material, and they subsequently tend to accumulate lipid, which may later become oxidized to a pigmented material called lipofuscin. In some long-lived cells (e.g., neurons, heart muscle, hepatocytes), large quantities of residual bodies (lipofuscin) accumulate with age.

Substances of extracellular origin that enter the cell by endocytosis do so by membrane-bound bodies. The cytoplasmic vacuole so formed by engulfing extracellular material may contain fluid with material in solution or suspension; this process is termed *pinocytosis*. If a relatively large, solid material such as a microorganism is included in the vacuole, the process is called *phagocytosis*. The vacuole so formed by internalization of materials from the exterior is referred to as a *phagosome* or *heterophagosome*. Another function of lysosomes concerns the turnover of cytoplasmic organelles. Primary lysosomes fuse with these structures and initiate the lysis of the enclosed cytoplasm. The resulting vacuole is known as an *autosome*, and the process is called *autophagy*. Fusion of a phagosome or autosome with a primary lysosome containing hydrolytic enzymes produces a secondary lysosome. Active enzymic digestion within the secondary lysosome breaks down the contents into small molecules that pass back across the lysosomal membrane into the

cytoplasm. Lysosomal enzymes may be released by exocytosis into the extracellular space, for example, in osteoclasts, cells involved in bone resorption. In some secretory cells when secretion is diminished or ceases, newly formed secretory granules may be passed directly into the lysosomal pathway to prevent overaccumulation of secretory material, this process being termed *crinophagy*.

*Tay-Sachs disease* is one of a group of several important genetic diseases involving lysosomes. If the enzymes in lysosomes fail to function, then substrates that should degrade accumulate in the cytoplasm to such a degree that proper cell activity is impaired. In Tay-Sachs disease, the enzyme galactoside is missing in nerve cells of the cerebral cortex, resulting in the accumulation of substances that the cells cannot break down. Electron micrographs show the diagnostic accumulation of laminated electron-dense bodies in these nerve cells. Lysosomes are implicated in many pathological processes; in extreme circumstances, their investing membranes may disrupt, causing cell destruction, as in post-mortem autolysis. Depending on which enzyme is missing, any one of a variety of substances may accumulate. The presence of abnormal accumulations in lysosomes interferes with normal cell functions and thereby causes the clinical manifestations of specific diseases, one example of which is mentioned previously.

Morphologically, lysosomes present a variety of appearances, as indicated earlier. All, of course, are membrane-bound. The primary lysosome has generally a finely granular or nearly homogeneous content and usually is spherical and 25 to 50 nm in diameter, with a limiting membrane 6 to 7 nm thick. Some lysosomes are ellipsoidal in shape, for example, in neutrophil leukocytes, and they occasionally contain more dense material in irregular crystalline arrays. Secondary lysosomes vary in size up to 0.4 μm or more in diameter, and the contents are pleomorphic. Because of the diverse morphology of secondary lysosomes, they are often given special names: (a) digestive vacuoles, resulting from phagocytosis of particles; (b) multivesicular bodies, membranous sacs containing numerous vesicles 50 nm in diameter; and (c) autophagic vacuoles, lysosomal structures containing intracellular membranes or organelles. And there are numerous others.

Lysosomes thus play an essential role in cellular

defense mechanisms, being the site for destruction of foreign bodies such as bacteria and fungi, and they also function in the normal replacement of cellular components and organelles. In cells that are damaged, the membranes bounding lysosomes may rupture or become permeable, thus exposing the general cytoplasm to the action of hydrolytic enzymes, resulting in lysis of the cell and cell death. Such a process occurs in neutrophil leukocytes during infections, when the cells are killed during phagocytosis of bacteria, and a similar process probably occurs during growth and remodeling of tissues.

### MITOCHONDRIA

Mitochondria studied by electron microscopy are perhaps the easiest cytoplasmic organelles to recognize (Figs. 1–25, 1–26, and 1–27). Characteristically, mitochondria are membrane-bound organelles that are quite pliant and lie free within the cytoplasm. On occasion, they appear contractile or motile. They are subject to swelling in certain physiological states. They are of great importance in energy metabolism as the major source of adenosine triphosphate (ATP) and are

the site of many metabolic reactions. The cytochrome electron-transfer system capable of fixing the energy obtained from the oxidations of the Krebs's cycle into ATP lies in the mitochondria. While not visible in routine H and E preparations, they can be demonstrated by Janus green B, pinacyanol, or other vital dyes that exist in either a colored oxidized form or a colorless reduced form. Because of their oxidative enzymes, mitochondria are able to maintain the dye in its oxidized form, whereas the rest of the cytoplasm is usually unable to do so. By phase-contrast microscopy of living cells, they appear as spheres, rods, ovoids, or thread-like bodies that move, change shape and size, divide, and fuse. The number and size of mitochondria are, in general, correlated with the level of oxidative phosphorylation. Hepatocytes may contain about 1000 or more mitochondria each. Mature erythrocytes, totally dependent for energy on glycolysis, contain none. They vary greatly in size and shape, from 0.1 to 0.5 μm wide with lengths up to 10 μm, but usually they are of similar size and shape in any single cell type.

Mitochondria generally have a characteristic structure under the electron microscope. They are

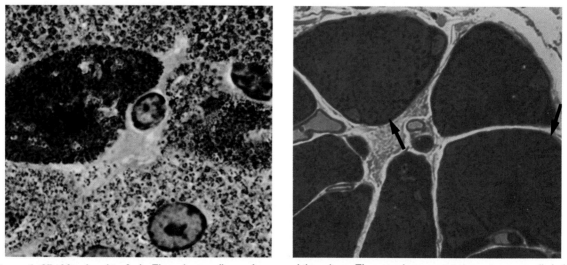

*Figure 1–25.* Mitochondria. Left: *These large cells are from amphibian liver. The cytoplasm contains numerous small dark-brown bodies, which are mitochondria. Nuclei are vesicular in type with prominent nucleoli. Liver. Plastic section. Osmic method. Oil immersion.* Right: *The muscle cells (fibers) are cut transversely. The pale (blue)-staining cytoplasm (sarcoplasm) contains myofibrils (not seen), and the dark-blue, small spherical profiles are mitochondria. In these cells, mitochondria are elongated in the length of the fiber; thus, here also they are cut transversely and therefore appear small. Nuclei in these cells are peripheral in location and are multiple—the cells (arrows) each contain two nuclei in the plane of section. Striated muscle. Plastic section. Toluidine blue. Oil immersion.*

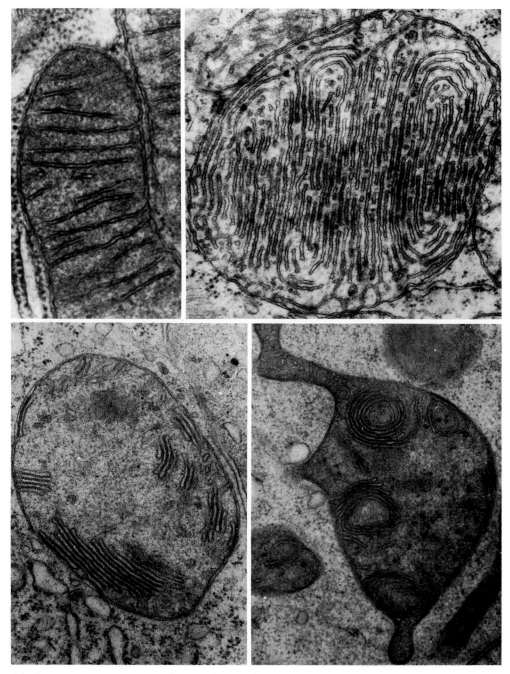

**Figure 1–26.** *Electron micrographs of mitochondria showing different morphological types.* Top left: *From a pancreatic acinar cell.* Top right: *From cardiac muscle.* Bottom left and right: *From interstitial cells of the human testis. All ×40,000.*

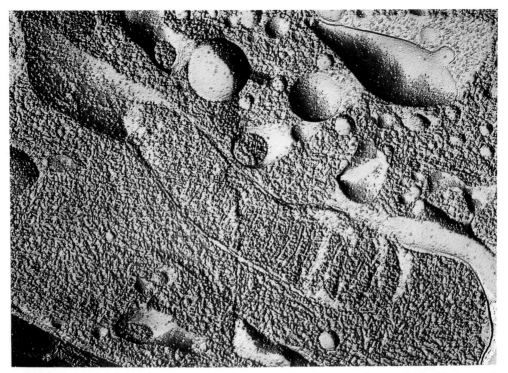

**Figure 1–27.** A freeze-fracture replica of mitochondrion from rat primary decidual cells. × 52,000. (Courtesy of Dr. H. N. Tung.)

composed of outer and inner mitochondrial smooth-surface membranes of 6 nm thickness, each showing the trilaminar unit membrane structure with an electron-lucent space of 8 nm between the membranes. The inner membrane projects folds into the interior of the mitochondria, which are termed *cristae mitochondriales*, which vary in form from transverse membranous plates to tubular or vesicular forms. Thus, two compartments are defined: the outer, between the two membranes, and the inner, or *matrix*, within the inner membrane, which is in turn penetrated by the cristae. Filling the space is a fine granular material of variable electron density. Most mitochondria have flat, shelf-like cristae in their interiors, whereas cells that secrete steroids (e.g., adrenal and gonadal cells) frequently contain tubular cristae. The cristae increase the internal surface area of mitochondria, and it is on these structures that enzymes and other compounds involved in the oxidative phosphorylation and the electron transport systems are located. The matrix also contains electron-opaque intramitochondrial

dense granules (30 to 40 nm in diameter) consisting of divalent cations, some ribosomes (25 nm in diameter), and fine strands of DNA, here lying as circular threads. Attached to the inner (matrix) surface of the inner membrane are closely packed particles 8.5 nm in diameter, "elementary" particles that appear club-shaped, with a short stem (5 nm long and 3 nm wide) attaching them to the cristal membrane (Fig. 1–28). These contain an enzyme, F1 coupling factor (ATPase), and are visible only after treatment by special techniques.

The outer membrane of the mitochondrion is permeable to water and ions, the inner membrane (bounding the matrix) is not, so that transport across this membrane requires active carrier mechanisms.

Mitochondria show a conformational change, the appearance as previously described being the *orthodox* form. This is typical of mitochondria in tissue section, since the methods of preparation usually result in low levels of ADP with the mitochondria inactive in oxidative phosphoryla-

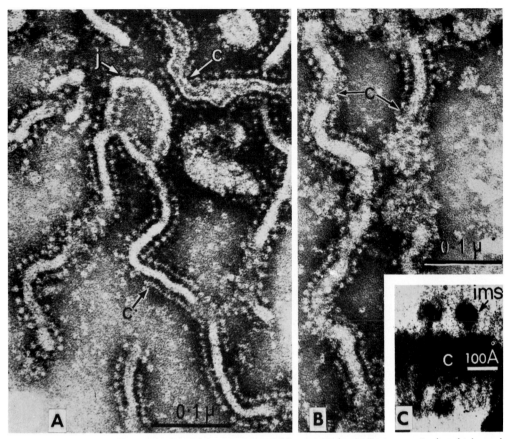

**Figure 1–28.** Electron micrograph of the subunit (elementary particle) associated with the inner mitochondrial membranes (or cristae) of mouse liver. A, A few cristae (c) consisting of long filaments that sometimes branch (j). The surfaces of the cristae are covered with projecting subunits. × 192,000. B, Similar cristae with subunits. × 192,000. C, Higher magnification showing a few subunits (ims) with spherical heads having a diameter of approximately 90 Å and stems 30 to 35 Å wide and 45 to 50 Å long. The center-to-center spacing is 100 Å. Reversed print, × 770,000. (Reproduced with permission from Parsons, D. F.: Mitochondrial structure: Two types of subunits on negatively stained mitochondrial membranes. Science 140:985, 1963; copyright 1963 by the American Association for the Advancement of Science.)

tion. If, however, oxidative phosphorylation is induced in isolated mitochondria, a *condensed* conformation is revealed. In this form, the volume of the outer chamber is increased, and the inner chamber is reduced in volume.

Within cells, mitochondria vary in location with functional requirements. For example, in muscle cells, they lie adjacent to contractile elements; in protein-secreting cells, they are found near the ribosomes and granular reticulum; and in the kidney tubule cells, they lie basally in the cytoplasm to provide energy for active transport mechanisms.

The functions of mitochondria are localized precisely within the organelle, although most of the activity occurs in the inner compartment via enzymes located either in the matrix (citric acid cycle) or on the inner mitochondrial membrane (electron transport and oxidative phosphorylation). As indicated, mitochondria are the major energy source of cells. Additionally, they concentrate calcium and maintain a general calcium environment within the cytoplasm.

## PEROXISOMES

Like the mitochondrion, the peroxisome is a major site of oxygen utilization (Fig. 1–29). Peroxisomes, or *microbodies*, are similar to lysosomes in structure but do not contain lysosomal

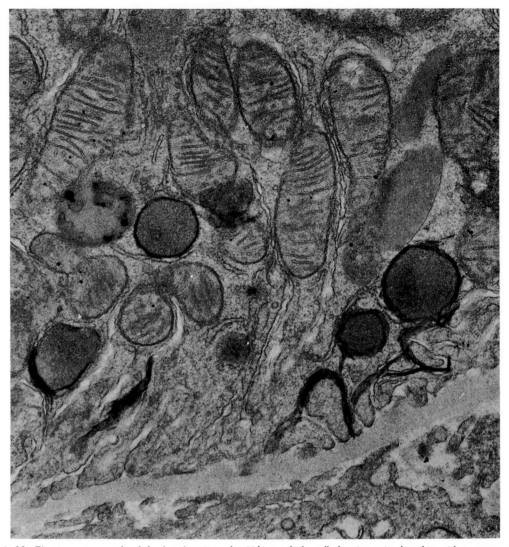

**Figure 1–29.** *Electron micrograph of the basal region of a kidney tubule cell showing mitochondria with transverse cristae, several microbodies (peroxisomes), and a lysosome. This is a special preparation in which the benzidine reaction product is localized at the periphery of the peroxisomes. The lysosome (left edge) shows a few dense granules.* × *22,000. (Preparation courtesy of Drs. S. Goldfischer and E. Essner.)*

hydrolases. They are membrane-bounded organelles, somewhat larger than primary lysosomes, and may be continuous with the tubules of smooth endoplasmic reticulum. They are 0.3 to 1.5 μm in diameter, usually with a finely granular homogeneous content but sometimes containing a crystalline body or nucleoid. Peroxisomes are relatively numerous in hepatocytes, in renal tubular cells, and in macrophages.

Peroxisomes are formed in the granular endoplasmic reticulum and contain several enzymes involved in the production (urate oxidase and other oxidases) or destruction (catalase) of hydrogen peroxide. The latter reaction is sometimes considered a safety device that prevents a dangerous accumulation of the strong oxidizing agent hydrogen peroxide in the absence of a sufficient supply of hydrogen donors. Important to peroxisome function is the fact that its membrane is unusually permeable, permitting inorganic ions and low-molecular-weight substances up to the size of sucrose to pass with ease. The large peroxisomes in liver and kidney cells are thought to be important in detoxifying various molecules. However, the function of these bodies remains obscure. Hydrogen peroxide is highly toxic to cells, and, persumably, it is advantageous to limit reactions that produce it to an organelle where it can be broken down as soon as it is formed.

## MICROTUBULES

The cytoplasm of many cells appears to contain a considerable array of very small, hollow, cylindrical, unbranched tubules called microtubules (Fig. 1–30). Microtubules are 25 nm in diameter and of indeterminate length. They run a straight course in the cytoplasm, and this implies that they have some degree of stiffness. Microtubules consist of molecules of tubulin, a globular polypeptide of 50,000 daltons being composed of $\alpha$ and $\beta$ tubulin molecules. These tubulin molecules have closely related amino acid sequences that assemble into microtubules by forming protofilaments that spiral along the wall of the microtubule in a left-handed helix. Usually 13 such protofilaments are arranged side by side around a central core that appears to be empty in electron micrographs. In very few specific locations, microtubules may be of smaller overall diameter, with only 12 protofilaments in the wall, or larger, with 15 protofilaments. Microtubules are present in nearly all cells and often occur as single elements randomly scattered in the cytoplasm, in groups in parallel array, or partially fused in two's and three's to form doublets and triplets. The adjacent microtubules at the areas of fusion in doublets and triplets share three or four subunits. This is discussed later in reference to centrioles and cilia.

Microtubules probably have several functions. They represent the main supporting elements of the cell. Microtubules serve as an internal skeleton for the cell, preserving its size and shape. In mitosis, microtubules form the cell spindle and appear to guide the movement of the chromosomes. Their relation to cilia (motile cell processes) as both structural and force-generating elements and to centrioles and the process of mitosis is discussed later. Microtubules as skeletal

elements are particularly prominent as bundles at the cell periphery in blood platelets, where they maintain the discoid shape. In addition, there are bands of microtubules in the axons of nerve cells (*neurotubules*), beneath the plasma membrane of many cylindrical or asymmetric cells, and within the endoplasm of such cells as macrophages. The relation of microtubules to cell movement is less well established. In all probability, they do not generate motile forces but interact with other cellular components, such as filaments, to determine the direction of cytoplasmic movement. For example, cells in tissue culture exhibit motility that, after the addition of colchicine (which destroys microtubules), is changed in character but not stopped. Microtubules of the cytoskeleton often appear to be associated with mitochondria. This association may determine the unique orientation and distribution of mitochondria in different cell types. Thus, the mitochondria of some cells form long, moving filaments, or chains, while in other cell types they are fixed in position near a site of unusually high ATP consumption. For example, they are packed between adjacent myofibrils in a cardiac muscle cell and are tightly wrapped around the flagellum in a sperm. Additionally, movements within the cytoplasm of organelles such as lysosomes and of inclusions (e.g., pigment granules) tend to be oriented parallel to bundles of microtubules (long saltatory movement), and these can be abolished by dispersing the microtubules. Microtubules influence the distribution of intermediate filaments in most cells in culture. If the cells are treated with colchicine, the microtubule network depolymerizes very rapidly, and over the next several hours the intermediate filament network gradually collapses into a dense filamentous cap lying adjacent to the nucleus. If colchicine is removed, the microtubules rapidly repolymerize, and the intermediate filaments slowly return to their normal distribution. It seems, then, that cytoplasmic microtubules determine the cell's polarity and coordinate the various parts of the cytoskeleton responsible for complex cell movements.

It should be emphasized that the cytoplasmic microtubules are plastic in the sense that they can be formed and can increase in length or, alternatively, can be dispersed. The formed or polymerized microtubule is, then, in equilibrium with a pool of unpolymerized tubulin lying in the

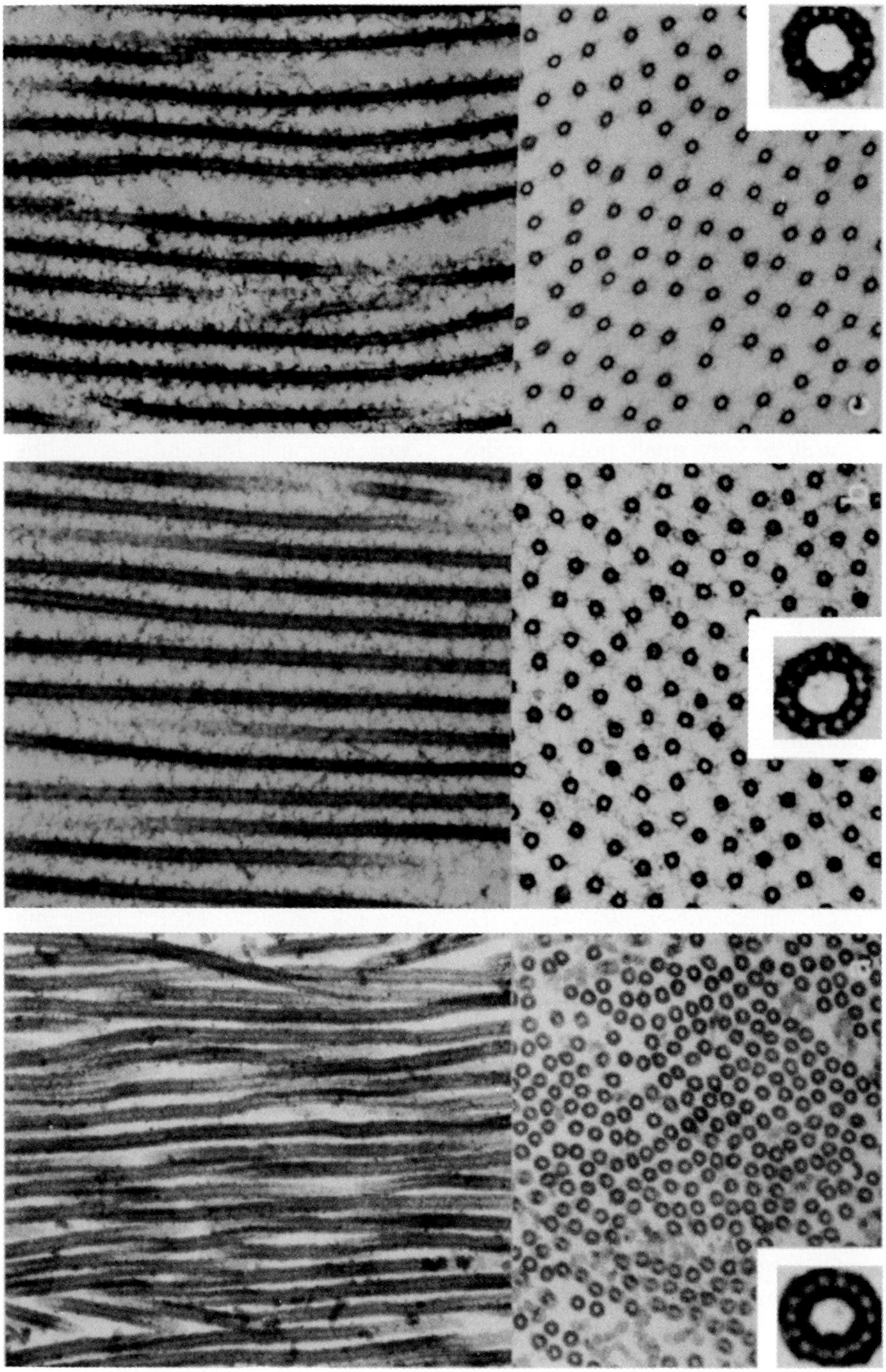

**Figure 1–30.** Thin sections of three different populations of microtubules assembled with and without MAPs (microtubule-associated protein). Top: Microtubules polymerized from tubulin only. Middle: Microtubules saturated with unfractioned MAPs. Bottom: Mictrotubules saturated with the purified MAP$_2$ fraction. All × 76,400. (From Rosenbaum, J. L., Kim, H., and Binder, L. I.: The periodic association of MAP$_2$ with brain microtubules in vitro. J Cell Biol 80:266–276, 1979. Permission of The Rockefeller University Press.)

cytoplasm. Microtubules are relatively easily dispersed by colchicine, vinblastine, or hydrostatic pressure. When such dispersing factors are removed, the subunits quickly reassociate to reform microtubules.

## CENTRIOLES

Centrioles appear by light microscopy as short rods or granules located near the nucleus, and in most interphase or nondividing cells there are two, called a *diplosome* (Fig. 1–31). Often the pair lies adjacent to the Golgi apparatus in a specialized area of the cytoplasm called the *centrosome*, or cell center, and may be surrounded by microtubules radiating out into the cytoplasm. Unlike other cytoplasmic structures, centrioles are duplicated before mitosis. The formation of each new centriole begins with the appearance of a *procentriole* (a ring-like condensation of granular material). This occurs next to an existing centriole and at right angles to it. The procentriole has essentially the same cross-sectional appearance as the parent centriole, but it is much shorter in length. Subsequent elongation of the tubules of the procentriole converts it into a mature centriole, a process that is not completed until after the ensuing mitosis. Centrioles also may replicate, pass to the cell surface, and form basal bodies (kinetosomes) from which cilia develop. Flagella arise in a similar fashion. Little is known as yet about the way in which centrioles and kinetosomes cause the formation of microtubules.

By electron microscopy, each centriole appears

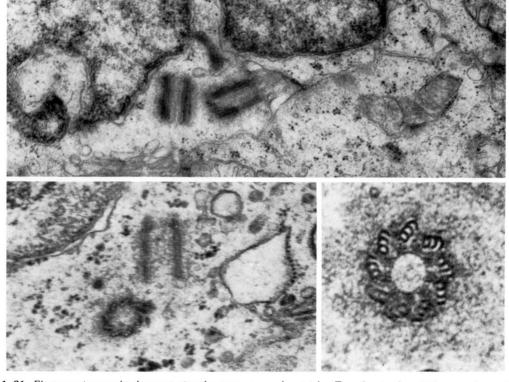

*Figure 1–31.* Electron micrographs demonstrating the appearance of centrioles. Top: A pair of centrioles near the nucleus (top left) of a supporting (Sertoli's) cell of the testis. Both are cut longitudinally but are oriented approximately at right angles to each other. × 35,000. Bottom left: A similar pair, but one centriole is cut in cross section and shows nine subunits in its wall. × 42,000. Bottom right: A centriole in cross section to show that each of the nine subunits is composed of triple microtubular elements. × 110,000.

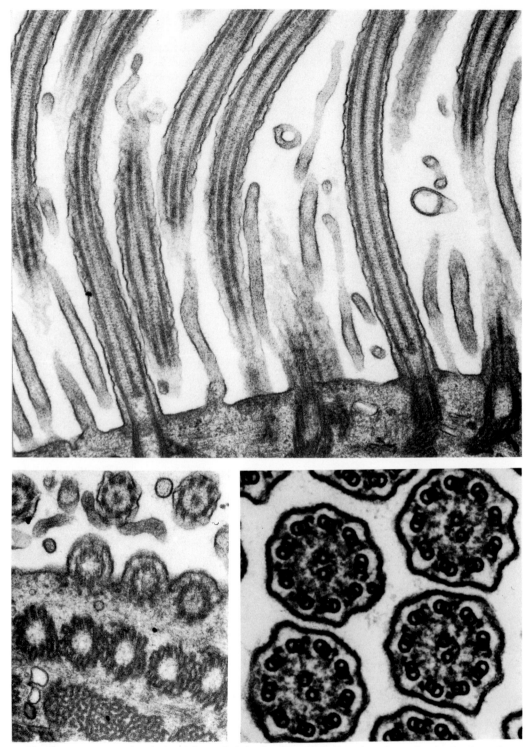

**Figure 1–32.** *Electron micrographs of cilia of the epithelial cells of bronchus. Top: Apical cytoplasm with cilia and microvilli in longitudinal section. Cilia show peripheral and central microtubules. × 36,000. Lower left: Cilia in transverse section at their bases. Note the lack of central tubules, and peripheral triplets in the profiles within apical cytoplasm. × 46,000. Lower right: Cilial shafts in transverse section. × 88,000.*

as a short cylinder 0.3 to 0.5 μm long and about 0.15 μm in diameter, with one "end" open and the other closed by dense material. The structure of centrioles has been remarkably conserved; with very few exceptions, centrioles contain nine evenly spaced fibrils, each of which appears in cross section as a band of three microtubules, designated the A, B, and C subfibrils, connected to the center of the organelle by a radial spoke. Subfibril A is the most central, or innermost. Each band of three microtubules is inclined at an angle to the surface of the structure, giving the centriole a characteristic pinwheel appearance. In the diplosome, the two centrioles usually lie at right angles to each other, and attached more or less directly to them are microtubules that radiate from them and from associated clumps of dense material called pericentriolar satellites. It is presumed that this dense material serves as a nucleation center for the initial formation of the microtubules.

## CILIA

Cilia are tiny hair-like appendages about 0.2 μm in diameter that contain a bundle of parallel microtubules at their core. They are very numerous in epithelial cells of the upper respiratory tract, parts of the male and female reproductive tracts, and the ependyma lining the cavities of the central nervous system (Fig. 1–32). Fields of cilia bend in coordinated, unidirectional waves. Each of the 250 or more cilia on the surface of a ciliated cell moves as a tiny whip. A forward active stroke, in which the cilium is fully extended and able to exert maximal force on the surrounding liquid, is followed by a recovery phase, in which the cilium

returns to its original position by an unrolling movement.

Each cilium is covered by an extension of the plasmalemma and consists of a long cylindrical shaft, a tapering tip, and a basal body, or *kinetosome*, located in the apical cytoplasm. By light microscopy, the basal body is visible as a dense granule at the base of the cilium. The ciliary core, or *axoneme*, is a complex structure composed entirely of microtubules and their associated protein (Fig. 1–33). The ciliary axoneme consists of nine doublet microtubules arranged in a ring around a pair of single microtubules. While each member of the pair of singlet microtubules (central pair) is a complete microtubule, each of the outer doublets is composed of one complete and one partial microtubule. In transverse sections, each complete microtubule (subfiber A) is seen to be formed from a ring of 13 protofilaments, while the incomplete microtubule (subfiber B) is formed from ten protofilaments, thus closing the "defect" in its wall. Associated with the microtubules of the axoneme are many other protein structures whose interactions provide the power for the ciliary motor. The most important of these are sets of arms that project from each subfiber A towards the subfiber B of the adjacent doublet (Fig. 1–34). The arm-like processes are spaced along the microtubule at regular 24-nm intervals and are composed of the protein *dynein*, a high-molecular-weight ATPase. At more widely spaced intervals, another protein, called *nexin*, forms "links" between the adjacent doublets. These are thought to be highly elastic links around the entire axoneme. Projecting inward from each doublet is a radial spoke, which ends in a globular portion

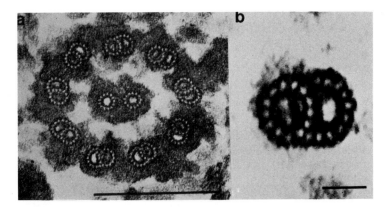

**Figure 1–33.** *Electron micrograph of the axoneme (a) of a cilium showing nine outer doublets and two central singlet microtubules and (b) one outer doublet demonstrating the A subfiber with 13 protofilaments and the B subfiber (C-shaped) with 11 protofilaments in its wall; a, × 165,000; b, × 360,000. (From Rosenbaum, J. L., and Binder, L. I.: The in vitro assembly of the flagellar outer doublet tubulin. J Cell Biol 79:500–515, 1978. Reproduced by copyright permission of The Rockefeller University Press.)*

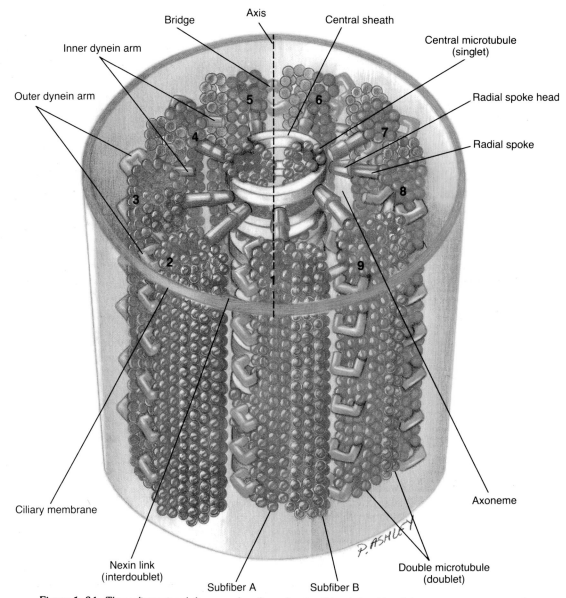

*Figure 1–34. Three-dimensional diagram of a cilium showing the relationship of the major components.*

very near the inner sheath. At the base of a cilium, the central pair of single microtubules terminates, and each of the peripheral doublets is continuous with a triplet of the kinetosome, a subfiber C being "added" to the doublet. With nine peripheral triplets, the kinetosome resembles a centriole, and, as in a centriole, the triplets lie tangential to the surface. In many cases, strands

of fibrous material extend from the basal body into apical cytoplasm (the "striated rootlets"), and other fibrous material may extend to the adjacent plasmalemma (Figs. 1–35 and 1–36). These structures are presumed to anchor the cilium firmly in apical cytoplasm.

Analysis of ciliary movement shows that the motile machinery is contained in the axoneme.

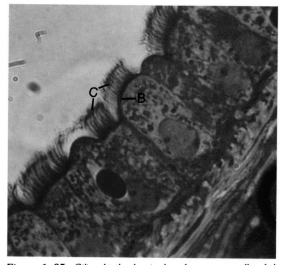

**Figure 1–35.** Cilia. At the luminal surface, most cells of the tracheal epithelium show the presence of cilia (C)—long, regular motile processes with basal bodies (B) in the apical cytoplasm, giving the appearance of a densely staining (red) line just beneath the apical surface. Trachea. Plastic section. H and E. Oil immersion.

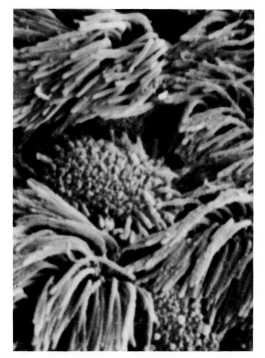

**Figure 1–36.** Scanning electron micrograph of cilia of tracheal epithelium. × 6000. (Courtesy of Dr. W. Krause.)

Indeed, an isolated axoneme will still propagate bending movements even after removal of its plasma membrane, provided that it is perfused with a salt solution containing ATP and calcium. Calmodulin, a calcium-binding protein, can regulate ciliary beating by removing this calcium from the ciliary axoneme. A cilium bends along the axis by a type of sliding filament mechanism between microtubules similar to that seen between myofilaments in striated muscle cells. In support of a sliding microtubule mechanism for ciliary movement, electron micrographs of cilia at various stages show that the microtubules do not change appreciably in length. Moreover, the rows of radial spokes show a relative displacement in the region of the bend that indicates that the microtubules slide relative to each other within the axoneme. Contact between dynein "arms" and a neighboring doublet is believed to activate ATP hydrolysis by the dynein and generate a sliding force between the microtubules. Accessory proteins, like nexin, bundle the ring of microtubule doublets together and limit the extent of their sliding. Relaxation is believed to be passive and perhaps due to the elasticity of the nexin links and enveloping plasmalemma.

## FLAGELLA

Flagella are whip-like processes similar in structure to cilia but considerably longer, being up to 15 to 30 µm in length, and usually there is only one or two associated with each cell (Fig. 1–37). They exhibit a quasi-sinusoidal wave type of movement. The motile tail of a spermatozoon is a flagellum and may be 70 µm or more in length. Flagella are found elsewhere in some epithelia (e.g., of the kidney and rete testis), where their function is uncertain. Single ciliary projections are also found associated with some sensory epithelial cells (e.g., the rods and cones of the retina and hair cells of the inner ear). Usually these are nonmotile and lack the central pair of single microtubules.

## MICROFILAMENTS AND INTERMEDIATE FILAMENTS

Although there are a variety of different types of filaments in a cell that can be visualized with the electron microscope, the term *microfilament* is generally reserved for a specific type of fibrous

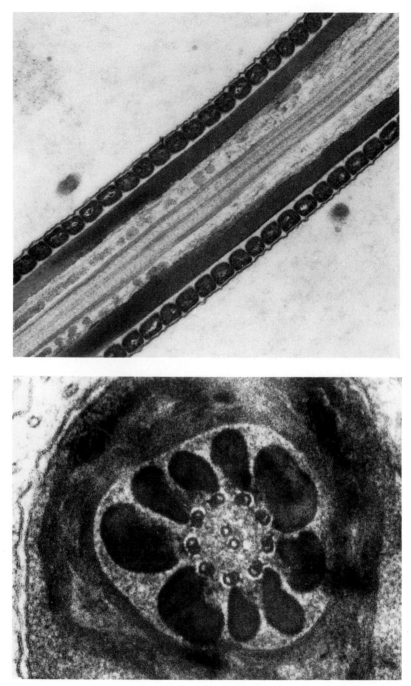

**Figure 1–37.** Electron micrographs of the flagellum of the rat spermatozoa. Top: Longitudinal section of the middle piece. × 50,000. Bottom: Transverse section of the middle piece showing an outer circumferentially oriented mitochondrial sheath, which tightly adheres to nine coarse fibers arranged in a helical pattern. The innermost core consists of an axoneme (9 + 2 pattern) of microtubules. × 138,000. (Courtesy of Dr. H. N. Tung.)

element—one that has a diameter of about 6 to 7 nm and is composed of the protein actin. Actin was identified as one of the major contractile proteins of muscle cells. In muscle cells, microfilaments are part of the actin-myosin system, which becomes contractile by sliding over myosin filaments—the other major contractile protein. Myosin is always present where actin filaments form contractile bundles in cells. Presumably, most microfilament-related activities depend upon the simultaneous presence of myosin. In nonmuscle cells, the basis of movement in many cellular processes (e.g., locomotion, cell division, pinocytosis, phagocytosis) appears to be contractile mechanisms, and it has become clear that the filamentous material involved in these processes is the same as that present in muscle cells. Many kinds of cellular extensions have a core of crosslinked actin filaments. Microvilli are the best known examples of such structures. The core of the microvillus contains about 40 actin filaments that run in a parallel bundle along its length. At the tip of the microvillus, the actin filaments are embedded in a cap of amorphous material, while at their base they extend into a network called the *terminal web* (Fig. 1–38). The terminal web contains both actin and myosin, and part of its function may be to create the tension required to maintain the stiff microvilli in their upright position. Bundles of actin filaments associated with nonmuscle myosin are found in specific regions of the cell where muscle-like contractions are needed, such as the contractile ring of a dividing cell and the belt desmosome at the apical region of an epithelial cell. In addition, in many cells near the cell surface (i.e., in ectoplasm), there is a network of 5- to 7-nm microfilaments that function in local movements of the surface membrane. Drugs that affect the state of actin polymerization can be shown to disrupt many cell movements. For example, cytochalasin B paralyzes many different kinds of vertebrate cell movements—inhibiting cell locomotion, phagocytosis, and cytokinesis. The cytochalasins act by binding specifically to one end of an actin filament, thereby preventing the addition of actin molecules to that end.

A second group of fine intracellular filaments that is stouter and represents a more diverse population of filaments than the microfilament is called *intermediate filaments.* Intermediate fila-ments are long, unbranched filaments that have a diameter of 8 to 10 nm, which is intermediate between that of microtubules and that of microfilaments. They are tough and durable protein fibers that appear as straight or gently curving arrays in electron micrographs. They are particularly prominent along the length of a nerve cell process, close to the spot desmosomes between adjacent epithelial cells, and throughout the cytoplasm of a smooth muscle cell. Unlike microfilaments and microtubules, the intermediate filaments are a chemically heterogeneous group of structures whose protein subunits can be divided into five major groups:

1. Cytokeratins, which are found in a wide variety of epithelial cells and consist of a network of 8-nm cytoplasmic filaments composed of a family of proteins (42,000 to 65,000 daltons) and very similar in structure to $\alpha$-keratin. These cytokeratins are often collected in bundles that make up the tonofilaments of the desmosomes.

2. Vimentin, a 57,000-dalton protein characteristic of cells of mesenchymal origin. In certain of the nucleated erythrocytes, vimentin-containing intermediate filaments can be demonstrated to be present in association with the inner surface of the plasma membrane, where they are presumed to participate in support of the cell and determination of its shape. Vimentin filaments can copolymerize in the cytoplasm with keratin filaments, glial filaments, and desmin filaments. Vimentin filaments are also often seen to interconnect the nuclear envelope and plasma membrane, and this has led to the suggestion that these intermediate filaments may play a role in supporting the nucleus and maintaining its position within the cell.

3. Desmin, which is composed of a 53,000-dalton protein in intermediate filaments that have a diameter of 10 nm and is found in muscle cells. It is found in the Z-disks of skeletal muscle cells, where it may play a role in linking the actin filaments of adjacent sarcomeres.

4. Glial fibrillary acid protein, which is characteristic of the cytoplasm of glial cells. These intermediate filaments are displayed in a scattered array of bundles of 8-nm filaments composed of a 55,000-dalton protein.

5. Neurofilaments, present in the cytoplasm of neurons and consisting of loosely packed bundles of 10-nm filaments. They are composed of three

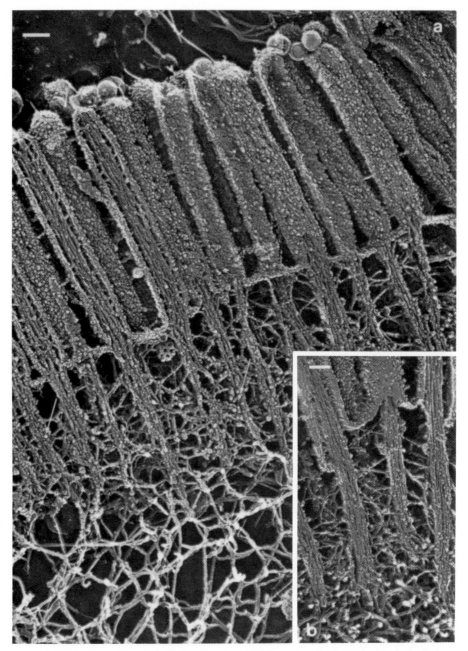

**Figure 1–38.** a and b: *The terminal web of a control brush-border preparation fixed, washed with distilled water, and quick-frozen. Tight bundles of actin filaments extend out of the microvilli to form straight "rootlets." In between the rootlets are found a number of delicate cross links, which appear as fine fibrils. Note that fibrils tend to form very complicated networks at the basal part of the rootlets. Small dots (arrows) on the rootlets appear to be the remnants of fine fibrils that were cross-fractured. The rootlets rest upon a tangle of thicker intermediate filaments located at the bottom of this field. Notice that the membrane covering the microvilli is studded with numerous, irregularly shaped bumps. Bar, 0.1 μm (a) × 97,000, (b) × 77,000. (From Nobutaka, H., Tilney, L. G., Fujiwara, K., and Heuser, J. E.: Organization of actin, myosin, and intermediate filaments in the brush border of intestinal epithelial cells. J Cell Biol 94:425–443, 1982 and reproduced with the permission of The Rockefeller University Press.)*

distinct proteins (68,000, 145,000, and 220,000 daltons) that copolymerize to form the intact filament.

## ANNULATE LAMELLAE

Annulate lamellae are visible only with the electron microscope (Fig. 1–39). The lamellae are flat, membranous, parallel cisternae with numerous pores or annuli. The organelle apparently is related to rough endoplasmic reticulum and the nuclear envelope, and, indeed, in structure it closely resembles the latter. The membranes of the lamellae are 7 to 9 nm thick, enclose a space 30 to 50 nm wide, and have pores 40 to 50 nm in diameter. Generally, the pores are spaced regularly at intervals of 100 to 200 nm. The pores appear to be closed by a single dense membrane, and, like those of the nuclear envelope, they have eight globular subunits around their peripheries with a small central granule in the membrane closing the pore. Lamellae occur singly and in parallel stacks in the cytoplasm and, in a few cells, are present within the nucleus. They are found in rapidly growing cells, such as germ, embryonic, and tumor cells, and in other cell types where they may be transitory during the life cycle. Lamellae are thought to be derived from the nuclear envelope, and, while their significance is uncertain, they may convey material from the nucleus to the cytoplasm, functioning in nucleo-cytoplasmic interactions. They often show direct connections to the endoplasmic reticulum.

## CYTOPLASMIC VITALITY

Very few, if any, cell types are static. Structurally and functionally, they constantly undergo changes. The probable constant breakdown and re-formation of microtubules is one example of this. By way of a further example and to emphasize the dynamic aspect of cells, the exchanges that occur between cytomembranes and their turnover are very interesting. For example, while the rat parenchymal liver cell probably lives for a period of six months, the life span of its cytomembranes is on the order of days. Membrane constantly is re-formed within a cell, and formed membranes can and do move from one site to another. Examples of such transfers have been indicated in the previous descriptions of cell or-

ganelles. They include the transfer of nuclear envelope in annulate lamellae formation, movement of endoplasmic reticulum membrane as transfer vesicles, membrane movement from the Golgi apparatus to the plasmalemma and to lysosomes, endocytotic vesicle and vacuole formation from the plasmalemma, and the formation of the multivesicular bodies and phagosomes. However, it must be remembered also that the cytomembranes vary in structure and function and, perhaps, particularly in associated enzymes. So membrane transfer implies a change in structure and function. Study of tissue sections and electron micrographs tends to give the false impression that cells and their components are static. The student can dispel this impression only by attempting constantly to correlate structure and function.

## INCLUSIONS

The cytosol of many cells contains inclusion bodies—particulate cytoplasmic regions that are not bounded by a membrane. Inclusions refer to materials such as stored foods, pigments, and some crystalline materials. Previously, inclusions were considered nonliving accumulations of metabolites, cell products resulting from synthesis, or materials from outside taken into the cell; many of them in fact are now known to participate in the normal functioning of the cell. In the form of granules and droplets, cells store food materials as well as products resulting from their metabolic processes. Bodies such as secretory granules or droplets were formerly considered cytoplasmic inclusions, but these are membrane-bound packets of enzymes and have been discussed in relation to the granular endoplasmic reticulum and Golgi apparatus. The following are some examples of cytoplasmic inclusions:

1. Stored foods in the form of carbohydrates and fats, which are stored in the cytoplasm as energy reserves (Fig. 1–40). Carbohydrate as a food material is absorbed from the intestine mainly as glucose and stored in the form of the polysaccharide glycogen. Glycogen is water-soluble and in ordinary histological preparations is removed, leaving a characteristic appearance of irregular, ragged spaces between strands of cytoplasm and thus giving a "moth-eaten" appearance to the cytoplasm (Fig. 1–41). It is stained

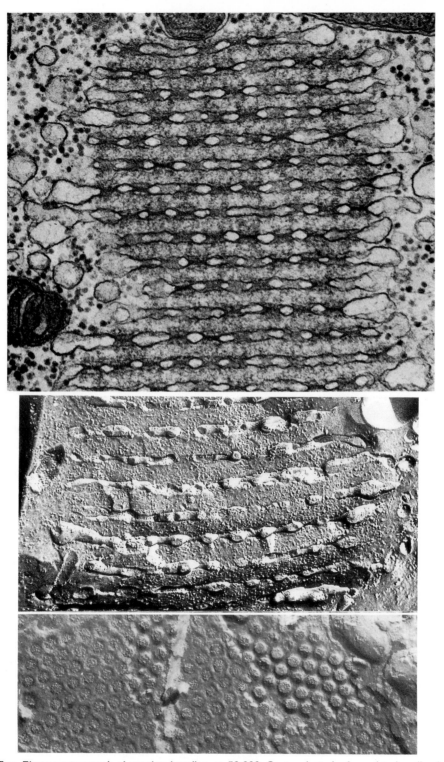

**Figure 1–39.** Top: *Electron micrograph of annulate lamellae.* × *50,000. Center: A stack of annulate lamellae freeze-cleaved perpendicularly to plane showing side view of pores.* × *60,000. Bottom: An en face freeze-etch preparation showing hexagonal packing of pores.* × *31,000. (Courtesy of Drs. R. G. Keesel, H. N. Tung, H. W. Beams, and R. Roberts.)*

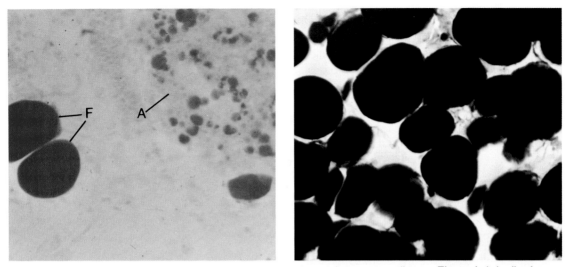

**Figure 1–40.** Lipid. Left: Fat is stained red by this method and is present here in two cell types. The epithelial cells of secretory units (alveoli) (A) contain several small globules of lipid, while in the surrounding connective tissue are fat cells (F), each containing a large single droplet. Lipid is normally removed in preparation, and this is a frozen section. Breast. Plastic section. Sudan IV. High power. Right: Fat cells, in which the content of fat has been preserved, appear closely opposed in this section of adipose tissue. No details of the protoplasmic envelope can be discerned. Fat cells. Osmic acid. Medium power.

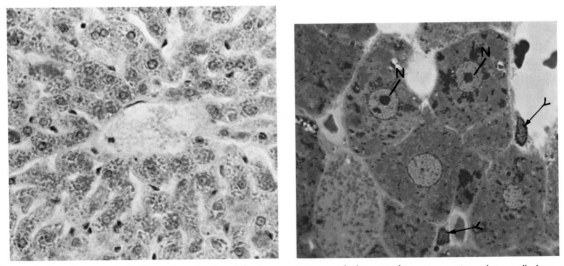

**Figure 1–41.** Glycogen. Left: Parenchymal cells of the liver contain stored glycogen, here seen as irregular, small clumps of red-staining material in the cytoplasm. Other inclusions and organelles are not seen, but nuclei are stained blue and appear vesicular with prominent nucleoli. Liver. Best's carmine. Medium power. Right: Nuclei of parenchymal cells are large, spheroidal, and located centrally in cells. They show a nuclear envelope; irregular chromatin clumps in the nuclear sap; and, in some cells, prominent, large nucleoli (N). Nucleoli may be multiple, and in these liver cells, two nuclei may be present—a condition called polyploidy. In the cytoplasm are irregular masses of pink-staining glycogen. A few small, irregular hyperchromatic or condensed nuclei (arrows) of cells associated with liver sinusoids also are seen. Liver. Plastic section. PAS, toluidine blue. Oil immersion.

magenta by the PAS reaction or Best's carmine method. In the electron microscope, glycogen is seen as free electron-dense particles 20 to 30 nm in diameter, often lying between tubular profiles of agranular endoplasmic reticulum. Two types of glycogen particles are visible in transmission electron microscopy: beta particles, which are round with an average diameter of 15–30 nm, and complexes of beta particles in the form of rosettes or alpha particles, which are about 50–100 nm in diameter. Fat is stored mainly in connective tissue as fat cells but, under certain conditions, by other cells as well, including hepatocytes. Fat is isolated in the cytoplasm as membrane-bound vacuoles and droplets containing neutral fats (triglycerides), fatty acids, cholesterol, and cholesterol esters. If frozen sections are stained with specific fat-soluble dyes or if the tissue is fixed in osmium tetroxide, the lipid droplets are retained and appear black. Fat droplets appear to arise in the Golgi apparatus or in relation to agranular reticulum and are bounded by a membrane 6 to 7 nm thick.

2. Pigments, which are materials that display color without having been stained (Figs. 1–42 and 1–43). Pigments may be either *exogenous*,

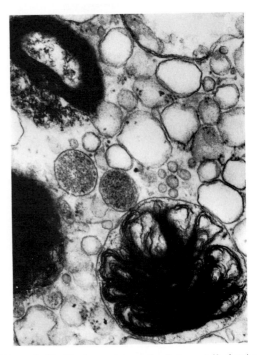

*Figure 1–43.* Electron micrograph of pigment (fuchsin) granules from the pigment epithelium of the rat retina. × 40,000.

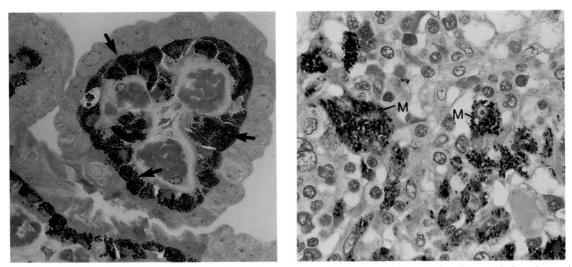

*Figure 1–42.* Left: Endogenous pigment (melanin) granules are present in the pigment layer of the ciliary epithelium (arrows), which rests on the stroma of the ciliary body. Ciliary body. Plastic section. H and E. High power. Right: Most cells present in this bronchial lymph node are small lymphocytes and plasma cells, but scattered among them are larger cells. These are macrophages (M) that have phagocytosed carbon, an exogenous pigment present here as black granules. Lymph node. H and E. Medium power.

that is, taken in by the organism from the environment, or *endogenous*, that is, formed in the organism. Exogenous pigments include carotenes, yellowish-red pigments of vegetables that are fat-soluble (lipochromes); dusts, that is, carbon, which is particularly prominent in the cells of the lungs and associated lymph nodes; and minerals, such as lead and silver. The most important endogenous pigment is hemoglobin and its breakdown products such as hemosiderin, which contains iron, and bilirubin (hematoidin), which does not. Melanin is an endogenous dark-brown or black pigment found in the skin and the eye. It is produced in sun tanning and is produced in large amounts in the epidermis of Negroid races. Lipofuscin (yellowish-brown granules) is now considered to be a membrane-bound, indigestible residue of lysosomal activity, as described previously in the section on lysosomes (Fig. 1–44). The amount of lipofuscin in cells increases with age. Since the cell is not able to get rid of it by exocytosis, it accumulates with time in the form of residual bodies.

3. Crystals and crystalloids, which occur in a few cell types (Fig. 1–45). Sertoli's cells (susten-

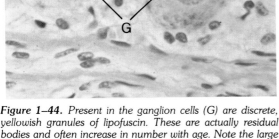

*Figure 1–44. Present in the ganglion cells (G) are discrete, yellowish granules of lipofuscin. These are actually residual bodies and often increase in number with age. Note the large nuclei of the ganglion cells, each showing a nuclear envelope; nuclear sap with fine, speckled chromatin masses; and a prominent nucleolus. Autonomic ganglion, lipofuscin. H and E. High power.*

tacular) and interstitial cells of the testis store these materials in the cytoplasm as non–membrane-bound packets. Crystalloids also occur in eosinophilic leukocytes, in some microbodies (peroxisomes), and occasionally within mitochondria associated with the cristae.

## Nucleus

The nucleus (or nuclei, if multiple) of the cell is a rounded or elongated structure, usually in the center of the cell. It is found in all cells except mature erythrocytes and platelets of the blood. The nucleus usually is in the range of 3 to 14 $\mu$m in diameter, although it can be 25 $\mu$m or more in the ovum and in some ganglion cells. Certain cell types have many nuclei or are polyploid. Hepatocytes may develop two or more nuclei, while skeletal muscle cells and osteoclasts are multinucleate. Osteoclasts may contain 25 or more nuclei. The nucleus may be cup-shaped or show indentations, and in a few cells it is lobated. The nucleus may also vary in shape in the same cell, corresponding to the different phases of activity (Fig. 1–46). In the nucleus is found the genetic material of the cell, deoxyribonucleic acid (DNA). Characteristically, the nucleus stains blue, that is, it is basophilic because of its content of nucleic acids and basic protein (histones), but it also contains some acid proteins. The weakly stained areas in the nucleoplasm are due to the presence of soluble DNA and various granular components that are only visualized by electron microscopy. The content of DNA accounts for the strongly positive reaction when stained with the Feulgen technique. The volume of the nucleus is related to its DNA content (and therefore, the number of chromosomes), and there is evidence that the volume increases with synthetic activities of the cell. The nucleus is that portion of the cell that contains the genetic material and manufactures molecules (ribosomal RNA, transfer RNA, messenger RNA) that control the synthetic activities of the organelles in the cytoplasm. The nucleus is essential for the life of the cell; if it is removed experimentally, protein synthesis in the cytoplasm ceases, and the cell soon dies. Erythrocytes are cells that lack a nucleus and as such are incapable of protein synthesis, cannot

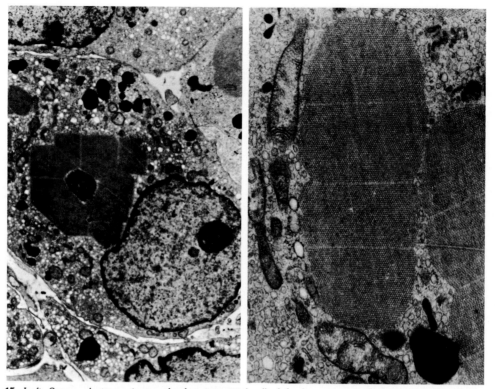

**Figure 1–45.** Left: *Survey electron micrograph of an interstitial cell of the human testis. Contained in the cytoplasm near the nucleus are a large crystalloid (gray) and several lipid inclusions (black).* × *4200.* Right: *A higher magnification of a crystalloid from a similar cell. The crystalloid shows a regular lattice pattern. There also is a lipid inclusion (bottom right).* × *28,000.*

undergo cell division, and have limited metabolic activity. There is a constant exchange of material between the nucleus and the cytoplasm. All the information necessary to initiate and control the metabolic activities of each individual cell is contained in the nucleus.

The nucleus is composed of a nuclear envelope, or nuclear membrane, and nucleoplasm (karyoplasm) and contains nuclear chromatin and a nucleolus.

### NUCLEAR ENVELOPE

The nuclear contents (the nucleoplasm) are separated from the cytoplasm by the membranes of the nuclear envelope (Figs. 1–47 through 1–50). The nuclear envelope is a double membrane composed of two lipid bilayers separated by a gap of about 20 nm in width known as the perinuclear space or cistern. On electron microscopy, the outer nuclear membrane can be seen to be continuous with the endoplasmic reticulum, and, like the membrane of the rough endoplasmic reticulum, the outer surface of the outer nuclear membrane is studded with ribosomes. Since the lumen of the endoplasmic reticulum is continuous with the perinuclear space, both the perinuclear space and the outer nuclear membrane can be regarded as a small specialized region of the endoplasmic reticulum. Both the perinuclear space and cisternae of the endoplasmic reticulum may contain in their lumina dense secretory material. On the inner surface of the inner nuclear membrane, there is in some cell types a thin layer formed by fine filamentous material—the fibrous lamina—to which clumps of nuclear chromatin

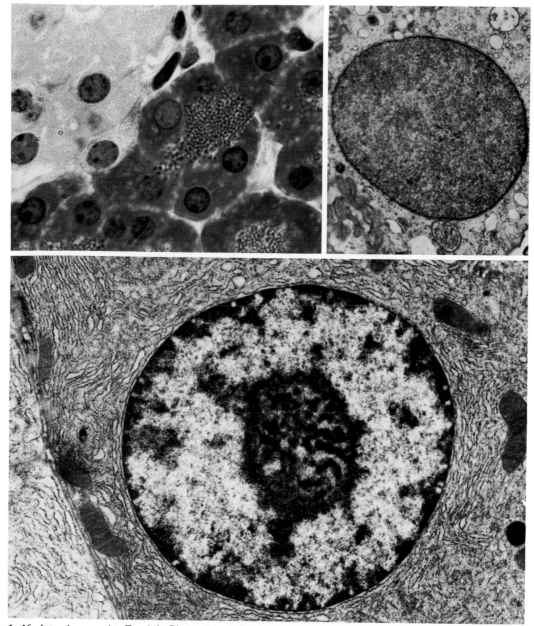

**Figure 1–46.** *Interphase nuclei.* Top left: *Photomicrograph of the pancreas showing nuclei of various types. In the exocrine basophilic cells, they are vesicular, spherical with prominent nucleoli. In islet (endocrine) cells, they are spherical and show speckled chromatin (top left), and two ovoid heterochromatic nuclei of connective tissue cells are seen at top center.* × 1100. Top right: *Electron micrograph of the euchromatic nucleus of a kidney tubule cell. No nucleolus or chromatin material is seen, but there is some increased density at the nuclear envelope that represents the fibrous lamina.* × 7000. Bottom: *Electron micrograph of the nucleus of a pancreatic exocrine cell. It is spherical and contains a large central nucleolus with chromatin masses (heterochromatin) dispersed mainly on the internal aspect of the nuclear envelope. The clear channels in the peripheral chromatin are at the sites of pores in the nuclear envelope.* × 10,500.

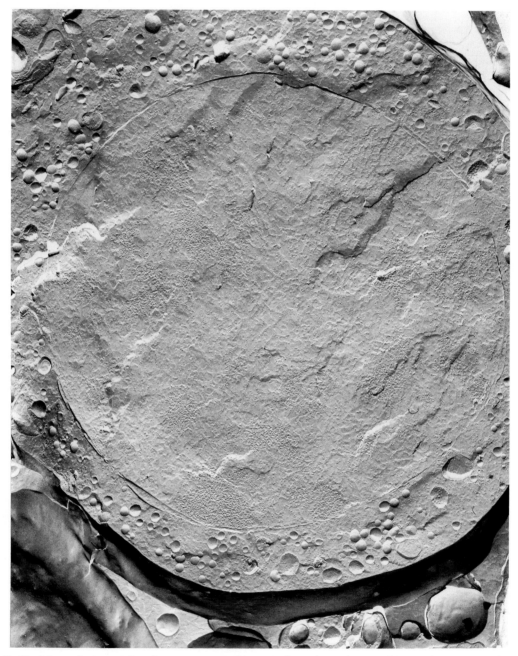

***Figure 1–47.*** *A freeze-fracture replica of a spermatocyte of rat testis shows the nuclear envelope, nuclear pores, and chromatin masses at the margin of the nucleus.* × *16,200. (Courtesy of Dr. H. N. Tung.)*

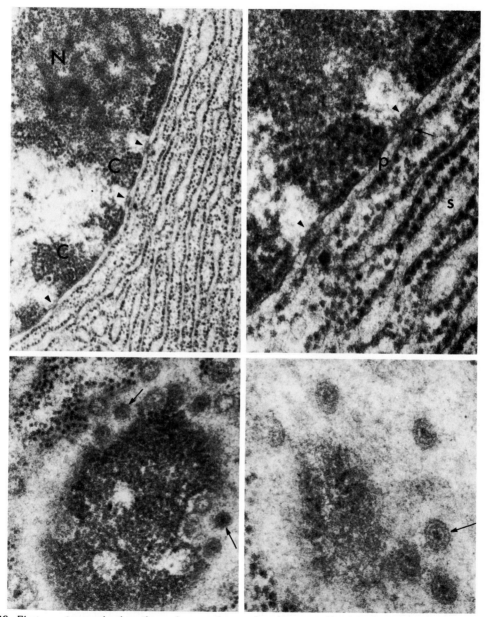

***Figure 1–48.*** *Electron micrographs show the nuclear envelope and nuclear pores. Top left: Three pores (arrowheads) are seen. N is the nucleolus and C is chromatin. × 26,000. Top right: A higher magnification of two of the the pores seen in the top left figure. Some fibrous material appears to traverse the pores, the upper of which shows a central dense granule (arrow). Note some flocculent material both within intracisternal spaces (s) of granular reticulum and in the perinuclear space (p) of the nuclear envelope. × 45,000. Bottom left: Tangential section of the nucleus illustrating close spacing of the pores, seen as circular profiles, some with a central dense granule (arrows), × 30,000. Bottom right: A higher magnification of the pores. × 45,000.*

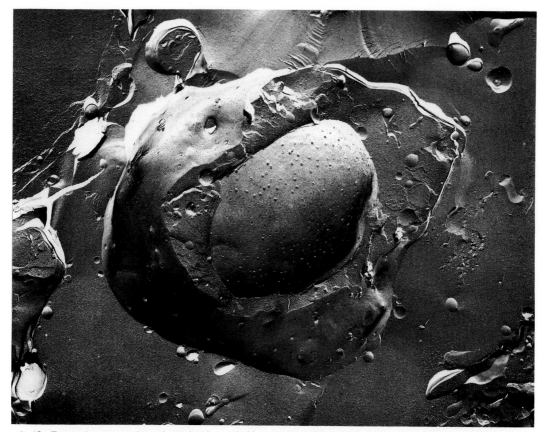

*Figure 1–49.* Freeze-fracture replica of rat decidua cell. Note a cleaved plane through the nucleus, cytoplasm, and plasma membrane (from the center outward). × 8200. (Courtesy of Dr. H. N. Tung.)

are attached. The fibrous lamina varies in thickness in different cells, and there is biochemical evidence that it plays a crucial role in organizing both the nuclear envelope and the underlying chromatin. The lamina polypeptides are probably instrumental in the dissolution and re-formation of the nuclear envelope that occurs during each mitosis.

At localized regions called nuclear pores (40 to 100 nm), the outer membrane is connected to the inner nuclear membrane. The pore is composed of eight granules that are arranged in precise symmetry on the annular perimeter. Eight radially distributed conical tips project from the annular perimeter into the pore lumen. A centrally located particle (granular or rod-like) may be present, and bundles of nucleoplasmic filaments are frequently seen attached to the granular components. The half of the nuclear "pore complex" facing the cytoplasm is, in some instances, decorated by large particles, similar in appearance and size to ribosomes. Pore formations with the same symmetrical architecture as that of the nuclear "pore complex" are observed in cytoplasmic cisternae of the endoplasmic reticulum. In sections perpendicular to the plane of the nuclear membranes, the edge of the pore complex is seen to cross the perinuclear space, bringing the two lipid bilayers of the inner and outer membranes together around the margins of each pore. These regions where the inner and outer nuclear membranes are continuous probably enable lipid-soluble materials dissolved in membranes to flow from the endoplasmic reticulum membrane, where they are synthesized, into the inner nuclear membrane. Apparently, the permeability of nuclear pores shows some variation with the functional state of the cell, and it is known also that

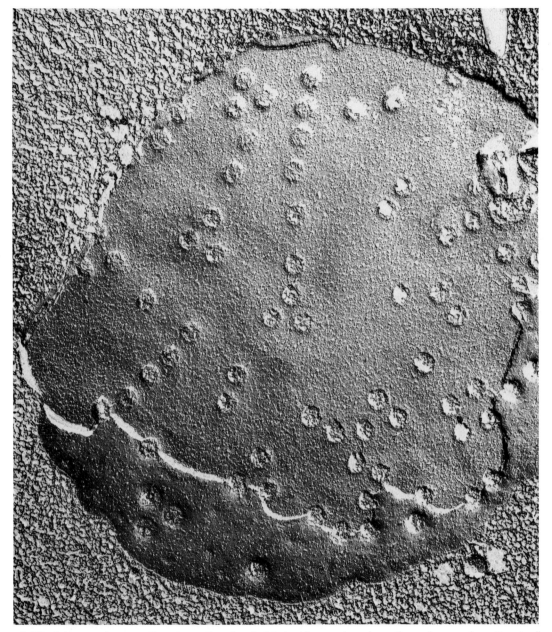

**Figure 1–50.** *A freeze-etch preparation of a portion of an isolated rat liver nucleus shows the nuclear envelope, its outer (lower edge) and inner membranes, and nuclear pores.* × *60,000. (Courtesy of Dr. G. G. Maul.)*

the number of pores varies with changes in nuclear activity. The nuclear pores thus act to shield the nucleoplasm from many of the particles, filaments, and large molecules that function in the cytoplasm.

## KARYOPLASM

Nuclear sap, or karyoplasm, is a term that describes the clear or apparently empty areas of the nucleus (i.e., those areas not occupied by nucleolus or chromatin). The karyoplasm is relatively electron-lucid on electron microscopy, although it contains dispersed chromatin, some small granules, and protein. Karyoplasm is a semifluid, colloidal solution in which the chromatin material and the nucleolus are suspended and serves as a medium for the diffusion of metabolites and larger macromolecules.

## NUCLEAR CHROMATIN

Chromatin is the designation for the DNA containing nuclear material and proteins and is the structural manifestation of chromosomes in interphase. Chromosomes in a dividing cell are simply threads of chromatin that at various sites along their course may be coiled, folded, or crumpled so as to form "condensed" masses that are visible by light microscopy. Chromosomes in the interphase nucleus are not visible, but in fact they remain intact. Chromatin is basophilic and stains Feulgen positive owing to its DNA content. During interphase, the chromatin exists in two forms: *euchromatin*, or extended chromatin, and *heterochromatin*, or condensed chromatin. Euchromatin is loosely packed and thus only lightly basophilic, with Feulgen staining. Here the genes are readily available for the transcription of messenger RNA. Heterochromatin is strongly basophilic, staining deeply with hematoxylin, and is formed by the tight coiling of the chromosomes. Because of the tight coiling, the genes are not available for the transcription of messenger RNA. Heterochromatic sections of the chromosome can be divided into two categories, *constitutive* heterochromatin and *facultative* heterochromatin, depending on whether the chromatin is always condensed or is condensed only under certain conditions. In most somatic cells, there is a mixture of the two states of chromatin; heterochromatin typically lies close against the inside of the nuclear envelope, leaving gaps at the nuclear pores, while the euchromatin occupies the more central region of the nucleus. The proportion of heterochromatin to euchromatin accounts for the variation from a light to dark appearance of the nucleus. The proportion or amount of euchromatin, usually associated with a large nucleolus (or nucleoli), can be used as an indication of the metabolic activity of a specific cell or cell type because euchromatin usually is active in RNA synthesis. Conversely, a high pro-

portion of heterochromatin indicates a cell with low metabolic activity. Thus, in nerve cells, the nuclei are large with very little visible chromatin in them, whereas lymphocytes have smaller and rather densely stained nuclei.

Nuclei themselves are basically of two types: *condensed*, or *hyperchromatic* (small, darkly staining nuclei with much stainable chromatin, e.g., of fibroblasts and some blood cells), and *vesicular* (larger paler-staining nuclei, e.g., of nerve cells and liver cells). In moribund cells, the heterochromatin is extremely dense, and the nuclei of such cells are called *pyknotic*.

Electron microscopy shows that chromatin consists of coiled strands of DNA bound to basic proteins (histones). These strands contain particles or beads called *nucleosomes*. A nucleosome consists of a disc-shaped histone core plus a segment of DNA that winds around the core. The nucleosome gives chromatin its "beads-on-a-string" appearance in electron micrographs taken after treatments that unfold the higher-order packing. This higher order of organization consists of adjacent nucleosomes packed into a helical secondary DNA-protein structure termed a *solenoid*. Chromatin released from the nucleus still in the solenoid form appears in electron micrographs as a thick (30 nm in diameter) fiber, in comparison with the thin (10 nm in diameter) fiber or beaded string. The internal arrangement of a solenoid is probably a chromatin fiber coiled into a helix containing six nucleosomes per turn; this structure has been referred to as a *chromatosome*. The solenoids may be further organized into giant "supercoiled" loops. These higher orders of coiling must be necessary, especially in the condensation of chromatin into chromosomes during mitosis and meiosis.

## NUCLEOLUS

As seen in the light microscope, the large, spheroidal nucleolus is the most obvious structure in the nucleus of a nonmitotic cell (Fig. 1–51). The number of nucleoli and the size (up to 1 μm in diameter or more) of the nucleolus are constant for any particular cell type. Unlike the cytoplasmic organelles, the nucleolus has no membrane to keep it together; instead, it seems to be con-

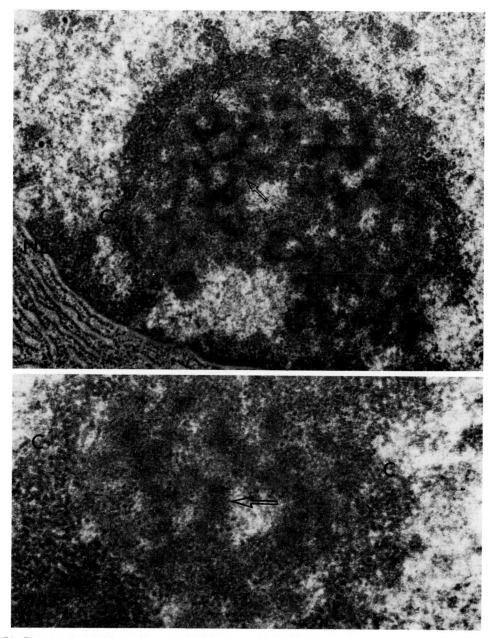

**Figure 1–51.** *Electron micrographs of the nucleolus.* Top: *Here lying adjacent to the nuclear envelope (NE), the nucleolus is sponge-like and consists of granules and fibrils arranged in a coiled cord (the nucleolonema) with areas of densely packed fibrils (the fibrillar centers, arrows) around less dense material. Surrounding the nucleolus is nucleolus-associated chromatin (C).* × 34,000. Bottom: *A higher magnification.* × 48,000.

structed by the specific binding of unfinished ribosome precursors to each other. Nucleoli are prominent and usually multiple in cells actively engaged in protein synthesis. The size of the nucleolus reflects its activity. The differences in size are due largely to contraction or expansion of the granular component, which is probably controlled at the level of ribosomal gene transcription. They are larger, more dense, and more regular in outline than masses of heterochromatin. They consist of 5 to 10 per cent RNA, with the rest protein and a small amount of DNA, and often are surrounded by a rim of condensed chromatin termed the *nucleolus-associated chromatin*. This chromatin consists of fibers with an average diameter of 25 nm containing loops of DNA that are protein-free and in the form of a double helix. Each nucleolus is produced from, and attached to, a specific *nucleolus-organizing region* located at a specific site on a specific *nucleolus-organizing chromosome*. In many cases, the nucleolus-organizing region is located near the terminus of a chromosome, and a small knob or *satellite* of the chromosome projects beyond this region. Staining varies with the relative proportions of RNA and basic protein, but usually they are basophilic owing to RNA content. Nucleoli may stain metachromatically with dyes such as toluidine blue and usually are Feulgen negative, although the rim of the nucleus-associated chromatin is strongly Feulgen positive. The use of special techniques also shows that the nucleolus possesses a definite internal structure, consisting of a coiled, thick filament called the *nucleolemma* embedded in an amorphous component.

The structural organization of the nucleolus reflects its chromosomal attachment and its functions in ribosome subunit production. By electron microscopy, four different components can be resolved:

1. *Granules* 12 to 15 nm in diameter, which represent ribosome subunits nearing completion.

2. *Fibrils* of RNA transcripts in nucleoprotein form, measuring about 5 nm in diameter.

3. *Chromatin* consisting of chromosomal loops, 10 nm wide, extending out from their point of attachment in the nucleolus-organizing region of the chromosome.

4. A *proteinaceous, amorphous matrix* in which all these materials are distributed. The matrix together with the chromatin filaments accounts for the less dense regions in the nucleolus, which vary in size and number depending on cell type.

The components may form a compact mass or may occur as a core of fibrils surrounded by a mass of granules; however, often fibrils and granules together form a thick, anastomosing cord (the nucleolemma) with patches along the cord formed either by granules or by fibrils. The nucleolus may enlarge in active cells and become reduced in size in inactive cells, principally as a consequence of expansion in the extent of the granular zone. These changes in dimensions undoubtedly result from different rates of ribosome subunit production in relation to cellular biosynthetic activities.

The static picture provided by stains or enzyme digestions can be animated by studies of the incorporation of labelled precursors during macromolecular synthesis. These studies show that proteins are not synthesized in the nucleolus or in any part of the nucleus. Mature ribosomes are absent from the nucleus, so no machinery is available for the synthesis of nuclear proteins. All the nuclear proteins are made at cytoplasmic ribosomes and must be transported across the nuclear envelope into the nucleus. The imported proteins become parts of chromosomes, ribosome subunits, nuclear lamina, and other nuclear structures, or they serve a catalytic or regulatory function in DNA replication and transcription.

## CELL CYCLE

The process of mitosis and *interphase* (the period between cell divisions) is termed the *cell cycle*. A cell cycle consists of three phases in which the macromolecular syntheses take place, plus the phase of mitosis in which the genomes are delivered to daughter cells. The three phases of biosynthesis are *G1*, when preparations are initiated for chromosome replication; *S*, when chromosomes replicate; and *G2*, when preparations are made for actual delivery of the genomes, which occurs in mitosis. At the termination of mitosis, the daughter cells enter the G1 stage, which lasts until DNA duplication occurs prior to the succeeding mitosis. Obviously, the length of the cell cycle varies with the cell type, for example, being short in the case of the epithelial cells lining the gut and much longer in liver cells. Although we know very few of the specific structural and catalytic molecules that are made or called into action during G1 and G2, we know that DNA replicates during the S phase and that histone proteins are synthesized at the same time.

## CHROMOSOMES

Chromosomes are vividly staining, rod-shaped bodies that are present between the two poles in dividing cells. As described earlier, chromosomes are made up of a stainable material called chromatin fibers. Chromatin fibers are complexes of DNA and proteins for the most part, although some small amounts of RNA may also be present. The chromatin fiber may be considered the basic structural unit of the eukaryotic chromosome.

### Fine Structure of Chromosomes

Each chromosome consists of a pair of chromatids, each of which is a fully replicated chromosome. The chromatin of these chromosomes on electron microscopy is a mixture or meshwork of fibrils about 30 nm in diameter. These fibrils probably represent a supercoiling or super helix of a beaded strand, only 2 nm in diameter, with chromatin subunits or *nucleosomes* 7 to 10 nm in diameter placed at intervals along the strand. The nucleosomes contain a double-stranded DNA fragment, 140 to 200 base pairs long, bound to an octamerous histone core. A flexible strand of "linker" DNA joins successive nucleosomes and contains about 60 base pairs. Chains of nucleosomes that encompass "linker" DNA may be coiled to form a more compact structure called a *solenoid*. The organization of the chromatin fiber as a chain of repeating nucleosome subunits provides a satisfactory explanation for the capacity of a rather stiff nucleoprotein fiber to be folded back on itself repeatedly and thereby occupy a space that may be little more than a few micrometers of chromosome length.

### DNA Structure and Replication

DNA consists of two parallel molecular chains in the form of a double helix (Fig. 1–52). Each chain is composed of a backbone of pentose sugar groups linked by phosphoric acid bridges. Each pentose group bears a nitrogen-carbon ring base, which is directed toward a corresponding group on the opposite chain. The bases of the two chains are connected by cross links. There are four such bases: the purines, adenine and guanine, and the pyramidines, cytosine and thymine. The pair bonding occurs always between adenine and thymine or between cytosine and guanine. During mitosis, the DNA content is doubled before division, ensuring each daughter cell an identical DNA content. The process is called DNA *replication* or *duplication* and corresponds to the S stage of the cell cycle. To achieve this conservation of genetic material during cell division, the DNA double helix unwinds, and each strand becomes a template for the assembly of a new molecular chain. In this process, the two chains of a DNA molecule separate from one another, and individual base-sugar-phosphate units (DNA nucleotides) attach to the exposed template DNA chains according to the comple-

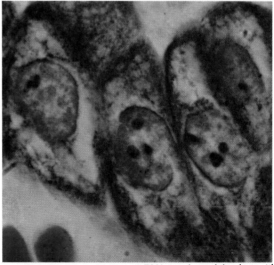

**Figure 1–52.** Both DNA and RNA are basophilic, but with azure B, DNA stains green and RNA stains purple. DNA is seen only in the nuclei, whereas RNA is present mainly in the cytoplasm but also in the nucleoli. Note that nucleoli may be multiple. DNA and RNA. Azure B. Oil immersion.

mentary base-pairing pattern. The base adenine always pairs with thymine and vice versa; cytosine always pairs with guanine and vice versa. Each daughter double helix, therefore, is composed of one strand, or chain, from the parent and one new strand, and the linear array of genes is copied exactly.

A *gene* is a triplet (i.e., three bases in a row), and this corresponds to a single amino acid in the protein that is formed. A single polypeptide (a chain of amino acids) is encoded by a sequence of several triplets, this sequence being called a *cistron*.

### Chromosome Numbers

There are 46 chromosomes in each of the human *somatic cells* (all cells except the reproductive cells) (Figs. 1–53 and 1–54). Two of these are *sex chromosomes* (two X chromosomes in females; one X and one Y chromosome in males). The remaining 44 chromosomes are called autosomes. Cells with two complete sets of chromosomes (46 chromosomes) are said to be *diploid cells*. In the gonads, the sex cells (ova or spermatozoa) contain half this number, or 23 chromosomes. Such cells are called *haploid cells* and cannot be produced by the normal process of mitosis. A second type of cell division, a *reduction division* known as meiosis, is responsible for the production of haploid reproductive cells. Thus, each ovum, or female sex cell, contains 22 autosomes and one X chromosome, and each spermatozoon, or male sex cell, contains 22 autosomes and one X or Y chromosome. After fertilization (i.e., after union of the sex cells), the fertilized ovum, or gamete, will contain either 44 autosomes plus two X chromosomes (a combination that develops into female) or 44 autosomes plus one X and one Y chromosome (a combination that develops into a male).

In some cases, human somatic cells may not have the correct number of chromosomes. In humans, most of the disorders of chromosome number arise because of *nondisjunction* (one daughter cell gets both homologue chromosomes, and the other daughter cell gets neither). *Poly-*

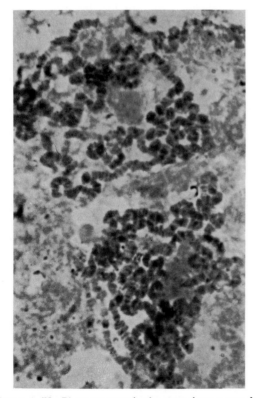

**Figure 1–53.** *Photomicrograph of a giant chromosome from a salivary gland of the fruit fly (Drosophila). A smear preparation.* × *850.*

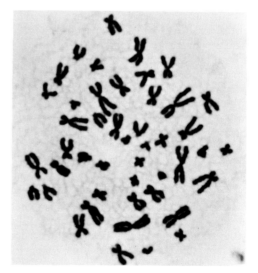

**Figure 1–54.** *Photomicrograph of human (male) chromosomes from a squash preparation. Notice the various positions of the centromeres.* × *1250. (Courtesy of Dr. M. L. Barr.)*

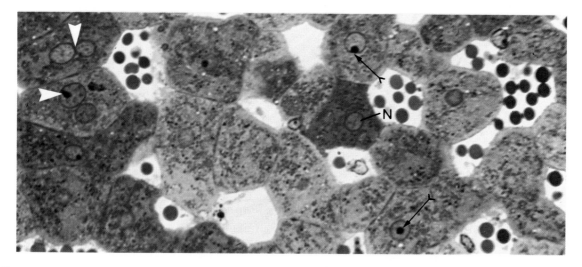

**Figure 1–55.** *Anastomosing cords of epithelial (parenchymal) cells are present with vascular, sinusoidal spaces between the cords; these contain erythrocytes that appear as round profiles staining dark blue and are non-nucleated. In the liver cells, cell borders are seen, and the cytoplasm is abundant and shows small dense particles that are mitochondria. Small, spherical, clear spaces represent dissolved lipid. Nuclei (N) are vesicular, often with prominent nucleoli (arrows), and polyploidal or binucleate cells (arrowheads) are common. Liver. Plastic section. Toluidine blue. High power.*

*ploidy* is a condition in which cells contain multiples of the haploid number of chromosomes (e.g., a tetraploid cell contains four times the haploid number of chromosomes, or 92) (Fig. 1–55). Polyploidy may occur normally in certain somatic cells. It is quite common in liver cells and results in the presence of a larger nucleus. Such normally occurring polyploid cells arise by doubling of the chromosome number without a subsequent karyokinesis. *Aneuploidy* is a condition in which a cell contains either less than the normal diploid number of chromosomes or a greater number that is not a multiple of it. Not surprisingly, substantial changes in the number and arrangement of chromosomes often result in serious abnormalities. Humans must have two and only two copies of each autosomal chromosome in order to be normal. Embryos that accidentally inherit only a single copy of one of the autosomes are not viable, and those individuals who survive with three copies of one autosome (*trisomy*) are always strikingly abnormal. Individuals with trisomy of chromosome 21 (Down's syndrome) can survive but are mentally retarded. Abnormal numbers of sex chromosomes also occur. These chromosome abnormalities do not produce such gross deformities as do abnormal numbers of autosomes.

Individuals with XXY and XXXY karyotypes develop as males (because of the presence of Y) but are sterile. The condition is known as Klinefelter's syndrome.

### Sex Chromatin (Barr's Body)

All female mammalian cells contain two X chromosomes, while the male cells contain one X and one Y chromosome. Presumably because a double dose of X chromosome products would be lethal, the female cells have evolved a mechanism for permanently inactivating one of the two X chromosomes in each cell. The single X chromosome in males is almost entirely euchromatic, as is one of the two X chromosomes in females. The second X chromosome in females condenses to the heterochromatic state very early in embryonic development and remains condensed thereafter in all cell lineages. This compact chromosome is seen in the light microscope during interphase as a distinct structure known as *Barr's body* and commonly occurs lying against the inner aspect of the nuclear envelope in a planoconvex form (epithelial cell nuclei) (Figs. 1–56 and 1–57). In some cells (neutrophil granular leukocytes), it

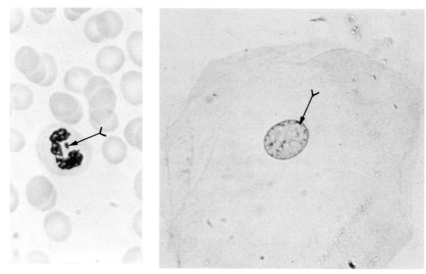

**Figure 1–56.** Barr's body. Left: In this blood smear many non-nucleated erythrocytes (red blood corpuscles) are present with one nucleated cell. This is a neutrophil, or polymorphonuclear leukocyte, and shows a large, irregularly lobated nucleus. Attached to one lobe of the nucleus by a fine strand of chromatin is a small nuclear appendage, or Barr's, body (arrow). This "drumstick" probably represents the sex chromosome and is found in only about 3 per cent of neutrophils in female blood. Neutrophil. Sex chromatin. Giemsa. Oil immersion. Right: This is a buccal smear, squamous epithelial cells having been scraped gently from the inside of the cheek and smeared onto a microscope slide. The nucleus shows a nuclear envelope, karyoplasm, and nuclear chromatin. Associated with the inner aspect of the nuclear envelope is a small, planoconvex, densely staining body (arrow). This is the Barr's body, or sex chromatin, and indicates the presence of two X chromosomes, that is, female sex. One X chromosome in an interphase nucleus is dispersed, that is, uncoiled. The other X chromosome of a female nucleus remains tightly coiled (i.e., heterochromatic) and is visible as the Barr's body. Oral smear. Barr's body. Aceto-orcein. Oil immersion.

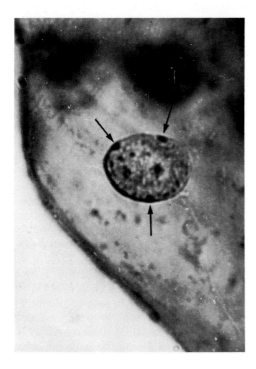

**Figure 1–57.** Photomicrograph of cells from the buccal smear of a two-month-old mentally retarded child. The somatic cells of this child, presumably a Klinefelter's syndrome patient, contain 22 times 2 autosomes plus XXXXY. The nucleus illustrated contains three female sex chromatin, or Barr's bodies. × 1200. (Courtesy of Dr. B. Smith.)

is seen as a "drumstick" or slender protrusion of the nucleus. It may appear as a small body associated with the nucleolus (nucleolar satellite) in nerve cells. It is not seen in normal male somatic cells. Males who show one or more Barr's bodies have one or more extra X chromosomes. This is correlated with the physical symptoms of Kline-felter's syndrome (sterility, small testicles, and enlarged breasts). Women with only one X chromosome (XO) exhibit the physical symptoms of Turner's syndrome (sterility, small stature, and underdeveloped breasts). No Barr's bodies are seen, although the individual is female. Females have no Y chromosome but have one or more X chromosomes. The complete absence of X chromosomes is a lethal condition because many essential genes are located on the X chromosome. The absence of the Y chromosome is obviously not lethal. In all these cases, the number of Barr's bodies plus one provides a direct count of the number of X chromosomes in the nucleus. The Y chromosome is male-determining in mammals.

## CELL DIVISION

During embryonic development most cells are undergoing repeated division as the body grows in size and complexity. As a particular cell matures, it becomes differentiated with respect to its structure and function. Some cell populations lose the ability to divide and do not undergo DNA synthesis (e.g., neurons). Other cell populations are expanding, and in this sense only a small proportion of the cells undergo DNA synthesis and cell division to permit growth (e.g., liver, kidney, and some glands). Finally, some cell populations contain stem cells capable of dividing throughout life to replace dying cells, for example, in bone marrow (forming blood cells), in the epithelium of the intestinal tract, and in the epidermis.

The process by which cells divide involves two basic events: division of the cytoplasm (cytokinesis) and division of the nucleus (karyokinesis); they are usually, but not always, coupled. Karyokinesis can occur without cytokinesis, resulting in the formation of a cell that is binucleate (or multinucleate after several karyokineses). This occurs in liver cells, megakaryocytes, and perhaps osteoclasts. In somatic cells, division of the nucleus occurs in mitosis. As already indicated, new DNA is synthesized during the S phase of interphase, so that in normal diploid cells, the amount of DNA has doubled by the onset of mitosis to the tetraploid DNA value, although the chromosome number is still diploid. The DNA replication ensures that each daughter cell has a DNA genetic content identical to that of the parent cell. The development of gonadal cells (ova and spermatozoa) involves a kind of cell division named meiosis. Meiosis results in the halving of a particular chromosome number, the haploid number. By fertilization, the haploid nuclei from the male and female gamete unite, and the diploid chromosomal number is restored to that present in somatic cells.

### Mitosis

The process of redistributing somatic genetic material into two new nuclei, each containing the same number and kind of chromosomes as the original nucleus, is called mitosis. The period between active cell divisions is called *interphase*. During interphase, the DNA molecules that comprise the genetic material appear only as distinct chromatin threads or granules in the nucleus. One of the principal events that occurs during interphase is DNA replication, that is, DNA molecules serve as templates for the replication of additional DNA molecules. By the end of interphase, the cell contains twice the amount of DNA it contained when it entered interphase. During this phase there is an active synthesis of protein and RNA and the nucleus and cytoplasm enlarge. Because the activities that occur in the cell change as the cell approaches mitosis, interphase is divided into three phases:

1. *G1 phase* immediately follows the completion of cell division.

2. *S phase* follows the G1 phase. The most notable event that occurs is the synthesis of DNA molecules. The new DNA is located in separate chromatin strands within the old chromosomes.

3. *G2 phase* follows the completion of DNA synthesis. The metabolic activities of the cell decrease in preparation for mitosis.

For descriptive purposes, mitosis is divided into

four stages: *prophase, metaphase, anaphase,* and *telophase.* However, mitosis is a continuous event and not a series of discrete steps (Figs. 1–58 through 1–61).

**Prophase.** During prophase, the pair of centrioles, usually adjacent to the nucleus of the interphase cell, start to duplicate, a daughter centriole forming adjacent to each, and the pairs of centrioles begin to move toward opposite poles of the cell (Fig. 1–62). The cell's original pair of centrioles replicates by a process that begins just prior to the S phase and gives rise to two pairs of centrioles. Each centriole pair now becomes part of a *mitotic center* that forms the focus for a radial array of microtubules, the *aster* (the complex of astral fibers, or rays, and centrioles). Other longer microtubules develop between the asters as *spindle fibers.* Some of these will extend from aster to aster as continuous microtubules, but these are complete only after disappearance of the nuclear envelope.

The transition from the G2 phase to the changes in preparation for mitosis (which is sometimes called the *M phase*) is not a sharply defined event. The chromatin fibers, which are diffuse in interphase, become condensed (shortened and thickened) so that the chromosomes become visible as short, dark rod-like structures. Each chromosome has duplicated during the preceding S phase and consists of two sister *chromatids* joined at a specific point along their length by a region known as the *centromere.* In fact, as a result of DNA duplication, each chromatid is a completely replicated chromosome, although it is not so called at this stage. While the chromosomes are condensing, the nucleolus begins to disassemble and gradually disappears.

Finally, the nuclear envelope starts to disintegrate in conjunction with the penetration into the chromosomal mass by the mitotic spindle. The envelope becomes less obvious and thinner as a result of movement of chromatin material away from its inner surface, and then it breaks down into vesicles indistinguishable from elements of the granular endoplasmic reticulum. These vesicles remain visible around the spindle during mitosis. The spindle, which has been lying outside the nucleus, can now enter the nuclear area.

**Metaphase.** By the beginning of metaphase, the nuclear envelope has disappeared completely. All the chromosomes (pairs of chromatids) move to the center of the cell in relation to the spindle

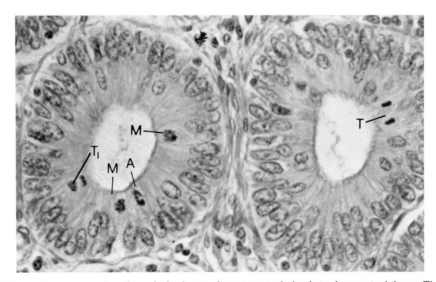

**Figure 1–58.** *This is a transverse section through the bases of two intestinal glands in the terminal ileum. The tubular glands are lined by simple columnar epithelium. Severe "mitotic figures" (cells undergoing mitosis) are seen. For cell division, which is active in the intestinal lining, cells round up, pass toward the lumen, and undergo mitosis to form two daughter cells. The visible stages are a late telophase (T), metaphase plates (M), an anaphase (A), and an early telophase (T₁). Intestinal glands, mitosis. H and E. High power.*

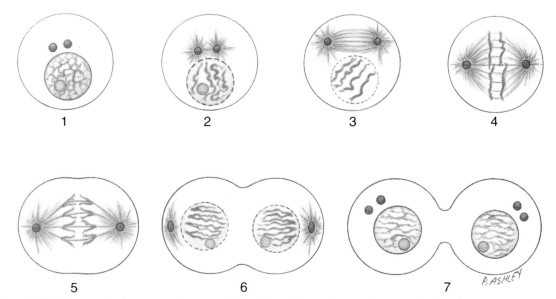

**Figure 1–59.** *Diagram of the stages of mitosis.* 1, Interphase: *The nuclear envelope, nucleolus, chromatin, and a pair of centrioles are illustrated.* 2, Early prophase: *Two centrioles are forming asters, the nuclear envelope and nucleolus are dispersing, and chromosomes are becoming visible.* 3, Late prophase: *A spindle is formed between the two centrioles. The nuclear envelope has virtually disappeared, and the nucleolus is broken up and dispersed over the chromosomes, four of which are illustrated, each split into two chromatids, and each joined only at a centromere.* 4, Metaphase: *The chromosomes (pairs of chromatids) are arranged at the equator of the spindle.* 5, Anaphase: *The chromosomes have split, and the chromatin of each pair is moving toward one pole of the cell.* 6, Early telophase: *The chromatids (now chromosomes) of each daughter cell are becoming uncoiled; a nuclear envelope and nucleolus are re-forming, and the centriole is duplicating.* 7, Late telophase: *The plasma membrane is constricting, and two new daughter cells are formed.*

and are arranged at the equatorial plate (parallel axis along which cytokinesis will occur). Specialized structures called *kinetochores* develop on either face of the centromeres and become attached to a special set of microtubules, the so-called chromosome microtubules. These microtubules radiate in opposite directions from each side of each chromosome and interact with the fibers of the bipolar spindle. One set of chromosomal microtubules thus extends from the kinetochore of one chromatid to the pole of the cell. The chromosomes are thrown into agitated motion owing to the interactions of their chromosomal microtubules. Further development of the microtubules of the spindle also occurs, in that spindle fibers from each pair of centrioles, having met in the region of the equatorial plate to form continuous microtubules, continue to elongate and thus move the pairs of centrioles further apart. However, it is the chromosomal microtubules (kinetochore microtubules) that seem to be re-

sponsible for aligning the chromosomes with their long axes at right angles to the spindle axis.

Finally, at the end of metaphase, a total split of the two chromatids of each chromosome occurs at the centromere, the kinetochores separating. In determining the number of chromosomes, one counts the number of centromeres and not the number of strands. Therefore, during prophase a chromosome consists of two chromatids, but following metaphase each chromatid is considered to be a chromosome, and thus the metaphase cell has a tetraploid number (92) of chromosomes.

Colchicine, some derivatives of colchicine, and vinblastine block the assembly of microtubules as described earlier. In mitosis, therefore, spindle microtubule formation does not occur. If these drugs are administered to an experimental animal, any cell undergoing cell division will be arrested at the metaphase stage. This has proved to be a valuable technique for studying cell turnover rates

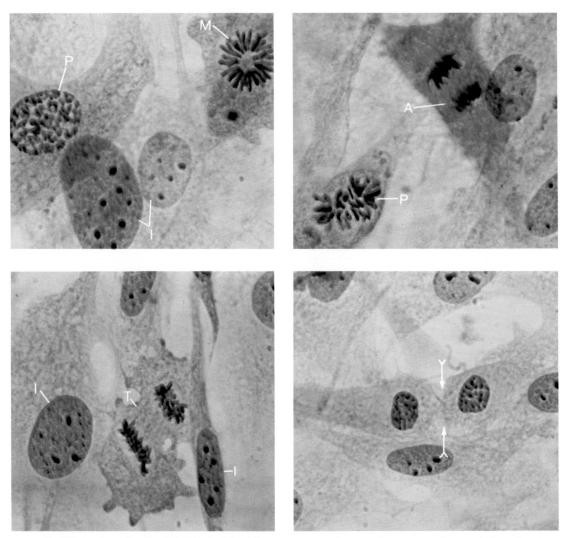

**Figure 1–60.** *Stages of mitosis. Top left: This and the following micrographs are cells in tissue culture and show the stages of mitosis. Interphase nuclei (I) and one early prophase (P) are seen. Here, the cell is "rounding up," that is, withdrawing its cytoplasmic process, and in the nucleus are irregular, darkly staining threads—these are the chromosomes. The cell at M shows a metaphase plate as seen from one pole of the cell. Chromosomes, or pairs of chromatids, lie at the equator of the cell, and the cell outline is defined clearly, that is, it has withdrawn its process. Pentachrome. Oil immersion. Top right: The cell at left (P) has rounded up, the nuclear membrane is disappearing, and chromosomes are clearly visible. This is a late prophase. The cell at A is somewhat elongated, and two groups of darkly staining daughter chromosomes are passing to opposite poles of the cell in anaphase. Pentachrome. Oil immersion. Bottom left: Apart from cells in interphase (I), the cell at T is in early telophase. Two daughter nuclei are commencing to re-form, although chromosomes still are visible; the cytoplasm is starting to constrict, the cleavage furrow deepening around the midbody. (The midbody is a mass of microtubules from the mitotic spindle located originally at the equator, now at the site of cytokinesis). Pentachrome. Oil immersion. Bottom right: In the center, two daughter cells have nearly separated completely at the cleavage furrow (arrows), and the daughter nuclei are complete. Nuclear envelopes are visible, and chromosomes have dispersed, leaving only a speckling of nuclear chromatin. This is late telophase. Pentachrome. Oil immersion.*

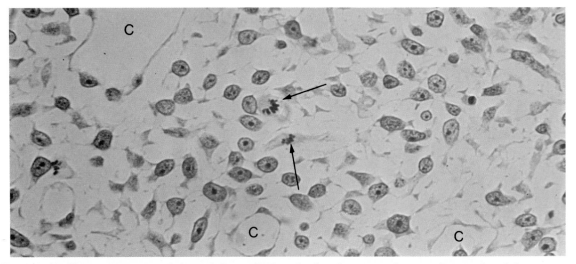

**Figure 1–61.** *The tissue is composed of irregularly spindle-shaped cells with processes that extend into a relatively homogeneous ground substance devoid of formed fibers. The cells show a spherical or ovoid nucleus with a distinct nucleolus. Two cells (arrows) are in the process of mitosis. The tissue is vascular, and portions of three small blood vessels (C), lined by a delicate endothelium, are present. Mesenchyme. Plastic section. H and E. High power.*

and for cytogenetic studies, since the chromosomes are most easily studied in the metaphase stage.

**Anaphase.** Anaphase begins abruptly as the paired kinetochores on each chromosome separate, allowing each chromatid to be pulled slowly toward a spindle pole (Fig. 1–63). During these anaphase movements, chromosomal microtubules shorten as the chromosomes approach the poles. At about the same time, the continuous microtubules elongate, and the two poles of the polar spindle move further apart.

Micromanipulation experiments demonstrate that chromosomal microtubules are most strongly attached to the spindle near the poles via a gel-like "net," which may generate the forces that move chromatids. The continuous microtubules have their free (fast-growing) ends near their area of overlap at the spindle equator, and the free ends elongate by addition of tubulin subunits. The sliding movements of the two sets of continuous microtubules seem likely to be caused by a dynein-like molecule that uses the energy of ATP hydrolysis. This is accompanied by a detachment from the two asters of the continuous microtubules and their movement to, and accumulation

in, the center of the cell near the region of ultimate cytokinesis. Here, the massing of microtubules forms a dense mass called the *midbody*. Toward the end of anaphase and extending into telophase, a band-like constriction occurs around the cell (the cleavage furrow) in the region of the midbody, and mitochondria and other cytoplasmic components are distributed evenly around the cell periphery.

**Telophase.** At each pole of the cell, the chromosomes detach from the chromosomal microtubules, and these microtubules disappear. The continuous microtubules elongate still further, and a new nuclear envelope re-forms around each group of daughter chromosomes. The nuclear envelope re-forms from cytoplasmic membranous vesicles, probably originating from granular endoplasmic reticulum. The nucleoli of each nucleus reappear in association with specific chromosomes. The condensed chromosomes expand and become less distinct, and eventually only portions of them remain tightly coiled as heterochromatin, the expanded regions being euchromatin. If mitosis and cytokinesis are occurring together, the membrane around the middle of the cell, perpendicular to the spindle axis and be-

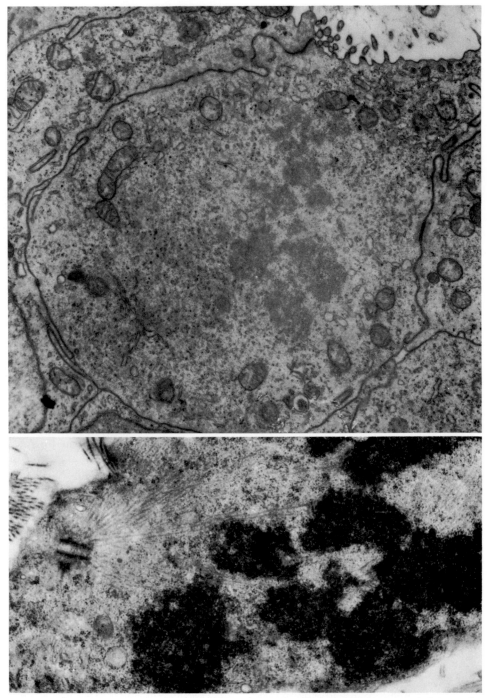

**Figure 1–62.** *Electron micrograph demonstrating mitosis.* Top: *A jejunal epithelial cell of the mouse in late prophase. The cell has rounded up, chromosomes are apparent, and the nuclear envelope has disappeared.* × *8500.* Bottom: *A fibroblast in metaphase with spindle fibers (microtubules) extending from the centriole (left) to chromosomes (chromosomal microtubules) and between them to the other pole of the cell (spindle fibers or continuous microtubules).* × *19,000.*

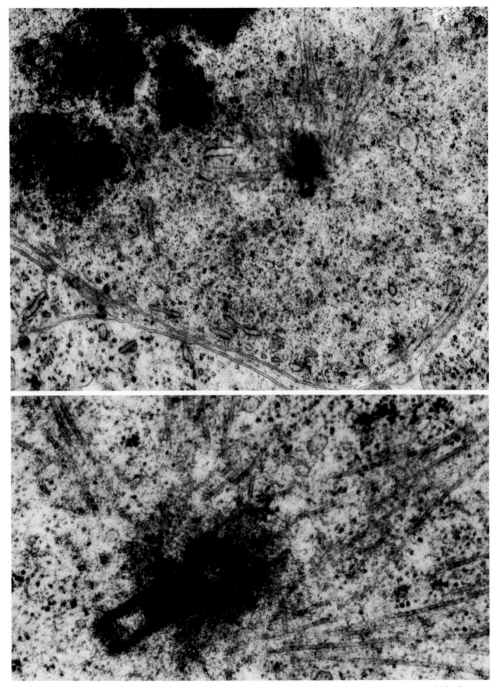

***Figure 1–63.*** *Electron micrographs (top and bottom) illustrating anaphase in an epithelial cell.* Bottom: *At higher magnification, a pair of centrioles with radiating microtubules is shown.* Top, × *19,000;* Bottom, × *60,000.*

tween the daughter nuclei, is drawn inward to form a *cleavage furrow*. This furrow deepens until it encounters the narrow remains of the mitotic spindle between the two nuclei. The narrow bridge, or midbody, may persist for some time before it breaks and two discrete daughter cells are formed. Cytoplasmic components are distributed equally between the two, and microtubules, formerly in the midbody, disintegrate or disperse.

In sections, cells undergoing division are recognized by the presence of *mitotic figures*, this term referring to any cell undergoing mitosis. Usually, the chromatin material, being more condensed, stains more densely than in an interphase nucleus, and of course, other features may be apparent, as described. In many cases, a cell changes its shape and moves its position when undergoing mitosis. For example, in simple epithelia, the cell becomes rounded and apparently moves toward the surface, losing its connection with the basal lamina.

## Meiosis

Cells with two complete sets of chromosomes (46 chromosomes) are said to be diploid cells. The formation of gametes, however, must result in the formation of cells that have only one set of chromosomes (23 chromosomes rather than 46). Such cells are called haploid cells and cannot be produced by the normal process of mitosis. A second type of division, a reduction division known as *meiosis*, is responsible for the production of haploid reproductive cells. This process consists of two successive nuclear divisions without an intervening period of DNA replication. In the first division, only one chromosome (pair of chromatids) from each homologous pair is passed to each daughter cell, thus halving the number of chromosomes to 23. The progeny of this division therefore contain a diploid amount of DNA but differ from normal diploid cells in that both of the two DNA copies of each chromosome derive from only one of the two homologous chromosomes present in the original cell. In the second division of meiosis, the two chromatids of each chromosome are separated, thus producing finally four

nuclei each with a haploid number of chromosomes and haploid amount of DNA content. When male and female gametes unite, the diploid number is regained. Meiosis allows a great deal of genetic diversity in the make-up of sperm and ova. The chromosomes that originally came from the individual's male or female parent, for example, do not necessarily all line up toward one centriole pair during the synapsis of chromosomes that occurs in the first division sequence of meiosis. Rather, a mixture of positions is assumed so that the resulting daughter cells each receive some chromosomes derived from the individual's male parent and some from the female parent in a random assortment. Further genetic diversity can occur by the exchange of segments of homologous chromosomes while the chromosomes are synapsed during the reduction division.

**First Meiotic Division.** The *prophase* of this division takes much longer than the prophase of mitosis and is divided into four stages. In *leptotene*, the chromosomes appear as fine threads in diploid number. Later, the homologous chromosomes (one paternal and one maternal) arrange themselves lengthwise in pairs close together, with corresponding sites on the two in register. This is termed *zygotene*. This kind of pairing of the chromosomes is designated a *synapsis*. In *pachytene*, the chromosomes become shorter and thicker. Each homologous pair, or bivalent, consists of four chromatids (two paternal and two maternal). In *diplotene*, the chromosomes begin to separate. This separation is not complete, since they remain connected at particular sites where they cross one another in areas of contact. These sites of crossing are called *chiasmata*, and here an exchange of chromosomal segments takes place between one chromatid from each homologue. The separation of chromosomes continues in *diakinesis*. The nuclear envelope starts to disappear along with the nucleolus, which fragments and also disappears.

In *metaphase*, the chromosome pairs now arrange themselves in the equatorial plate. In *anaphase*, no division of centromeres or kinetochores of the bivalents occurs, with the result that whole chromosomes, each consisting of two sister chromatids, move to opposite poles of the cell.

**Second Meitoic Division.** This begins with *prophase*, after a short period called interkinesis has occurred. During interkinesis, the 23 double-stranded chromosomes of the daughter cell do not duplicate themselves. During prophase, a spindle forms, the nuclear envelope breaks down, and the chromosomes move to the equator to form a *metaphase* plate. A division of kineto-chores in each bivalent results in the release of sister chromatids, which are now converted to daughter chromosomes. The latter move to opposite poles in *anaphase* and form daughter nuclei and daughter cells in *telophase*. The entire process results in four daughter cells with haploid nuclei. In the meiosis of male germ cells, cytokinesis results in four viable germ cells, one of the 23 chromosomes is either an X or a Y chromosome. In the female, cytokinesis results in one viable germ cell, one of the 23 chromosomes is an X chromosome.

## CELL DIFFERENTIATION

In the development of the embryo, a single cell (the fertilized ovum) divides, eventually forming all cells of the body. The body is constructed from a rather limited number of distinguishable cell types—about 200 in a vertebrate. This process of cell proliferation leads to cell differentiation, with various cell types being specialized for different functions. The cell types are distinct essentially because each makes a different set of specialized proteins: keratin in epidermal cells, hemoglobin in red blood cells, digestive enzymes in gut cells, crystallins in lens cells, and so on. Since the cell types differ in that they contain different sets of gene products, one may ask whether this is simply because they contain different sets of genes. The lens cell, for example, might have lost the genes for hemoglobin, keratin, and so on, while retaining those for crystallins; or they might have selectively amplified the number of copies of the crystallin genes. There are several lines of evidence to show that such is not the case, and that all differentiated cell nuclei possess identical and complete chromosome—and therefore gene—sets (the genome, which is to be found in the fertilized egg). The cells of the body appear to differ not because they contain different genes but because they express different genes. Gene activity is subject to control: Genes can be switched on and off. It is evident that most of the genome in the highly differentiated cells is repressed (i.e., most of the genes do not express themselves). This may occur because the means whereby a gene can express itself are not present in the cell, and, certainly, some control over cellular synthetic mechanisms resides in the cytoplasm. However, while the components mainly responsible for gene regulation and gene repression have not been identified, repression undoubtedly is controlled chiefly by the activities of the genetic material, that is, the DNA together with nucleoproteins and nucleic acids that form the chromatin of the interphase nucleus. As cells develop, some regions of the genome become active, others become inactive.

## PROTEIN SECRETION AND TRANSCRIPTION OF DNA

The major use of cellular energy is the synthesis of molecules required for cell growth. The nucleus is the portion of the cell that contains the genetic material and manufactures molecules that control the synthetic activities of the organelles in the cytoplasm. Most cells contain a single nucleus. Cells that lack a nucleus are unable to synthesize proteins. The information required for protein synthesis is coded into different sequences of the four nucleotides making up DNA molecules of the nucleus (Fig. 1–64). Two primary kinds of information are stored in the DNA sequences. The directions for making proteins are spelled out by a code that uses the four DNA nucleotides, three at a time, in all possible combinations. Each three-nucleotide codeword stands for an amino acid. Reading the codewords in sequence along the DNA spells out the sequence of amino acids in a protein. These protein-encoding regions are duplicated into RNA copies, called messenger RNAs (mRNAs), that carry the directions for making proteins to the cytoplasm. Other DNA regions store directions for making two types of accessory DNAs that act in parts of the protein synthesis mechanism. One is ribosomal RNA (rRNA), that forms a part of the ribosomes, the RNA-protein structures that assemble amino acids into proteins in the cytoplasm. The second, transfer RNA (tRNA), binds directly to amino acids during protein synthesis and provides the necessary link

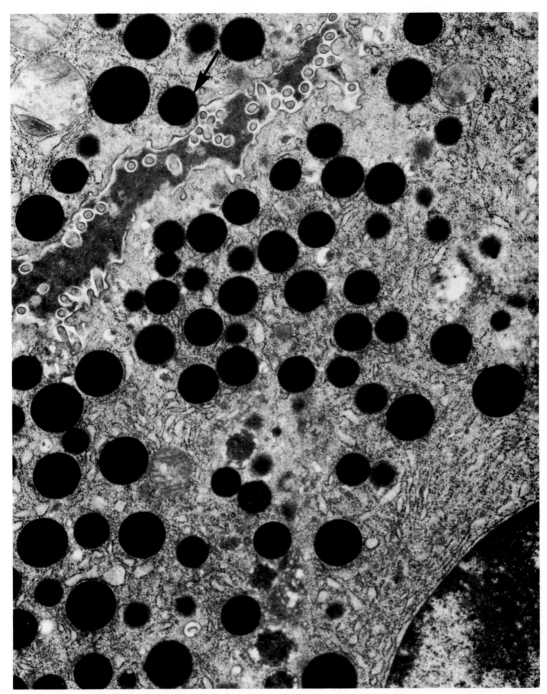

**Figure 1–64.** Electron micrograph of the apical portion of a pancreatic acinar cell to demonstrate the dynamic process of protein secretion. Part of the nucleus limited by the nuclear envelope lies at bottom right, with part of the nucleolus at the internal aspect of the nuclear envelope. In the apical cytoplasm is a mass of granular endoplasmic reticulum with some mitochondria, portions of Golgi apparatus at lower center and near the right edge of the micrograph just above the center, condensing vacuoles or prezymogen granules in relation to the Golgi apparatus, and zymogen granules. The last are very dense, spherical, and membrane-bound. At top left is part of the lumen of the acinus with microvilli in transverse and longitudinal section. The lumen contains discharged, electron-dense secretory material. The zymogen granule or droplet at arrows is in the process of fusing with the apical plasmalemma and discharging its contents (exocytosis). × 18,000.

between the nucleic acid code and the amino acid sequences of proteins.

## Transcription of DNA

In the process of transcription, one strand of the DNA duplex serves as a template for the synthesis of a complementary single-stranded RNA polymer. The reactions are catalyzed by the enzyme RNA polymerase, and the resulting transcript molecule is mRNA, which moves from its site of synthesis along the DNA template out to the cytoplasm. This process is crucial for the transfer of information from DNA to protein. In principle, any region of the DNA could be copied into two different mRNA molecules—one from each of the two DNA strands. In fact, only one is copied. The "factor" that indicates the strand to be copied is a promotor DNA sequence that is present in a particular *cistron*, or structural gene, of the master strand. This promotor (the start signal) is oriented in such a way that it sets the RNA polymerase off in a particular direction across a given genetic region, and this automatically determines which of the two strands will be read. Upon this exposed template, a strand of RNA is constructed. The RNA strand is similar to that of DNA, and the process of formation of the RNA strand is similar to that of DNA replication, but there are three differences:

1. The RNA strand is single and not double as in DNA.

2. It contains ribose and not deoxyribose groups.

3. The base uracil replaces thymine, the other three bases being adenine, cytosine, and guanine.

As in DNA, base-pairing occurs between cytosine and guanine, but in RNA, uracil instead of thymine pairs with adenine. The DNA triplets are thus transcribed into complementary triplets, or *codons*, of RNA by the RNA polymerase.

After binding to the DNA promotor, the RNA polymerase unwinds about one turn of the DNA helix to expose a short stretch of single-stranded DNA that will act as a template for complementary base-pairing with incoming ribonucleotides. The enzyme continues to add nucleotides until it encounters a second special sequence of DNA, the termination signal, at which point the polymerase releases both the DNA template and the newly made mRNA chain.

## Protein Synthesis

Once in the cytoplasm, mRNA attaches to one or more ribosomes (Fig. 1–65). The ribosomes then assemble amino acids into proteins, using the information (codons) carried in the attached mRNA as a guide. The ribosomes are nonspecific in the sense that they simply form any protein (or polypeptide chain) on "orders" from mRNA. In this synthesis, called *translation*, a ribosome starts at one end of an mRNA molecule and then moves along the sequence of nucleotides in the mRNA until it reaches the other end. As it moves along the mRNA, it assembles amino acids into a gradually lengthening polypeptide according to the directions coded into the mRNA. At any instant, several ribosomes may be at different places on a single mRNA strand (150-Å filament), engaged in reading the message and assembling protein chains. In this way, each mRNA molecule may serve as a template for many identical protein molecules.

Protein synthesis involves a "carrier" in the form of tRNA; tRNA molecules function as a "dictionary" in the translation mechanism. Each kind of tRNA corresponds to one of the 20 amino acids used in protein synthesis. The tRNAs are also capable of recognizing and binding to the coding triplets in mRNA specifying their attached amino acid.

Binding of tRNAs and their attached amino acids to mRNA coding triplets takes place on ribosomes. As a ribosome encounters an mRNA coding triplet specifying a given amino acid, the tRNA carrying the amino acid binds to the ribosome. This binding places the amino acid in its correct location in the protein chain growing from the ribosome. The ribosome then moves to the next mRNA coding triplet, causing the next tRNA–amino acid complex specified by the code to bind. As each successive amino acid arrives at the ribosome, it is split from its tRNA carrier and linked into the gradually lengthening protein chain. The process repeats until the ribosome reaches the end of the message and completes assembly of the protein.

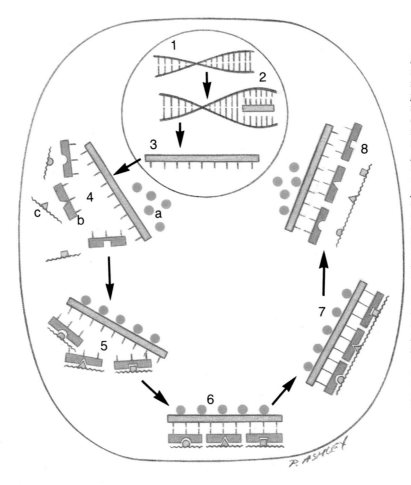

**Figure 1–65.** *Diagrammatic representation of the steps involved in the synthesis of a three–amino acid protein. 1, DNA molecule. 2, Synthesis of a messenger RNA molecule from the DNA. 3, Release of the messenger RNA molecule and its transfer from nucleus to cytoplasm. 4, Messenger RNA molecule in the cytoplasm and its association with (a) ribosomes, (b) three transfer RNA molecules, and (c) three amino acids. 5, Linkage of amino acids to transfer RNA molecules and association of ribosomes with the messenger RNA molecule. 6, Transfer of amino acids by transfer RNA to messenger RNA and correct alignment. 7, Linkage of amino acids to form a polypeptide. 8, Release of the polypeptide and dissociation of ribosomes from messenger RNA. The newly synthesized protein (polypeptide) then is transported in the channels of the endoplasmic reticulum to the Golgi region where it is membrane-wrapped and either stored or transported to the cell surface for release.*

Synthesis of the mRNA, rRNA, and tRNA copies of DNA, called transcription, occurs within the cell nucleus. Following transcription, the RNA copies pass through the nuclear envelope and enter the cytoplasm.

In summary, the ribosomes are nonspecific as to which type of protein they synthesize. They are, as it were, for hire. Specificity is determined by mRNA, carrying the message directly from DNA of the nucleus; tRNA acts simply as a carrier of amino acids.

If destined for secretion, the newly formed protein passes into canals of the endoplasmic reticulum and thence by transfer vesicles to the Golgi apparatus. Here it is concentrated, a carbohydrate moiety may be added, and it then leaves the Golgi apparatus as a condensing vacuole, which progresses to a secretory granule.

Such granules are stored in the apical cytoplasm until released by the cell.

## THE FOUR PRIMARY TISSUES

The body is composed of only three basic elements (i.e., cells, intercellular substances, and body fluids). During development, the embryo consists of three cellular layers (ectoderm, mesoderm, and endoderm). In all three germ layers, cells continue to divide and gradually specialize functionally and structurally. Specialized cells frequently carry out their functions as multicellular aggregates of like cell types called tissues. A primary, or basic, tissue may be defined as a collection of cells and associated intercellular ma-

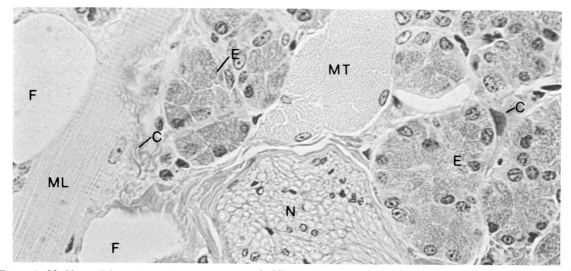

**Figure 1–66.** Here, all four primary tissues are seen, each differing in appearance and function from the others. Epithelium (E) is represented by secretory units (acini)—groups of cells containing numerous pink-stained secretory droplets or granules. Connective tissue is present as strands of collagen (C) between acini and around groups of acini and as fat cells (F). Muscular tissue occurs as striated muscle fibers cut in longitudinal (ML) and transverse (MT) sections, showing cytoplasmic fibrils (myofibrils). These cells have peripherally located nuclei. Nervous tissue is seen as a transverse section of a peripheral nerve (N), a bundle of nerve fibers (nerve cell processes), and supporting tissue. All organs are formed from these four basic tissues, often all four being present in the same organ, as here. Tongue, primary tissues. Plastic section. H and E. High power.

terials specialized for a particular function or functions. In turn, organs are formed from these tissues, and, usually, all four basic tissue types are present in a single organ. The construction of the organism, consisting of only four basic tissues, makes the study of histology much easier, since a thorough knowledge of the basic tissues simplifies the study of the structure of the organs.

The four primary tissues are *epithelium, connective tissue, muscle,* and *nervous tissue* (Fig. 1–66). The subdivisions and varieties of these primary tissues can be classified according to structure and function (Table 1–1).

**Epithelium.** The cells lie very close together without intervening intercellular substances. They are arranged as sheets covering or lining surfaces or as masses of cells in glands.

**Connective Tissue.** The cells usually are widely separated by an abundant intercellular matrix. This group includes certain specialized tissues such as blood and blood-forming tissues, bone, and cartilage.

**Muscle.** There are three types; cells are elongated, contain cytoplasmic filaments, are relatively closely associated, and are separated by fine, vascular connective tissue.

**Nervous Tissue.** This consists of cells, some of which are very large, and their elongated processes, which are usually grouped as relatively isolated masses or bundles.

## FUNCTIONAL SUMMARY

All living organisms are made up of one or more living units or cells. The living material of a cell is called protoplasm. Protoplasm has a variety of physiological properties that indicate the functions of the cell. Every living cell must have and maintain an intact plasma membrane if it is to survive. This plasma membrane serves as the interface between the machinery in the interior of the cell and the watery fluid that bathes all cells. Plasma membranes are selectively permeable boundaries organized as a mosiac of protein in and on a relatively fluid bimolecular layer of amphipathic phospholipids. Substances move through the membranes of a cell selectively by free diffusion, transport, or cytosis. Membranes and other cellular structures are in a constant state of turnover, during which new components replace existing ones. One economical means of replacing membranes is by transforming from one membrane type to another. The transformation of rough endoplasmic reticulum to Golgi membranes, and Golgi membranes to plasma membrane is one such pathway. The folded membranes of the endoplasmic reticulum provide a system for the distribution of proteins made at ribosomes attached to one surface of the rough endoplasmic reticulum. Endoplasmic reticulum without attached ribosomes, smooth endoplasmic reticulum, is the site of lipid and steroid synthesis, drug detoxification, glycogen catabolism, and calcium regulation in muscle. Proteins are delivered by transfer vesicles to the Golgi apparatus, which acts as a packaging and processing station for various cell secretions and for other kinds of proteins that remain within the cell. Other important roles of the Golgi apparatus are production of hydrolytic enzymes to lysosomes and cell coat and adding carbohydrate groups to glycoprotein molecules.

As indicated, lysosomes are also made at the Golgi apparatus. Lysosomes contain hydrolytic

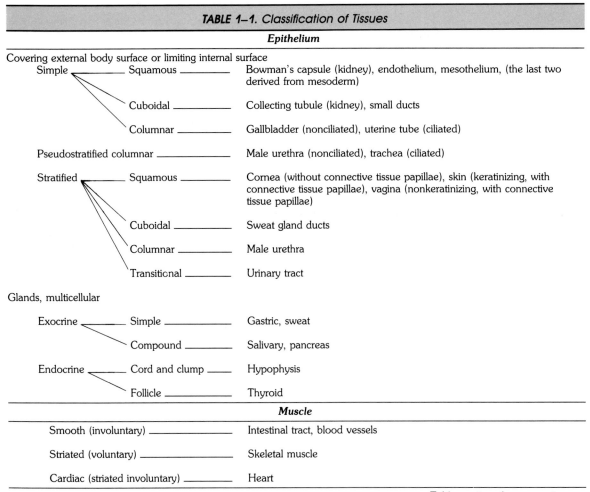

**TABLE 1–1. *Classification of Tissues***

| Epithelium | | |
|---|---|---|
| Covering external body surface or limiting internal surface | | |
| Simple | Squamous | Bowman's capsule (kidney), endothelium, mesothelium, (the last two derived from mesoderm) |
| | Cuboidal | Collecting tubule (kidney), small ducts |
| | Columnar | Gallbladder (nonciliated), uterine tube (ciliated) |
| Pseudostratified columnar | | Male urethra (nonciliated), trachea (ciliated) |
| Stratified | Squamous | Cornea (without connective tissue papillae), skin (keratinizing, with connective tissue papillae), vagina (nonkeratinizing, with connective tissue papillae) |
| | Cuboidal | Sweat gland ducts |
| | Columnar | Male urethra |
| | Transitional | Urinary tract |
| Glands, multicellular | | |
| Exocrine | Simple | Gastric, sweat |
| | Compound | Salivary, pancreas |
| Endocrine | Cord and clump | Hypophysis |
| | Follicle | Thyroid |
| Muscle | | |
| Smooth (involuntary) | | Intestinal tract, blood vessels |
| Striated (voluntary) | | Skeletal muscle |
| Cardiac (striated involuntary) | | Heart |

*Table continued on opposite page*

**TABLE 1–1. Classification of Tissues (Continued)**

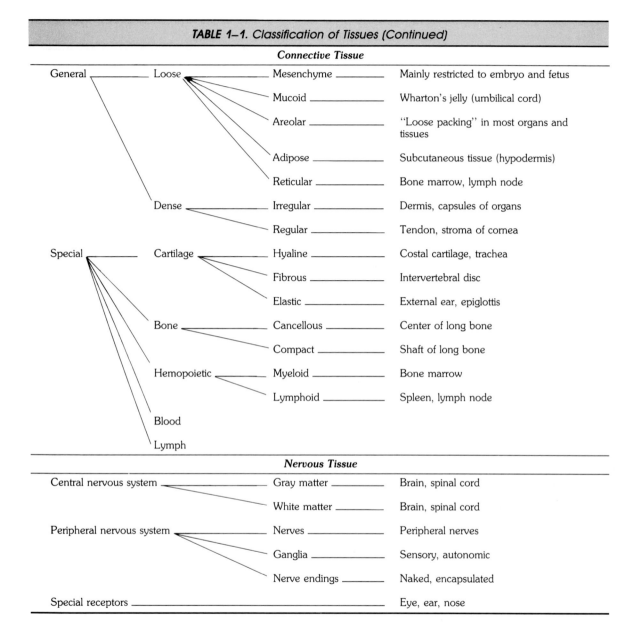

*Connective Tissue*

| General | Loose | Mesenchyme | Mainly restricted to embryo and fetus |
| | | Mucoid | Wharton's jelly (umbilical cord) |
| | | Areolar | "Loose packing" in most organs and tissues |
| | | Adipose | Subcutaneous tissue (hypodermis) |
| | | Reticular | Bone marrow, lymph node |
| | Dense | Irregular | Dermis, capsules of organs |
| | | Regular | Tendon, stroma of cornea |
| Special | Cartilage | Hyaline | Costal cartilage, trachea |
| | | Fibrous | Intervertebral disc |
| | | Elastic | External ear, epiglottis |
| | Bone | Cancellous | Center of long bone |
| | | Compact | Shaft of long bone |
| | Hemopoietic | Myeloid | Bone marrow |
| | | Lymphoid | Spleen, lymph node |
| | Blood | | |
| | Lymph | | |

*Nervous Tissue*

| Central nervous system | Gray matter | Brain, spinal cord |
| | White matter | Brain, spinal cord |
| Peripheral nervous system | Nerves | Peripheral nerves |
| | Ganglia | Sensory, autonomic |
| | Nerve endings | Naked, encapsulated |
| Special receptors | | Eye, ear, nose |

enzymes that can dismantle virtually every organic substance of biological importance. Lysosomes serve on the front line of defense against disease, since they fuse with incoming endocytic vesicles containing particles and digest them. Digested residues are expelled from the cell by exocytosis, but vesicles containing undigested residues (residual bodies) may remain within the cell. Consumption of parts of the cell itself may take place within autophagic vacuoles.

The major system for energy transformations in cells is aerobic respiration, which takes place in mitochondria. Mitochondria have two enveloping membranes, of which the innermost is folded into tubular invaginations called cristae. Mitochondria produce most of the cell's ATP and can renew themselves through division. Their matrix contains DNA, RNA, ribosomes, and calcium granules.

Peroxisomes are organelles bounded by a single membrane and are believed to arise as vesicles pinched off parts of the smooth endoplasmic reticulum. These enzymes play a role in disposing of hydrogen peroxide and in the conversion of noncarbohydrate precursors to glucose.

Microtubules and microfilaments are fibrous protein structures that contribute to all directed motion of living cells. Microtubules participate in intercellular transport, chromosome movement during mitosis, and the beating of cilia and flagella. Centrioles contain nine sets of microtubule triplets and are found in many kinds of cells at the base of cilia or flagella and at the poles of dividing cell nuclei. Microfilaments contribute to the "skeleton" of the cell and correspond to thin filaments of skeletal muscle. Both protoplasmic movements of saltatory motion and streaming appear to depend on microfilament systems. Different kinds of intermediate filaments are also present and function in a stress-bearing or supportive capacity.

The nucleus is the control center of the cell. Contained within the nuclear envelope (a two-membrane system) enclosure are chromosomes, one or more nucleoli, and granular nucleoplasm. Ribosomes stud the cytoplasm-facing surface of the outer nuclear membrane.

The nucleolus is a condensation of the nucleolus-organizing chromosome and is located at the nucleolus-organizing region of this chromosome. Ribosome subunit precursor particles assemble within the nucleolus.

There is one chromatin fiber in each unreplicated chromosome. Each chromatin fiber is a deoxyribonucleoprotein strand with genes housed within the duplex DNA molecules. Histone as well as numerous nonhistone proteins are associated with the DNA molecule. The most widely accepted model of a chromatin fiber is that of a flexibly jointed chain in which nucleosome units are spaced like beads on a string. The chromatin exists in two forms: euchromatin, or extended "active" chromatin, and heterochromatin, or condensed "inactive" chromatin.

The cell cycle, which characterizes populations capable of nuclear division, is subdivided into G1, S, and G2 phases of the interphase stage between mitoses, and the M phase of mitosis itself. The G1 phase, before DNA replication in S, is the most variable. The G2 phase, after DNA replication, is less variable in duration than is G1. Besides being the time for DNA replication, interphase is the time of most active metabolism in general.

Mitosis is the mechanism for distributing replicated chromosomes into daughter nuclei. Mitosis is arbitrarily divided into the stages of prophase (when chromosomes condense and begin to move toward the equatorial plane of the spindle), metaphase (when chromosomes are aligned at the spindle equator), anaphase (when sister chromosomes move toward opposite poles), and telophase (when nuclear reorganization takes place). Mitosis ensures that a full set of genes is distributed into the daughter nuclei.

Meiosis consists of two sequential nuclear divisions that take place in the germ cells. The reduction division process leads to nuclei with half the number (haploid) of chromosomes and half the DNA content of the parental nucleus. The chromosome number is reduced by one half in the first division, and the DNA content is reduced to one half by the end of the second division. The regularity of synapsis during the zygotene sequence of the prophase stage of meiosis I and subsequent stabilizing of the paired homologous chromosomes by synaptonemal complex formation in pachytene provide the basis for understanding cross-over and recombinations in species.

The genetic information for making proteins is coded in the four DNA nucleotides. Each three-nucleotide codeword stands for a particular amino acid. These protein-encoding regions are duplicated in RNA copies called mRNA, which carry the directions for making proteins to the cytoplasm. DNA also directs the synthesis of two accessory RNAs. One is ribosomal (rRNA), which assembles amino acids into proteins that pass into canals of the rough endoplasm. The second is transfer RNA (tRNA), which provides the necessary link between the nucleic acid code and the amino acid sequence of proteins. The information contained in the protein-encoding regions of DNA both initiates and regulates the activities of the cell and thereby controls the growth, differentiation, maturation, and metabolic activities of each cell.

# Epithelium

## INTRODUCTION

Epithelial tissues are formed by closely apposed cells with little or no intercellular material and occur as *membranes* and as *glands* (Figs. 2–1 and 2–2).

Membranes are sheets of cells that cover an external surface or line an internal surface. Glands, composed of cells mainly specialized for secretion, develop from epithelial surfaces by downgrowths or ingrowths into underlying connective tissue. In most, the connection to the surface remains as the duct of the gland, and these are the *exocrine* glands. In some, the surface connection is lost, and the gland secretes into the vascular system, the secretion being a hormone. These are the *endocrine* glands. In both types of gland and in membranes, the epithelial cells are supported by connective tissue containing vessels and nerves but are separated from subjacent connective tissue by a *basal lamina* (see page 135). There are no blood vessels within epithelium itself, and metabolism thus depends upon diffusion of oxygen and metabolites from blood vessels in the supporting connective tissue.

Functionally, epithelial membranes forming the coverings or linings of surfaces are involved in protection, absorption, secretion, excretion, digestion, and sensation. All materials that enter or leave the body do so through an epithelial membrane, the membrane serving as a selective barrier between the exterior (or interior cavity) and the connective tissue. The main function of glands is secretion.

2

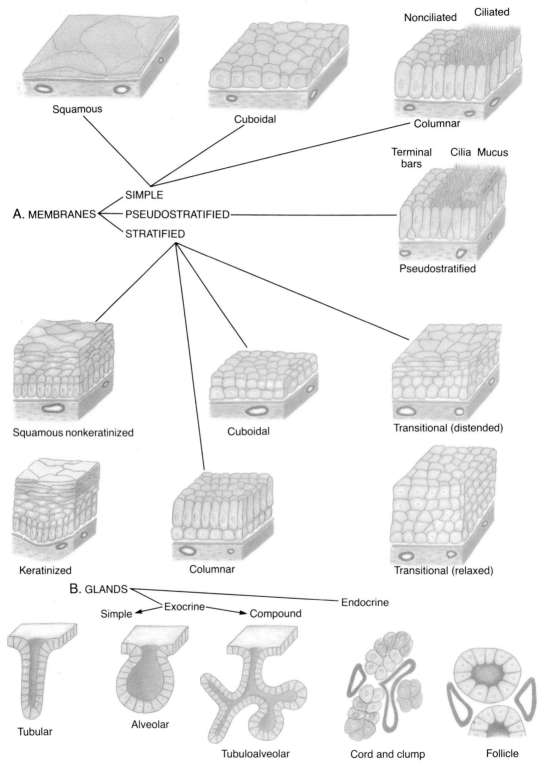

*Figure 2–1.* Diagram illustrating the classification of epithelia with membranes (A) (above) and glands (B) (below).

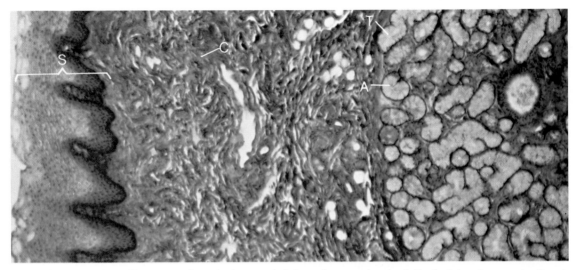

**Figure 2–2.** *Lip, epithelia. This section shows both an epithelial membrane and a gland. To the left is the inner (oral) surface lined by a thick stratified squamous epithelium (S) supported by connective tissue (C), the two forming a mucous membrane. To the right is part of a labial (salivary) gland. This is a compound tubuloalveolar mucous gland with both alveolar (acinar) (A) and tubular (T) secretory units, and among them lies a duct (D). Iron hematoxylin, aniline blue. Medium power.*

## MEMBRANES

**Classification.** Most epithelial cells, being closely packed, are polygonal in outline, but some may be highly irregular. Basically, classification depends upon two factors—the shape of the cells and their arrangement into layers. Only three cell shapes are used in the classification:

1. *Squamous*—cell height is much less than width.

2. *Cuboidal*—height and width are approximately equal.

3. *Columnar*—height exceeds width.

In all, nuclear shape conforms to that of the cell and thus is flattened in squamous cells, spheroidal in cuboidal cells, and ovoid in columnar cells.

In membranes, cells are arranged in one or more layers. *Simple* epithelia show cells in a single layer, whereas *stratified* epithelia show cells in two or more layers, only the cells of the deepest or basal layer contacting the basal lamina. *Pseudostratified* epithelia are those in which all cells contact the basal lamina but not all reach the surface. Thus, it really is a simple epithelium, with several cell types present in a single layer but with nuclei at different levels, giving the false appearance of several layers. By combining the two factors of shape and layering, thus we classify

simple squamous, simple cuboidal, and simple columnar epithelia. In stratified epithelia, only the surface layer of cells is utilized to determine the classification of stratified squamous, stratified cuboidal, and stratified columnar. A special type of stratified epithelium is called transitional. This lines the urinary tract and can accommodate to distention, the surface layer varying from squamous to cuboidal with the degree of distention. Pseudostratified columnar epithelium may be ciliated or nonciliated. Additionally, specific names are applied to certain epithelia. Endothelium lines the vascular system, and mesothelium lines the walls and covers the contents of the pleural, pericardial, and peritoneal cavities. Both are varieties of simple squamous epithelia. Mesothelium, with its basal lamina and supporting connective tissue is called a *serous membrane*, or serosa. Most epithelial membranes line wet cavities and, in these locations, are one component of *mucous membranes*. A mucous membrane, or mucosa, is the moist inner lining of viscera formed by an epithelial membrane, its basal lamina, and a layer of areolar connective tissue (the lamina propria) with, in some locations, a layer of smooth muscle (the muscularis mucosae). The epithelium (epidermis) of skin is exceptional in that the surface is dry, and here the stratified squamous epithelium is keratinized, the flat surface cells undergoing a transformation into a tough, resistant, nonliving layer of material called keratin.

It is not feasible to classify epithelia on the basis of embryological origin, for all three germ layers give rise to epithelia—those of skin and oral and anal regions being of ectodermal origin, those lining respiratory and digestive tracts of endoderm, and others such as those of the urinary tract derived from mesoderm.

Most epithelia have a capacity for renewal, cell replacement occurring by mitosis. The rate of renewal varies with the location and type of epithelium but, for example, is very rapid in the epithelium lining the small intestine.

As cells lie in epithelial membranes, for descriptive purposes the surface abutting the lumen is termed the *apical surface*, that adjacent to basal lamina the *basal surface*, and the surfaces between adjacent cells as *lateral surfaces*. Most cells show polarity in respect of organelles; for example, mitochondria and cytoplasmic basophilia lie basally or infranuclearly, the Golgi apparatus is supranuclear, and any secretory material is apical. Cell adhesion and specializations of the cell surface are discussed later.

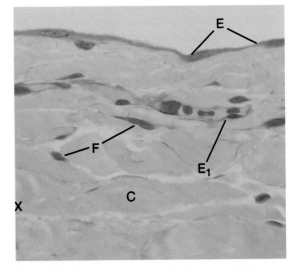

*Figure 2–3. Simple squamous epithelium—mesothelium and endothelium. Above lies the mesothelium (E) of the epicardium that covers the outer surface of the heart, a type of simple squamous epithelium but derived from mesoderm. Also of the simple squamous type is endothelium ($E_1$) lining a blood capillary with erythrocytes (red) in its lumen. In the supporting connective tissue are collagen fibers (C) and nuclei of fibroblasts (F). Methylene blue, basic fuchsin. Oil immersion.*

## Simple Epithelia

*Simple squamous epithelium* is composed of thin, flat cells of irregular outline fitted closely together and has the appearance, from the surface, of a tiled floor (Figs. 2–3 through 2–5). In section, the cells show attenuated cytoplasm with local protuberances where the cytoplasm contains nuclei. Examples are found in the parietal layer of Bowman's capsule and the loop of Henle in the kidney (Fig. 2–6), lining pulmonary alveoli, and in the inner and middle ear. The description also covers endothelium and mesothelium, these two being of mesodermal origin.

*Simple cuboidal epithelium* shows polygonal cells in a surface view; in vertical section, it shows box-like or cube-like cells with central spherical nuclei. This type is found in the ducts of many glands and covering the surface of the ovary.

*Simple columnar epithelium* appears similar to the simple cuboidal type in surface view but in

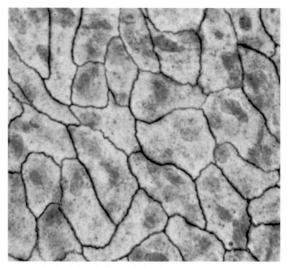

*Figure 2–4. Mesothelium. This flat preparation of the peritoneum shows mesothelial (squamous) cells clearly outlined, flat and irregular in shape, their nuclei stained blue. Silver technique. Oil immersion.*

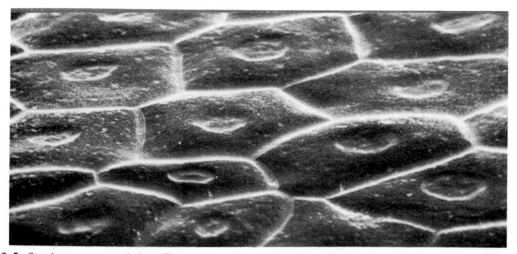

*Figure 2–5.* Simple squamous epithelium. This scanning electron micrograph (SEM) shows a surface view of a simple squamous epithelium, × 800. (See also Figure 2–4.) (Courtesy of Dr. W. J. Krause.)

perpendicular section shows tall cells with ovoid nuclei usually at the same level and located nearer to the basal than to the apical surface (Fig. 2–7). This type is found as the absorptive-secretive lining of the digestive tract and in larger ducts and, while nonciliated, may show an apical brush or striated border of numerous microvilli, and often the membrane also contains mucus-secreting "goblet cells." (These will be discussed later.) Simple ciliated columnar epithelium is similar to the nonciliated type, but the free surface of the cells is covered with cilia: It is found lining the uterine tubes, ductuli efferentes of the testis, and small bronchi.

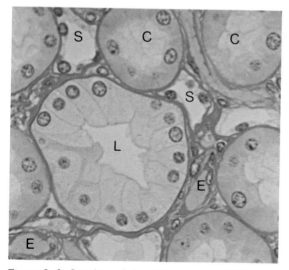

*Figure 2–6.* Simple epithelia, kidney. Kidney tubules, here cut in transverse section, are surrounded by basal laminae (dark pink) and show the three main types of simple epithelia—squamous (S), cuboidal (C), and columnar (L). Also present are blood capillaries lined by endothelium (E). H and E, PAS. Oil immersion.

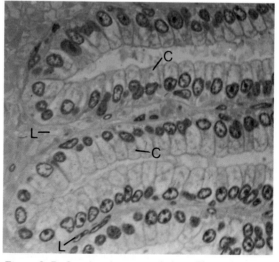

*Figure 2–7.* Simple columnar epithelium. The mucous membrane of the seminal vesicle is formed by the loose connective tissue of the lamina propria (L) and simple columnar epithelium (C), complexly folded. The columnar cells show clear cell interfaces, basal nuclei, and extensive, pale-staining apical cytoplasm. H and E. High power.

### Pseudostratified Epithelia

*Pseudostratified columnar epithelium* contains cells of several types, all of which contact the basal lamina. Not all reach the lumen, and nuclei lie at various levels, giving a false impression of stratification. This type lines larger excretory ducts and parts of the male urethra but more commonly is ciliated, usually in association with goblet cells, and is found lining the larger respiratory passages and in excretory ducts of the male reproductive system (Figs. 2–8 and 2–9).

### Stratified Epithelia

All stratified epithelia can resist more trauma than the simple types but are not membranes through which absorption can occur readily because of their thickness.

*Stratified squamous epithelium* is a thick membrane, only the more superficial layers being flat, with the deeper cells varying from cuboidal to columnar. The basal layer often shows considerable irregularity. While the epithelium of the cornea (of the eye) lies upon connective tissue with a smooth, regular surface, in other locations the underlying connective tissue is raised into ridges

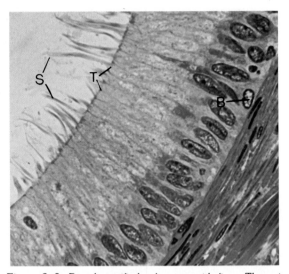

**Figure 2–9.** *Pseudostratified columnar epithelium. The epithelium of the ductus epididymidis is formed mainly by tall columnar cells, with apical stereocilia (S) with some basal cells (B), and nuclei lie at different levels. Note the dark-pink–staining terminal bars (T) on interfaces near the lumen. H and E. High power.*

and folds that appear as papillae or finger-like processes in perpendicular section, for example, in the vagina, esophagus, and skin (Fig. 2–10). The epithelial surface is moist in most locations, and the epithelium is nonkeratinized: The skin, however, is dry, and here the epithelium is keratinized (Fig. 2–11). This process is discussed later (see Chapter 10), but it is important to appreciate that keratinized epithelium is resistant to friction, is relatively impervious to bacterial invasion, and is waterproof.

*Stratified cuboidal epithelium* is limited to the ducts of sweat glands and consists of two layers of cuboidal cells. In that it lines a tube, the cells of the superficial layer are smaller than those of the basal layer when seen in cross section.

*Stratified columnar epithelium* is relatively rare also and is found in parts of the male urethra, some larger excretory ducts (Fig. 2–12), and the conjunctiva of the eye. Usually, the basal layer or layers are formed of low, irregularly polyhedral cells, and only the cells of the superficial layer are columnar.

*Transitional epithelium* is so termed because originally it was believed to represent a transition between the stratified squamous and stratified columnar types. It lines the urinary tract from the

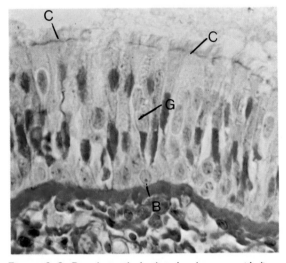

**Figure 2–8.** *Pseudostratified ciliated columnar epithelium. This epithelium lines the trachea and shows several cell types—columnar ciliated cells (C), goblet cells (G) (unicellular glands), and small basal cells (B). Nuclei lie at different levels, giving a false appearance of a stratified epithelium. Mallory. Oil immersion.*

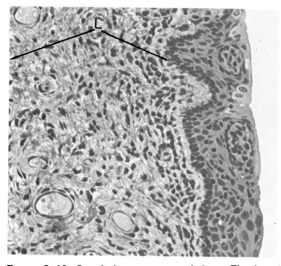

*Figure 2–10. Stratified squamous epithelium. The lamina propria (L) of the vaginal mucosa has an irregular interface with the nonkeratinizing epithelium. In the epithelium, the basal layer is of cuboidal cells. Then there are several layers of polygonal cells that become progressively more squamous, and the surface cells are squamous. H and E. Medium power.*

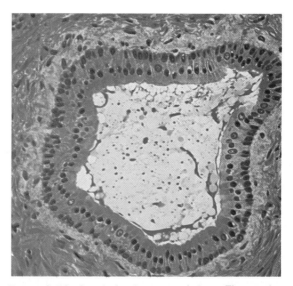

*Figure 2–12. Stratified columnar epithelium. This two-layered epithelium shows a basal layer of cuboidal cells and an apical layer of columnar cells. It lines a lobar duct of the sublingual salivary gland. H and E. High power.*

renal pelvis to the urethra, where it is exposed to variations in internal pressure and capacity and thus its appearance varies with the degree of distention (Fig. 2–13). The basal layer is cuboidal

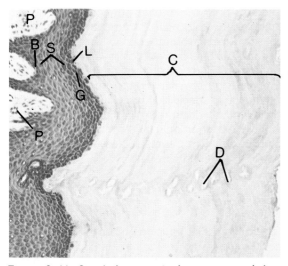

*Figure 2–11. Stratified squamous keratinizing epithelium. The interface between connective tissue (dermis) of the skin and the dry epithelium (epidermis) is irregular, with pegs and ridges (P) of dermis protruding into epidermis. Several layers, or strata, of the epidermis are seen—stratum basale (B), stratum spinosum (S), stratum granulosum (G), stratum lucidum (L), and a thick stratum corneum (C). Cells die in the stratum lucidum and become keratinized, dead, scale-like cells in the stratum corneum, later to be shed. The duct of a sweat gland (D) also is seen. H and E. Medium power.*

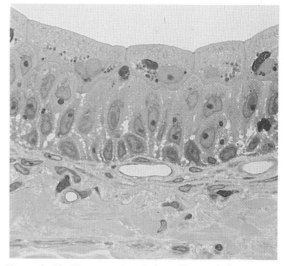

*Figure 2–13. Transitional epithelium. This epithelium is composed of several layers. It lines the urinary tract and is subject to variations in internal pressure and capacity. Here, in the urinary bladder, the surface cells vary from cuboidal in the relaxed organ (as seen here) to squamous in the distended organ. Methylene blue, basic fuchsin. High power.*

or columnar, intermediate layers are cuboidal and polyhedral, and the superficial layers vary from cuboidal (relaxed) to squamous (distended). Cells of the superficial layer are often binucleate.

## CELL ADHESION IN EPITHELIAL MEMBRANES

Within epithelia, cells not only are closely opposed but also usually show a firm cell-to-cell adhesion capable of resisting distracting forces. Spaces between cells are narrow, of the order of 15 to 20 nm, the spaces occupied by glycocalyx, which provides some adhesion. This material also contains cations, particularly calcium, that likewise are important in cell adhesion. In many cases, adjacent plasma membranes are not parallel but show reciprocal tongues and grooves as "zipper" or "jigsaw" interlockings. Additionally, by light microscopy, *terminal bars* are seen to be present in many epithelia (Figs. 2–14 and 2–15). These appear in perpendicular section as dark, dot-like

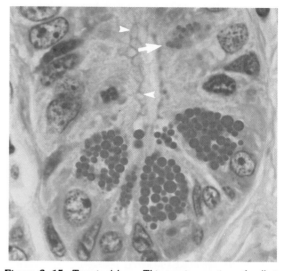

**Figure 2–15.** *Terminal bars. This grazing section of cells in the base of a jejunal gland demonstrates that the terminal bars extend fully around the apices of the columnar cells (arrowheads). The cells at the bottom of the gland with discrete, pink-staining secretory droplets are Paneth cells—cells that are to be classified as serous, producing lysozyme. The arrow indicates an immature Paneth cell. H and E. Oil immersion.*

structures near the luminal surface; in horizontal section of the cells near the luminal surface, they are seen to surround entirely the cell apices, appearing as bars between cells—hence the term. By electron microscopy, terminal bars are seen to be formed by specializations of the cell surface, or *junctional specializations* (Fig. 2–16). These specializations occur also in tissues other than epithelia and not only are concerned with cell adhesion but also permit cells to interrelate functionally in several ways.

### Cell Junctions

Specialized cell junctions are of several types, and two factors are utilized in classifying them.

1. The shape and extent of the contact area. If this is spot-like and of limited extent, it is termed a *macula*; if it passes around the entire cell like a belt or crown, a *zonula*; or if it appears as a strip or sheet-like area, a *fascia*.

2. The relative closeness and the nature of the cell contact (Figs. 2–17 and 2–18). In *occluding* or *tight* junctions, the outer surfaces of the two plasma membranes appear to be in contact or

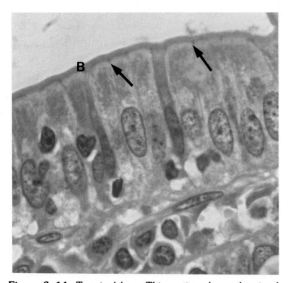

**Figure 2–14.** *Terminal bars. This section shows the simple columnar epithelium of the jejunum as it covers a villus. The columnar cells have a brush border (B) and at lateral cell interfaces near the lumen show dark pink dots (arrows)—the terminal bars. On electron microscopy, they are formed by zonula occludens, zonula adherens, and scattered maculae adherentes. H and E. High power. (See also Figure 2–9.)*

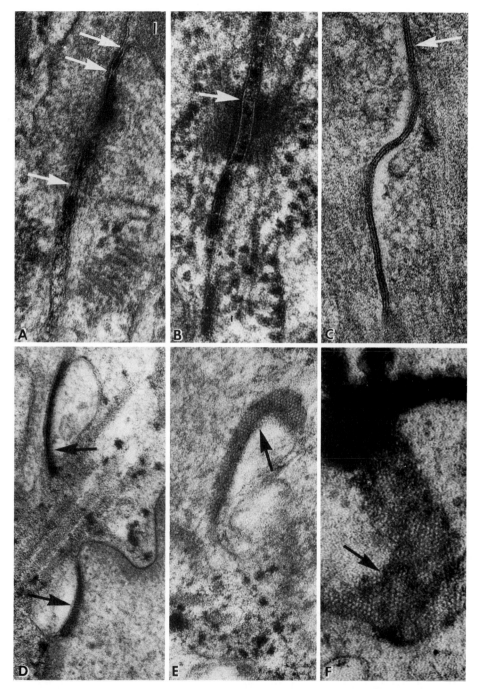

**Figure 2–16.** Junctional specializations, as seen with the lanthanum tracer technique. A, The apical interface between two pancreatic acinar ·cells shows the lumen (l) and a zonula occludens with three sealing strands (arrows). × 110,000. B, The electron-lucid transverse lines (arrow) represent transmembrane linkers in this macula adherens. Note associated tonofilaments in adjacent cytoplasm. × 120,000. C through F, Nexuses (gap junctions) of smooth muscle in different planes of section. In transverse section note pentalaminar structure with interruptions in the central dense lamina (C, arrow), transverse dense lines representing spaces between connexons in oblique section (D, arrow), and pale connexons outlined by dense tracer (E, F, arrows) in tangential (grazing) sections. C, D, E, × 100,000; F, × 170,000.

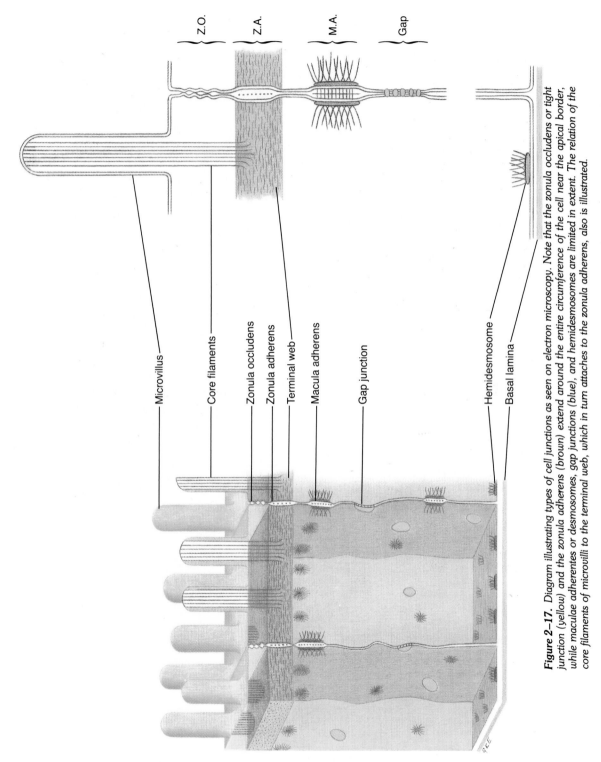

**Figure 2–17.** Diagram illustrating types of cell junctions as seen on electron microscopy. Note that the zonula occludens or tight junction (yellow) and the zonula adherens (brown) extend around the entire circumference of the cell near the apical border, while maculae adherentes or desmosomes, gap junctions (blue), and hemidesmosomes are limited in extent. The relation of the core filaments of microvilli to the terminal web, which in turn attaches to the zonula adherens, also is illustrated.

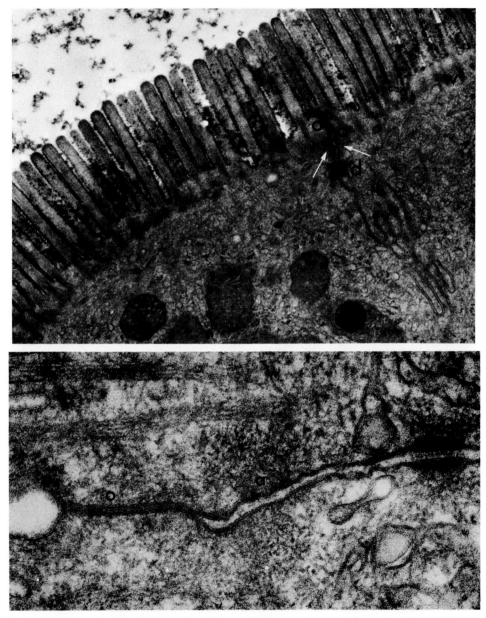

**Figure 2–18.** *Junctional complex.* Top: *In intestinal epithelial cells, the components of the terminal bar on light microscopy are seen on electron microscopy to consist of zonula occludens (o) and zonula adherens (a) with a macula adherens (d). Note apical microvilli of the brush border with core filaments (f) passing into the terminal web (w) that passes to zonula adherens (arrows).* Bottom: *A higher magnification of a junctional complex. Top:* × *22,000. Bottom:* × *110,000.*

fused, with obliteration of the intercellular space. In *adhering* (adherens) junctions, the intercellular space is 20 to 25 nm wide, with dense material in it and associated with the cytoplasmic surfaces of the opposed membranes. In the *gap* junction, there is an intercellular gap of about 2 nm, and this type is concerned with intercellular communication rather than adhesion.

## TIGHT OR OCCLUDING JUNCTIONS

The *zonula occludens* is in the form of a belt completely encircling a cell near its apical border and, on electron microscopy, may show a pentalaminar structure, that is, three dense lines separated by two electron-lucent lines with apparent fusion of the outer leaflets of the two plasmalemmae of the adjoining cells. Freeze-fracture studies show that fusion occurs as a network of linear ridges and complementary grooves, each ridge formed by a double row of 3- to 4-nm particles

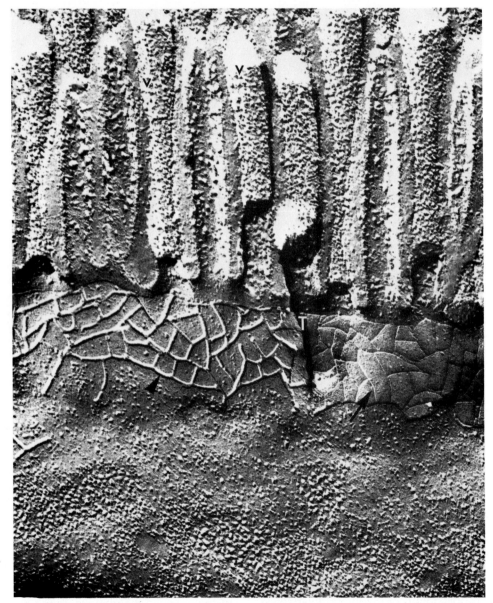

**Figure 2–19.** *Zonula occludens (tight junction). This freeze-fracture electron micrograph is of mouse intestinal epithelial cells showing apical microvilli (v) and below them a zonula occludens. The zonula occludens is here fractured to show to the left (on the P face) a network of ridges (arrowhead) and on the right (on the E face) a network of furrows (arrow) with transition (T) of the fracture face between the two appearances. × 10,800. (Courtesy of Dr. S. Bullivant.)*

(Fig. 2–19). These particles are integral membrane proteins, one row arising from each plasmalemma, effectively obliterating the intercellular space at the ridges. The ridges, or *sealing strands*, physically bar the passage of molecules and fluid through the intercellular space. The number and complexity of sealing strands vary with the type of epithelium—the more impervious junctions showing more points of fusion, for example, in the epithelium of the urinary bladder. A *fascia occludens* is similar in structure but limited in extent, being strip-like in form. This type is found between endothelial cells lining some blood capillaries.

## ADHERING JUNCTIONS

The *zonula adherens*, or belt desmosome, like the zonula occludens, also completely encircles the cell but lies just below it (i.e., to the basal side) (Fig. 2–18). There is a regular intercellular space of 20 to 25 nm containing some filamentous material, and the cytoplasmic surfaces of inner leaflets of the two plasmalemmae show some electron-dense material associated with filaments. These filaments are 7 nm in diameter and are composed of actin. In cells with a microvillus border, such as those lining the intestine, the filaments pass as a flat, horizontal band from the zonula adherens into the terminal web (to be described later). Zonulae adherentes of epithelia and other tissues (e.g., cardiac muscle) function in mechanical attachment and, perhaps, transmit forces generated in cells.

A *macula adherens*, or spot desmosome, is a small, discoid structure about 410 by 250 nm located at various levels on lateral cell interfaces (see Figs. 2–16 and 2–17). At a macula adherens, the intercellular space is 20 to 30 nm wide, filled with filamentous material, and bisected by a linear density (the central stratum) (Fig. 2–20). Fine filaments, the connecting strands, appear to cross the space as transmembrane linkers. On cytoplasmic surfaces of the two adjacent plasma membranes are dense plaques, to which 10-nm tonofilaments are attached. They arise within cytoplasm, pass into the dense plaque, and loop back into cytoplasm. Maculae adherentes are found in many cell types but are particularly numerous in epithelia subject to mechanical stress and abrasion. In epidermis, for example, during

fixation cells tend to separate but are held at numerous focal attachment points that appear on light microscopy as slender *intercellular bridges* (Fig. 2–21). These bridges, in fact, are the sites of desmosomes that provide firm cell adhesion. *Hemidesmosomes* lie on basal surfaces adjacent to the basal lamina and, as the name suggests, are half desmosomes, showing tonofilament bundles extending into the cytoplasm from attachment plaques (thickening of the inner cytoplasmic leaflet of the plasma membrane). Some show connecting strands between the plasma membrane and the basal lamina. Hemidesmosomes are found in cells where mechanical stress occurs (e.g., the basal surface of stratified squamous epithelia).

## GAP JUNCTIONS

At gap junctions, the intercellular space is only 2 to 3 nm and, in grazing sections, is seen to contain a hexagonal array of 7- to 9-nm particles or connexons, each particle being in the form of a short, hollow cylinder with a central channel (Figs. 2–22 and 2–23). Freeze-etch studies reveal that gap junctions vary from discoid, macula-like structures to belt- or strip-like regions with densely packed particles or reciprocal pits. These particles appear to be formed by six subunits arranged around a central channel 1.5 nm in diameter, the cylindrical units of the two opposing plasmalemmae being in register and their central canals confluent, thus permitting direct cell-to-cell interchange. Not only do gap junctions permit small molecules and ions to pass directly between cells, but also they are regions of low electrical resistance. They are distributed widely in the body, being absent only in blood cells and skeletal muscle. In tissues such as smooth and cardiac muscle (where usually they are called *nexuses*), gap junctions transmit electrical impulses and permit synchronization of activity between cells that are electrically coupled.

*Terminal bars* have been described above as seen by light microscopy (see Figs. 2–14 and 2–15). By electron microscopy, they are seen to be formed by a zonula occludens lying near the luminal surface with, more basally, a zonula adherens, both extending around the entire cell perimeter like a crown, with scattered maculae adherentes lying closer to the cell base. The term

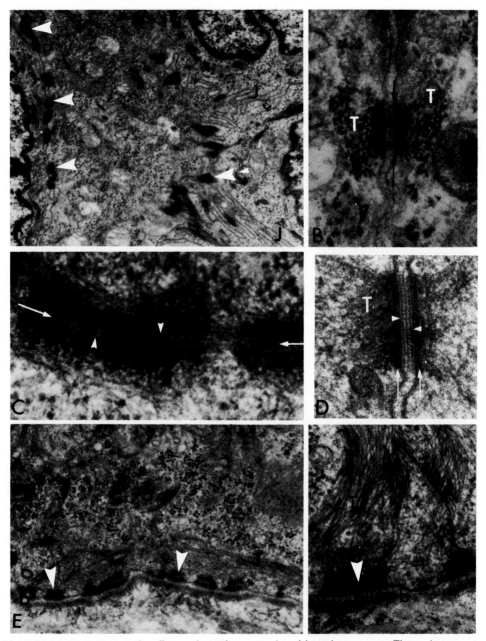

**Figure 2–20.** *Adhering junctions: macula adherens (spot desmosome) and hemidesmosomes. These electron micrographs of the stratum spinosum of the epidermis show the following. A, Desmosomes (arrowheads) and complex cell interfaces or jigsaw interlocking (J), × 5000. B, The central stratum (arrows) of a desmosome and associated tonofilaments in transverse section (T), × 88,000. C, An extensive desmosome with central stratum (arrows) and thin transmembrane linkers (arrowheads) passing between plasma membranes, × 100,000. D, Desmosome showing transmembrane linkers (arrowheads), dense cytoplasmic plaques (arrows), and associated tonofilaments (T), × 100,000. E and F, Hemidesmosomes (arrowheads) at the base of the cells in relation to the basal lamina (b) and associated tonofilaments (T). E, × 20,000; F, × 80,000.*

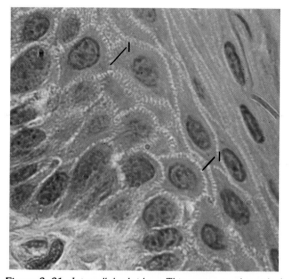

**Figure 2–21.** *Intercellular bridges. This section is of stratified squamous epithelium of the tongue. In the deeper layers of stratum basale and stratum spinosum, the cells are connected by intercellular bridges (I). There is no cytoplasmic continuity between cells, and each bridge is formed by short cytoplasmic processes of adjacent cells that meet at a desmosome, or macula adherens. H and E. Oil immersion.*

"junctional complex" also is used to describe the appearance on electron microscopy.

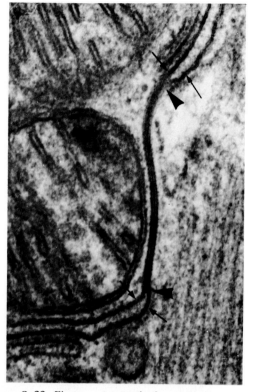

**Figure 2–22.** *Electron micrograph of a gap junction or nexus between two cardiac muscle cells of the rat atrium. Plasmalemmae of adjacent cells (arrows) form an extensive nexus extending between the arrowheads.* × *80,000.*

## SURFACE SPECIALIZATIONS IN EPITHELIA

Many of these specializations have been described briefly in Chapter 1, but they generally are prominent in epithelial cells and include microvilli, stereocilia, cilia, and basal infoldings.

### Microvilli

Microvilli are small, slender, finger-like projections of the apical cell surface formed by tube-like evaginations of the apical plasma membrane, with a core of cytoplasm containing microfilaments of actin. These filaments are anchored to the plasma membrane at the tip and sides of the microvillus and pass down into apical cytoplasm to mesh into a network of other filaments called the "terminal web" (Figs. 2–24 and 2–25).

Microvilli vary in length and number and provide an increase in surface area. Generally, the number and shape correlates with the absorptive capacity of the cell, so that cells with little absorptive function show few, poorly developed microvilli, not visible by light microscopy. However, cells with a principal absorptive function, such as intestinal and kidney tubule epithelia, show closely packed, long, parallel microvilli on their apical surfaces, visible by light microscopy as a *brush*, or *striated*, border. In these cells, the *terminal web* also is well-developed and appears as a horizontal network of microfilaments lying in cytoplasm just below the bases of the microvilli and extending peripherally to the zonula adherens. Actin filaments lie superficially in this network and pass to the zonula; more deeply are 10-nm tonofilaments that pass to spot desmosomes at

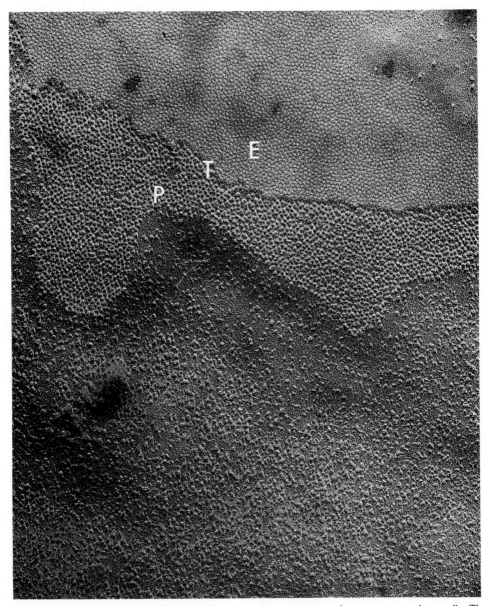

***Figure 2–23.*** *A freeze-fracture electron micrograph of an extensive gap junction between mouse liver cells. The polygonal arrangement of pits of the gap junction is seen above (E, or E face), and below a fracture face transition (T) is an area of closely packed particles of the gap junction (P, or P face). The rest of the P face (bottom) is nonjunctional. Direction of shadowing is from below. × 108,000. (Courtesy of Dr. S. Bullivant.)*

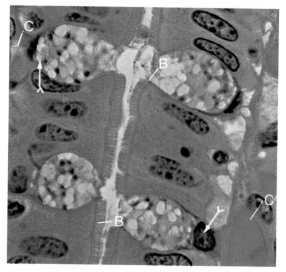

**Figure 2–24.** *Microvilli. In the jejunum, as throughout the small intestine, the mucosa is thrown into finger-like processes, or villi, each with a connective tissue (C) core of lamina propria covered by epithelium. The tall columnar cells of this simple epithelium show a brush border (B) composed of regular, closely packed microvilli. (See also Figures 2–17 and 2–18.) Scattered among the columnar cells are goblet cells (unicellular glands) with a flask shape, basal irregular nuclei (arrows), and apical cytoplasm filled with pale-staining mucigen droplets. H and E. Oil immersion.*

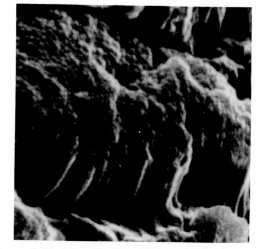

**Figure 2–25.** *Microvilli. This SEM shows closely packed microvilli of the brush border of duodenal epithelium. × 17,000. (Courtesy of Dr. W. J. Krause.)*

regular and contain bundles of core filaments. They are found only in these two locations, being absorptive in function in the epididymis and serving as a receptor in the hair cells.

the cell periphery. Myosin also is present in the terminal web, and an actin-myosin interaction is believed to result in shortening of microvillus core bundles and contraction of microvilli in an oscillating manner to aid the absorptive process. The terminal web provides rigidity to permit this actin-myosin interaction. Where fully developed, the terminal web can be seen by light microscopy utilizing, for example, the tannic acid, phosphomolybdic acid, amino black technique.

### Stereocilia

By light microscopy, stereocilia appear as long, slender, sometimes branching, processes of the apical surface that are nonmotile. In the epididymis of the male reproductive tract, by electron microscopy they are seen to be composed of groups of extremely long, slender, often branching microvilli (Fig. 2–26). In the sensory epithelia ("hair" cells) of the inner ear, they are more

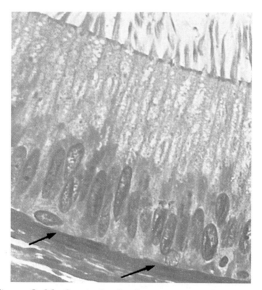

**Figure 2–26.** *Stereocilia. In the pseudostratified columnar epithelium of the ductus epididymidis, the tall columnar cells show apical stereocilia. Also present are some basal cells. H and E. High power. (See also Figure 2–9.)*

### Cilia

The structure of cilia has been described previously (page 61) as fine, hair-like processes of the free apical surface of some epithelial cells. They may be very numerous, for example, in respiratory epithelial cells where they function to transport material (mucus) in one direction along the surface of the membrane, each cilium undergoing a rapid forward beat with a slower recovery stroke (Fig. 2–27). Cilia also are found in maculae and cristae of the inner ear and in rods of the retina where they are receptors. In other cell types, they occur singly and function possibly as chemoreceptors. The single flagellum of spermatozoa is similar in structure to a cilium and also motile.

### Basal Infoldings

Some epithelial cells show numerous infoldings of the basal plasma membrane, thus forming "pockets" of basal cytoplasm. These infoldings

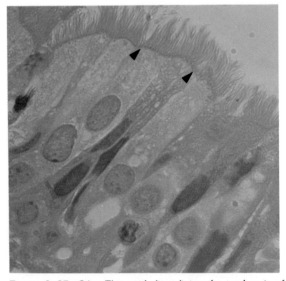

**Figure 2–27.** *Cilia. This epithelium lining the trachea is of the pseudostratified ciliated columnar type. Most of the cells are columnar with apical cilia—long, motile processes with basal bodies (dark pink; arrowheads) in apical cytoplasm. H and E. Oil immersion. (See also Figure 2–8.)*

are a method of increasing surface area at the base of a cell, just as microvilli increase surface area at the apex; indeed, often both specializations are present in, for example, the convoluted tubules of the kidney (Fig. 2–28). Such epithelia show rapid absorption and/or secretion of fluid. Similar infoldings of lateral plasmalemmae also occur in some epithelia, again in cells involved in fluid transport.

## GLAND EPITHELIUM

**Classification.** The cells of many epithelial membranes secrete material in addition to their other functions such as protection and absorption, but the function of secretion often is of secondary importance. Additionally, the surface area of the epithelial surfaces of the body is inadequate to accommodate the numbers of secretory cells required. Thus, a system of glands is developed, and, as outlined above, they are divided into two main groups, exocrine and endocrine (see Fig. 2–1). Exocrine glands pass their secretion to a surface, usually via a duct system (i.e., their secretion is external). In a few glands, the secretion characteristically contains intact, living cells (e.g., the sex glands that secrete germ cells). Endocrine glands pass their secretions directly into the blood or lymph as internal secretions (hormones), which then are transported throughout the body to the target organ or organs.

In general, exocrine glands can be classified by the manner in which their secretory product is elaborated.

1. *Holocrine.* In these glands, examples of which are sebaceous and tarsal glands, the cell elaborates and accumulates secretory product in its cytoplasm, dies, and is discharged as the secretion. In that cells are lost in the process, cell division in such a gland is rapid to replace them.

2. *Apocrine.* Here, secretory product accumulates in apical cytoplasm, which then is pinched off, the cell losing part of its cytoplasm in the process. Examples of apocrine glands are the mammary gland and certain types of sweat glands. Although electron microscopy has not demonstrated loss of apical cytoplasm in apocrine glands, the term is retained.

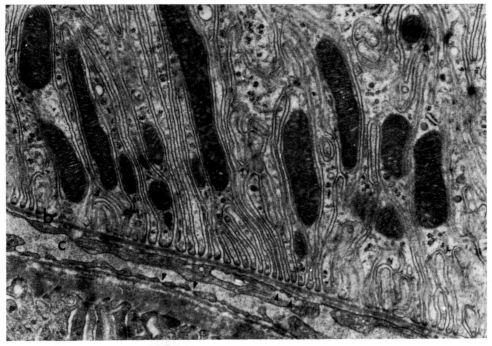

**Figure 2–28.** Basal infoldings. This electron micrograph of the distal convoluted tubule of the kidney shows basal infoldings of the basal plasmalemma as it lies upon the basal lamina (b). A capillary blood vessel (c) is lined by fenestrated endothelium, the pores indicated by arrowheads. Such infoldings are prominent in epithelia involved actively in fluid transport. × 24,000.

3. *Merocrine.* Most glands (e.g., salivary glands and the pancreas) are merocrine, that is, the secretory product is formed in and discharged from the cell by exocytosis without the loss of any cytoplasm.

### Exocrine Glands

#### UNICELLULAR GLANDS

Unicellular glands are single cells lying in a columnar or pseudostratified columnar epithelium, these being *goblet* cells that produce mucus (Fig. 2–29). Characteristically, they resemble a goblet or wine glass in shape, with the nucleus in the basal stem and apical cytoplasm distended with a mass of mucigen droplets. The mucin is a proteoglycan complex that, when mixed with water, forms mucus, a slimy lubricating fluid. While goblet cells are exocrine, isolated (single) endocrine cells of several types are found in the gastrointestinal mucosa. These cells secrete hormones and are termed "enteroendocrine" cells.

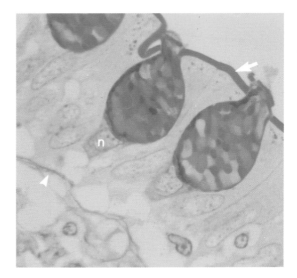

**Figure 2–29.** Goblet cells, unicellular glands. Mucus-secreting goblet cells are found in many epithelia as unicellular glands. Here, in the ileum, the section has been stained to demonstrate the proteoglycan mucin (pink) distending apical cytoplasm of these cells, with nuclei (n) in the basal stem. The stain also demonstrates the brush border (arrow) of columnar epithelial cells and, faintly, the basal lamina (arrowhead). PAS stain. Oil immersion. (See also Figure 2–24.)

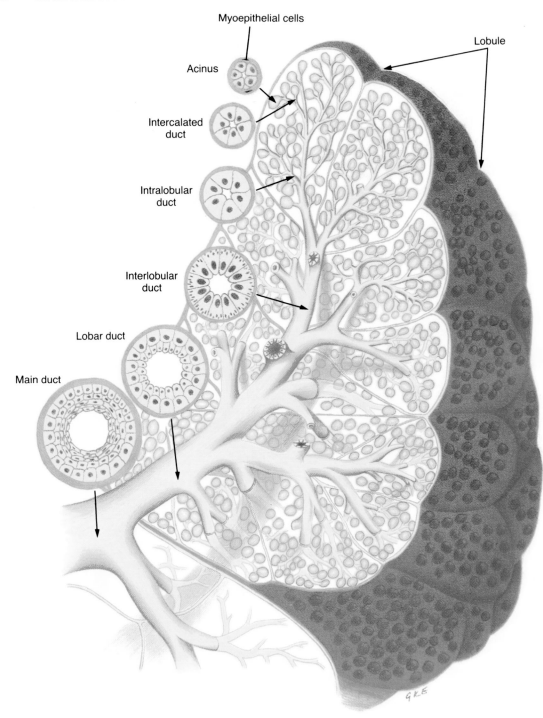

**Figure 2–30.** *Multicellular gland. This diagram illustrates part of an exocrine gland. One lobe and part of another (below, left) are shown, each lobe divided into lobules. Acini and smaller ducts lie within lobules, and the organization of the duct system is illustrated.*

## MULTICELLULAR GLANDS

*Multicellular* glands consist of more than one cell and are classified further according to the presence or absence of branching in the duct system and on the arrangement of the cells in the secretory units (Figs. 2–30 and 2–31).

In *simple* glands, the duct is unbranched and may be coiled or not.

In *compound* glands, the duct branches.

In respect of secretory units, which lie at the termination of a duct in simple glands or a small branch of a duct in a compound gland, they may be either *tubular* (Fig. 2–32) or flask-shaped, this type being called *alveolar* or *acinar* (like a hollow vessel or like a berry). In many glands, secretory units are mixed, and the gland then is termed *tubuloalveolar*. If the acinar or flask shape is very large (i.e., formed by many cells), the unit may be called *saccular*.

The nature of the secretion may be either *mucous* (thick) or *serous* (watery), and the secretory units that form them differ in appearance (Fig. 2–33). If both types are present, then the gland is *mixed*. Additionally, both serous and mucous cells may be found in one acinus, which is called a *mixed acinus* (Fig. 2–34).

Structurally, a compound exocrine gland is composed of three main elements—connective tissue, ducts, and glandular (secretory) units. Each gland usually has a connective tissue capsule from which septa extend into the gland, the major septa dividing it into lobes, with each lobe sub-

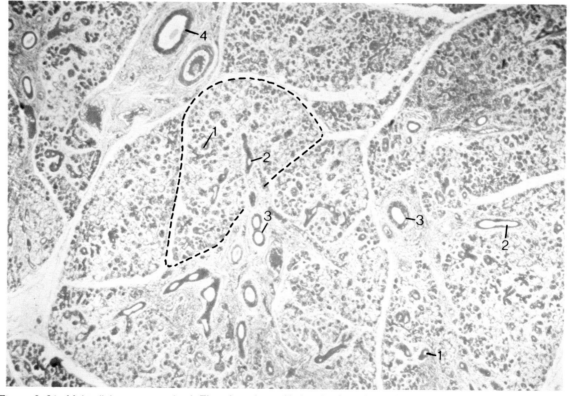

**Figure 2–31.** *Multicellular exocrine gland. This, the submandibular gland, is classified as a compound, tubuloalveolar mixed gland, which means that the duct system is branched (compound), the secretory units are both tubular and alveolar in shape (tubuloalveolar), and both mucous- and serous-secreting cells are present (mixed). In fact, some acini are serous, some mucous, and some mixed (mucous acini with serous crescents). Parts of several lobes are seen with relatively dense (interlobar) connective tissue between them, each containing several lobules, one of which is outlined by the interrupted line. Ducts are labeled as intralobular (1), lobular (2), interlobular (3), and lobar (4).*

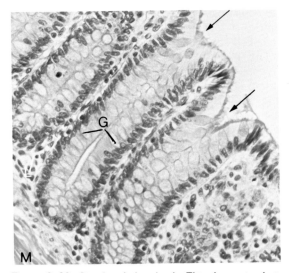

**Figure 2–32.** Simple tubular glands. This shows simple tubular glands of the colon passing from the surface (arrows) into the underlying connective tissue of the lamina propria (L) with part of the muscularis mucosae (M) (below, left). Thus, all three components of a mucous membrane, or mucosa, are seen. The epithelium is simple columnar in type, with numerous pale-staining goblet cells (G). H and E. High power.

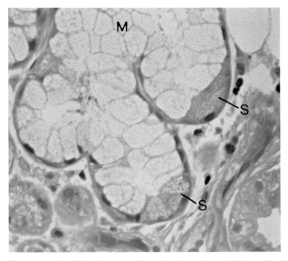

**Figure 2–34.** Mixed acini. Here, in the submandibular gland, a branching mucous acinus (M) is composed of pale-staining cells with condensed basal nuclei and shows two serous crescents, or demilunes (S), formed by cells with pink-staining, discrete apical droplets. Also seen at lower right is part of an intralobular duct lined by simple, high cuboidal epithelium. Masson. Oil immersion.

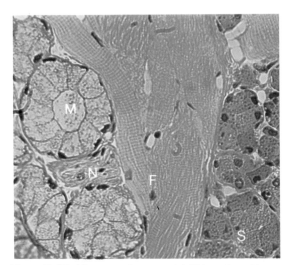

**Figure 2–33.** Mucous and serous acini. This section of tongue shows mucous acini (M) with pale-staining cells, "foamy" cytoplasm and dense, irregular nuclei compressed against the basal lamina, and serous acini (S) with discrete pink secretory droplets in apical cytoplasm and basally located, spherical, vesicular nuclei. Also present are striated muscle fibers (F) and a small peripheral nerve (N). H and E. Oil immersion.

divided by finer connective tissue into lobules. Within the lobule, thin connective tissue forms a meshwork in which lie the secretory units and ducts. The amount and density of connective tissue vary greatly, being, for example, relatively profuse and dense in salivary glands but much thinner and less dense in the pancreas. Blood vessels, lymphatics, and nerves lie in the connective tissue, entering the gland through its capsule and then being distributed along interlobar and interlobular septa. Small arteries pass from interlobular septa into the lobule, where they break up into a capillary network lying in the intralobular, slender connective tissue between secretory units.

The duct system of compound glands is to be compared to a tree, the secretory units being the leaves, the smallest ducts the twigs, and the main duct being the trunk. The smallest ducts are termed *intercalated*, indicating that they are inserted between (and therefore connect) secretory units and intralobular ducts. *Intralobular* ducts are small ducts lying in the lobule and, usually, lined by small cuboidal cells. Several intralobular ducts join to form a larger *lobular* duct, this also lying

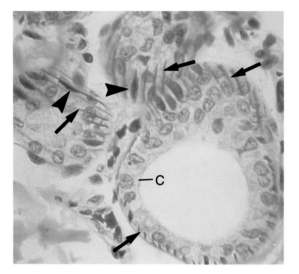

**Figure 2–35.** *Myoepithelial cells. The ducts of labial mucous glands seen here are lined by pale-staining, simple cuboidal epithelium (C). Myoepithelial cells are seen as dark-pink slips of cytoplasm (arrows), some containing nuclei (arrowheads). They lie within the basal lamina, are contractile, and have an octopus-like shape. Masson. Oil immersion.*

among secretory units. Lobular ducts pass into interlobular septa, where they unite to form an *interlobular duct*. At the apex of a lobe, the interlobular ducts of that lobe unite to form a *lobar* duct, and, finally, all lobar ducts unite to form (usually) a single *main* duct that drains the entire gland. Progressively, from smaller to larger ducts, the epithelium increases in height from squamous (intercalated duct) through cuboidal (intralobular and lobular) to columnar (interlobular) and variations of stratified columnar or even stratified squamous in the larger ducts. Also, the supporting connective tissue increases in amount.

In *serous* secretory units, the cells generally show a pink or pinkish-purple cytoplasm with H and E stain, with some basophilia at the base and apical secretory (zymogen) granules that are often eosinophilic. Nuclei are regularly spheroidal or ovoid, often with prominent nucleoli. The lumen of the unit usually is small but definite. *Mucous* cells stain much lighter with H and E, and the cytoplasm has a foamy appearance with nuclei usually dark, thin, and flattened against the basal plasma membrane. The lumen of mucous acini is small and often irregular. As already mentioned, mixed glands contain both serous and mucous secretory units. A *mixed* acinus is basically a mucous acinus, usually tubular in type, with a few serous cells at its termination arranged in a crescent or half-moon shape. Cells of these *serous*

*demilunes* pass their secretion into tiny intercellular canals between adjacent mucous cells to reach the acinar lumen.

**Myoepithelial Cells**

All acini are surrounded by a thin extracellular basal lamina, and between acinar cells and the basal lamina lie myoepithelial, or basket, cells (Fig. 2–35). They usually appear as small dark nuclei with little surrounding cytoplasm, but from the central area, long, thin arms of cytoplasm extend around the acinus to grasp it in the form of a basket or like the arms of an octopus. These cells show fibrillar cytoplasm and have many features of smooth muscle, including contractility, although they are of epithelial origin. By their contraction, they aid in expelling secretion from the gland. They are located also around smaller ducts of many glands, for example, around ducts of sweat glands.

### Endocrine Glands

Histologically, endocrine glands are much simpler than exocrine glands. Usually, there is a thin connective tissue capsule from which incomplete septa extend internally to divide the gland into lobes. Within the gland, the supporting tissue is thin and sparse and associated with a very rich blood capillary or sinusoidal network, with groups of epithelial cells lying between the fine blood channels. Each cell is adjacent to a fine blood vessel into which it passes its hormonal secretion. Based on cell grouping and the method of hormone storage, two types of endocrine gland are classified. In most cases, the cells are arranged in anastomosing cords and clumps between dilated blood capillaries, and storage of hormones is intracellular—this is the *cord and clump* type (Fig. 2–36). In a few cases (e.g., the thyroid), a group of cells forms a vesicle or follicle with a central cavity into which the secretory product is passed and stored. When required, the hormone passes back through the cells and into blood capillaries located between follicles—this is the *follicle* type (Fig. 2–37).

In the body, many glands are mixed, having both exocrine and endocrine functions. In the liver, each cell not only formulates bile that it passes into a duct system as an exocrine secretion but also secretes internal secretions directly into the blood system. However, in most mixed glands (e.g., the pancreas, testis, and ovary), one group of exocrine cells secretes into a duct system and another group, of endocrine cells, secretes directly into the blood system.

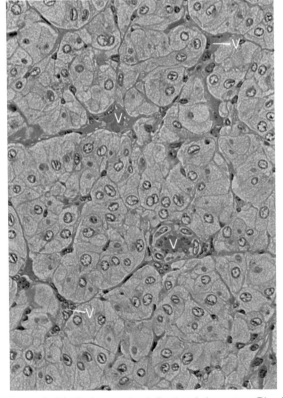

**Figure 2–36.** *Endocrine gland. Cord and clump type. Blood vessels (v), mainly sinusoidal capillaries, lie around and between groups of epithelial cells arranged in short, anastomosing cords. These are cells of the suprarenal medulla. They have large vesicular nuclei and cytoplasm that shows numerous, clear droplets, these droplets, or granules, representing the secretory product, the catecholamine hormones epinephrine and norepinephrine. Thus, this type of endocrine gland shows cells in cords and clumps, the cells storing the hormone to be secreted. H and E. High power.*

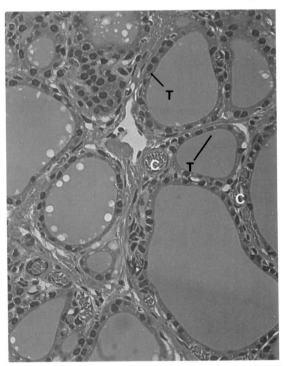

**Figure 2–37.** *Endocrine gland, follicle type. In the thyroid gland, the epithelial cells are arranged in follicles, the walls formed by low cuboidal cells (T) surrounding central cavities filled with stored, secretory hormone. When needed, the hormone passes back through the cells to numerous blood capillaries (C) located in the sparse connective tissue that lies around and between the follicles. The stored material in the follicles stains pink and is called colloid. H and E. High power.*

## Summary Table 2–1. Epithelial Membranes

| Classification | Cell Type | Example | Function |
|---|---|---|---|
| Simple (one layer of cells) | Squamous | Parietal layer of Bowman's capsule and loop of Henle (kidney) | Bounding (limiting) membrane Fluid absorption |
| | | Pulmonary alveoli | Gaseous exchange |
| | | Endothelium, lining blood vessels | Active transport, pinocytosis |
| | | Mesothelium, covering/lining body cavities | Aids visceral movement |
| | Cuboidal | Ducts of many glands | Secretion, absorption |
| | | Ovary, surface | Protection |
| | | Lens capsule | Formation of lens fibers |
| | Columnar | Surface epithelium of stomach | Secretion (mucus), protection |
| | | Gallbladder | Secretion, absorption |
| | | Small intestine (brush border) | Absorption, secretion, protection |
| | | Uterine tubes, ductuli efferentes (ciliated) | Transport, protection |
| Pseudostratified (Nuclei at different levels: All cells contact basal lamina, not all reach lumen) | Columnar | Trachea and bronchi (ciliated with goblet cells) | Transport, secretion, protection |
| | | Male urethra (nonciliated) | Protection |
| | | Epididymis (stereocilia) | Absorption, secretion |
| Stratified (More than one layer of cells) | Squamous | Vagina, esophagus, cornea (nonkeratinizing) | Protection |
| | | Epidermis (keratinizing) | Protection, prevents water loss |
| | Cuboidal | Sweat glands | Protection, secretion |
| | Columnar | Large excretory ducts | Secretion, absorption, protection |
| | | Conjunctiva | Protection, secretion |
| | Transitional | Urinary tract | Protection, distensibility |

## Summary Table 2–2. Epithelial Glands

| Type of Gland | Classification | Duct System | Secretory Unit | Example |
|---|---|---|---|---|
| Unicellular | Exocrine | — | — | Goblet cell |
| | Endocrine | — | — | Enteroendocrine |
| Multicellular | Exocrine | Simple (unbranched) | Tubular | Intestinal glands (crypts of Lieberkühn) |
| | | | Tubular, coiled | Sweat glands |
| | | Simple (branched) | Tubular | Fundic (stomach) glands, glands of Bowman |
| | | | Acinar (saccular) | Meibomian glands |
| | | Compound | Tubular | Gastric cardia, labial glands |
| | | | Tubuloalveolar, serous | Pancreas, parotid, lacrimal |
| | | | Tubuloalveolar, mucous | Bulbourethral, labial |
| | | | Tubuloalveolar, mixed | Submandibular |
| | | | Acinar (saccular) | Prostate, mammary |
| | Endocrine | — | Cord and clump | Adrenal medulla, pars distalis (hypophysis) |
| | | | Follicular | Thyroid |

Manner of secretion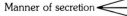
Holocrine—the entire cell breaks down (e.g., sebaceous glands)
Apocrine—release of secretory product involves loss of apical cytoplasm (e.g., mammary gland)
Merocrine—secretory product discharged by exocytosis, no loss of cytoplasm (most glands)

# Connective Tissue Proper

## INTRODUCTION

During embryological development, the ectoderm and endoderm become separated by the third germ layer, the mesoderm. The embryonic tissue formed by cells of the mesoderm is termed *mesenchyme* (*mesos*, middle; *enchyma*, infusion), and it is from mesenchyme that the connective (supporting, communicative) tissues of the body develop. These include the connective tissue proper, cartilage, bone, blood, and the lymphatic and hemopoietic tissues.

Mesenchyme is typically a loose spongy tissue, which in early embryonic life occurs as packing between structures developing from other germ layers; it later penetrates the developing organs and structures. It is composed of stellate and fusiform cells that form an open network and of an amorphous intercellular substance containing a few scattered fibrous elements.

Mesenchymal cells are multipotent and are able to differentiate along several different lines to produce many different kinds of connective tissue cells. Thus, the tissues that have a

**3**

common origin from mesenchyme are known as *mesenchymal tissues*, or *connective tissues*.

Connective tissues differ from the other tissue types (epithelium, muscle, and nerve) by the presence of abundant intercellular material, or *matrix*. Matrix is composed of an amorphous ground substance and fibers. The proportions of cells and intercellular material show considerable variation and form the basis of classification. It must be recognized, however, that the classification is inexact, since various types are linked by transitional forms.

In a discussion of any type of connective tissue there are three elements to consider: the amorphous ground substance, the fibers, and the cells. These elements are bathed in tissue fluid and will be discussed in detail before any consideration is given to the features of the various types of connective tissue.

## TISSUE FLUID

The blood vascular system is responsible for transporting oxygen and food materials to, and removing waste products from, the cells. However, it must be appreciated that the great majority of cells is situated external to, and some distance removed from, blood vessels. Thus, it is necessary for oxygen and nutritive materials to leave the blood, pass through the thin walls of small blood vessels, and enter the intercellular spaces to reach the cells. Waste materials follow a similar route in a reverse direction. The small blood vessels (capillaries) have walls that allow the ready passage through them of a watery fluid containing crystalloids, dissolved oxygen, and food materials. This filtrate of the blood, the *tissue fluid*, is formed by simple diffusion and occurs at the arterial end of a capillary (i.e., toward the heart). The drainage of tissue fluid back into a capillary is accomplished by *osmosis*, the thin endothelial lining of the blood capillary functioning as a living selectively permeable membrane.

In the intercellular spaces, tissue fluid is related closely to the intercellular substances, and this relationship varies with the type of intercellular material. In tissues where the amorphous intercellular substance is in the form of a sol, and fluid or semifluid in nature, it is the tissue fluid that

functions as the dispersion medium. In sites where the intercellular substance is present as a rigid or semirigid gel, there is a high content of bound water derived from tissue fluid at the time of formation of the intercellular substance. Such a gel is readily permeable because diffusion occurs through the bound water. At sites where the intercellular substance not only is gelled but also becomes impermeable owing to impregnation with calcium and other salts (e.g., in bone matrix), tiny channels exist in the matrix to permit passage of tissue fluid. Thus, cellular metabolism, although dependent on the blood vascular system, occurs by the exchange of material with tissue fluid. Tissue fluid sometimes is termed "extracellular fluid" or "intercellular fluid," as opposed to "intracellular fluid" within the cells.

Tissue fluid contains those constituents of blood that can diffuse readily through capillary walls. Blood consists of a fluid component, the *plasma*, which contains both crystalloids and colloids, and cellular elements. Only the crystalloid component of plasma can diffuse readily through the capillary wall to enter the tissue fluid, the cells and the great majority of the colloids remaining within the blood vessels. The volume of tissue fluid varies from tissue to tissue, and within any tissue there are physiological and pathological variations also.

The volume of tissue fluid that is drawn back into the blood capillaries by osmosis is much less than that which passes out through the capillary walls. Tissue fluid, however, also returns to the blood vascular system indirectly through the lymphatic capillaries, which originate blindly in the tissues. Tissue fluid passes through the endothelial walls of these lymphatics and, once inside, is called *lymph*. These small vessels drain into larger lymphatic vessels that finally open into veins near the heart to return the contained lymph to the right atrium and thus to the blood vascular system. Together, these two methods of absorption balance the rate of formation of tissue fluid.

In permanent histological preparations, tissue fluid is removed and therefore cannot be seen as such under the microscope. However, in all organs there are small empty spaces and slits, and, although most of these are caused by shrinkage of tissues in preparation and therefore are artifacts, they do represent to some extent the tissue spaces that in life are occupied by tissue fluid. One common pathological condition, *edema*, oc-

.curs when there is a considerable increase in the volume of tissue fluid. It is characterized histologically by the presence of enlarged spaces within the tissues caused by the increased volume of fluid.

## INTERCELLULAR SUBSTANCES

The intercellular substances are nonliving and form the matrix, or mold, in which cells live. They provide the strength and support of tissues and also act as a medium for the diffusion of tissue fluid between blood capillaries and cells to permit cellular metabolism. In addition, they have an important role in tissue differentiation. They are widely distributed throughout all tissues of the body.

Two main types of intercellular substances are present, *amorphous* (nonformed) and *fibrous* (formed).

### Amorphous Intercellular Substances

The amorphous intercellular substances (ground substances) are transparent, colorless, and homogeneous. They occupy the spaces between the cells and fibers of connective tissue and function principally as a medium through which tissue fluid containing nutrients and waste products can diffuse between capillaries and cells.

The amorphous substances of connective tissue are composed principally of *glycosaminoglycans* and *glycoproteins*. Glycosaminoglycans, which in the past were referred to as acid mucopolysaccharides, are linear polymers of repeating disaccharide units composed of a hexosamine and a uronic acid. The hexosamine is either D-glucosamine or D-galactosamine, and the uronic acid is D-glucuronic acid or L-iduronic acid. With the exception of hyaluronic acid, all glycosaminoglycans are sulfated in varying degrees and are linked covalently to protein as *proteoglycans*. The principal glycosaminoglycans of the matrix are *hyaluronic acid, chondroitin sulfate, dermatan sulfate, keratan sulfate*, and *heparan sulfate*. These differ in molecular weight, the nature of their disaccharide units, and the length of chain.

Hyaluronic acid is the largest glycosaminoglycan and is the only one lacking sulfate groups. It is present in nearly all the connective tissues and is a major component of synovial fluid, the vitreous body of the eye, and *Wharton's jelly* of the umbilical cord. It readily binds water, and this has an important influence on the exchange of material between tissue cells and blood plasma. In addition, because of its viscosity, it is an effective lubricant in the synovial fluid of the joints. The enzyme hyaluronidase hydrolyzes it, reducing its viscosity, and thus increases permeability of certain tissues.

Chondroitin sulfate is the most abundant of the sulfated glycosaminoglycans and predominates in cartilage, bone, intervertebral discs, and large blood vessels. Dermatan sulfate, which can be viewed as an isomer of chondroitin sulfate, is widely distributed and occurs in high concentration in skin, tendon, and heart valves. Two forms of keratan sulfate are known, type I being found exclusively in the cornea and type II being associatd with tissues of skeletal origin, including cartilage and intervertebral discs. Heparan sulfate is structurally related to heparin and generally is present in the form of a high-molecular-weight proteoglycan in relation to cell surfaces and basal laminae.

Glucosaminoglycans and proteoglycans can be stained with basic dyes such as hematoxylin, owing principally to the presence of sulfate groups. They also exhibit metachromasia with such dyes as toluidine blue and crystal violet. They appear as dense matrix granules, 10 to 20 nm in diameter, in electron micrographs.

The structural glycoproteins are proteins with one or more heterosaccharide chains containing hexosamine, galactose, and other sugars. They differ from the proteoglycans in their high proportion of protein and in the fact that their carbohydrate moiety frequently is a branched structure. Several glycoproteins have been isolated, and they include *fibronectin, chondronectin*, and *laminin*.

Fibronectin is a major surface glycoprotein of the fibroblast. As the name implies, it binds to other proteins such as collagen and fibrin, and it has been isolated from cultures of fibroblasts and from the dermis. It occurs also in the blood plasma, where it is called *cold-insoluble globulin* or *plasma fibronectin*, and in the α granules of blood platelets. Fibronectin generally is thought to have a biological role in linking cells, collagen, and glycosaminoglycans. It cannot be visualized in routine histological preparations, but immunocytochemical localization with fluorescent antibody gives an indication of its wide distribution.

Chondronectin is more restricted than fibronectin in its distribution. It has been isolated from cartilage and appears to promote adhesion of mature cartilage cells to collagenous substrates, a role that is similar to that of fibronectin in relation to fibroblasts. Laminin also is restricted in its distribution and has been isolated from basal laminae. It is composed of at least two large polypeptide chains and appears to be involved in the attachment of epithelial sheets to their underlying lamina propria.

### Fibrous Intercellular Substances

The function of providing tensile strength and support for tissues is performed mainly by the fibrous intercellular substances. Three types of formed fibers exist—*collagenous, reticular*, and *elastic*—and they are distinguished by their appearance and chemical reactions (Fig. 3–1). All are complex proteins formed by long chains of amino acids with peptide linkages (i.e., polypeptide chains), and all are comparatively insoluble in neutral solvents. Thus, they exist as formed fibers in the fluid internal environment of the body. The characteristics of each type of fiber now will be considered.

#### COLLAGENOUS FIBERS

Collagenous fibers are found in all types of connective tissue and consist of the protein collagen. They are extremely tough. In bulk in the fresh state (e.g., in tendons and aponeuroses), they appear white and, hence, are termed "white" fibers.

**Physical Properties.** Collagenous fibers vary from 1 to 20 micrometers (μm) in diameter and are of indeterminate length. The fibers have a straight or slightly wavy course and may be loosely or densely packed, depending upon the

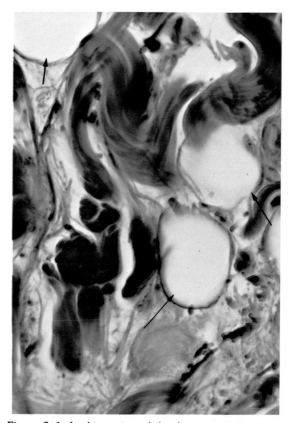

**Figure 3–1.** In this section of the dense connective tissue beneath the epithelium of the lip, the presence of abundant intercellular material is clearly apparent. Two types of fibrous intercellular substance, collagenous and elastic, are demonstrated. Collagenous fibers (dark blue) generally are coarse and show a faint longitudinal striation owing to their component fibrils. Elastic fibers (black) are less numerous and more delicate than collagenous fibers and appear homogeneous. Although tissue fluid and the amorphous intercellular substances have been largely removed during preparation, they are represented by the small empty spaces and slits between the fibers. Apart from scattered fat cells (arrows), very few cells are present in this tissue. Iron hematoxylin, aniline blue. High power.

location and functional need. In the fresh state, collagenous fibers are soft and flexible, relatively inelastic, and of high tensile strength. The fibers are transparent and homogeneous but, at high magnification, show a faint longitudinal striation. In tissue sections, collagenous fibers are acidophil and are stained pink by eosin, red by van Gieson's picrofuchsin, blue-purple by the aniline blue of

Mallory's connective tissue stain, and green by Masson's trichrome stain. They are birefringent under polarized light, indicating a longitudinal orientation of subunits, or *fibrils* (Fig. 3–2). The fibers may branch and recombine owing to the interchange of fibrils between one fiber and another.

The finest strand of collagen visible by light microscopy is the *fibril*, about 0.3 to 0.5 μm thick. As indicated earlier, a fiber is composed of the parallel aggregation of several fibrils. In turn, a fibril is composed of still smaller units of diameters from 20 nm to 100 nm, averaging 75 nm. These are the *microfibrils*, or *unit fibers*, of collagen (Fig. 3–3). Newly formed microfibrils are only about 20 nm in diameter, and there is evidence that they increase in size with age, although in certain areas of the body the microfibrils show a uniform diameter throughout life. The microfibrils are visible only with the electron microscope and show a characteristic cross-banding with a major periodicity of 64 nm.

When collagenous material is denatured by boiling, it becomes hydrated and softens, yielding gelatin. The fibers can be digested by pepsin in acid solution and by the enzyme collagenase. After treatment with salts of heavy metals or tannic acid, collagen forms an insoluble product. This is the basis of the "tanning" process in the preparation of animal hides (leather), which consist principally of collagen.

Following treatment with dilute acids and alkalis, collagen fibrils swell and disintegrate into fibrillar units or macromolecules of *tropocollagen*, each 1.5 nm wide and 280 nm long. The tropocollagen molecule in turn is composed of three polypeptide chains, twisted around each other to form a right-handed superhelix. Each individual polypeptide chain is formed by about a thousand amino acids linked together and twisted into a left-handed helix, or spiral. Collagen is rich in glycine, proline, hydroxyproline, and hydroxylysine, the latter also forming strong cross links between adjacent tropocollagen molecules within a microfibril. In the microfibril, tropocollagen molecules lie end to end in parallel chains or rows, all molecules facing the same direction, and between rows there is an overlap of about one quarter of the length of the tropocollagen molecule. The 64-nm major periodicity of microfibrils is caused by this 25 per cent overlap (4 times 64

is 256, approximately the length of a tropocollagen molecule).

In addition to the microfibril with the periodicity of 64 nm characteristic of native collagen, collagen can exist also in a long-spacing form with a periodicity of about 240 nm. There are two varieties of this: the fibrous long-spacing (FLS) form found in the trabecular meshwork of the eye and aging cartilage, and the segment long-spacing (SLS) form. Each type can be dissolved readily and reprecipitated into either of the other two forms. FLS collagen is formed by rows of tropocollagen units lying end to end in parallel-antiparallel array without overlap, and SLS collagen is formed by lateral and lengthwise aggregation of similar units.

**Types of Collagen.** In the past, collagen was considered to be a unique protein, but improvements in methodology have revealed that it is a family of closely related proteins produced by many different cell types. All types possess the triple helical structure, but they differ from each other in the primary structure of their constituent polypeptide chains. The chains can be separated into two classes, alpha-1 and alpha-2, which differ slightly in amino acid sequence and composition. Many types of collagen have been described in recent years, and the most important are collagen types I, II, III, IV, and V.

*Type I.* The most ubiquitous form of collagen, known as type I, accounts for about 90 per cent of the collagen in the body and consists of two alpha-1 (type I) chains and one alpha-2 (type I) chain. This collagen is found in the dermis of the skin, tendons, bone, teeth, and virtually all the connective tissues. Cells responsible for synthesis of type I collagen include fibroblasts, osteoblasts, and odontoblasts.

*Type II.* Type II collagen, synthesized by chondroblasts, consists of three alpha-1 (type II) chains and is the principal constituent of cartilaginous matrix.

*Type III.* In this type, there are three alpha-1 (type III) chains. This type of collagen is found early in the development of a number of different connective tissues and later is largely replaced by type I collagen. In the adult, it persists in reticular networks in association with the skin, blood vessels, uterus, and gastrointestinal tract. In the skin, it is synthesized by fibroblasts and in the other regions by smooth muscle cells.

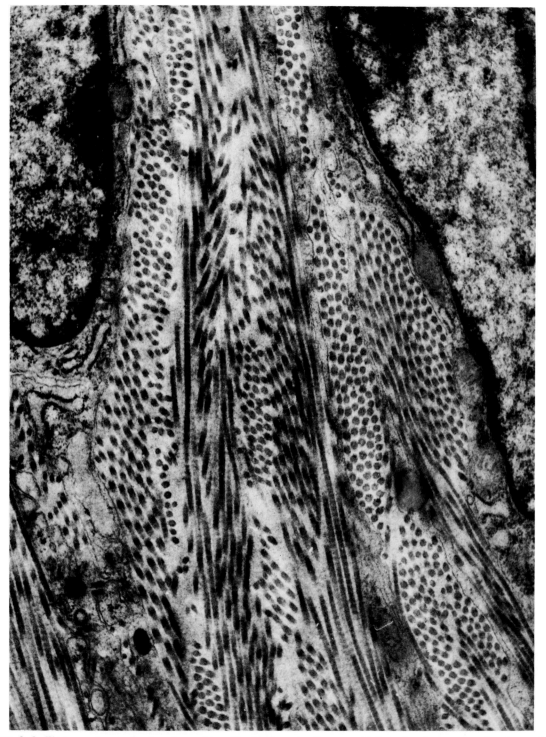

**Figure 3–2.** Electron micrograph of portions of two fibroblasts and collagenous fibrils in the dense connective tissue of the epididymis. The fibrils are cut in both cross and longitudinal section and, in the latter, show cross-banding. × 40,000.

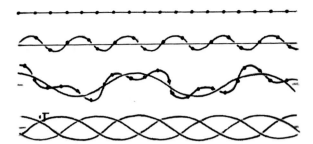

Molecular chain of amino acids

Single chain molecular helix

Single chain coiled helix

Triple chain coiled helix

forming a

Tropocollagen molecule

Tropocollagen molecules

forming a

Collagen microfibril

(Unit fiber)

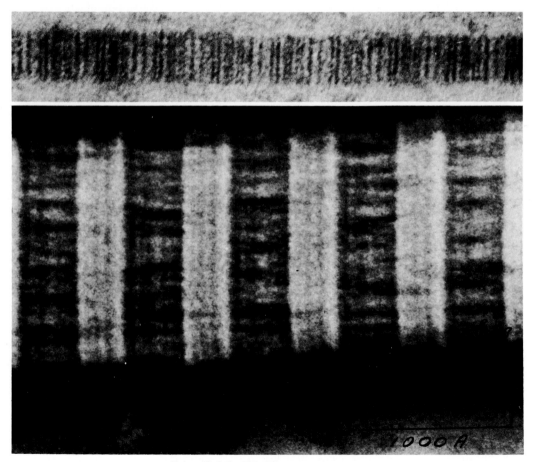

*Figure 3–3* See legend on opposite page

***Type IV.*** Type IV collagen, consisting of three alpha-1 (type IV) chains, is present in basal laminae and is thought to be a product of cells directly associated with the laminae, principally epithelial and endothelial cells.

***Type V.*** Type V collagen, the structure of which still is the subject of controversy, is present in thin laminae beneath fetal membranes and in blood vessels.

To identify the various genetic species of collagen *in situ*, immunological techniques are utilized. Specific antibodies have been prepared against each of the common molecular types and are used to locate the collagens in tissue sections by standard immunohistochemical methods.

As mentioned earlier, the diameter of collagen fibrils varies greatly, depending upon the tissue. For example, type I collagen of tendon forms thick, uniform fibrils up to 200 nm in diameter packed in parallel bundles, whereas type I collagen of bone is a weave of finer fibrils that are heavily mineralized. Collagen type II in cartilage occurs as delicate fibrils but does not form fibers. Collagen type III in the adult appears as fine networks of fibrils, and collagen types IV and V, mostly restricted to basal laminae, do not form fibrils or fibers.

**Formation of Collagen.** Collagen synthesis has been studied principally in fibroblasts, but the process probably is identical in other cell types capable of producing collagen. It involves the following steps, some occurring within the synthesizing cell and others extracellularly.

1. Polypeptide alpha chains are assembled on polyribosomes bound to endoplasmic reticulum and then are transferred into the cisternae. These polypeptide chains are longer than the alpha chains of mature collagen and are called *pro-alpha-chains*.

2. Hydroxylation of proline and lysine occurs before the chains are completed within the cisternae of the endoplasmic reticulum. This is necessary for the future formation of the triple helix and for the stability of the future cross links between the chains.

3. Assembly of procollagen begins in the cisternae, and the procollagen molecules then are transported to the Golgi complex and from there to secretory vacuoles. The latter fuse with the plasma membrane to discharge the precursor molecules.

4. Outside the cell, a specific protease, *procollagen peptidase*, cleaves off the extra lengths to create tropocollagen from procollagen.

5. The tropocollagen molecules aggregate in a specific manner to form unit fibers of collagen.

6. Formation of cross links between the tropocollagen molecules. This process is catalyzed by the enzyme *lysyl oxidase* and is necessary for the tensile strength of the whole fiber.

### RETICULAR FIBERS

Reticular fibers are very fine collagenous fibers, the collagenous component of which is principally type III collagen (Fig. 3–4). Generally, they are arranged to form a net-like supporting framework, or reticulum. They occur as fine networks around muscle fibers, nerve fibers, fat cells, and small blood vessels; in the fine partitions of the lung; and, particularly, at boundaries between connective tissue and other tissue types. Beneath epithelial membranes, for example, reticular fibers form dense networks as components of basal laminae. They also are found in myeloid and lymphoid tissues in association with reticular cells (see Chapter 9). They are difficult to visualize in routine H and E sections but can be demonstrated by silver impregnation methods (e.g., Bielschowsky's method) where they become visible as thin, dark lines, collagenous fibers proper being colored yellow or brown.

The coloration of reticular fibers by silver impregnation has led to the term "argyrophil." They stain more darkly red with the periodic acid–Schiff (PAS) technique than do collagenous fibers but, on electron microscopy, show the periodicity of 64 nm characteristic of collagenous fibers. The staining differences between the two types of fiber probably result from the high content of hexoses

---

*Figure 3–3. Collagen structure.* Top: *The diagrams illustrate the formation of a collagen microfibril. (After Gross, J. Biophys Biochem 30:59, 1966.) The electron micrograph (center) is of a single collagen microfibril stained positively with uranyl acetate.* × 185,000. Bottom: *The micrograph is of a single microfibril stained negatively with phosphotungstic acid.* × 430,000. *(Photograph courtesy of Dr. R. Borasky.)*

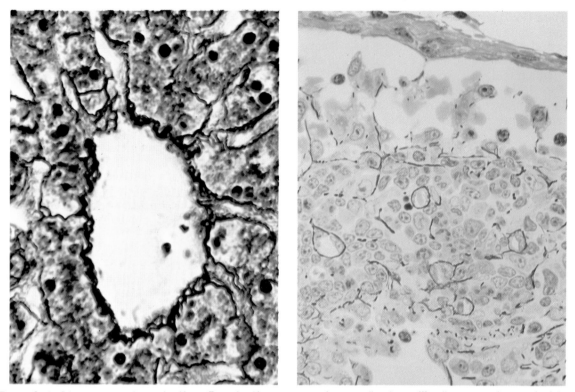

*Figure 3–4.* Silver staining of reticular fibers. Reticular fibers, composed principally of type III collagen, are distinguished from other collagenous fibers by their small size, homogeneity, their arrangement in fine networks, and the fact that they are argyrophil. Left: This section shows the central vein of a liver lobule with radiating columns of liver cells (hepatocytes). The black-staining reticular fibers are concentrated around the central vein and extend between the columns of liver cells in relation to blood vascular spaces (sinusoids). High power. Right: Delicate reticular fibers (brown-black) are present within the capsule of a lymph node (top) and in relation to a concentration of lymphocytes (center). The space beneath the capsule, the subcapsular sinus, contains numerous lymphocytes and a delicate network of reticular fibers. Wilder's silver method. High power.

in reticular fibers—6 per cent or more as opposed to 1 per cent in collagen.

### ELASTIC FIBERS

Elastic fibers are present in loose fibrous connective tissue and are seen as long, thin, highly refractile, cylindrical threads or flat ribbons that branch to form networks (Fig. 3–5). They are thinner than collagenous fibers, ranging in size from less than a micrometer to 4 μm in diameter, although in some elastic ligaments, they may reach a diameter of 10 to 12 μm. In contrast with collagenous fibers, by light microscopy they appear homogeneous and not fibrillar in nature. They may form extensive, fenestrated lamellae

(e.g., in the walls of major blood vessels). In the fresh state, adult elastic tissue in bulk has a yellowish color.

Elastic fibers stain erratically with eosin but can be stained selectively with orcein (brown), resorcin-fuchsin (dark blue–purple), and aldehyde-fuchsin (black). If fresh tissue is treated with dilute acid solutions, collagenous fibers swell and become transparent, whereas elastic fibers become visible as highly refractile, homogeneous, shining threads.

Elastic fibers are composed of the albuminoid *elastin*, which shows a remarkable resistance to most agents. It is not affected by hot or cold water or by dilute solutions of acids or alkalis and is not digested by trypsin. However, it is easily hydro-

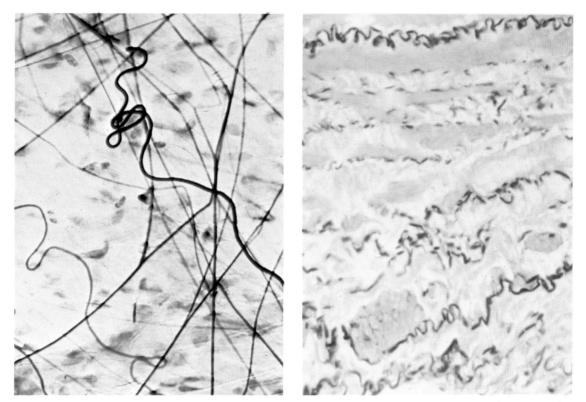

**Figure 3–5.** Elastic fibers. Left: *This is a spread preparation, not a section of mesentery. Elastic fibers (dark brown-black) are thin, homogeneous threads that, in such a preparation of loose connective tissue, can be seen to branch and anastomose, forming an open network. Most fibers appear straight (under tension), but some are curled into loose spirals (relaxed). Verhoeff's elastic stain. Medium power.* Right: *Section of a vein. Elastic fibers, stained brown, are concentrated in relation to the lumen of the vein (above) as a convoluted, complete internal elastic lamina and appear as individual fibers, often sectioned transversely or obliquely, in the underlying coats of the venous wall. Weigert's stain. Medium power.*

lyzed by the pancreatic enzyme *elastase*. As indicated by the name, elastic fibers can be stretched and return to their former length when tension is released.

On electron microscopy, elastic fibers show two components. The *microfibrils* are 10 to 12 nm in diameter and tubular, with a light central core. The *amorphous component* usually lies centrally, surrounded by a group of microfibrils. In embryonic tissues, the microfibrils appear first, synthesized by fibroblasts and smooth muscle cells, and later small clumps of amorphous material are formed within the groups of microfibrils (Figs. 3–6 and 3–7). With age, the microfibrils are reduced in number, and the amorphous component increases. The amorphous component chemically is elastin, which contains the amino acids desmosine and isodesmosine not found in collagen. The microfibrils consist of a connective tissue protein that is neither collagen nor elastin and is rich in hydrophilic amino acids.

## BASAL LAMINAE

Basal laminae are sheets of extracellular material present under the basal surface of epithelial cells, around muscles, nerves, capillaries, and fat cells, and situated between these elements and the underlying or surrounding connective tissue (Fig. 3–8). Thus, they are distributed widely, and, in many organs, the connective tissue elements virtually are limited by basal laminae.

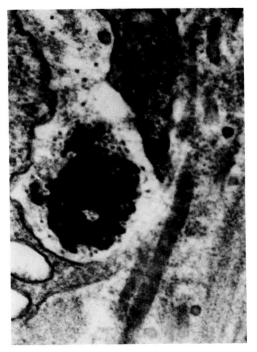

**Figure 3–6.** Electron micrograph of transverse section of an elastic fiber (center), surrounded by branching fibroblast processes. The elastic fiber shows an amorphous component surrounded by groups of microfibrils. A few collagenous fibrils also are present (lower right). × 55,000.

material. This external layer is called the *reticular lamina*. All three elements—basal lamina, reticular fibers, and ground substance—constitute the *basement membrane*, seen with the light microscope. Although the terms basal lamina and basement membrane commonly are used synonymously, this practice does not distinguish between these two different structures.

The PAS technique probably stains the basal lamina itself and the reticular fibers on the connective tissue surface. The basal lamina consists largely of type IV collagen, laminin, and proteoglycans rich in heparan sulfate. The reticular lamina contains type III collagen and varying amounts of fibronectin. External to the reticular lamina, there are thicker fibers of type I collagen.

Basal laminae are synthesized by the related cells and provide for a strong connection between epithelia and underlying connective tissues, and between muscle and connective tissue, by the intermingling of fibrillar elements between basal laminae and connective tissue. Basal laminae also act as filtration barriers to substances moving between the parenchymal cells and the connective tissue space, holding back molecules on the basis of their size, shape, and electrostatic charge. Additionally, they provide a scaffold for migration of cells during embryogenesis and regeneration.

Basal laminae vary in thickness and stain intensely with the PAS and silver techniques but are poorly demonstrated in H and E preparations. On electron microscopy, the basal lamina appears as two zones, a thin, electron-lucent zone adjacent to the cellular elements, the *lamina rara*, and one adjacent to the connective tissue matrix, the *lamina densa* (Fig. 3–9). The latter consists of a dense feltwork of fine fibrillar material 4 nm in diameter and is about 30 to 70 nm thick. On its external or connective tissue side, the lamina densa blends with fine reticular fibers and microfibrils of collagen, often also with some elastic

## CONNECTIVE TISSUE CELLS

The description of the cells is based upon their appearance in areolar (loose) connective tissue, which is the principal "packing" material in the adult, and which may be considered as the prototype of the connective tissues (Fig. 3–10). Some cells of loose connective tissue, such as fibroblasts and fat cells, represent a relatively stable population of fixed cells, whereas others, including macrophages, mast cells, and leukocytes, are mobile, wandering cells that may be transient

---

**Figure 3–7.** Electron micrographs of elastic fibers; a and b, respectively, are longitudinal and transverse sections from the ligamentum nuchae of a three-month fetal calf, and c and d are from a calf at term (nine months). Note the tubular fibrils (t) surrounding a core of amorphous material (e). With increasing age, the amorphous component increases in amount. There is evidence that the central amorphous component is elastin, the tubular fibrils being an as yet unidentified protein. Unit fibrils of collagen (f) also are present; a, × 50,000; b, × 80,000; c, × 25,000; d, × 45,000. (All courtesy of Russel Ross.)

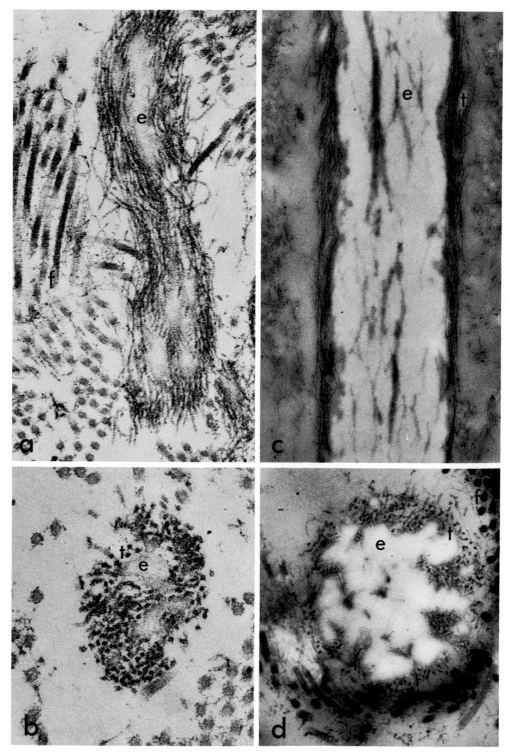

*Figure 3–7* See legend on opposite page

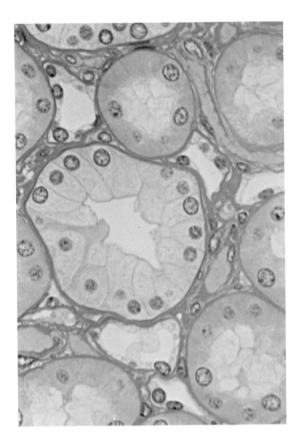

*Figure 3–8. Kidney, medulla. The red-staining material that surrounds each cross section of the kidney tubules and blood capillaries represents a basal lamina and the associated reticular fibers (basement membrane). It is a complete thin layer intimately related to the epithelial cells or to the endothelium of the capillaries. PAS and hematoxylin. High power.*

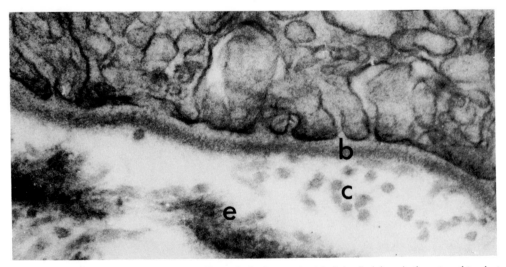

*Figure 3–9. Electron micrograph of a basal lamina. Beneath the bases of epithelial cells (above), there is a thin electron-lucent zone (the lamina rara) and the lamina densa (b), these two constituting the basal lamina. External to the basal lamina, there are microfibrils of collagen (reticular fibers) (c) and some elastin (e) within the ground substance. Together with the basal lamina, the reticular fibers and ground substance form the basement membrane visualized with the light microscope. × 80,000.*

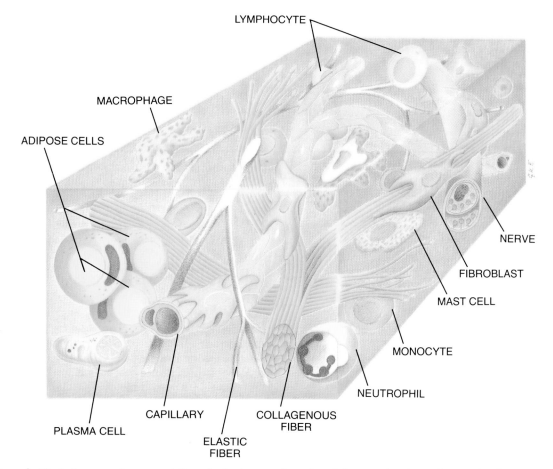

**Figure 3–10.** *A diagrammatic representation of subcutaneous, loose (areolar) connective tissue, showing the characteristic cell and fiber types. These are suspended in the homogeneous amorphous ground substance.*

inhabitants of connective tissue. It must be appreciated that there is a dynamic equilibrium between connective tissue proper and specialized connective tissues such as circulating blood and lymph.

### Fibroblasts

These are one of the two most numerous cells of areolar connective tissue, the other being macrophages. Fibroblasts, as their name suggests, are considered to be responsible for the production of collagenous, reticular, and elastic fibers and for the synthesis of the glycosaminoglycans and glycoproteins of the amorphous intercellular substance. They are large, flat, branching cells that appear spindle-shaped or fusiform in profile. The

branching processes are slender and inconspicuous in most preparations. The nucleus is oval or elongated and has a delicate nuclear membrane, one or two distinct nucleoli, and a small amount of finely granular chromatin. In connective tissue spreads, the nucleus appears pale, whereas in sectioned material it usually appears shrunken and deeply stained with basic dyes (Fig. 3–11). Since the outlines of the cell are indistinct in most histological preparations, the nuclear characteristics are of considerable value in identification.

In young fibroblasts, which are actively engaged in protein synthesis for the production of intercellular substances, the cytoplasm appears relatively homogeneous and is basophilic owing to the high concentration of granular endoplasmic reticulum (Fig. 3–12). Mitochondria appear as

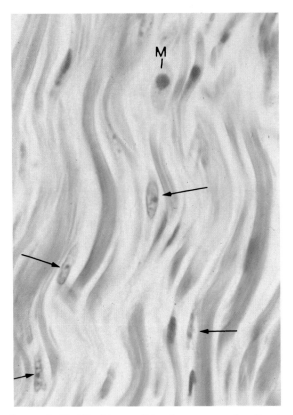

*Figure 3–11. Fibroblasts within dense connective tissue. Coarse collagenous fibers are sectioned longitudinally and exhibit a faint longitudinal striation. A few cells, mostly fibroblasts (arrows), lie within the matrix between fibers. Generally, although the outlines of the cells are indistinct, they appear fusiform and show a pale nucleus, with a distinct nucleolus, and little cytoplasm. A macrophage (M) exhibits a distinct cell outline and a spherical nucleus that is smaller and denser (heterochromatic) than that of the fibroblasts. H and E. High power.*

Fibroblasts are regarded as fixed cells of connective tissue, but they retain throughout adult life a capacity for growth and regeneration. They rarely undergo division, but mitoses can be observed in fibroblasts within connective tissue that is damaged. Some authors, however, believe that in such situations fibroblasts arise from cells somewhat less differentiated than themselves.

### Undifferentiated Mesenchymal Cells

Most authorities believe that some embryonic cells persist in the adult. They are difficult to distinguish from active fibroblasts but, in general, are smaller and stellate in shape and possess elongated nuclei with coarse chromatin. Whereas fibroblasts are seen usually in close association with collagen fibers, undifferentiated mesenchymal cells often are located along the walls of blood vessels, particularly capillaries, where they are referred to as *perivascular*, or *adventitial, cells* or *pericytes*. Their recognition with the light microscope is difficult. However, numerous observations of their responses to certain stimuli indicate that they are capable of differentiation either into the usual cell types found within loose connective tissue or into other cell types such as smooth muscle cells following injury to, or pathological conditions within, blood vessels. Additionally, many investigators consider these cells, rather than fibroblasts, to be the precursors of adipose cells. Probably they should be considered pluripotential cells, similar in many respects to the primitive reticular cells of blood-forming tissue (see Chapter 5).

### Fat Cells

Fat cells are a normal component of areolar tissue. They are large cells and may be 100 μm or more in diameter. They occur singly or in clumps along small blood vessels. If they accumulate in large numbers, the tissue is transformed into *adipose tissue* (Fig. 3–13). Fat cells are spherical if they occur singly, but they appear polyhedral in adipose tissue, where they are crowded together.

In fresh tissue, fat cells have the appearance of glistening droplets of oil surrounded by an ex-

slender rods, and the Golgi apparatus is well developed and located near the nucleus. Microtubules also are present and are thought to be required for the translocation of secretory vesicles.

In old and relatively inactive fibroblasts, the cytoplasm is sparse and only weakly basophilic or even acidophilic, since the granular endoplasmic reticulum is scanty. Such mature and relatively inactive fibroblasts sometimes are called *fibrocytes*. If adequately stimulated, as in wound healing, fibrocytes may revert to the fibroblast state.

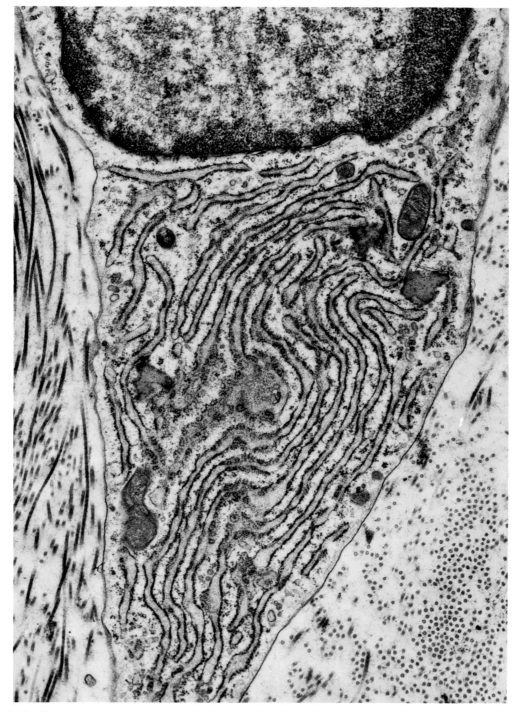

**Figure 3–12.** *Electron micrograph of a portion of a fibroblast. Note the marked development of granular endoplasmic reticulum within the cytoplasm and the close association of collagenous fibrils with the cell membrane.* × *35,000. (Courtesy of Russel Ross.)*

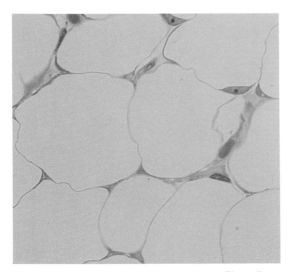

*Figure 3–13. Fat cells within the omentum. The cells are closely packed in this adipose tissue, and each cell shows a thin rim of cytoplasm (red) surrounding the large fat globule, which has dissolved during preparation. Occasional nuclei (blue), with distinct nucleoli, may be seen within the thin rim of cytoplasm. Because of the large size of fat cells, nuclei are not seen in many cells. Plastic section. H and E. High power.*

ceedingly thin rim of cytoplasm. Each mature cell contains a single large droplet of oil, and the thin rim of cytoplasm contains in one area the flattened nucleus (Fig. 3–14). The thicker portion of cytoplasm in relation to the nucleus contains scattered, filamentous mitochondria, a Golgi apparatus, free ribosomes, and a few elements of granular endoplasmic reticulum. In relationship to the large lipid droplet, which is not surrounded by a membrane, the thin rim of cytoplasm possesses occasional mitochondria and microtubules and numerous pinocytotic vesicles. In fresh or formalin-fixed tissue, the fat droplet can be stained with osmic acid or with Sudan dyes, but in most histological preparations, the lipid has been extracted, leaving only the delicate protoplasmic envelope. Individual fat cells are surrounded by a fine network of reticular (argyrophil) fibers.

Fat cells are fully differentiated cells and are incapable of mitotic division. New fat cells, therefore, which may develop at any time within connective tissue, arise as a result of differentiation of more primitive cells (Fig. 3–15). Although fat cells, before they commence to store fat, resemble fibroblasts, it is likely that they arise directly from undifferentiated mesenchymal cells that are pres-

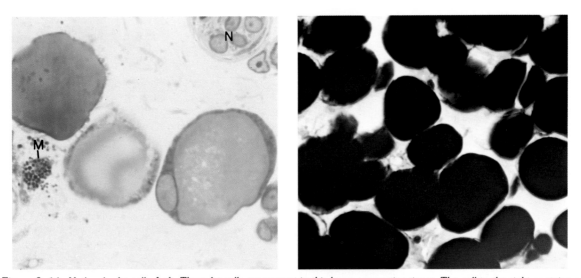

*Figure 3–14. Unilocular fat cells. Left: Three fat cells are present in this loose connective tissue. The cell to the right contains a single large droplet of fat surrounded by a thin rim of cytoplasm that contains a distinct ovoid nucleus. Because this tissue was fixed in osmic acid, the fat has been preserved. This section also shows a transverse section of a small nerve (N) and a mast cell (M), from which some granules have escaped into the surrounding matrix. Plastic section. Toluidine blue. High power. Right: Unilocular fat cells, in which the content of fat has been preserved, appear closely opposed in this section of white adipose tissue. No details of the protoplasmic envelope can be discerned. Osmic acid. Medium power.*

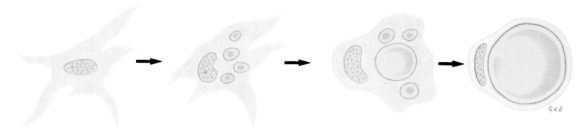

**Figure 3–15.** *Diagram illustrating the development of a fat cell.*

ent within the body, commonly as pericytes in relation to small blood vessels. Initially, small droplets of fat make their appearance within the cytoplasm. The droplets increase in size and finally coalesce to form a single large droplet, and the cytoplasm is reduced to a thin encompassing layer. The nucleus is compressed and flattened.

When fat is utilized, it leaves the cell as free fatty acids and glycerol (the same form in which it enters), and the cell takes on a wrinkled appearance. The mobilization of the stored fat is influenced by neural and hormonal factors, including the activation of lipase by norepinephrine.

### Macrophages

Often termed *histiocytes,* macrophages are almost as numerous as fibroblasts in loose connective tissue and are most abundant in richly vascularized areas. They may be either attached to the collagenous fibers of the matrix (*fixed macrophages*) or free within the amorphous ground substance (*free* or *wandering macrophages*). These two designations refer to different functional phases of cells of the same lineage. When stimulated, fixed macrophages detach from the collagenous fibers and migrate as free macrophages to sites of bacterial invasion or tissue injury.

Generally, macrophages are irregularly shaped cells with processes that usually are short and blunt. Occasionally, they may exhibit long, slender branching processes. When stimulated, macrophages are capable of ameboid movement, and in this phase, they are very irregular in outline with pseudopodia extending in numerous direc-

tions. The plasma membrane becomes pleated and exhibits numerous folds and delicate processes. These surface irregularities participate in spreading, cell movement, and phagocytosis.

Macrophages, which measure from 10 to 30 μm, possess a nucleus that is ovoid or indented and is smaller and more heterochromatic than that of the fibroblast. Nucleoli are inconspicuous. The cytoplasm is faintly basophilic and may contain a few small vacuoles that stain supravitally with neutral red. These cells, when they are activated, can be distinguished readily from fibroblasts, owing to their ability to ingest particulate matter. Sections of tissue from animals that have received injections vitally of colloidal carbon or of colloidal dyes, such as trypan blue, show macrophages with accumulations of the dye within vacuoles in the cytoplasm (Figs. 3–16 and 3–17). Fibroblasts contain little or none of the dye.

During phagocytosis, there is uptake of particulate matter by an invagination of the cell membrane. Once the phagocytosed particle, enclosed within the invaginated cell membrane, becomes detached and moves into the cytoplasm, it is referred to as a *phagosome.* Ingested organic material is destroyed by the action of the intracellular proteolytic enzymes, derived from primary lysosomes. The latter fuse with phagosomes to form secondary lysosomes, which later, as lysis proceeds, become residual bodies. Inert foreign material that resists digestion may remain in the cytoplasm indefinitely. An example of this is the inhaled carbon particles that accumulate within macrophages of the lung.

Macrophages are important agents of defense. Because of their mobility and phagocytic activity, they are able to act as scavengers, engulfing

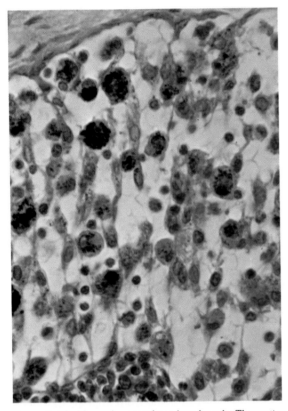

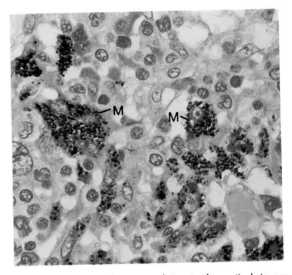

*Figure 3–17.* Macrophages in relation to the cortical sinuses of a lymph node. Most cells present in the cortex of this bronchial lymph node are small lymphocytes and plasma cells, but scattered among them are larger cells of irregular outline. These are perivascular macrophages (M) of the sinusoids that have phagocytosed carbon, an exogenous pigment present here as black granules. These macrophages (histiocytes) constitute an important component of the mononuclear phagocyte system. H and E. Medium power.

*Figure 3–16.* Macrophages within a lymph node. The section here shows a portion of the subcapsular sinus, which is bridged by reticular cells that are interconnected by delicate cytoplasmic processes. The macrophages are large and show accumulations of carbon particles within their cytoplasm. This particulate matter has been ingested by the cells from the surrounding lymph. H and E. High power.

stances, including enzymes such as lysozyme, elastase, and collagenase.

## MACROPHAGES AND THE MONONUCLEAR PHAGOCYTE SYSTEM

extravasated blood cells, dead cells, bacteria, and foreign bodies. When macrophages encounter large foreign bodies, they eventually fuse together to form multinucleated *foreign body giant cells*.

Macrophages also contribute to the immunological reactions of the body. They ingest, process, and store antigens and pass specific information to neighboring immunologically competent cells (lymphocytes and plasma cells). During infection, stimulated T lymphocytes produce a variety of *lymphokines* that attract macrophages to areas where they are needed, and proceed to activate them. Such activated macrophages are highly phagocytic. Macrophages also are secretory cells that produce and secrete several important sub-

The use of the word "system" here is somewhat unfortunate, since it refers to physiological and pathological considerations rather than to a discrete anatomical entity. It is a collective term for a widespread system of highly phagocytic cells. The cells possess no morphological characteristics that distinguish them with certainty from other cells. All cells of this system are derived from precursor cells within the bone marrow and are transported in the blood as monocytes. They migrate through the walls of small blood vessels and reside within tissues throughout the body. Classical histologists described this system of highly phagocytic cells as the *reticuloendothelial system*, but recent re-examination of these cells, particularly with regard to their origin and to cytokinetic studies, has led to the current concept of the mononuclear phagocyte system.

Cells of this system are found in the following situations:

1. In peripheral blood, where they are represented by the monocytes.

2. In connective tissues, where they correspond to the macrophages or histiocytes just described. They occur in large numbers in relation to small blood vessels and lymphatics of the subserous connective tissue of the pleura and peritoneum. In the latter situations, these pleural and peritoneal macrophages may be aggregated into small patches known as *milky spots.*

3. In the liver, lining the sinusoids, where they are known as *Kupffer's cells.*

4. Perivascular macrophages of sinusoids of the spleen, lymph nodes, and bone marrow.

5. In the lungs, as alveolar macrophages.

6. In the central nervous system, where they are termed *microglia.*

7. In bone, where they exist as multinucleated giant cells, the *osteoclasts.*

Because of their phagocytic and ameboid properties, these cells are active in the defense of the body against microorganisms. Additionally, they are intimately involved, along with other cells, in the antigen-antibody response and have receptor sites for immunoglobulins and complement upon their cell membranes.

### Mast Cells

Mast cells are widely distributed in connective tissues but tend to occur in small groups in relation to blood vessels. They are particularly common in connective tissue of rodents.

Mast cells, which exhibit several of the cytological and functional characteristics of basophil leukocytes, are identified easily by their content of cytoplasmic granules (Figs. 3–18 and 3–19). They are irregularly oval in outline and occasionally have short pseudopodia, an indication of their slow mobility. The nucleus is small and inconspicuous, often masked by the crowded granules. In most preparations, the cell membranes of many mast cells are ruptured, and their granules escape into the surrounding tissue.

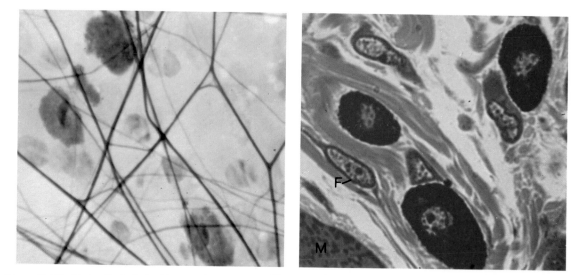

**Figure 3–18.** Mast cells. Left: *In this spread preparation of loose areolar connective tissue, elastic fibers (black) are slender and form a branching three-dimensional network. The mast cells are large, ovoid, darkly staining cells, the nuclei of which are masked by large numbers of cytoplasmic granules. H and E, orcein. High power.* Right: *Mast cells lie within the connective tissue between skeletal muscle fibers (M) of the tongue. They are ovoid and show large numbers of granules that stain metachromatically (dark purple). The nucleus of each cell appears as a pale-staining area, although, commonly, nuclei are masked by the crowded granules. Also present are collagenous fibers and a fibroblast (F). Plastic section. Toluidine blue. High power.*

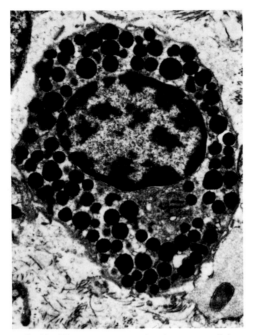

**Figure 3–19.** *Electron micrograph of a mast cell from rat omentum. The dense granules appear homogeneous in this species.* × 5500.

The granules are refractile and water-soluble and stain with basic dyes. Neutral red stains them supravitally a dark red-brown, and they exhibit metachromasia with basic aniline dyes such as methylene blue or azure A because of their content of heparin, a sulfated glycosaminoglycan. The granules also show a positive staining reaction with the periodic acid–Schiff reagent. In electron micrographs, the granules average 0.5 μm in diameter and are bounded by a unit membrane. The granular content varies with the species; in humans, it is quite heterogeneous and in the form of membranous whorls.

Mast cell granules contain several active substances. Quantitative studies have shown that tissues and organs in which mast cells are most numerous contain more heparin than do structures containing few mast cells. Mast cell tumors possess a heparin content many times greater than that of liver, which is used as a commercial source of the anticoagulant. Similar evidence has demonstrated that mast cells also contain and secrete histamine, which causes contraction of smooth muscle (mainly within the bronchioles), produces dilation of blood capillaries, and in-creases the permeability of blood capillaries. The mast cell granules of some species also contain serotonin, a vasoconstrictor.

In addition, mast cells release other pharmacologically active mediators, such as the eosinophil chemotactic factor of anaphylaxis (ECF-A) and the slow-reacting substance of anaphylaxis (SRS-A). ECF-A induces eosinophils to migrate from the blood to sites where activated mast cells are situated, and SRS-A produces slow contractions of smooth muscle and increases the permeability of small blood vessels.

The release of the chemical mediators from mast cells promotes the allergic reactions known as "immediate hypersensitivity reactions," including such phenomena as edema, shock, pain, hypercoagulation, and fever. Mediator release initially involves the invasion of the body by antigens. This stimulates the formation by plasma cells of antibodies belonging to immunoglobulin class E (IgE). Most IgE molecules are attached to the surface of mast cells and blood basophils. When the sensitized cells later are exposed to the same antigens, the antigens react with the IgE molecules and trigger the degranulation of the mast cells and the release of the chemical mediators.

The release reaction is an active process. Membranes of peripheral granules fuse with the cell membrane and discharge their contents. Simultaneously, membranes of granules more centrally placed fuse with each other, creating channels that connect with the cell surface. The process of degranulation is energy-dependent, requires calcium, and appears to involve microfilaments, since release is inhibited by cytochalasin, a compound that restrains their activity. Mast cells are not damaged by the process of extrusion and later proceed to synthesize new granules.

### Blood Leukocytes

Although leukocytes are transported by the blood stream, they perform their principal functions extravascularly, and thus it is not surprising that they are encountered within connective tissue. The two most frequently encountered leukocytes within normal connective tissue are lymphocytes and eosinophils, and a brief description of them follows. They are discussed in more detail in Chapter 5.

**Lymphocytes.** Lymphocytes are the smallest of the free cells of connective tissue, the majority being only 6 to 8 μm in diameter. They possess a spherical, darkly staining nucleus that occupies most of the cell. Around the nucleus is a thin rim of homogeneous cytoplasm that is basophil.

Lymphocytes are not seen in large numbers in connective tissue generally, but they are numerous in the connective tissue (lamina propria) that supports the epithelial lining of the respiratory and gastrointestinal tracts. Most lymphocytes present in loose connective tissue are thought to emigrate there from the blood stream.

The lymphocytes of connective tissue represent two distinct populations of cells, one with a brief life span and the other living for months or years. Functionally, at least two types are recognized: *T lymphocytes*, which are long-lived and responsible for initiating cell-mediated immune responses, and *B lymphocytes*. The latter are short-lived cells that, when stimulated by an antigen, are capable of active division and differentiation into plasma cells that synthesize antibodies against the stimulating antigen.

**Eosinophils.** These cells, like lymphocytes, emigrate from the blood stream into the connective tissue. They are not numerous in human connective tissue generally but are plentiful in connective tissue of the lactating breast and of the respiratory and gastrointestinal tracts. The nucleus is usually reniform or bilobed, and the cytoplasm contains spherical granules that are highly refractile and stain with acid dyes.

Eosinophils accumulate in the blood and in the tissues in allergic and subacute inflammatory conditions resulting from parasitic diseases. They are attracted to antigen-antibody complexes, which they later phagocytose, although they are relatively inactive in the phagocytosis of bacteria and foreign particles.

## Plasma Cells

These cells bear a resemblance to lymphocytes but generally are larger, with a diameter of 10 to 20 μm (Fig. 3–20). They possess more cytoplasm, which, like that of the lymphocytes, is basophil, and a nucleus that usually is eccentric in position. Within the nucleus, chromatin occurs in coarse clumps peripherally and often is arranged in a pattern suggestive of the spokes of a

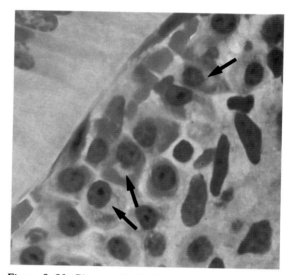

**Figure 3–20.** Plasma cells. In this section of the mucosa of the gastrointestinal tract, the epithelium is of the tall columnar type (upper left), and the loose areolar tissue of the lamina propria (center and lower right) is very cellular and contains numerous plasma cells. The cells generally are large and ovoid, with a densely staining nucleus that is eccentrically placed. Clumping of chromatin at the margin of the nucleus is apparent in most cells. The extensive cytoplasm is basophil and, in some cells, shows a negative Golgi image in a juxtanuclear position (arrows). Plastic section. H and E. High power.

wheel or the hours on a clock. Accordingly, the nucleus is described as having a cartwheel or clockface appearance. Adjacent to the nucleus, the cytoplasm contains a clear, rounded area that is the site of the centrosphere and the large Golgi apparatus. An extensive endoplasmic reticulum with associated ribosomes is the most conspicuous fine structural feature of the cytoplasm (Fig. 3–21).

Plasma cells are rare in connective tissue generally, but they are found frequently in serous membranes, lymphoid tissue, and the lamina propria of the gastrointestinal tract and are plentiful in sites of chronic inflammation. They represent a special differentiation of the lymphocyte, and their principal function is the production of antibodies, which are synthesized within the granular endoplasmic reticulum. The antibodies, immunoglobulins, are transported to the Golgi apparatus and, from there, to the cell surface in small vesicles. This is unusual, since protein-secreting cells normally package and store the secretion in large cytoplasmic granules.

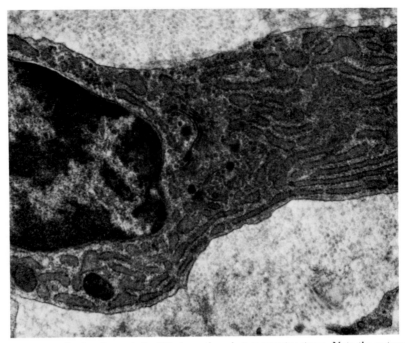

**Figure 3–21.** Electron micrograph of a plasma cell within loose (areolar) connective tissue. Note the extensive development of granular endoplasmic reticulum, many cisternae of which are dilated, and the coarse pattern of heterochromatin within the nucleus. × 24,000.

Occasionally, acidophil inclusions called *Russell's bodies* are present in the cytoplasm of plasma cells. Most authors believe that they do not represent the sites of large accumulations of secretory material but are indicative either of an aberrant state or of cellular aging and degeneration.

### Pigment Cells

Cells containing pigment (*chromatophores*) are rare in loose connective tissue but are found commonly in the dense connective tissue of the skin, in pia mater, and in the choroid coat of the eye. Other pigment cells, the *melanocytes*, which are derived from embryonic neural crest, also occur within the dermis of the skin. Typically, such cells have irregular cytoplasmic processes that, like the general cytoplasm, contain small granules of pigment, the *melanosomes*. In addition to melanocytes, the dermis may also contain *melanophores*, which are macrophages that have

phagocytosed melanosomes from disintegrating or aging melanocytes.

### TYPES OF CONNECTIVE TISSUE PROPER

The character of connective tissue varies greatly in different parts of the body. The appearance depends upon the relative proportions and arrangement of the cellular, fibrous, and amorphous components. The major subdivision in the classification of connective tissues is determined by the concentration of fibers. Connective tissues that show an abundance of compactly arranged fibers are referred to as *dense connective tissues*. In *loose connective tissues*, there are fewer fibers and relatively more cells. Loose connective tissues may be further subdivided into those that are present only in the embryo (*mesenchyme* and *mucous connective tissue*) and those that are found in the adult. The latter include *loose areolar connective tissue*, *adipose tissue*, and *reticular tissue*.

## Loose Connective Tissues

### MESENCHYME

Mesenchyme, as mentioned in the introduction to this chapter, is the typical, unspecialized connective tissue of the early weeks of embryonic life. Subsequently, it disappears as such when component cells undergo differentiation. It is composed of mesenchymal cells, whose branching processes often appear to join, although they do not form a true syncytium, and of a ground substance that is a coagulable fluid in the earliest stages but later contains fine reticular fibers (Fig. 3–22). The reticular fibers gradually are replaced by collagenous fibers as the mesenchyme develops and differentiates into the adult connective tissues.

### MUCOUS CONNECTIVE TISSUE

This is the transient type of tissue that appears in the normal development and differentiation of the connective tissues. It occurs also as Wharton's jelly in the umbilical cord, where it does not differentiate further (Fig. 3–23).

Component cells are large, stellate fibroblasts whose processes often appear to fuse with those of neighboring cells. A few macrophages and wandering lymphocytes are encountered occasionally. The ground substance is especially abundant and is soft and jelly-like. It gives a mucin reaction and stains metachromatically with toluidine blue, and contains a delicate meshwork of fine collagenous fibers.

### LOOSE (AREOLAR) CONNECTIVE TISSUE

Loose connective tissue is formed by the direct differentiation of mesenchyme (Fig. 3–24). It is a loosely arranged, fibroelastic connective tissue and is encountered in almost every microscopic section of the body, since it is the packing and anchoring material and the embedding medium of many structures, including nerves and blood and lymphatic vessels. It binds other tissues, organ components, and organs together and allows, owing to its flexibility, a considerable degree of mobility between such parts.

All the structural elements, amorphous ground substance, fibers, and cells, previously described, are present within it. The two most common cell types are fibroblasts and macrophages. Collagenous fibers are most prominent; elastic fibers, which form a continuous branching network, are relatively inconspicuous. Reticular fibers are repre-

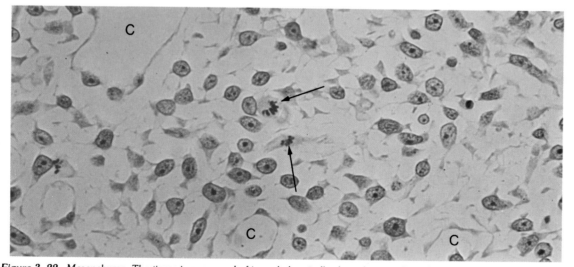

**Figure 3–22.** Mesenchyme. The tissue is composed of irregularly spindle-shaped mesenchymal cells with processes that extend into a relatively homogeneous ground substance containing sparse reticular fibers (not visible here). The cells show a spherical or ovoid nucleus with a distinct nucleolus. Two cells (arrows) are in the process of mitosis. The tissue is vascular, and portions of three small blood vessels (C), lined by a delicate endothelium, are present. Plastic section. H and E. High power.

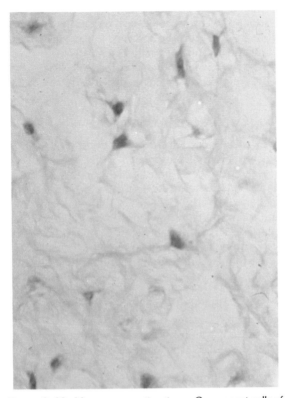

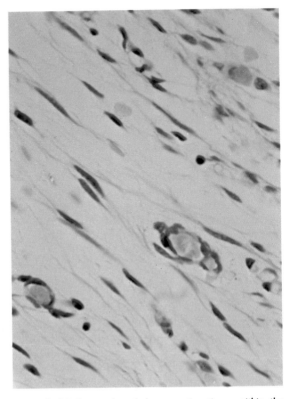

*Figure 3–23. Mucous connective tissue. Component cells of this tissue, present within the umbilical cord, are large, stellate fibroblasts with spherical or ovoid nuclei. Delicate collagenous fibers (pink) form a loose network within the ground substance and show no definite spatial organization. H and E. Medium power.*

*Figure 3–24. Loose (areolar) connective tissue within the fetal hypodermis. Early during fetal life, the hypodermis is composed of mesenchyme. As development proceeds, differentiation into loose connective tissue occurs. In this section fibroblasts constitute the principal cell type. They appear fusiform; since they generally have been sectioned on the side, their nuclei appear slender and densely stained. Collagenous fibers are delicate, and elastic fibers are not visualized. The tissue is vascular and shows numerous small blood vessels, sectioned transversely. H and E. Medium power.*

sented also but are abundant only where areolar tissue borders upon other structures. The ground substance is relatively fluid-like and occupies many little areas (*areolae*) in which no structure ordinarily can be seen in sectioned material. The tissue generally is richly vascularized.

Areolar connective tissue is studied usually in two different types of histological material. It can be found in most sectioned material and can be examined also in spread preparations of subcutaneous tissue and of mesentery. Study of sectioned material alone, although it reveals many important cytological details, does not easily demonstrate the three-dimensional organization of areolar connective tissue. In spread preparations, unlike sectioned material, whole cells are viewed, and the pattern of the fiber networks can be discerned.

## WHITE ADIPOSE TISSUE

Fat cells are scattered in areolar connective tissue. When fat cells form large aggregations and are the principal cell type, the tissue is designated adipose tissue. Since each fat cell contains a single large droplet of oil, the tissue often is termed *unilocular* adipose tissue (Fig. 3–25).

Each fat cell is surrounded by a web of fine reticular fibers; in the spaces between are fibroblasts, lymphoid cells, eosinophils, and occasional macrophages and mast cells. The closely packed fat cells form *lobules*, separated by fibrous septa. There is a rich network of blood capillaries in and between the lobules. The richness of the blood

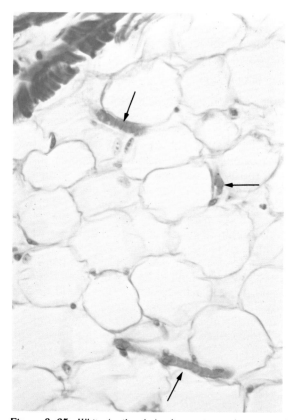

*Figure 3–25.* White (unilocular) adipose tissue. A portion of a lobule of adipose tissue is shown, and a fibrous septum, composed principally of collagenous fibers (blue), is present at the top left. The adipose tissue exhibits its characteristic meshwork appearance, and each space represents the site of the single large droplet of lipid removed during preparation. The blue-stained material surrounding each space is the thin rim of cytoplasm together with some intervening connective tissue, principally reticular fibers. Occasional nuclei (red) may be seen within the thin rim of cytoplasm. Blood capillaries (arrows), containing red blood cells, indicate the rich vascularity of this tissue. Mallory's stain. Medium power.

supply is indicative of the high metabolic acitivity of adipose tissue.

It should be appreciated that adipose tissue is not static. There is a vital balance between deposits and withdrawals of fat. Fat contained within fat cells may be derived from three sources:

1. Fat cells, under the influence of the hormone insulin, can synthesize fat from *carbohydrate.*

2. Fat cells also can produce fat from *fatty acids,* which are derived from the breakdown of dietary fat and which are brought to the cells as *chylomicrons* from the small intestine.

3. Fatty acids may be synthesized from *glucose* in the liver. The resulting triglycerides are transported to the fat cells as very low-density *lipoproteins.*

Fat from different sources differs chemically. Dietary fat may be saturated or unsaturated, depending upon the individual diet. Fat that is synthesized from carbohydrate is mostly saturated.

Withdrawals of fat result from enzymic hydrolysis of stored fat and release of free fatty acids and glycerol in the blood stream. If there is a continuous supply of glucose, withdrawals are negligible. The normal balance is affected by hormones (principally insulin) and by the autonomic nervous system. Insulin accelerates the conversion of glucose into triglycerides by the fat cells. Norepinephrine, on the other hand, activates the lipases that break down the triglyceride molecules during mobilization of fat from adipose tissue.

Adipose tissue may develop almost anywhere areolar tissue is plentiful, but in humans, the most common sites of fat accumulation are in the subcutaneous tissues (where it is referred to as the *panniculus adiposus*), in the mesenteries and omenta, in bone marrow, and around the kidneys. The distribution and density of adipose deposits within the subcutaneous tissues differ in the two sexes and, in part, account for the differences in body form. In the female, principal areas of fat accumulation are the breasts, the buttocks, and the anterior and lateral aspects of the thighs. In the male, subcutaneous fat is preferentially located in areas overlying the shoulder and upper arm, the nape of the neck, the buttocks, and the lumbosacral region. In addition to the primary function of storage and metabolism of neutral fat, in subcutaneous areas the adipose tissue also acts as a good shock absorber and insulator to prevent excessive heat loss or gain through the skin.

### BROWN ADIPOSE TISSUE

Brown adipose tissue is a special type of adipose tissue that is concerned with heat production, particularly important in newborn and in young animals exposed to cold. It is common in mammals that hibernate. In humans, it is relatively common in the fetus and in children, but in the adult it is restricted in its distribution to the neck and to regions around the abdominal aorta and kidney.

The extremely rich blood supply of brown adipose tissue, together with the presence of abundant cytochromes in the mitochondria of its cells, gives the tissue its color (Fig. 3–26). The fat cells are smaller than those of white adipose tissue, and their cytoplasm contains multiple lipid droplets of varying size that do not coalesce. These droplets generally appear as vacuoles after routine histological preparation: Thus, brown adipose tissue is referred to as *multilocular* in contrast with unilocular white adipose tissue. Mitochondria are large and numerous, and their cristae are closely packed and extend completely across the organelles.

The fat cells are directly innervated by sympathetic adrenergic neurons, the naked axons of which frequently are encountered in close relationship with the surface of the fat cells. Unlike white fat, brown fat is not readily affected by changes in the nutritional state of the animal, but lipid is mobilized from the fat cells and heat is generated following stimulation by the sympathetic nervous system.

## RETICULAR TISSUE

This is a primitive type of connective tissue that is characterized by the presence of a network of reticular fibers associated with *primitive reticular cells* (Fig. 3–27). These cells are stellate and have long cytoplasmic extensions that appear to join with those of other cells. In appearance they are not unlike mesenchymal cells. They have large, pale nuclei, with distinct nucleoli, and abundant basophil cytoplasm.

Although reticular fibers are distributed widely in the body in association with fibroblasts, reticular fibers in association with reticular cells (i.e., reticular tissue) are limited to certain sites. Reticular tissue forms the framework of lymphoid organs, bone marrow, and liver. In appearance it resembles embryonic mesenchyme but is largely inconspicuous, since the interstices of the tissue nor-

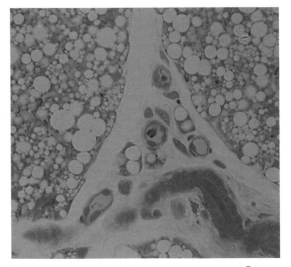

**Figure 3–26.** *Brown (multilocular) adipose tissue. Portions of two lobules of brown adipose tissue are shown, separated by loose connective tissue containing numerous small blood vessels (bottom center). The fat cells are closely packed, and their cell boundaries are indistinct. Each cell shows a spherical nucleus and contains numerous lipid droplets, here removed during preparation, that do not coalesce. Thus, brown adipose tissue is referred to as* multilocular, *in contrast to unilocular white adipose tissue. Plastic section. H and E. Medium power.*

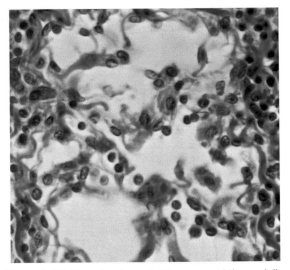

**Figure 3–27.** *Reticular tissue. In this section of the medulla of a lymph node, the majority of the field is occupied by reticular tissue. Reticular cells, interconnected by delicate cytoplasmic processes, form a network that delineates irregular medullary sinuses. The cells are supported by reticular (argyrophil) fibers, not stained specifically in this preparation. At the periphery (left and right), there are concentrations of small lymphocytes that form medullary cords. Mallory's stain. Medium power.*

mally are crowded with other cell types, principally lymphocytes and other blood cells.

## Dense Connective Tissues

Dense connective tissues are characterized by the close packing of their fibers. Cells are proportionally fewer than in loose connective tissues, and there is less amorphous ground substance. In areas where tensions are exerted in multiple directions, the fibers are interwoven and without regular orientation and the tissues are termed *irregularly arranged*. In structures subject to tension in one direction, the fibers have an orderly parallel arrangement, and the tissues are designated *regularly arranged*. In most regions, collagenous fibers are the principal component, but in a few ligaments, elastic fibers predominate.

### DENSE IRREGULAR CONNECTIVE TISSUE

This tissue occurs in sheets, its fibers interlacing to form a coarse, tough feltwork (Fig. 3–28). Dense irregularly arranged connective tissue forms the basis of most fascias; the dermis of the skin; the fibrous capsules of some organs, including testis, liver, and lymph nodes; and the fibrous sheaths of bone (*periosteum*) and of cartilage (*perichondrium*) (Fig. 3–29).

Although coarse collagenous fibers are the main component, elastic and reticular fibers, particularly within the dermis, are present also. There is little ground substance, and the cells, principally fibroblasts, located among the densely packed fibers, are difficult to identify.

### DENSE REGULAR CONNECTIVE TISSUE

This tissue contains fibers that are densely packed and lie parallel to each other, forming structures of great tensile strength. This group includes tendons, ligaments, and aponeuroses (Fig. 3–30). The latter two are less regularly arranged than tendons but, in general, have a similar organization.

In *tendons*, the collagenous fibers, or *primary tendon bundles*, run parallel courses (Fig. 3–31). Each fiber or bundle is composed of a large number of fibrils of varying sizes. Fibroblasts, or *tendon cells*, are the only cell type present, and in longitudinal sections of tendon, they are aligned

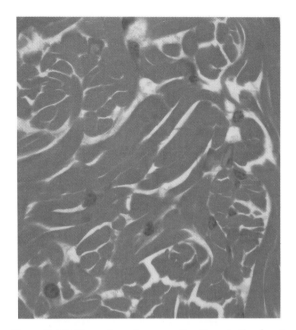

*Figure 3–28.* Dense irregular connective tissue in the dermis of the skin. The coarse collagenous fibers are randomly oriented. There is little ground substance and few cells, principally fibroblasts, that are difficult to identify. H and E. High power.

in rows between the collagenous fibers. Cytoplasm of the cells often is indistinct. In cross sections, the cells appear stellate with cytoplasmic processes extending between the collagenous bundles.

Each primary bundle is covered by a small amount of loose areolar (fibroelastic) connective tissue, termed the *endotendineum*. Generally, several primary bundles are grouped together into secondary bundles or fascicles bounded by a coarser type of connective tissue, the *peritendineum*. The tendon itself, composed of a number of fascicles, is ensheathed by thick connective tissue called the *epitendineum*.* Nerves and blood vessels course in the major connective tissue septa but do not invade the fascicles.

*Ligaments* are similar to tendons, but the collagenous elements are somewhat less regularly arranged. *Aponeuroses* have the same composi-

---

*Note on terminology: The prefixed "endo-," "peri-," and "epi-" indicate a progression in size. They also are used in reference to muscle with the word stem "-mysium" and to nerve with the word stem "-neurium."

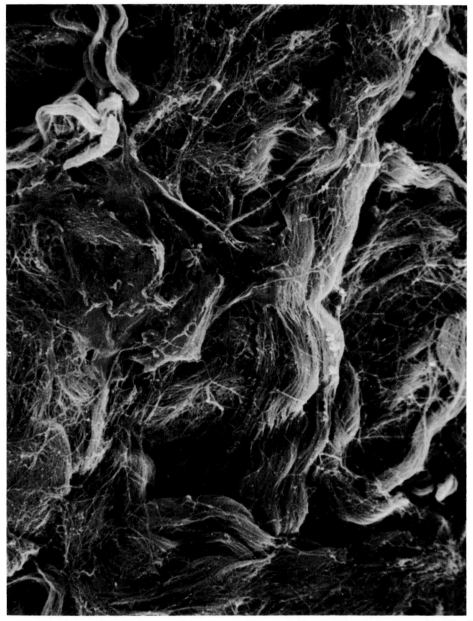

**Figure 3–29.** A scanning electron micrograph of dense, irregularly arranged connective tissue. Note the network of delicate fibrils and coarse collagenous fibers in association with a fibroblast (f). × 1500. (Courtesy of Dr. P. M. Andrews.)

tion as tendons and ligaments but are broad and flat. Generally, the collagenous fibers are arranged in multiple sheets or layers, with those in one layer running at an angle to those of neighboring layers. The layers often interweave, and an isolation of the layers seldom is possible. Most ligaments have a similar composition, but a few are composed almost entirely of elastic fibers.

**Figure 3–30.** *Dense regular connective tissue. Tendon, here sectioned longitudinally, is an example of dense regular connective tissue in which the principal fibrous component is collagen. Each collagenous fiber (pink), or primary tendon bundle, possesses a longitudinal striation, since it is composed of a large number of fibrils. The fibers tend to follow a wavy course. Fibroblasts, or tendon cells, are aligned in rows between the collagenous fibers. Their cytoplasm is indistinct, and only the elongated nuclei (blue-purple) are seen. The collagenous fibers are grouped into fascicles or secondary bundles, each bounded by a more cellular connective tissue, the peritendineum (arrows). H and E. Medium power.*

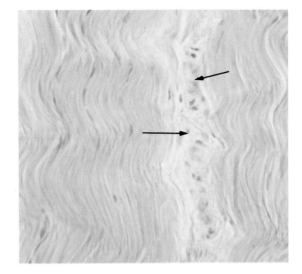

## ELASTIC TISSUE

In *yellow elastic ligaments*, coarse parallel fibers of elastic tissue are bound together by a small amount of delicate connective tissue, in which typical fibroblasts are present (Fig. 3–32). The elastic fibers, 10 to 15 μm in diameter, branch frequently and fuse with one another. Individual fibers are surrounded by a delicate network of reticular fibers. Yellow elastic ligaments show numerous oval or elongated nuclei of fibroblasts, with little associated cytoplasm, between the parallel elastic fibers. This is one feature of elastic

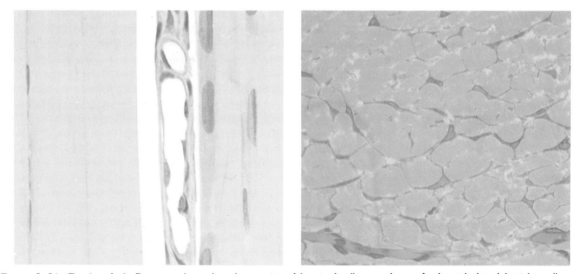

**Figure 3–31.** *Tendon. Left: Portions of two fascicles, sectioned longitudinally, are shown. In the right-hand fascicle, collagen fibers are separated by fibroblast nuclei that appear ovoid. No associated cytoplasm is visible. In the left-hand fascicle, fibroblast nuclei are sectioned on the side and appear dense and elongated. A portion of the cellular peritendineum, containing small blood vessels, occupies the center of the field. Right: Tendon, sectioned transversely. The fibroblasts, or tendon cells, appear stellate with delicate cytoplasmic processes extending between the large collagenous fibers. Blood capillaries lie within a connective tissue septum (bottom). Plastic sections. H and E. High power.*

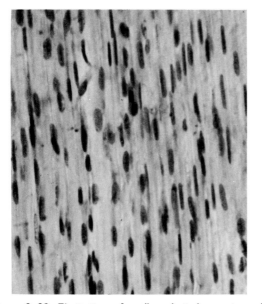

**Figure 3–32.** *Elastic tissue. In yellow elastic ligaments, such as this ligamentum nuchae of ox sectioned longitudinally, the large, parallel elastic fibers are separated by numerous ovoid or elongated nuclei of fibroblasts, with little associated cytoplasm. Fibroblasts are much less frequent in tendons. Compare with Figure 3–30. H and E. High power.*

ligaments that distinguishes them histologically from tendons and collagenous ligaments, in which fibroblasts are sparse and their nuclei markedly flattened.

The most typical form of yellow elastic ligament is found in the ligamentum nuchae of quadrupeds. In humans, examples are found in the ligamenta flava of the vertebrae, the suspensory ligament of the penis, and the true vocal cords.

## SUMMARY

The basic function of connective tissues is mechanical. The connective tissues provide the supporting framework for the body and bind together and compartmentalize other tissues and organs. All connective tissues develop from mesenchyme, and their component cells are embedded within a matrix composed of an amorphous ground substance and fibers. These elements are bathed in tissue fluid, which allows transport in solution of oxygen, nutritive materials, carbon dioxide,

and waste products between blood capillaries and cells to permit cellular metabolism and excretion.

The amorphous ground substance is composed principally of glycosaminoglycans and glycoproteins. The principal glycosaminoglycans are hyaluronic acid, chondroitin sulfate, dermatan sulfate, keratan sulfate, and heparan sulfate. With the exception of hyaluronic acid, all are sulfated and are linked covalently to protein as proteoglycans. The glycoproteins, which differ from proteoglycans in their higher proportion of protein and in the branching nature of their carbohydrate moiety, include fibronectin, chondronectin, and laminin.

The fibrous intercellular substances provide support and tensile strength for the tissues. Three types of formed fibers exist—collagenous, reticular, and elastic—and all are complex proteins formed by long polypeptide chains. Collagenous fibers are composed of macromolecules of tropocollagen, each consisting of three polypeptide chains that form a superhelix. There are two classes of chains, alpha-1 and alpha-2, and the various types of collagenous fibers differ from each other in the primary structure of their constituent polypeptide chains. The most important types of collagen are summarized in Summary Table 3–1. Reticular fibers are fine collagenous fibers, the collagenous component of which is principally type III collagen. They are stained black by impregnation with silver salts, and thus they are termed argyrophil. Elastic fibers, composed of the albuminoid elastin, can be stained selectively with orcein, resorcin-fuchsin, and aldehyde-fuchsin. They allow connective tissues to undergo considerable expansion or stretching and permit recovery to the original dimension or shape on removal of the deforming force. Basal laminae, present beneath epithelia and around muscles, nerves, and capillaries, consist largely of type IV collagen, laminin, and proteoglycans. They provide a strong connection between epithelia and the underlying connective tissue and act as filtration barriers.

The cells found within connective tissues are of many different types. Some are responsible for the production and maintenance of the amorphous and fibrous intercellular substances, and others make a significant contribution to the defense mechanisms of the body. Fibroblasts, one of the two most common cell types, elaborate the

| Collagen Type | Molecular Formula | Morphological Features | Distribution | Site of Synthesis |
|---|---|---|---|---|
| | | **Summary Table 3–1. Characteristics of the Different Collagen Types** | | |
| I | Two alpha-1 (type I) and one alpha-2 (type I) | Thick-banded fibrils | Widespread: dermis, tendon, bone, teeth, fascias, capsules, fibrocartilage | Fibroblast, osteoblast, odontoblast, chondroblast |
| II | Three alpha-1 (type II) | Delicate, banded fibrils | Cartilaginous matrix | Chondroblast |
| III | Three alpha-1 (type III) | Small-diameter banded fibrils, argyrophilic reticular fibers | Reticular networks in skin, blood vessels, uterus, liver, spleen, gastrointestinal tract | Fibroblast, smooth muscle cells, reticular cells |
| IV | Three alpha-1 (type IV) | Feltwork of nonbanded material | Basal laminae | Endothelial and epithelial cells |
| V | Insufficient data | Feltwork of nonbanded material | Basal laminae | Insufficient data |

amorphous and fibrous intercellular substances and are responsible for their maintenance. Undifferentiated mesenchymal cells, located in the adult principally as pericytes in relation to the walls of small blood vessels, represent a reserve of undifferentiated cells that serve as a source of new connective tissue cells, principally fibroblasts, and

smooth muscle cells. Fat cells may be either unilocular (white) or multilocular (brown). The former are the major energy reservoir of the body, whereas the latter cells, prominent in the newborn and in hibernating animals, help maintain body heat. Macrophages, almost as numerous as fibroblasts in loose connective tissue, are intensely

| Type | Location | Principal Components |
|---|---|---|
| | | **Summary Table 3–2. Types of Connective Tissue Proper** |
| **LOOSE CONNECTIVE TISSUES** | | |
| Mesenchyme | Primarily in embryo | Mesenchymal cells, ground substance, and scattered reticular fibers |
| Mucous connective tissue | Umbilical cord | Stellate fibroblasts, abundant ground substance, fine collagenous fibers |
| Loose (areolar) connective tissue | Widespread as packing and anchoring material | All connective tissue cells, but principally fibroblasts and macrophages, ground substance, and collagenous, elastic and reticular fibers |
| White adipose tissue | Subcutaneous tissues, omenta | Unilocular fat cells, fine reticular fibers; arranged in lobules |
| Brown adipose tissue | Embryo, neck, abdomen | Multilocular fat cells; richly vascularized |
| Reticular tissue | Lymphoid organs, bone marrow | Reticular cells, reticular fibers |
| **DENSE CONNECTIVE TISSUES** | | |
| Irregularly arranged | Dermis, fascias, capsules of organs, periosteum, perichondrium | Fibroblasts, collagenous fibers |
| Regularly arranged | Tendons, ligaments, aponeuroses | Collagenous fibers (primary tendon bundles), fibroblasts (tendon cells) |
| Elastic tissue | Yellow elastic ligaments: ligamentum nuchae, ligamenta flava | Elastic fibers, fibroblasts |

phagocytic cells that are important agents of defense. They are derived from monocytes and constitute a significant component of the mononuclear phagocyte system. Mast cells possess metachromatic cytoplasmic granules that contain several pharmacologically active substances, including heparin and histamine. They degranulate in response to interaction of an antigen with IgE bound to their surface. Blood leukocytes found within the connective tissues include lymphocytes of two types and eosinophils. T lymphocytes initiate cell-mediated immune responses, and B lymphocytes are capable of differentiating into plasma cells. Plasma cells, which possess an eccentric nucleus with a cartwheel or clockface appearance, contain an extensive granular endoplasmic reticulum and produce antibodies, immunoglobulins, against stimulating antigens.

Connective tissues proper may be subdivided into two types: dense connective tissues, which contain an abundance of fibrous intercellular substances, and loose connective tissues, in which there are fewer fibers and relatively more cells. Loose connective tissues include mesenchyme, mucous connective tissue, loose areolar connective tissue, adipose tissue, and reticular tissue. In dense connective tissues, component fibers may be irregularly arranged, as in most fascias and in the dermis of the skin, or regularly arranged, as in tendons, ligaments, and aponeuroses. The principal fibrous component of most dense connective tissues is collagen, but in yellow elastic ligaments, elastic fibers predominate. The main features of the various types of connective tissue proper are summarized in Summary Table 3–2.

# Specialized Connective Tissue: Cartilage and Bone

## GENERAL ORGANIZATION

Cartilage and bone, the skeletal tissues, are specialized types of supporting tissues. Like connective tissue, they consist of *cells*, *fibers*, and *ground substance*. The latter two constitute the intercellular substance, or *matrix*. They differ from the connective tissues discussed previously in the rigidity of their matrices. Cartilage ground substance consists principally of proteoglycans (chondroitin sulfate) and glycoproteins. The connective tissues that have been described up to this point all have thin or, at most, semisolid matrices. With a firm matrix, such as chondroitin, cartilage is able to function as a structural support. At the same time, the presence of fibers in the matrix imparts a certain amount of flexibility to cartilage. In bone, the ground substance has become modified through impregnation with certain inorganic materials. The most important of these

4

salts are calcium phosphate, which is the most abundant, calcium carbonate, calcium fluoride, and magnesium chloride; the last two named being present only in small quantities.

## CARTILAGE

Cartilage develops from mesenchyme, as do the other supporting tissues (Fig. 4–1). In an area where cartilage will develop, mesenchymal cells round up and become closely packed, and collagenous fibrils are deposited within the intracellular substance. The original fibers and matrix of cartilage are formed by cells called *chondroblasts*. Each chondroblast becomes surrounded by the fibers and matrix that it produces. As a result, the cartilage-forming cells eventually occupy small spaces called *lacunae*. As cells differentiate further

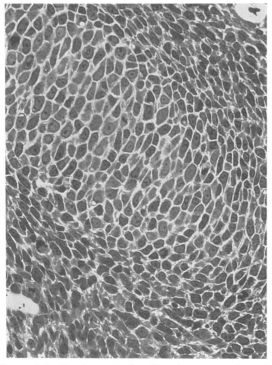

*Figure 4–1. Development of cartilage from mesenchyme in rat embryo. The mesenchyme (above and below) gradually merges into the protochondral tissue with interstitial substance (center). H and E. Medium power.*

and gradually become more separated as a result of elaboration of matrix around them, they acquire the characteristics of mature cartilage cells, or *chondrocytes*. They accumulate vacuoles, lipid, and glycogen. The matrix is nonvascular—that is, it does not contain blood vessels. The only blood supply to cartilage is provided by blood vessels found in the inner layer of the *perichondrium*—a fibrous connective tissue membrane, derived from the mesenchyme, surrounding the enlarging mass of cartilage. The perichondrium merges gradually into the cartilage on one side and into the surrounding connective tissue on the other. Vessels and nerves enter the perichondrium from the surrounding loose connective tissue. For nourishment, then, chondrocytes depend on the diffusion of nutrients through the matrix from capillaries located in the perichondrium or from the synovial fluid of joint cavities. Similarly, waste materials must diffuse from the cells to the vascular perichondrium. As growth and development proceed, the amount of matrix between cells increases, pushing them farther apart, so that ultimately the condition is reached in which the cells lie in lacunae scattered through a relatively large amount of intercellular substance. For a time, growth may be effected *interstitially* (or *endogenously*) by the division of cartilage cells and the laying down of matrix around each daughter cell. Later, however, the increasing solidity of the matrix renders this type of growth more difficult, and increase in size of the cartilage plate is caused by the addition of new layers at the periphery by the cells of the perichondrium (*appositional* or *exogenous* growth). It results from activity within the inner layer of the perichondrium. Fibroblasts in the perichondrium multiply by division, and some transform into cartilage cells and surround themselves with intercellular substance. These, in time, become overlaid by still newer cells and matrix added from the perichondrium. In adult cartilage, one may find two or four lacunae close together separated by very thin walls of matrix. These indicate that interstitial growth is proceeding with difficulty.

Cartilage forms the skeleton of the embryo and is exemplified in the adult by the tracheal rings. The matrix contains collagenous or elastic fibers that increase the tensile strength and elasticity, respectively, and adapt the tissue to the mechanical requirements of different regions of the body.

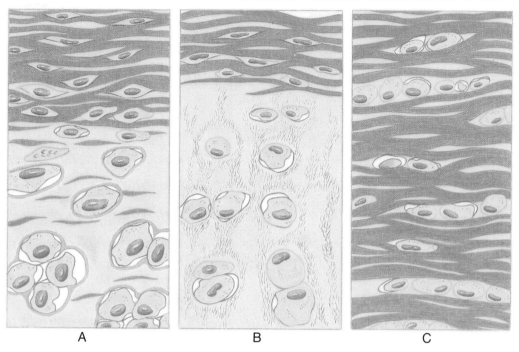

*Figure 4–2.* Diagram of the three types of cartilage. The diagrams of hyaline (A) and elastic cartilage (B) show perichondrium above. Note that intercellular elastic and collagenous fibers are prominent, respectively, in elastic cartilage (B) and fibrocartilage (C). A also illustrates both appositional (above) and interstitial (below) forms of growth.

The differences in the kind and abundance of fibers incorporated within the matrix form the basis of classification. There are three generally recognized varieties of adult human cartilage: *hyaline cartilage, elastic cartilage,* and *fibrocartilage* (Fig. 4–2). It is stressed that this terminology is artificial and that a continuous spectrum of intermediate cartilage tissue types is frequently observed. Pathological tissues surely do not respect classifications, and, accordingly, the student must be prepared to recognize mixtures of these types. Hyaline cartilage is the most prevalent and widespread type; the others are variations upon this basic theme, varying in fiber content, biochemical constitution, and biophysical function.

### Hyaline Cartilage

In the adult, hyaline cartilage is found covering the articular surfaces of most joints and in the costal cartilages, the nasal cartilages, and the walls of the respiratory passageways. The word "hyaline" is derived from the Greek *hyalos,* meaning glass. Hyaline cartilage appears as a translucent, bluish-white mass in the fresh condition. It is more widespread in the fetus, forming the basis for most of the skeleton, where it is gradually replaced by bone in the process of endochondral ossification. With the exception of the articular cartilages, this tissue is always covered by perichondrium. Hyaline cartilage lacks both blood vessels and nerves. This tissue is relatively cellular.

**The Cells.** The *cartilage cells,* or *chondrocytes,* are present in the lacunae of the matrix (Fig. 4–3). They are large, reaching diameters of 40 μm. The young cells are flattened or elliptical, with their long axis parallel to the surface. Toward the interior, they become oval or hypertrophied and lie within *cell nests* or isogenous groups (Fig. 4–4). The chondrocytes undergo a great deal of shrinkage during the technical preparation and, therefore, seldom conform to the shape of the lacunae.

The nucleus is ovoid, and one or two nucleoli are present. The cytoplasmic organelles of chondrocytes are similar to those found in fibroblasts, which also synthesize extracellular matrix (Fig.

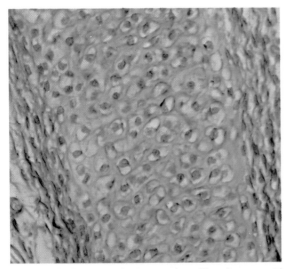

*Figure 4–3.* Embryonic hyaline cartilage. Chondrocytes, with spherical nuclei (red) and a vacuolated cytoplasm, are closely packed and generally uniform in size. They are separated by little intercellular substance (pale blue). At the periphery of the cartilage mass, the surrounding mesenchyme is concentrated as the perichondrium (left and right). Component cells here are elongated and are associated with concentrations of collagenous fibers (dark blue). The perichondrium merges gradually into the cartilage on one side and into the surrounding mesenchyme on the other. Mallory's stain. Medium power.

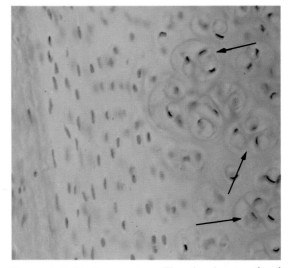

*Figure 4–4.* Hyaline cartilage. The chondrocytes that lie centrally within mature hyaline cartilage are large and tend to be arranged in groups, or cell "nests" (arrows). Each group represents the offspring of a single parent chondrocyte (interstitial growth). Peripherally, the cells are smaller and individually arranged. All chondrocytes occupy lacunae within the matrix, which appears homogeneous and stains blue-gray. Collagenous fibers within the matrix are not readily apparent. The perichondrium (left) is composed of fibroblasts, with dense, elongated nuclei, and of elastic and collagenous fibers (pink). Next to the cartilage, the perichondrium appears more cellular and merges into cartilage. This appearance indicates that cells of the inner zone of perichondrium may transform into cartilage cells and surround themselves with intercellular substance (appositional growth). H and E. Medium power.

4–5). There is an abundance of granular endoplasmic reticulum and a prominent Golgi complex. The cytoplasm of cartilage cells is basophilic and may be vacuolated; lipid droplets, glycogen, mitochondria, and pigment are present (Figs. 4–6 through 4–8). Secretory vesicles are associated with the Golgi region and secrete material into the surrounding matrix. The mature cartilage cells are generally found toward the center of the cartilage mass. The latter cells show less abundant rough endoplasmic reticulum and Golgi region with large accumulations of cytoplasmic glycogen. In fetal cartilage, the cells often are flattened, and cell nests are seen rarely.

**The Matrix.** Although the matrix appears homogeneous in the fresh condition and after ordinary fixation, it contains considerable quantities of both formed and amorphous kinds of intercellular substance. The formed kind is represented by collagenous fibers that form a feltwork that permeates the stiff, gelatinous ground substance of the matrix. The collagenous fibers are not

visible in fresh preparations, because most are in the form of submicroscopic fibrils and have a refractive index very close to that of the surrounding ground substance. However, these fibers may be readily visualized either by removing the gelatinous ground substance by tryptic digestion or by polarized light microscopy. They can be seen readily in electron micrographs. These micrographs reveal that the fibers and fibrils of cartilage matrix are finer than those of fibrous or dense connective tissue. Bundles of collagen have been seen only in articular hyaline cartilage. The collagen of cartilage differs from that of tendon and skin in that it consists of triple helices of three alpha-1 (type II) proteins. These collagen fibers have a variable periodicity and fail to show the characteristic 640 A banding seen in connective tissue and bone. The collagen present in most

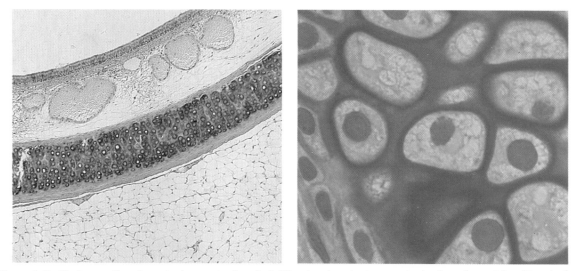

*Figure 4–5.* Hyaline cartilage from the human trachea. Left: The chondrocytes increase in size from the perichondrium to the interior of the cartilage. H and E. Low power. Right: This section shows a narrow band of hyaline cartilage surfaced by perichondrium (lower left). Lacunae within the matrix, occupied by chondrocytes, are not readily apparent, since the chondrocytes completely fill and conform to the shape of the lacunae. The cells show a finely granular cytoplasm that contains discrete vacuoles, which represent the sites of fat droplets lost during preparation. The matrix surrounding chondrocytes is rich in proteoglycans and stains intensely (territorial matrix of the cartilage capsules). Plastic section. Alcian blue. High power.

hyaline cartilage is probably less polymerized than other types of connective tissue. However, when cartilage cells are cultured at low density, they undergo a fundamental change. They cease to make type II collagen and, instead, begin to make type I collagen, which is characteristic of fibroblasts. It seems that the chondrocytes have been converted into fibroblasts. The switch must occur abruptly, since very few cells are ever observed to make both types of collagen simultaneously.

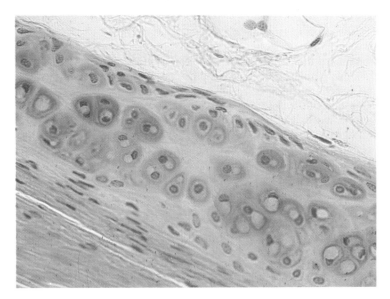

*Figure 4–6.* Hyaline cartilage from human trachea. Cell nests and cartilage capsules are evident within the interior of the cartilage. The large vacuoles within the cytoplasm of many chondrocytes represent the sites of fat droplets lost during preparation. An intact perichondrium is present at the lower surface. H and E. Medium power.

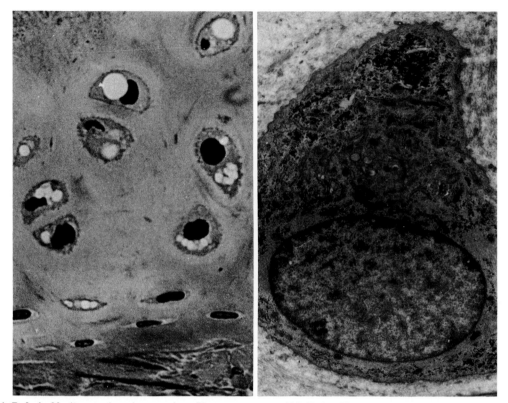

**Figure 4–7.** Left: *Hyaline cartilage from trachea. Plastic section.* × *600.* Right: *Electron micrograph of a chondrocyte from tracheal cartilage. The dark granular mass in the cytoplasm (above) is glycogen.* × *5800.*

The extracellular matrix that a cell secretes would seem to help maintain the cell's differentiated state.

The ground substance of cartilage is markedly basophil owing to its content of proteoglycans, which are molecules composed of polysaccharide glycosaminoglycans covalently linked to a large protein core of about 250,000 molecular weight. The collagen fibers are embedded in a ground substance that is a highly hydrated, gel-like material formed by the proteoglycan molecules. The collagen fibers strengthen and organize the extracellular matrix, and the aqueous phase of the proteoglycan gel permits nutrients, metabolites, and regulatory substances to diffuse readily between cartilage cells and the blood stream. The proteoglycans are believed to bind cations and thereby play an important role in the transport of water and electrolytes within the matrix. The numerous long, unbranched glycosaminoglycan chains of proteoglycans are highly hydrophilic, so

that hydrated gels are formed at low concentrations of carbohydrate. The compressive resistance of this hydrated gel and the resistance to stretching by the embedded collagen fibers account for the great resilience and padding properties of many connective tissues. Very little is known about the organization of glycosaminoglycans or proteoglycans in the extracellular matrix, beyond their ability to bind to collagens and other macromolecular components of the matrix.

Proteoglycans are abundant throughout the matrix of embryonic cartilage, but in mature cartilage, they are unevenly distributed. The area immediately surrounding the lacunae is called the *territorial matrix* (or the cartilage capsules). This region around cells is rich in proteoglycans and exhibits an intense basophilia, metachromasia with toluidine blue, and a strongly positive periodic acid–Schiff (PAS) reaction. The less basophilic matrix located between lacunae is known as *interterritorial matrix.* Radioautographic studies

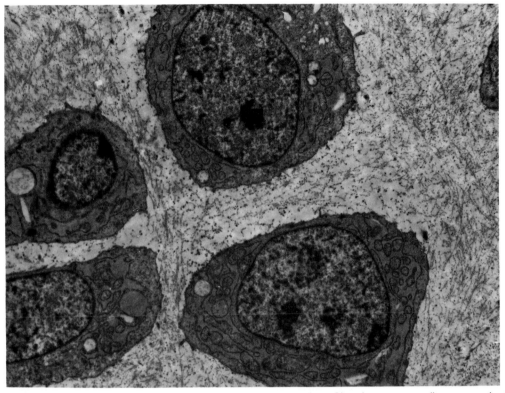

**Figure 4–8.** *Electron micrograph of hyaline cartilage from developing trachea. Chondrocytes generally appear spherical, and their cytoplasm contains small fat droplets, mitochondria, and granular endoplasmic reticulum. Collagenous fibrils form a fine feltwork within the surrounding ground substance.* × *5500.*

have shown that the chondrocytes are responsible for the formation both of collagenous fibrils and of the ground substance. The protein component of the proteoglycans is synthesized on granular endoplasmic reticulum. Sulfation and packaging next occurs in the Golgi complex with subsequent release of secretory vesicles. The specific proteoglycans present in all cartilage are chondroitin 4-sulfate and 6-sulfate, keratan sulfate, and some hyaluronic acid.

**Perichondrium.** The *perichondrium* is a tough layer of dense connective tissue that demarcates the cartilage boundary, except over articular cartilage. It is composed of elastic and collagenous type I fibers and spindle-shaped cells that are similar in appearance to fibroblasts. The outer layer of the perichondrium, called the *fibrous layer*, is adjacent to the blood vessels from the surrounding connective tissue with which it blends. The inner layer of the perichondrium,

called the *chondrogenic* layer, is more cellular. At the inner border of the chondrogenic layer, a condition is reached in which individual fibers are no longer distinguishable, their identify being obscured by the solid matrix in which they are embedded. The cells are no longer free, as in the fluid matrix of the perichondrium. They surround themselves with matrix and become incorporated into the cartilage as typical chondrocytes.

**Nutrition.** In general, cartilage is devoid of blood vessels, lymphatics, and nerves. The great fluid content of the matrix permits dissolved gases, nutrients, and waste products to diffuse readily to and from capillaries located outside the perichondrium. This limited diffusion is adequate for cartilage, since chondrocytes function mainly by glycolytic metabolism as an adaptation to their slightly anaerobic environment. Diffusion becomes increasingly difficult as the matrix matures, gels, and becomes more dense. If the cartilage becomes too dense, the cartilage cells become necrotic. Articular cartilage is unusual in that its cartilage cells derive their nutrition from synovial fluid.

**Retrogressive Changes.** With old age, cartilage loses its translucency and becomes less cellular, and the matrix shows less basophilia owing to the loss of proteoglycans and an increase in noncollagenous proteins. In certain forms of degenerating cartilage, parallel groups of fibers are deposited in the matrix. These fibers are not collagenous. Since these fibers are shiny and glossy, resembling asbestos, this type of cartilage degeneration has been called *asbestos cartilage.*

The most important retrogressive change within cartilage is *calcification.* While calcification normally occurs as a temporary strengthening expedient during the process of longitudinal bone growth, it occurs elsewhere without connection with growth processes. This latter incidence seems to be related to the aging of cartilage and consequent nutritional difficulty. Calcification occurs in widely scattered areas as depositions of minute granules of calcium carbonate and calcium phosphate in the intercellular substance near cells. Later, they tend to coalesce as they increase in size and are found in the general matrix. The

cartilage becomes hard and brittle. The most noticeable histological feature is hypertrophy and subsequent death of chondrocytes, as a result of the lack of ready diffusion of nutrients to the cells. With their death, the calcified matrix undergoes a slow process of reabsorption.

**Regeneration.** The ability to regenerate an area of adult cartilage that has been lost or damaged is low. Repair depends on the transformation of neighboring connective tissue elements (perichondrium) into cartilage. Tissue from the perichondrium proliferates and fills in the defect. Some of the connective tissue cells slowly differentiate into cartilage cells and gradually may be converted to cartilage in a manner similar to appositional growth. Fractured mature cartilage is usually united by dense fibrous tissue that may eventually be replaced by bone.

### Elastic Cartilage

Elastic cartilage is similar to hyaline cartilage except that it has numerous elastic fibers in its matrix in addition to many fine collagenous fibers (Fig. 4–9). The matrix is yellowish in the fresh

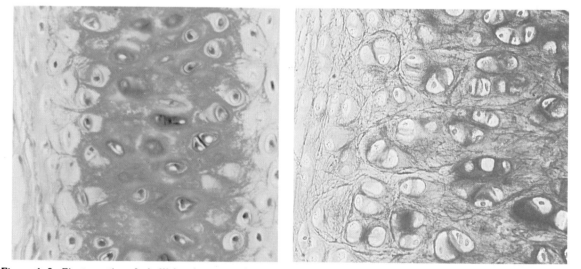

*Figure 4–9. Elastic cartilage.* Left: *Within the matrix, there are extensive networks of specifically stained elastic fibers. Generally, the fibers are large and densely packed within the interior of the cartilage. Chondrocytes also are large within the interior and tend to be smaller toward the perichondrium (left and right). Verhoeff's elastic stain. Medium power.* Right: *The arrangement of elastic fibers (purple) within the matrix is clearly apparent. They are concentrated in the matrix immediately in relation to the lacunae. Chondrocytes tend to be large and arranged in small cell nests centrally but are smaller and individually aligned toward the periphery (left). Weigert's stain. High power.*

condition, owing to the presence of elastic fibers, and is more opaque than hyaline cartilage, of which it is a modification. The belief that elastic cartilage is a typical hyaline cartilage, differing only in the presence of elastic fibers, is borne out by the conditions existing in the arytenoid cartilages of the larynx. The bodies of these cartilages consist of a type of hyaline cartilage, then elastic fibers begin to appear as the cartilage extends into the vocal processes, and the processes themselves become definitely elastic in character. Component cells of elastic cartilage, however, show less accumulation of fat and glycogen than do those of hyaline cartilage. This cartilage is also surrounded by a perichondrium, and growth oc-

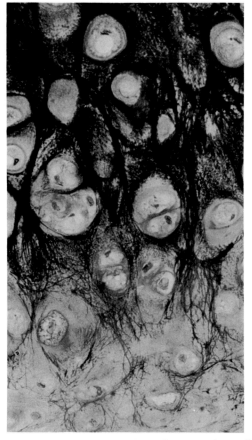

**Figure 4–10.** *Elastic cartilage from the external ear. This preparation is similar to that in Figure 4–9. There is a profusion of elastic fibers within the ground substance (above). Fewer elastic fibers surround chondrocytes close to the perichondrium (below). High power.*

curs both interstitially and by apposition from the perichondrium. Elastic cartilage is less likely to undergo retrogressive changes, principally calcification, than is hyaline cartilage.

The elastic fibers form a more or less dense network in the deeper portions of the matrix. They are less abundant at the periphery of the cartilage, from which they may be traced into the surrounding perichondrium (Fig. 4–10). This type of cartilage occurs in locations where support with flexibility is required, as in the external ear, auditory tube, epiglottis, and certain cartilages of the larynx.

### Fibrocartilage

This type of cartilage occurs where a tough support or tensile strength is required. Fibrous cartilage is to be found in the intervertebral disc. It is the cartilage that borders the glenoid fossa of the shoulder and the acetabulum of the hip and is found in the interarticular joints of the sternum and clavicle and of the clavicle and acromion process; the articulation of the jaw; and the symphysis pubis. It never occurs alone but merges gradually into the neighboring hyaline cartilage or with dense fibrous tissue. Unlike elastic cartilage, it cannot be considered a modification of hyaline cartilage. Fibrocartilage is a transitional type between hyaline cartilage and dense fibrous connective tissue of tendons and ligaments. The cells tend to be grouped in capsules, separated from each other by thick bundles of collagenous fibers. The cells are enclosed in capsules of hyaline cartilaginous matrix. There is no true perichondrium.

Fibrocartilage develops in a manner similar to that of ordinary connective tissue, and initially only fibroblasts, separated by considerable amounts of fibrillar material, are present. Later the cells are transformed into chondrocytes and surround themselves with a thin layer of cartilaginous matrix (Fig. 4–11). The density of this matrix increases with age, demonstrated by the fact that it acquires a bluish tinge when stained with hematoxylin and eosin instead of being clearly transparent as in the earlier condition.

A small body of tissue bearing a slight resemblance to degenerating cartilage, and known as

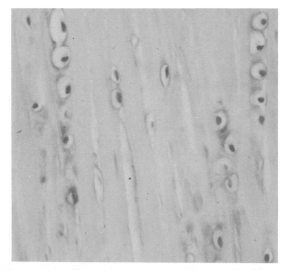

*Figure 4–11.* Fibrocartilage is composed principally of bundles of dense collagenous fibers (pink) that are regularly arranged. Between the bundles are chondrocytes that lie in lacunae within small regions of hyaline cartilaginous matrix. The chondrocytes typically occur in short rows between the collagenous bundles. H and E. Medium power.

the *nucleus pulposus*, is found in the center of the intervertebral disc. Its position corresponds to that of the notochord of the embryo.

## BONE

Bone, or osseous tissue, represents the highest differentiation among supporting tissues. It is a rigid tissue that constitutes most of the skeleton of higher vertebrates. It consists of cells and of an intercellular matrix. Its primary organic component, collagenous fibers, forms a strengthening framework, invisible in preparations by the usual methods but demonstrable with special stains. These fibers are united in bundles about 5 μm thick by a cementing substance. The inorganic salts that are responsible for the hardness and rigidity of bone include calcium phosphate (about 85 per cent), calcium carbonate (10 per cent), and small amounts of calcium fluoride and magnesium fluoride. Collagenous fibers contribute greatly to the strength and resilience of bone. The bone mineral, the composition of which is mainly hydroxyapatite, is found within collagenous fibrils

as apatite crystals. The crystals are of submicroscopic size, the largest measuring about 400 Å in length and 30 Å in thickness. The mineral content of bone increases in the course of development, reaching 65 per cent of bone in adult human beings.

If a longitudinally split long bone is examined grossly, it is at once evident that two types of bony tissue are present: a hard, outer investing layer of *compact (dense)* bone and a loose, *spongy (cancellous)* type of tissue formed by pieces of bone that anastomose to form a latticework of bony tissue on the inside of compact bone (Figs. 4–12 and 4–13). No sharp boundary may be drawn between the two types of osseous tissue, and the differences between them depend merely upon the relative amount of solid matter and the size and number of spaces in each. They both contain the same histological elements. The relative proportions of these two types of bone vary according to the needs for strength or lightness of weight. In a typical long bone, the shaft (*diaphysis*) is chiefly compact bone surrounding a medullary (or bone marrow) cavity. The dilated extremities, or *epiphyses*, of long bone consist of spongy bone covered with a thin layer of compact

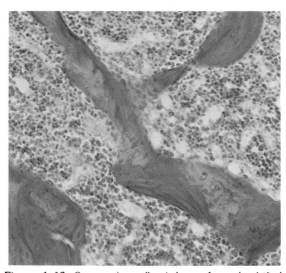

*Figure 4–12.* Spongy (cancellous) bone. In a decalcified section such as this, details of the matrix are not apparent. It appears homogeneous (pink), and the small dark areas within it are lacunae occupied by osteocytes. The spicules of bone are separated by bone marrow. Decalcified section. H and E. Low power.

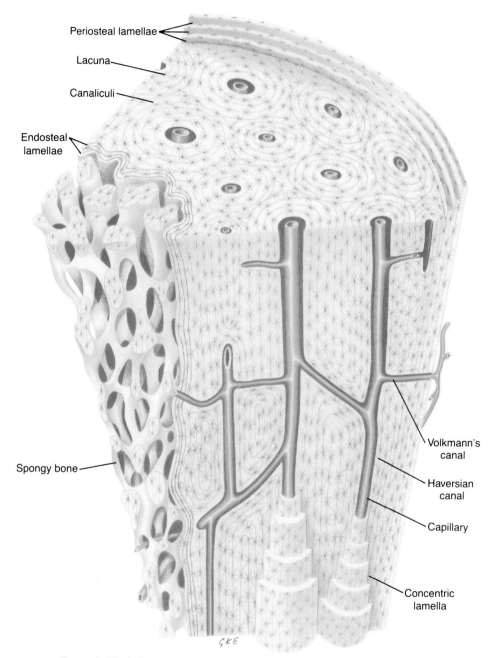

Periosteal lamellae

Lacuna

Canaliculi

Endosteal lamellae

Spongy bone

Volkmann's canal

Haversian canal

Capillary

Concentric lamella

**Figure 4–13.** *A diagrammatic representation of a small portion of compact bone.*

bone. The cavities of the spongy bone are continuous with the bone marrow cavity of the diaphysis. In flat bones of the skull, special terms are applied to comparable structures. The two parallel layers of compact bone are the outer and inner tables. The spongy bone between them is called the *diploë*. Most irregular bones (vertebrae) consist of a compact exterior and a spongy interior. The compact bone is usually in the form of a thin shell.

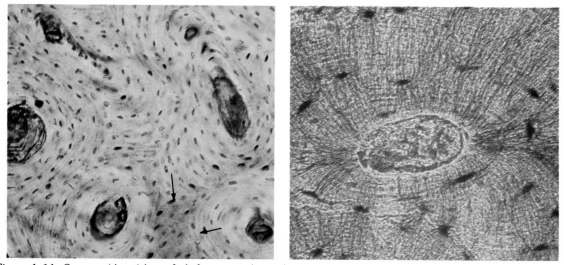

**Figure 4–14.** Compact (dense) bone. Left: In compact bone, the arrangement of lamellae is determined by the distribution of blood vessels, which lie in channels within the matrix. Volkmann's canals enter the bone and communicate with Haversian canals that run in the longitudinal axis of the bone. Each Haversian canal is surrounded by a number of concentric lamellae. The lamellae, the cells, and the central canal constitute the Haversian system. Here, several Haversian systems are sectioned transversely. Each Haversian canal is surrounded by lamellae, and lacunae, which in life contain osteocytes, occur between the lamellae. At the lower right (arrows), there is a small group of interstitial lamellae. These represent the remnants of Haversian systems that were partially destroyed during internal reconstruction of the bone. Ground section. Medium power. Right: The central portion of one Haversian system, or osteon, in transverse section is shown. The Haversian canal (center) is surrounded by concentric lamellae, with lacunae (black) between the lamellae. In life, the lacunae contain osteocytes. Fine canaliculi radiate from them to interconnect all lacunae with the central canal, thus permitting nutrition of all osteocytes by vessels in the canal. Ground section. High power.

The outer surface of compact bone, except over its articular surfaces, is covered by a connective tissue called the *periosteum*. The *endosteum* lines the marrow cavity, and it covers the spongy bone that lines the cavity. Each layer has the histogenetic capacity to form bone.

Bone tissue is pervaded by vascular canals and spaces, around which the matrix is arranged in closely apposed sheets, or *lamellae* (Figs. 4–14 and 4–15). The bone cells, or *osteocytes*, are flattened oval bodies with finely branching processes. These cells lie in slit-like *lacunae* between sheet of *bone matrix* (the calcified intercellular substance), their processes occupying tiny *canaliculi*, which penetrate the lamellae. The processes of certain of the cells have direct access to the vascular canals, and, as the processes of all cells contact their neighbors, a system of communicating canaliculi is set up throughout the matrix. It is by diffusion along these channels that the cells effect their exchanges of material with the blood, the diffusion through the matrix itself being prevented by the presence of the inorganic salts.

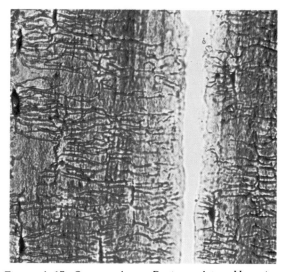

**Figure 4–15.** Compact bone. Portions of two Haversian systems are separated by an artifactual gap, representing a Haversian canal. Although lamellae, lacunae, and canaliculi are well defined, the concentric nature of the lamellae is not apparent in longitudinal sections. Ground longitudinal section. High power.

## Structural Elements

In a histological study of bone, it must be borne in mind that, owing to its inorganic component, bone cannot be examined in routine histological preparations. The intimate nature of this combination can be shown by several special methods of tissue preparation. If one of the long bones is treated with an acid solution, the inorganic salts are dissolved (*decalcification*), and the organic constituents alone remain. When this has been completed, the bone retains its original size, shape, and characteristic markings, although it can be readily bent and twisted. It should be noted that the cells in decalcified bone tend to be shrunken, and details of the matrix are blurred owing to swelling of osteocollagenous fibers by the reagents used. On the other hand, when the organic material has been removed by exposing the bone to intense heat (*calcification*), the size, form, and markings of the bone remain as before, but it has a chalky appearance and texture and shows a marked tendency to crumble. In *ground bone* sections, which are prepared by taking a thin piece of bone and grinding it down with abrasives until a section thin enough to be viewed under the microscope is obtained, details of matrix structure are well preserved. However, bone cells are removed by this method and lacunae appear empty. From these observations, it is evident that bony hardness is attributed to the inorganic salts, strength and resiliency to organic collagen and its matrix.

## Bone Cells

Four cell types peculiar to bone are recognized: *osteoprogenitor cells, osteoblasts, osteocytes,* and *osteoclasts.*

**Osteoprogenitor Cells.** Osteoprogenitor cells constitute a population of stem cells that are derived from mesenchyme. These cells have a capacity for mitosis and further differentiation into mature bone cells. Osteoprogenitor cells are spindle-shaped with oval or elongated nuclei and inconspicuous cytoplasm. They are found near bone surfaces, in the inner portion of the periosteum, in the endosteum, and within the vascular canals of compact bone. Two types of osteoprogenitor cells can be recognized by electron mi-croscopy: one type (preosteoblast) has some endoplasmic reticulum and a poorly developed Golgi region and gives rise to the osteoblast, and the other (preosteoclast) has more mitochondria and free ribosomes and gives rise to the osteoclast.

**Osteoblasts.** Osteoblasts, as their name implies, are associated with bone formation and are invariably found on the margin of growing bones where osseous matrix is being deposited (Fig. 4–16). During the period of growth, they are arranged in an epithelioid layer of cuboidal or low columnar cells. The cells can be shown to be in contact with each other by means of short, slender processes. The large nucleus, usually located in the basal region, exhibits a prominent nucleolus. The cytoplasm is extremely basophilic owing to the presence of ribose nucleoprotein, which is probably concerned with the synthesis of organic components of bone matrix (i.e., collagen and glycoprotein) (Fig. 4–17). By appropriate staining methods a diplosome and well-developed Golgi apparatus can be observed adjacent to the nucleus. Mitochondria are numerous and usually elongated. The cytoplasm contains PAS-staining granules that probably contain precursors of the glycosaminoglycans of the matrix. The role of osteoblasts in secreting bone collagen has been well documented. This newly synthesized, not yet calcified matrix near the osteoblasts is termed *osteoid*. Osteoblasts contain the enzyme *alkaline phosphatase*, which would suggest that they are concerned not only with the elaboration of matrix but also with its calcification. This enzyme is believed to break down local inhibitors of calcification in the matrix and to release phosphate ions from the substrates. Osteoblasts are polarized cells in which the extrusion of synthesized materials takes place at the cell surface at the points of contact with bone matrix. When they cease to produce particular products, they flatten, and concurrently, the cytoplasmic basophilia declines as does the amount of alkaline phosphatase. Osteoblasts have many microfilament-rich, finger-like cytoplasmic processes that extend into the developing bone matrix to contact cell processes from neighboring osteoblasts. These processes are more evident when the cell begins to surround itself with bone matrix.

**Osteocytes.** Once imprisoned in hard matrix, the original bone-forming cell, now called the *osteocyte*, has no opportunity to divide or to

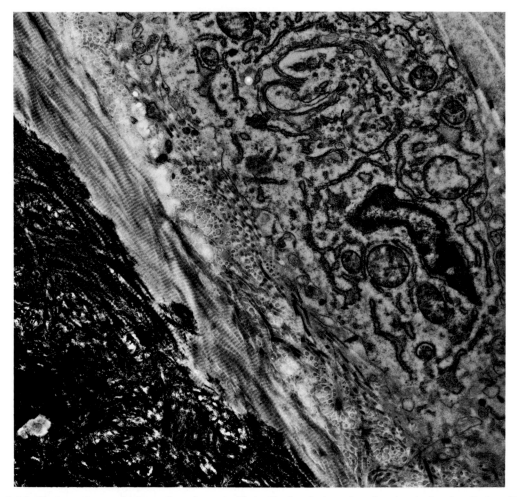

**Figure 4–16.** *Electron micrograph of a portion of an osteoblast with abundant rough-surfaced endoplasmic reticulum. Note the unmineralized matrix, containing collagen fibrils, running obliquely across the center of the figure, and mineralized matrix at left. × 18,400. (Courtesy of R. R. Cooper.)*

secrete matrix in appreciable quantities. The osteocyte, like the chondrocyte, occupies a small cavity or lacuna in the matrix, but unlike the chondrocyte, it is not isolated from its fellows. Osteocytes do not divide as evidenced by the fact that only one cell is ever found in a lacuna. They have a faintly basophil cytoplasm, which can be shown to contain fat droplets, some glycogen, and fine granules similar to those present within osteoblasts. The nucleus exhibits a condensed nuclear chromatin and is darkly staining. There is a significant reduction in rough endoplasmic reticulum and Golgi complex as compared with os-

teoblasts. Osteocytes are often somewhat shrunken in preparation, but their normal configuration can be inferred from the shape of the lacunae that they occupy. The young osteocytes are found nearer bone surfaces and are in round lacunae. The old osteocytes are in oval or lenticular lacunae. The cell processes of osteocytes extend for considerable distances in canaliculi, which radiate out from the lacunae. Gap junctions (maculae communicantes) are present at points of contact between osteocytic processes in the canaliculi. This finding explains how the cells can survive in such an isolated environment. This

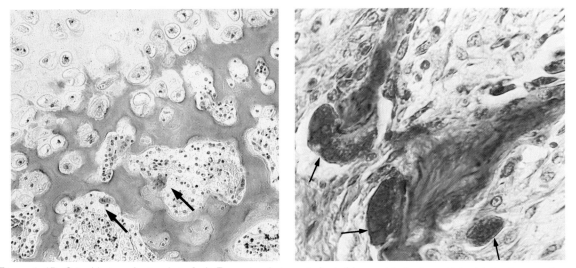

**Figure 4–17.** *Osteoblasts and osteoclasts. Left: Two osteoclasts are indicated (arrows) in the immediate vicinity of spongy bone. H and E. Medium power. Right: Two spicules of bone (blue), developing in mesenchyme, are shown. Numerous osteoblasts, cuboidal or pyramidal, form an almost continuous row in relation to the surface of the bony trabeculae. They have large nuclei and a markedly basophil cytoplasm. Three large osteoclasts (arrows) also occur in relation to the developing bone. These are multinucleated giant cells with a granular cytoplasm. Azan. High power.*

coupling is thought to provide for the passage of ions and small molecules through the gap junctions of adjoining cell processes. In the mature bone, the processes are withdrawn almost completely, but the canaliculi remain to provide an avenue for the exchange of nutrients and of waste products between the blood stream and the osteocytes. Electron microscopy has shown that osteocytes can periodically remove and replace perilacunar bone—a narrow amorphous zone of a unique form of bone surrounding the cells and their processes to the depth of about 1 μm. This zone of amorphous material probably acts as an additional medium for the exchange of metabolites, as evidenced by the variation in the size of the lacunae and incorporation of tetracycline (a bone marker) in perilacunar amorphous material.

**Osteoclasts.** While bone matrix is deposited by osteoblasts, it is eroded by *osteoclasts.* These large (20 to 100 μm in diameter) multinucleated (2 to 50 nuclei) cells are a type of macrophage. Like other macrophages, they develop from monocytes that originate in the hemopoietic tissue of the bone marrow. These precursor cells are released into the blood stream and collect at sites of bone reabsorption, where they fuse to form the multinucleated osteoclasts, which cling to surfaces of the bone matrix and eat it away. They are found in close association with the surface of bone, often in shallow excavations known as *Howship's lacunae.* The cytoplasm is often foamy in appearance and appears faintly basophil and granular. These numerous granules stain with acid phosphatase, the marker enzyme for lysosomes. Electron micrographs show that the surface of the osteoclast facing the matrix has numerous cytoplasmic projections and microvilli, described as a *ruffled border,* that apparently facilitate bone reabsorption. The ruffled border is surrounded by an actin filamentous zone that seems to be the site of adhesion of cell to bone surface. In the genetic disease *osteopetrosis,* the osteoclasts lack ruffled borders and are not capable of reabsorbing bone. It would seem that the actin filamentous zone of the ruffled border is required to maintain a microenvironment conducive to bone reabsorption. Osteoclasts secrete collagenase and other proteolytic enzymes that attack the bone matrix and liberate the calcified ground substance. Once the reabsorption process is complete, the osteoclasts disappear—probably either by degeneration or by reversion to their parent cell type.

## Bone Matrix

Although the intercellular substance of bone is apparently homogeneous, it has a well-ordered structure. The two major constituents are organic matrix and inorganic salts.

The organic portion (comprising about 35 per cent) consists mostly of osteocollagenous fibers united into bundles about 5 μm thick by a *cementing substance*. This substance consists mainly of glycosaminoglycans (protein-polysaccharides). Bone collagen is composed of type I collagen and is similar to that found in tendons, skin, and fascia. The collagen molecules in the fibrils are arranged in a staggered manner, resulting in a 400-Å pore, or gap, between the collagen molecules. About 50 per cent of the hydroxyapatite crystals are deposited in these pores. The fibers are difficult to see in ordinary preparations but can be revealed by special methods. The amorphous ground substance contains sialoproteins, phosphoproteins, acid-containing proteins, and a smaller amount of sulfated polysaccharides (chondroitin sulfates) that is present in cartilage. Thus, the bone matrix generally is acidophil, unlike cartilage, which is basophil and metachromatic. The highly acid nature of the amorphous ground substance components is associated with high calcium-binding properties and aggregation tendencies and may influence the mineralization process. The inorganic component is located solely in the cement between osteocollagenous fibers and accounts for 65 per cent of the weight of bone in adults. The minerals are deposited as dense particles within the gaps of the osteocollagenous fibers at intervals of about 600 Å along their length. The amorphous ground substance interacts and stabilizes these hydroxyapatite crystals and brings about the hardness and rigidity that is so characteristic of bone. These bone crystals are principally calcium phosphate in the form of the hydroxyapatite $[Ca_{10}(PO_4)_6 (OH)_2]$. The bone crystals are not pure and may contain carbonate, citrate, sodium, magnesium, and variable quantities of trace elements. The hydration shell associated with the outer portion of the bone crystal facilitates the exchange of ions with the body fluid. It is to be noted that lacunae and canaliculi are bordered by a layer of special organic cement, which differs from the rest of the intercellular substance in that it lacks fibrils.

Bone matrix is arranged in layers or lamellae 3 to 7 μm thick. Within lamellae, component fibers are arranged in a radial manner, those of one lamella at approximately a right angle to those of the neighboring one, so that lamellae have a helical fibrous framework in which the pitch of the adjacent spirals alternates. When viewed with polarized light, the successive lamellae appear alternately dark and light. This alternating arrangement in fiber direction explains why lamellae appear to be so distinct, one from another. In one lamella, collagenous fibers will appear elongated on section; in the next, the fibers are sectioned transversely and appear granular.

## Architecture of Bone

In compact bone, the lamellae are regularly arranged in a manner determined by the distribution of blood vessels that nourish the bone. The lamellae are concentrically disposed around vascular channels (*Haversian canals*) to form cylindrical units of structure called *Haversian sys-*

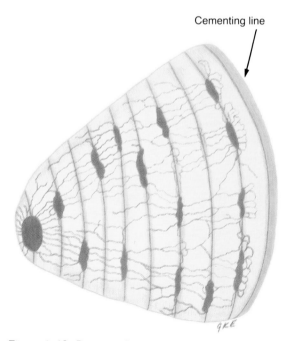

Cementing line

**Figure 4–18.** *Diagram of a segment of a Haversian system in cross section illustrates the arrangement of osteocytes, canaliculi, and lamellae.*

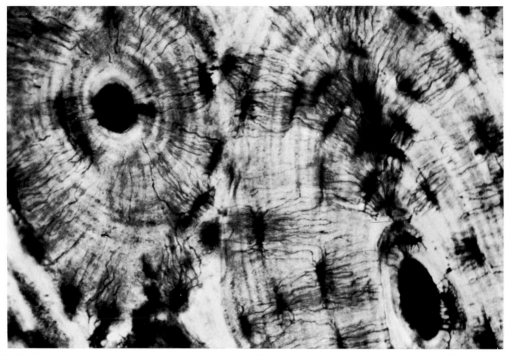

**Figure 4–19.** *High-power photomicrograph of portions of two Haversian systems transversely sectioned. Note the arrangement of lacunae and canaliculi. High power.*

*tems,* or *osteons* (Fig. 4–18 through 4–20). The lamellae of the bone matrix, the cells, and the Haversian canal constitute the osteon, the unit of structure of compact bone. Each osteon consists of from 5 to 20 lamellae that surround the central Haversian canal. in which blood vessels and nerves are present. The vessels within the Haversian canal run longitudinally, but they connect with the vessels of the marrow cavity and periosteum by means of lateral branches that course as the *Volkmann's canals* (or nutrient canals). The latter run either obliquely or at right angles to the Haversian canals. Thus, there is a continuous and complex system of canals that contains the blood vessels and nerves of bone. Adjacent lamellae of any series alternate in fiber direction, and thus lamellae appear to be distinct from one another. The boundaries of adjacent lamellar systems are sharply delineated by a thin layer of refractile, modified matrix (*cement line, cement membrane*). *Interstitial lamellae* are angular pieces of lamellar bone of different sizes and shapes present among the various Haversian systems. These are the remnants of Haversian systems partly de-

stroyed during internal reconstruction of the bone. At the periphery and on the internal surface in relation to the marrow cavity, there are several layers that extend around the shaft. These are the outer (periosteal) and inner (endosteal) *circumferential* or *general* lamellae. In addition to the osteocollagenous fibers contained within lamellae, there are coarse bundles of collagenous fibers, called *Sharpey's fibers* (Fig. 4–21). These latter fibers have their origin in the outer layers of bone (periosteum) and penetrate the outer circumferential lamellae to end among the Haversian systems and interstitial lamellae. They are not found in the lamellar systems or in the internal circumferential lamellae. They are surrounded by a narrow zone of uncalcified or partially calcified matrix. They serve to anchor the periosteum to bone and are most readily seen at the sites of attachment of tendons and ligaments. Canaliculi project from all surfaces and pass in a perpendicular direction through lamellae. Canaliculi that border upon a Haversian canal communicate with its cavity and thus bring all lacunae (flattened openings present within but mainly between two

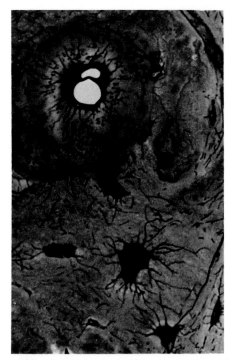

*Figure 4–20.* A portion of one Haversian system obliquely sectioned. One osteocyte, which fills its lacuna, shows numerous branching processes that lie within canaliculi. Note also the Haversian canal (top left) and a portion of a cement line (top right). Undecalcified plastic section. High power.

tissue known as the *periosteum*. It consists of collagenous fiber bundles intermingled with numerous elastic fibers. Its close connection with bone depends upon the presence of Sharpey's fibers. It consists of two layers that are not sharply defined. The fibers of the outer layer form a dense connective tissue and blend with the surrounding connective tissue. They give support to numerous blood vessels and lymphatics. The inner layer is composed of more loosely arranged connective tissue, some component collagenous fibers of which enter the bone as Sharpey's fibers. When bone is injured, the cells of the inner layer become osteoblasts and restore the bone that has been removed or destroyed in the injured area. This is sometimes referred to as the *osteogenic layer*. Under normal conditions, the cells of this layer remain inactive (osteoprogenitor cells) in the adult bone and are seen as spindle-shaped connective tissue cells.

**Endosteum.** The *endosteum* is a delicate layer composed of osteoprogenitor cells that line the marrow cavity and are present as a lining of cells in the canal system of compact bone. Since endosteum has a very small amount of reticular connective tissue, it is considerably thinner than the periosteum. Endosteum has both osteogenic and hemopoietic potencies.

### Development and Growth of Bone

Certain unique qualities of bone must be emphasized before an appreciation of bone development and growth can be fully grasped. Four essential points to be discussed are the bone canalicular system, bone vascularity, bone growth, and bone architecture.

1. Bone has a canalicular system that contains the slender processes of osteocytes. This system rises perpendicularly to the lacunae and anastomoses with the canaliculi from neighboring lacunae and with vessel-containing channels in the bone. At the bony surfaces, they open into the tissue spaces. The tissue fluid in these spaces becomes continuous with the fluid in the canalicular system. The osteocytes in this way are able to exchange substances with the blood by diffusion through tissue fluid that surrounds the cytoplasmic processes in the canaliculi. By this mechanism, cells of the bone remain alive even though

lamellae) of a lamellar system into continuity with the canal. Canaliculi at the periphery of a lamellar system do not cross the cement line but instead form loops and return to their own lacunae.

The structure of trabeculae or plates of spongy bone is similar to that of compact bone. The small trabeculae lack lamellar systems, for they are not penetrated by blood vessels but are surrounded by vascular marrow spaces. The network or pattern of these trabeculae is directly related to the mechanical functions of individual bones. Its lamellae contain lacunae with osteocytes and a system of intercommunicating canaliculi. In prenatal spongy bone, the lamellae are indistinct, since the osteocollagenous fibers form an irregular network. This is characteristic of rapid bone development and is referred to as *woven bone*. Isolated examples of this bone can be seen in the adult and during repair of fractures.

**Periosteum.** Applied to all parts of bone, except the articular surfaces, is a layer of connective

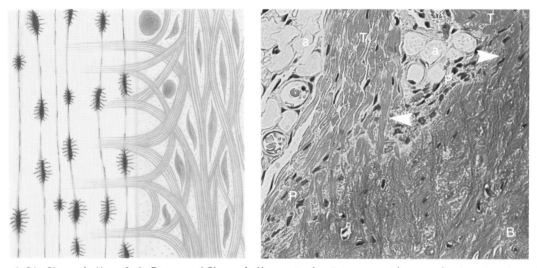

**Figure 4–21.** *Sharpey's fibers.* Left: *Diagram of Sharpey's fibers extending into compact bone as direct continuations of the fibers of the periosteum.* Right: *At lower right is bone (B) with osteocytes (dark blue) in lacunae. The bone surface is covered by periosteum (P). Above are two bundles of collagenous (tendon) fibers (T), which penetrate the periosteum (arrowheads) to enter bone matrix as Sharpey's fibers, thus anchoring the tendon firmly to bone. Around the tendon and between the two bundles is adipose tissue (a). H and E. Medium power.*

surrounded by an intercellular substance through which diffusion is impossible because of calcification.

2. Bone is vascular. For proper functioning of bone as a tissue, osteocytes must be as close as possible to the blood vessels. The canalicular system cannot operate effectively if it is more than about 0.5 mm removed from a capillary. Hence, bone is richly supplied with medullary and periosteal vessels that branch into narrow arteries that flow into fenestrated capillaries of Haversian and Volkmann's canals to ensure circulatory exchange for bone cells. Arterial pressure drives blood from the endosteum to the periosteum. The intravascular pressure is about 60 mm Hg on the endosteal side and 15 mm Hg on the periosteal side.

3. Bone can increase in size by appositional growth. Cartilage grows by interstitial and appositional growth. Bone grows by deposition of mineral salts on the surface of connective tissue elements, but never from within. Interstitial growth is impossible in bone because the presence of inorganic salts in the matrix prevents expansion within the interior.

4. Bone architecture is not static. Through life, bone is constantly being molded and reshaped. Bone is destroyed locally and re-formed repeatedly, adapting to changes brought about by external stresses, aging, and hormonal imbalances. Thus, there is a continuous process of reconstruction to consider.

According to the embryological origin, there are two types of bone development, *intramembranous* and *endochondral* (or *intracartilaginous*). Certain bones arise directly within the membranes in which they are located and are called *membrane bones*. The process is termed intramembranous bone development. In the second type of bone development, endochondral bone development, the original membranous matrix is converted into cartilage, which in turn is removed and replaced by bone. The bone produced by these two methods is histologically the same; the terms merely indicate the method of development. The first bone formed by either method is woven, or immature bone, in which lamellae are indistinct owing to the irregular arrangement of collagenous fibers. This is temporary tissue and is soon replaced by the definitive mature lamellar variety of spongy bone, which may become compact, owing to internal remodeling of existing bony materials. Bone is not simply deposited on and on until adult size is reached, but growth is accomplished by a twofold process of construction and destruction. Therefore, during bone growth, areas of immature bone, reabsorption, and mature bone may appear alongside each other in a given histological preparation.

### INTRAMEMBRANOUS BONE FORMATION

The most typical examples of intramembranous ossification are to be found in the formation and growth of the bones of the cranial vault (frontal, parietal, and upper portions of the occipital bones) (Figs. 4–22 and 4–23). Immediately preceding the formation of bone, there is a tendency for the mesenchymal cells to group themselves together in elongated clusters throughout this area. These cells connect themselves to one another via their processes, which do not exhibit any cytoplasmic continuity. In the region where this change is taking place, the delicate collagenous fibrils within the semifluid intercellular spaces become swollen. With the vascularization of this mesenchymal

sheet, these primitive connective tissue cells change and assume a more or less cuboidal shape, and the cytoplasm takes on a more basophilic stain, which characterizes them as bone-forming cells, or osteoblasts. The osteoblasts produce certain changes in the ground substance in the form of thin bars of dense intercellular eosinophilic substances. This masks the connective tissue fibers already present within the matrix. These thin bars of dense matrix are not calcified and constitute the organic base for the bone called *osteoid*. Following the formation of the organic portion of the matrix, calcium salts in a finely granular condition are deposited in its substance by the osteoblasts. The calcium salts are not merely precipitated in the preosseous substance (as in the calcification of cartilage) but assume a regular intimate relation with the collagenous fibers. This is known as *ossification*. In this manner, a number of bony spicules are formed in the connective tissue. There often is a delay in the deposition of mineral salts in osteoid, and thus matrix at the periphery of growing bone stains less densely than the fully mineralized matrix at the center. The deposition of bone around the osteoblasts and their processes creates the lacunae and canaliculi. Since the cytoplasmic processes of adjoining osteoblasts are already in contact with each other within the preosseous substance, a primitive lacunar-canalicular system is already in place. As the bars of preosseous material thicken and mineralize, increasing amounts of preosseous material are deposited by the osteoblasts. Through this activity of the osteoblasts, the bone increases in thickness. Successive layers of matrix are added by apposition, which results in osteoblasts becoming entrapped within the young bone and transformed into osteocytes. These osteocytes remain in cytoplasmic continuity with their neighbors and surface osteoblasts. The number of osteoblasts on the surface is maintained by mitosis and by formation of osteoblasts from osteogenic cells within the surrounding connective tissue.

At this stage of ossification, initially the bone consists of a network of spicules and trabeculae of woven bone. Later, some of this spongy bone is replaced by compact bone as the areas between trabeculae are filled in with concentric lamellar bone, thus creating inner and outer plates. Between the plates, spongy bone remains (as the diploë), and the intertrabecular spaces within it

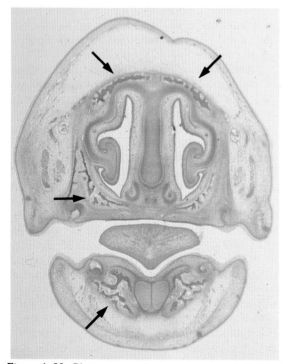

*Figure 4–22.* Photomicrograph of a section through the skull from an embryo showing intramembranous bone formation (arrows). H and E. Low power.

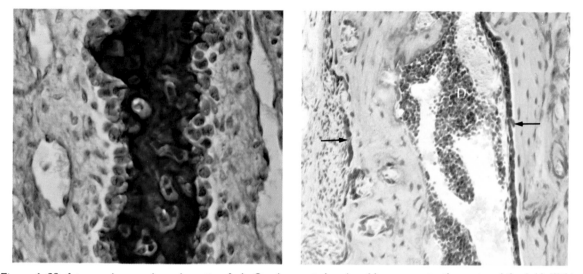

**Figure 4–23.** *Intramembranous bone formation. Left: One bar, or trabecula, of bone occupies the center of the field. Within the bone matrix (deep blue), a few osteocytes, each within a lacuna, are present. The bone is surrounded by a continuous layer of osteoblasts, which generally appear cuboidal, with large nuclei and a basophil cytoplasm. The surrounding mesenchyme contains numerous blood vessels. Through the activity of osteoblasts, the bone increases in thickness. Successive layers of matrix are added by apposition, and osteoblasts, which initially lie on the surface, become included within the matrix as osteocytes. Azan. Medium power. Right: This section of the developing calvarium shows two plates of bone separated by a marrow cavity of diploë (D). The dense concentrations of osteoblasts on the outer surface of one plate and on the inner surface of the other (arrows) indicate active addition of bone matrix at these sites. Decalcified section. H and E. Low power.*

constitute the *primary marrow cavities*. In the intertrabecular spaces, the connective tissue differentiates into myeloid, or the *hemopoietic,* tissue of the bone marrow. The portion of the connective tissue layer that does not undergo ossification gives rise to the periosteum and the endosteum of intramembranous bone.

### ENDOCHONDRAL (INTRACARTILAGINOUS) BONE FORMATION

This type of ossification, involving the replacement of a cartilage model by bone, is best observed in a long bone (Figs. 4–24 and 4–25). The cartilages that form the early embryonic skeleton, moreover, serve to give direction to the growth of the bone by which they are replaced, and, to a certain extent, influence their form. During development, the cartilage is replaced by bone except on the articular surfaces of the bone, but this is a slow process that is not achieved until the bone has reached its full size, and growth has ceased. The cartilage model is surrounded by functional perichondrium. Growth of the model occurs by perichondrial apposition and by interstitial chondrocytic mitosis. Endochondral bone

development begins with the transformation of the perichondrium into the bone-producing periosteum. The perichondrium becomes richly vascularized and assumes an osteogenic function with the gathering of osteoblasts on the inner surface of the periosteum. As a result, the cartilage of the diaphysis becomes encased by a *periosteal bone ring*, or *collar*, of compact bone laid down on the cells of the periosteum (Fig. 4–26). These latter changes result in typical intramembranous bone formation and produce a collar of bone that increases rapidly in length along the shaft in both directions while thickening only slightly. The periosteum becomes increasingly vascular, providing the necessary prerequisites for continued bone formation.

Simultaneously with the appearance of the bony collar, changes are taking place in the center of the cartilage within the shaft of the long bone. In the center of the diaphysis, the cartilage has become honeycombed by the removal of some of the cartilage between the spaces occupied by the hypertrophied cartilage cells. In the meantime, the cells and fibers of the osteogenic layer of the periosteum, accompanied by blood vessels, organize to form a *periosteal bud*. This forms a

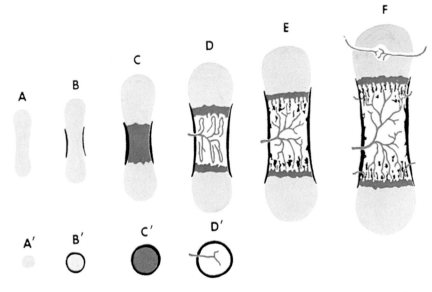

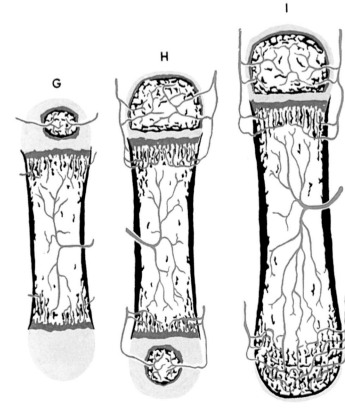

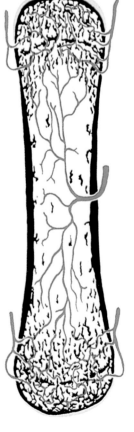

*Figure 4–24* See legend on opposite page

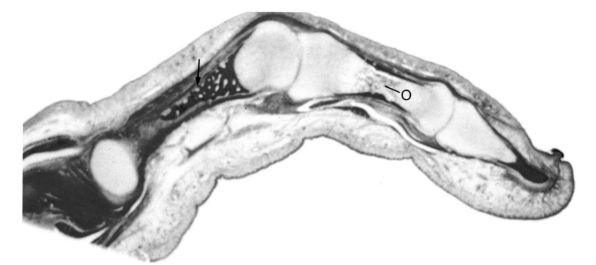

**Figure 4–25.** *Endochondral bone formation in the finger. The three phalanges of a finger are shown. The process of endochondral bone formation is seen best in the intermediate phalanx. The cartilage model (pale gray) is surrounded by perichondrium (dark blue), later to become periosteum, except over the joint surfaces. Around the center of the diaphysis, a periosteal bony collar (dark purple) has formed. Centrally within the diaphysis, a primary center of ossification (O) is present. In the proximal phalanx, the process of ossification is more advanced (arrow). The section shown here is tangential and passes obliquely through the bony collar (dark purple), demonstrating the spongy nature of the bone at this stage. Mallory-Azan. Low power.*

channel through the intervening bone collar and cartilage by the removal of their substance and breakdown of the thin walls of the lacunae. The cavities thus formed are the *primary marrow spaces.* From the tissue of the periosteal bud is derived the cells and constituents of the *primary bone marrow,* which soon fills the primary marrow space. As the periosteal bud invades the bone and cartilage, it carries with it the potential bone-forming cells, or osteoblasts. The walls of the primary marrow cavity are irregular owing to the spicules of calcified cartilage that still remain and project into it. The osteoblasts arrange themselves along the cartilaginous substrates and deposit bone upon them in the same way as bone was deposited along the fiber bundles in intramembranous bone formation. This deposition of bone in the center of the diaphysis constitutes the *primary ossification center* (Fig. 4–27). This erosive process extends in both directions, keeping pace with the linear increase of the bony collar. The bony collar becomes thicker and widens towards the epiphyses. It assists in maintaining the strength of the shaft, which otherwise would be weakened by the removal of cartilage within the diaphysis. Thus, the periosteal bone collar acts as a buttress to support the central zone of reabsorbing cartilage prior to its replacement by bone. The calcification of the cartilage, with the accompanying changes in the cells, results in the

**Figure 4–24.** *Diagram of the development of a typical long bone as shown in longitudinal sections (A to J) and in cross sections A', B', C', and D' through the centers of A, B, C, and D. Pale blue, cartilage; purple, calcified cartilage; black, bone; red, arteries. A, Cartilage model. B, Periosteal bone collar appears before any calcification of cartilage. C, Cartilage begins to calcify. D, Vascular mesenchyme enters the calcified cartilage matrix and divides it into two zones of ossification (E). F, Blood vessels and mesenchyme enter upper epiphyseal cartilage, and the epiphyseal ossification center develops in it (G). A similar ossification center develops in the lower epiphyseal cartilage (H). As the bone ceases to grow in length, the lower epiphyseal plate disappears first (I) and then the upper epiphyseal plate (J). The bone marrow cavity then becomes continuous throughout the length of the bone, and the blood vessels of the diaphysis, metaphyses, and epiphyses intercommunicate. (From Bloom, W., and Fawcett, D. W.: A Textbook of Histology, 11th ed. Philadelphia, W. B. Saunders Co., 1986.)*

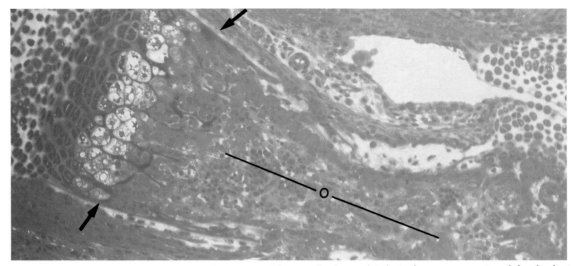

**Figure 4–26.** Endochondral bone formation. The periosteal bony collar (arrows) is limited to one extremity of the diaphysis, but the primary marrow cavity (O) is extensive. To the left of this, the cartilage model shows definite zones of activity and the establishment of cartilage columns and calcification of the matrix (dark blue). Details of the zones are depicted in Figures 4–28 through 4–30. Plastic section. H and E. Low power.

formation of other primary marrow spaces, which are finally joined into a single large cavity in the diaphysis, known as the *secondary marrow cavity.* When this process has extended to the subperiosteal bone, this latter structure forms the outer boundary of the secondary marrow cavity.

With the continued growth of cartilage in the epiphyses, the entire cartilage model increases in

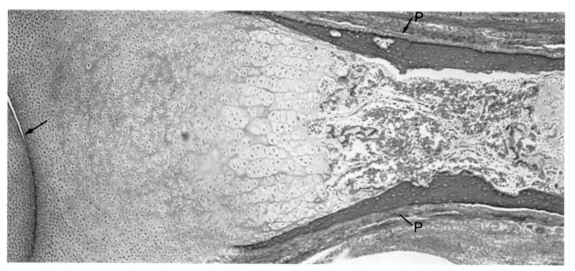

**Figure 4–27.** Endochondral bone formation. A more advanced stage of ossification than that shown in Figure 4–25. The periosteum (P) covers the developing bone, and a wide periosteal collar of spongy bone (dark blue) encloses the diaphysis. In the primary ossification center (right center), which appears red owing to the marked vascularity, cells of the original periosteal bud have opened up wide cavities, the primary marrow spaces. In the epiphysis (left), there is a reserve, or quiescent, zone of hyaline cartilage, and, toward the diaphysis, the cartilage cells become larger and the region appears pale. A joint cavity (arrow) is present beyond the epiphysis. Mallory-Azan. Low power.

size. As a result of this and of the extension of the primary ossification centers, definite zones become apparent within cartilage. Of course, each zone changes character as ossification advances toward it. This epiphyseal cartilage is now the important site for continued longitudinal growth of bone. It is as if the original cartilage anlage were restricted to the ends of the bone. Beginning at the ends of the cartilage and passing toward the ossification center in the diaphysis, the following zones, which illustrate the continuing process of endochondral bone formation, can be recognized (Fig. 4–28 through 4–31).

1. *Quiescent, or reserve, zone* is an extensive zone initially, but it becomes shorter as ossification proceeds. It is composed of primitive hyaline cartilage and is present nearest to the ends of the bone. It is the zone that shows growth in all directions, with cells undergoing repeated randomly oriented mitoses.

2. *Zone of proliferation* is an active zone showing numerous directional mitoses. Cells of the quiescent zone divide and produce daughter cells

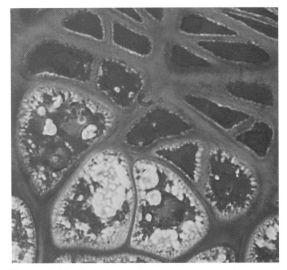

*Figure 4–29.* Endochondral bone formation. Above, the cartilage cells of the epiphysis are aligned in rows in the zone of proliferation. Below, the cells are large and vesicular as a result of the accumulation of glycogen within their cytoplasm; this is the maturation zone. Plastic section. H and E. High power.

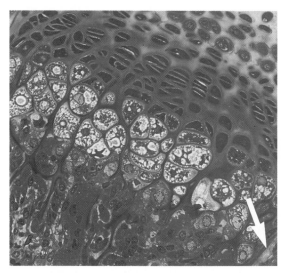

*Figure 4–28.* Endochondral bone formation. Details of the zones of activity within the cartilaginous epiphysis are shown. The quiescent, or reserve, zone (top right) gives way to a zone of proliferation where cartilage cells are aligned in distinct rows. Below this zone, there is maturation of cells and calcification of the matrix (dark blue) surrounding the cells. The zone of retrogression occupies the lower left part of the field. A small portion of the periosteal bony collar appears to the right (arrow). Plastic section. H and E. Medium power.

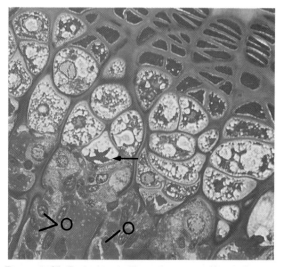

*Figure 4–30.* Endochondral bone formation. Above, the zone of proliferation gives way to the maturation zone. Below this, there is the zone of calcification, where the matrix appears deeply basophil, and the narrow zone of retrogression, where cartilage cells die and undergo dissolution (arrow). The lower left part of the field shows the ossification zone. Here, bone matrix (pink) is being deposited upon the surface of the remnants of calcified cartilage matrix by osteoblasts (O). Plastic section. H and E. High power.

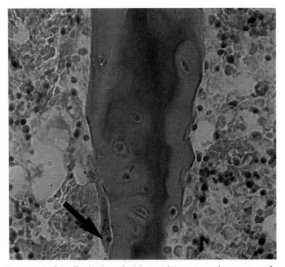

**Figure 4–31.** *Endochondral bone formation. A portion of a trabecula in the ossification zone is shown. Bone matrix (pink) has been deposited upon the calcified cartilage matrix (purple). A few osteocytes within lacunae are present within the bone matrix. The presence of an osteoclast (arrow) indicates that bone resorption also is occurring here to enlarge the primary marrow spaces that surround the trabecula. Decalcified section. H and E. Medium power.*

that align themselves in distinct rows or columns parallel with the long axis of the cartilage model. The lacunae and cells are flattened at right angles to the longitudinal axis. A row grows principally by addition of cells at the distal free end in relation to the previous zone. This is the zone in which the directional mitoses effectively produce elongation of the cartilage.

3. *Maturation zone* is a zone of hypertrophy of cartilage cells with no further mitoses. The enlargement of lacunae adds further to the length of the cartilage in this region. The cytoplasm of the cartilage cells contains glycogen, and the reabsorbed matrix appears as thin bars between these cells.

4. *Zone of calcification* is an area in which the matrix between adjacent longitudinal columns becomes impregnated with minerals and stains deeply basophil.

5. *Zone of retrogression* contains cartilage cells that show degenerative signs and eventually die. The thicker plates of matrix between rows of cells remain virtually intact. The deepest regions exhibit

an erosion of matrix related to vascular invasion by capillaries from the marrow cavity. Many calcified longitudinal bars of matrix are left.

6. *Zone of ossification* contains endosteal osteoblasts that gather on the exposed struts of calcified cartilage and now begin osteogenesis. This results in the formation of a number of cancellous trabeculae whose cores contain calcified matrix.

7. *Zone of reabsorption* represents the last gradient of maturation of epiphyseal hyaline cartilage. As ossification advances towards the ends of the cartilage, the marrow cavity increases in size, owing to the reabsorption of bone in the center of the diaphysis. As a result, the length of spongy bone remains nearly constant.

Concurrently with the growth in length within the epiphyseal cartilage, the periosteal collar grows in both length and diameter. The increase in extent of the periosteal collar compensates for the loss, by reabsorption, of endochondral bone centrally. By the reabsorption of the internal surface of this collar, the medullary cavity grows in width. The zone of reserve cartilage is maintained by cell division and provides for a continued growth in length by the plate of cartilage that remains between the diaphysis and epiphysis of bone. It becomes reduced in length as ossification of the diaphysis proceeds.

The epiphyses of the long bones retain their cartilaginous condition until after birth. Blood vessels, accompanied by osteogenic tissue, invade the cartilage and form *secondary centers of ossification (epiphyseal centers)* from which the process of ossification extends in all directions (Fig. 4–32). Several of these centers are formed in the epiphyses of longer bones; in smaller bones, only a single center is present. Ossification spreads peripherally until there is replacement of cartilage by bone except in two regions. Cartilage remains over the free end as articular cartilage and as a plate between the epiphysis and the diaphysis. This is the *epiphyseal plate* or *disc* (Figs. 4–33 and 4–34).

Since the ossification of both the diaphysis and the epiphysis takes place before the bones have attained their adult condition, provision is made for their continued growth in length by the epiphyseal disc that remains between them. The continued growth of the bone in length is accom-

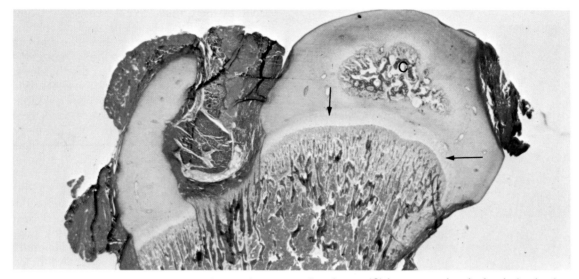

**Figure 4–32.** Secondary ossification center. A secondary center of ossification (C) has appeared in the head of a developing femur. Below is the diaphysis, with a periosteal collar of bone (dark blue) and a marrow cavity containing a few spicules of spongy bone. Above right, small bony trabeculae are present within the secondary ossification center. This center is surrounded by hyaline cartilage of the original cartilage model. The epiphyseal disc (arrows) appears as a pale band between the epiphysis and the shaft. Above left, the greater trochanter is composed solely of hyaline cartilage; a secondary ossification center has yet to appear within it. Azan. Low power.

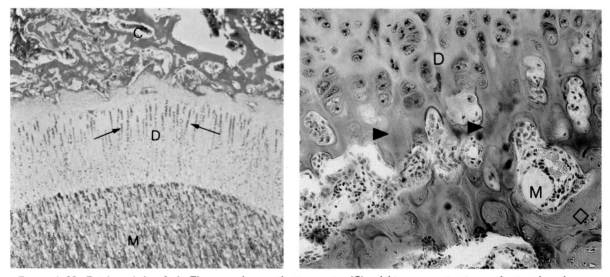

**Figure 4–33.** Epiphyseal disc. Left: The secondary ossification center (C) exhibits more extensive ossification than the one shown in Figure 4–32. Ossification has spread peripherally, and cartilage remains only as articular cartilage over the free surface (not shown) and as a plate, the epiphyseal disc (D), between the epiphysis and the diaphysis. The formation of cartilage columns (arrows), the calcification of cartilage, and the deposition of bone continue here as earlier in the shaft. Below is the marrow cavity (M) of the diaphysis. Azan. Medium power. Right: Lower portion of the epiphyseal disc (D), showing the zone of calcification (arrowheads), marrow cavity (M), and zone of ossification ( ◊ ). H and E. High power.

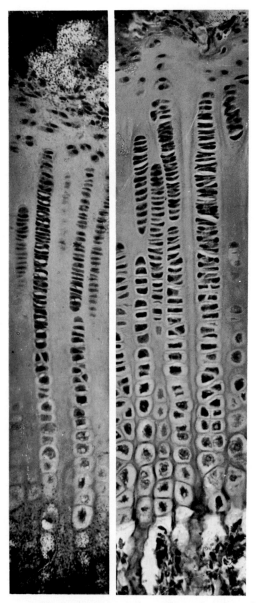

*Figure 4–34. Sections of growth cartilages of upper end of tibias of two-month-old (left) and three-month-old (right) rabbits. Radioactive calcium was injected 30 hours before killing, and the undecalcified sections were dipped in photographic emulsion and developed after several weeks. Silver grains overlie the secondary ossification center (above) and the calcifying ends of the cartilage columns (below), in continuity with the primary bony trabeculae. Medium power. (Courtesy of F. W. Fyfe.)*

plished by the formation of the cartilage columns, the calcification of the cartilage, and the continued deposition of bone here as earlier in the shaft. Proliferation of cartilage and bony replacement occur at about the same rate, so the thickness of the epiphyseal disc remains constant. When growth ceases, there is no further proliferation of cartilage, and the epiphyseal disc is ossified. The position of this cartilaginous disc is indicated on the surface in the adult by a dense accumulation between epiphysis and diaphysis called the *epiphyseal line*.

As the periosteal bone about the diaphysis increases in thickness by intramembranous bone formation, the process of reabsorption becomes active on its endosteal surface with the consequent enlargement of the diameter of the marrow cavity. The thickness of bone does not increase at the same rate since, as bone is added progressively to the periosteal surface, bone in lesser amounts is reabsorbed from the endosteal surface. This process of growth and reabsorption of the bone about the diaphysis continues until it has attained its adult size and condition.

### Remodeling and Reconstruction of Bone

As a bone enlarges in size, its structure is complicated by internal reconstruction and by remodeling. *Remodeling* results from reabsorption in certain areas and deposition of new bone elsewhere. Reabsorption is associated with the appearance of osteoclasts. At the electron microscopic level, it has been shown that the surface of the cell adjacent to the bone appears to be characterized by numerous infoldings of the cell membrane, giving rise to clefts or striations. Evidence suggests that bone salt crystals are loosed from the bone matrix by enzymic activity and taken up by the folds in the surface, then by vesicles in the cytoplasm, where they undergo demineralization by proteolytic enzymes elaborated by the osteoclasts. Bones have a remarkable ability to remodel their structure in response to local mechanical stresses. The stresses may act on the cells by giving rise to local electric fields to which the osteoclasts are sensitive. Collagen fibers in bone matrix are *piezoelectric*—that is, they become electrically polarized when subjected to mechanical stress. It seems likely that osteocytes are involved in the process of reconstruction, since any region of bone matrix whose osteocytes have been killed is promptly eroded.

In the growth of bone, we have been concerned so far with the deposition of spongy bone. In certain areas, this is replaced by compact bone. In this process, osteoblasts produce layer after layer of bone inward on the surface of the longitudinal cavities within the spongy bone until the cavities are reduced to narrow canals containing blood vessels. The system of concentric lamellae with its canal and blood vessels is called a *primitive Haversian* system.

**Development of Haversian Systems.** Compact bone is more regular in its arrangement than spongy bone. Its development may be described as follows (Fig. 4–35). The marrow spaces are penetrated throughout by a rich vascular network. The vessels of the periphery of the bone follow a more or less regular pathway parallel to the surface. In long bones, they run in the long axis of the bone. In places where compact bone is to be formed, erosion follows a definite plan, rounding out the marrow spaces so that they form cylindrical cavities around the blood vessels. After the marrow spaces have been thus reshaped, they are lined by successive concentric lamellae of new bone. The process continues until the space is almost filled with lamellae, and it eventually persists as a central canal containing blood vessels, nerves, and connective tissue. Such a grouping of layers of bone, with its central canal, is called a primary Haversian system. There is evidence suggesting that the normal mechanisms of internal bone reabsorption may occur under the influence of mature osteocytes. This process is referred to as *osteolysis*. The cells responsible for this activity are able to produce both alkaline phosphatase and protease. It is this lytic process, which is hormonally controlled, that results in the formation of cylindrical cavities containing blood vessels and embryonic marrow tissue. The overall

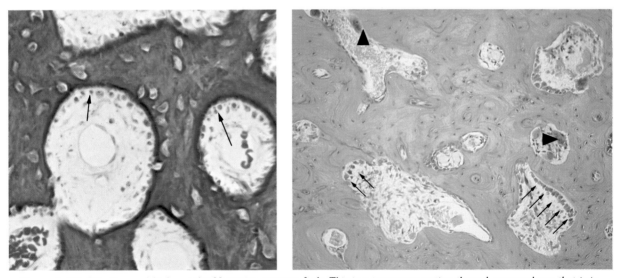

**Figure 4–35.** *Primitive and higher order Haversian systems. Left: This is a transverse section through spongy bone that is in the process of being transformed into compact bone. The spongy bone matrix (blue) contains numerous osteocytes within lacunae and shows no obvious lamellar pattern. Each large cavity contains a blood vessel centrally, embedded within a primitive connective tissue. Peripherally, osteoblasts (arrows) form an irregular row of cells directly in relation to the bone matrix. As this layer elaborates additional bone matrix and becomes incorporated within it, a further layer of osteoblasts will differentiate from the primitive connective tissue. In this way, there is a rhythmical deposition of concentric lamellae to form a primitive Haversian system. Mallory-Azan. High power. Right: Resorption cavities appear continuously, containing osteoblasts (arrows) and osteoclasts (arrowheads), and are replaced by higher orders of Haversian systems. H and E. Medium power.*

width of the osteon that forms depends on the diameter of the persisting tunnel and also on the maximum distance over which osteocytes can obtain nourishment via the canalicular system.

The remodeling of bone does not end when the primary Haversian systems are laid down but continues into adult life. The primary systems are partially destroyed to provide space for new ones in response to changes in mechanical requirements. The final result is a mass of bone composed of secondary and tertiary Haversian systems embedded in the remains of earlier systems. In the process, portions of former Haversian systems may escape destruction and become interstitial lamellae that fill in between new systems. These latter lamellae form the background for the Haversian systems that hold them together in a solid mass of material. As growth nears completion, the surface of the bone is formed by outer circumferential lamellae that have been laid down by the osteoblasts of the periosteal tissue. This region contains no Haversian systems. Endosteal circumferential lamellae of the same character line the shaft where it borders the marrow cavity.

In mature bone, therefore, the majority of the matrix is of intramembranous origin. Bone of endochondral origin perisists only as narrow trabeculae in the diaphysis and the metaphysis and as the central spongy bone of the epiphyses.

**Development of Irregular Bones.** The foregoing description is based upon conditions in a typical long bone. Irregular bones develop in a manner similar to that of the epiphyses of long bones. Ossification begins in the center and radiates out in all directions. The cartilage at the periphery serves as the proliferant zone until growth within it ceases, when it is replaced by bone. Further bone may be added by apposition from the periosteum.

### Repair of Bone

After bone fracture, the following events occur in connection with the repair of injured bone. First there is a hemorrhage, caused by the rupture of blood vessels, which is soon followed by the formation of a clot. Subsequently, fibroblasts and capillaries migrate into the area formed by the clot, resulting in the formation of granulation tissue, the *procallus*. The granulation tissue becomes infiltrated with dense fibrous tissue that is soon transformed to cartilage. The latter constitutes a temporary union or *callus* that unites the fractured bones. Osteoblasts develop from the periosteum and endosteum and lay down spongy bone, which progressively replaces the cartilage of the temporary callus in a manner similar to endochondral ossification. Finally, excess bone present in the callus is partially or completely reabsorbed, and a bony union of the fracture is achieved.

The repair of the bone is dependent on an adequate blood supply, on the activity of the bone-forming cells in the periosteum and endosteum, and also on adequate vitamin and mineral supplies. The sequence of events in the callus formation illustrates the multipotentiality of the cells of the periosteal and endosteal layers. The differentiation of these cells is dependent upon an adequate blood supply. Initially, the vascularity to the injured area is poor, and the differentiation of cells is in the direction of fibroblasts and of chondroblasts. After the ingrowth of blood vessels, osteoblasts make their appearance.

### Histophysiology of Bone

Both vitamins and hormones play an important role in ossification and the maintenance of bone. In vitamin D deficiency, there is a faulty absorption of calcium from foods and a diminished concentration of phosphate in the blood. This leads to widening of the epiphyseal growth plate, increased numbers of hypertrophic cartilage cells, and decreased longitudinal growth. There is a failure to reabsorb the growth plate, which appears to be related to defects in the mineralization process. The condition is called *rickets* in children. In adults the deficiency causes a retardation in the synthesis rate and the failure of the osteoid to mineralize. It is known as *adult rickets* or *osteomalacia*. Vitamin C deficiency results in the condition known as *scurvy*, which is characterized by an inability of tissues of mesenchymal origin to produce and maintain osteocollagenous fibers and ground substance. Impaired bone formation is caused by a decreased synthesis of collagen and of glycosaminoglycans. Formation of osteoid ceases because of the scarcity of osteoblasts, and fibroblasts predominate. Cartilage cells continue to show directional mitoses in the growth plate, but the matrix calcifies in the form of a brittle network. In vitamin A deficiency, bone matrix is not normally synthesized by the osteoblasts. There is a decrease in bone reabsorption and collagen synthesis and an interference with the process of remodeling and the balance between bone deposition and erosion. Excessive amounts of vitamin A stimulate the existing monocytic osteoprogenitor cells and thereby increase the number of osteoclasts.

Hormones profoundly influence the growth and maintenance of bones. The *growth hormone* of the anterior pituitary is essential for normal bone growth. It stimulates cell division and DNA, RNA, and mucopolysaccharide synthesis in cartilage. The oversecretion and undersecretion of growth hormone lead to *gigantism* and *dwarfism*, respectively. Parathyroid hormone regulates the reabsorption of bone and controls the release of calcium to the blood. The possible mechanisms for calcium mobilization may involve an acute increase in osteoclastic and osteocytic reabsorption and stimulation of calcium pump of osteoblasts. The action of parathyroid hormone appears to be in direct opposition to that of thyrocalcitonin, which inhibits reabsorptive activity and calcium mobilization. Thus, there is a balance between release and deposition of calcium to maintain the level of calcium in the blood. Male and female sex hormones regulate growth rates by controlling the appearance of ossification centers and the rate of maturation. Thyroxine promotes cartilage cell maturation and cartilage matrix synthesis.

It has been postulated that the extraordinary capacity of bone for growth, continuous internal remodeling and reconstruction, and regeneration may be due in part to the presence within bone matrix of *bone morphogenetic protein (BMP)* and of *bone-derived growth factors (BDGF)*. BMP induces differentiation of mesenchymal-type perivascular cells into osteoprogenitor cells. The osteoprogenitor cells occur in the mesenchyme of the fetus near ossification centers and in the endosteum and the deep layer of the periosteum postnatally. BDGF, secreted by the osteoprogen-

itor cells, are hydrophilic proteins that stimulate DNA synthesis and the proliferation of osteoprogenitor cells. Thus, BMP and BDGF appear to be coefficient in bone generation and regeneration.

## THE JOINTS

The sites where two or more components of the skeleton, whether bone or cartilage, meet are referred to as joints, or *articulations* (L. *articulatio,* a forming of vines). They may be either *temporary* or *permanent.* Temporary joints occur during the period of growth; for example, the epiphysis of a long bone is united to the bone of the shaft by hyaline cartilage of the epiphyseal disc. This functions to allow for growth of the participating skeletal parts and disappears when growth ceases and the epiphysis fuses with the shaft. Most joints, however, are permanent, and they may be classified on the basis of their structural features into three main types: fibrous, cartilaginous, and synovial (Fig. 4–36). The first two types frequently are termed *synarthroses* (*syn*, together; *arthron*, articulation), joints that are immovable or only slightly movable through an intervening deformable tissue. Synovial joints, which allow considerable freedom of movement, are referred to as *diarthroses* (*di*, two; *arthron*, articulation). Bones are joined together in continuity by synarthroses or in discontinuity by diarthroses.

## Fibrous Joints

These joints are united without an intervening cavity, being held together firmly by dense fibrous connective tissue, some of which is in the form of ligaments. If the union is extremely tight, the joint is termed a *suture.* Sutures occur only in the skull, and strictly speaking, they are not permanent, since the periosteum and collagen fibers run from one to the other, allowing for appositional growth to take place in the connective tissue spaces. When growth is complete, the connective tissue may undergo ossification, the result being a *synostosis.* Joints in which the participating bones are held together by a considerably greater amount of fibrous tissue than in the suture are called

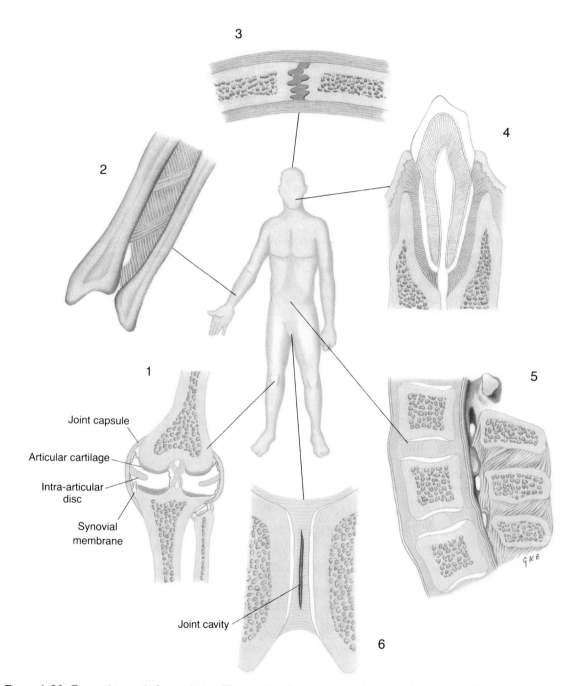

**Figure 4–36.** *Types of joints. 1, Synovial joint. Fibrous joints: 2, syndesmosis; 3, suture; 4, gomphosis. Secondary cartilaginous joints: 5, intervertebral disc; 6, symphysis. (From Leeson, C. R., and Leeson, T. S.: Human Structure: A Companion to Anatomical Studies. Philadelphia, W. B. Saunders Co., 1972, p. 26.)*

*syndesmoses.* A syndesmosis permits a certain amount of movement. Such joints, examples of which are the radioulnar and tibiofibular articulations, are held together by interosseous ligaments that allow a certain degree of displacement.

The third type of fibrous joint, the *gomphosis*, is a specialized articulation restricted to the teeth in the maxilla and mandible, where the uniting fibrous tissue constitutes the periodontal membrane (see Chapter 11).

### Cartilaginous Joints

These joints, often termed *secondary* cartilaginous to distinguish them from the *primary joints*, are best exemplified by the joints between the bodies of adjacent vertebrae. The surfaces of the bones are covered with sheets of hyaline cartilage, and these in turn are connected by a dense plate of fibrocartilage that radiates into the periosteum and the surrounding ligaments. *Symphyses*, such as the pubic and manubriosternal joints, are further examples of secondary cartilaginous joints.

They differ from the intervertebral discs in that a secondary cleft formation takes place. However, this joint cavity lacks the specializations of a synovial joint.

### Synovial Joints

In synovial joints, the participating bones are held together by an *articular capsule* that is a continuation of the periosteum. Each bone borders on a joint cavity and has at its end a cap of *articular cartilage* that baths in a lubricating *synovial fluid* (Fig. 4–37).

The articulating surfaces of the diarthrotic joint are always covered with cartilage, which is usually hyaline containing abundant collagenous fibers. In some situations in which shearing forces predominate, such as the margins of the glenoid fossa of the shoulder joint and the acetabulum of the hip joint, fibrous cartilage covers the articulating surfaces. The deepest layer of the articular cartilage, immediately above the compact bone, is calcified, and its cells lie in perpendicular col-

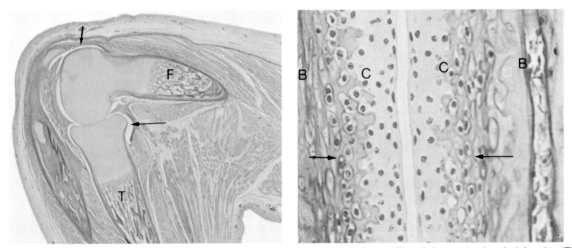

**Figure 4–37.** *Diarthroses. Left (knee joint): In this section, the distal end of the femur (F) and the proximal end of the tibia (T) are shown. The epiphyses of both these bones are cartilaginous at this stage, and there is no distinction between articular cartilage and the main mass of each epiphysis. The joint space between the epiphyses is limited by the joint capsule (arrows). No details of the capsule are apparent at this magnification, but the inner layer is becoming specialized as the synovial membrane, which lines the joint cavity, except over articular surfaces. Van Gieson. Low power. Right (articular cartilage): This is a section through the synovial joint between two of the small bones (ossicles) of the middle ear. The participating bones (B) are covered with articular (hyaline) cartilage (C). Near the joint surface, the nuclei of chondrocytes appear flattened and more densely stained than those within the interior of the cartilage. The interface between articular cartilage and the underlying bone (arrows) is irregular. H and E. High power.*

## Summary Table 4–1. Morphological Characteristics of Cartilage and Bone

| Classification | Cells | Fibers | Matrix |
|---|---|---|---|
| **CARTILAGE** | | | |
| Hyaline | *Chondroblasts* are elliptical and flattened, with rounded nuclei containing one to two small nucleoli. Cytoplasm contains lipid droplets. Forms sulfated protein polysaccharides of matrix. *Chondrocytes* are ovoid or spherical and occupy small cavities, or lacunae. Large central nucleus, one or two nucleoli, and cytoplasm basophil, vacuolated with glycogen and pigment granules and cytoplasmic processes. Group of cells in a lacuna called isogenous group, or cell nest. | Acidophilic collagenous, rarely in definite bundles forming a fine feltwork of type II collagen, absent around territorial areas. Masked by dense matrix (same refractive index) and can be visualized with polarized microscope. | Semisolid. Quantity great. Homogeneous and glassy in fresh preparations. Consists of sulfated glycosaminoglycans, keratan sulfate, and some hyaluronic acid. Territorial areas (cartilage capsules) are rich in proteoglycans, intensely basophil, and metachromatic with toluidine blue and show a strongly positive PAS reaction. Grows appositionally (exogenously) and interstitially (endogenously) except at articular surfaces. Avascular, with nutrients and oxygen reaching cells via long-range diffusion. With age, basophilia lessens and retrogressive calcification changes occur. |
| Elastic | Oval, few, and scattered. Same cell types as in hyaline but less accumulation of fat and glycogen. | Elastic elements vary in thickness and amount; predominate. In general, larger and more intensely packed in the interior. Stain black with Verhoeff's elastic tissue stain. | Semisolid. Quantity large and resilient owing to elastic fibers masking collagenous fibers. Grows appositionally and interstitially. Yellow color in the fresh state. More opaque than hyaline and less likely to undergo retrogressive changes. |
| Fibrous | Oval; few occurring singly; found in pairs or small groups or in linear rows between the fiber bundles. | Massive numbers of collagenous elements arranged in wavy parallel bundles. | Fluid. Small quantity. Grows interstitially only (lacks perichondrium). Reinforced by additional parallel bundles of collagenic fibers. |

*Table continued on opposite page*

umns. The outer cells tend to have the long axes of their lacunae parallel to the articular surface. The distribution and abundant amount of collagenous fibers is thought to be functionally determined. Articular cartilage possesses no nerve fibers or blood vessels, and its outer surface is not covered wiith a perichondrium. The replacement of the surface is by mitoses in deeper layers.

The joint capsule is composed of two layers, one external *fibrous layer*, which represents a continuation of the periosteum and forms the ligament of the joint, and one internal *synovial layer* or *membrane*, which lines the joint cavity, except over the articular cartilage and, when present, intra-articular discs.

The synovial membrane is a thin vascular membrane containing large blood vessels that are derived from a mass of capillary loops found near the margins of the cartilage. More deeply, a layer of loose connective tissue or fat may be present. The lining cells, *synovial cells*, consist of one to three cell layers of flattened or cuboidal cells. These cells originate in the mesenchyme and are separated from each other by a small amount of connective tissue ground substance. No basement membrane occurs beneath these lining cells, and the underlying capillaries therefore have no barrier separating them from the joint cavity. Observations made with the electron microscope reveal two cell types lining the synovial membrane; however, they may represent different functional stages of the same cell type. Type A cells (or M cells) are intensely phagocytic. They represent the predominant form and contain within their cyto-

| Summary Table 4–1. Morphological Characteristics of Cartilage and Bone Continued | | | |
|---|---|---|---|
| **Classification** | **Cells** | **Fibers** | **Matrix** |
| BONE | *Osteoprogenitor* are spindle-shaped, with pale-staining elongated nuclei and sparse cytoplasm. Two types: *preosteoblast* and *preosteoclast*.<br><br>*Osteoblasts* are bone-forming, cuboidal to pyramidal in shape, with delicate cytoplasmic processes. Oval eccentric nucleus with prominent nucleolus. Cytoplasm markedly basophil, containing fine granules and vesicles (alkaline phosphatase).<br><br>*Osteocytes* are ovoid-biconvex, faintly basophil, fat droplets, some glycogen and fine granules in cytoplasm. Nucleus darkly staining and cytoplasmic processes with gap junctions at points of contact.<br><br>*Osteoclasts* are resorptive in function, multinucleated (50–200) giant elements that lie in shallow indentations (Howship's lacunae). Cytoplasm is faintly basophil, granular, containing lysosomes (acid phosphatase) and extensive ruffled border abutting on bone. Also secrete collagenase and proteolytic enzymes. | Osteocollagenous (type I) masked by density of matrix. | Hard and dense. Large quantity of heavily calcified collagen. Vascular, tissue fluids and nutrients reach cells via canalicular system. Deposited by apposition only. Osteocollagenous fibers united by cementing substance (glycosaminoglycans). Amorphous ground substance has less chondroitin sulfate than cartilage—more acidophil. Arranged in lamellae (3–7 μm thick), with alternating pattern. Bone ash: calcium phosphate (85 per cent); calcium carbonate (10 per cent) and 5 per cent (calcium fluoride, manganese fluoride, magnesium fluoride).<br><br>Architecture: *Spongy (cancellous) bone* consists of trabeculae separated by marrow cavities. Prenatal (woven) spongy bone consists of irregular network of collagenous fibers. *Compact bone* consists of regularly arranged lamellae, pattern determined by blood vessels:<br><br>1. Haversian canals—longitudinal vascular channels.<br>2. Canaliculi—spaces (lacunae) that pass in perpendicular direction through lamellae.<br>3. Haversian system—concentric lamellae, bone cells, and central canal.<br>4. Volkmann's canal—enters bone at right angles to the long axis, communicates with Haversian canal.<br>5. Interstitial lamellae—angular pieces of bone among Haversian systems.<br>6. External circumferential lamellae—subperiosteal parallel lamellae.<br>7. Internal circumferential lamellae—subendosteal parallel lamellae.<br><br>Development: *Intramembranous ossification*—within condensation of mesenchymal tissue. *Endochondral ossification*—within a piece of hyaline cartilage whose shape resembles a small model of bone to be formed. |

plasm a large Golgi complex, numerous mitochondria and lysosomes, and micropinocytotic vesicles but only a small amount of rough endoplasmic reticulum. In type *B* synovial cells (or *F* cells), the cytoplasm contains a well-developed rough endoplasmic reticulum, and generally, the cells possess the cytological features of fibroblasts. The latter cells are more electron-dense than A cells. The internal surface of the synovial membrane may have microscopic finger-like projections that protrude into the joint cavity as coarse folds (*synovial villi*) and may evaginate through the fibrous layer of the capsule, between neighboring tendons and muscles, to form pockets known as *bursae*.

The synovial membrane produces a colorless, transparent, viscous fluid, rich in hyaluronic acid, called *synovial fluid*. The hyaluronic acid is strongly polymerized and is well suited as a lubricating fluid to facilitate the sliding of articular surfaces. This synovial fluid also supplies nutrients and oxygen to the avascular articular cartilage, since it represents a dialysate of the blood plasma and lymph. Much of the covalently bound protein present in this fluid derives from the blood plasma.

The joint cavity sometimes is partially or completely subdivided by *intra-articular discs*. These discs are derived from mesenchyme that later differentiates into fibrocartilage. At the periphery, the discs are connected to the fibrous layer of the capsule. It is thought that the discs function to improve the fit between the articular surfaces and as shock absorbers. These discs are fibrocartilaginous in nature because they are almost always found in joints where shearing forces are present.

# Specialized Connective Tissue: Blood

## INTRODUCTION

Blood is a specialized form of connective tissue, first formed in mesenchymal vascular spaces of human embryos at early somite stages. It consists of formed elements, or blood cells, and a fluid intercellular substance, the *blood plasma*. Blood is a circulating tissue, integrating one region of the body with another. Throughout life, it is kept in continual circulation through blood vessels (Chapter 8) by the pumping action of the heart. In this way, it acts as a transporting medium, conveying to the cells the substances essential to their life processes and removing from them metabolic wastes. The volume of blood in the healthy adult human is about 5 liters, and blood composes 8 per cent of the body weight. Because of the fluidity of plasma, blood cells have no definite spatial relationship. Cells of the blood are designated according to their appearance in the fresh unstained condition. The cellular, or formed, elements of the blood are:

5

the red corpuscles (*erythrocytes*), white cells (*leukocytes*), and blood platelets (*thrombocytes*).

The examination of the formed elements of blood is of clinical importance, since the morphology, numbers, and proportions of the different cell types are indicators of many pathological changes in the body. Although some features of the formed elements are visible in fresh blood, many others are seen only after fixation and staining. It is suggested that several standard atlases of blood cells be kept in the histological laboratory while blood is being studied. A great deal of time will be saved if students can have at hand excellent colored illustrations of all of the blood cells they are likely to meet here and in their subsequent work in clinical hematology.

The Romanovsky methods of staining, of which the Giemsa and Leishman stains are examples, are used extensively in histological and clinical laboratories. They involve staining in solutions that are mixtures of methylene blue and eosin. Additionally, it should be noted that figures given for cell dimensions and numbers are approximate ranges only and that, with the exception of the red blood cells, the dimensions of cells when measured in the fresh state are smaller than when measured in a dried and fixed smear of blood.

## ERYTHROCYTES

The erythrocytes, or *red blood corpuscles*, are highly specialized cells whose function is to carry oxygen from the lungs to the tissues and to bring back carbon dioxide. Erythrocytes are called corpuscles because, unlike the leukocytes, they do not possess a nucleus. However, a nucleus is present in the cells (*normoblasts*) from which the red corpuscles are derived. In a few mammals, and in many of the lower animals, the erythrocytes retain their nuclei throughout life. The red corpuscles are flattened, biconcave discs (Fig. 5–1). This biconcave shape offers the greatest possible surface area for the size of the cell. They appear dumbbell-shaped when cut in half and viewed edgewise. When viewed on its flattened surface, the corpuscle shows a thin central portion that appears lighter than the thickened margin portion. In certain diseases, human erythrocytes of altered shape are found in the circulation (Fig. 5–2). The corpuscles are elastic and are capable of considerable distortion, as evident in their ability to pass through capillaries of small caliber. While the biconcave disc shape is by far the most common seen in the circulating blood, bell- and cup-shaped cells have been described. These variations are most likely a modification of the biconcave form in response to external forces.

Corpuscles average about 7.6 μm in diameter and 1.9 μm in greatest thickness in dried smears. The living hydrated corpuscle has a diameter larger than this (about 8.5 μm), and in sectioned material, the diameter is smaller (about 7 μm). The corpuscle is a handy measuring stick for estimating the size of adjacent structures in histological sections.

Erythrocytes are the most numerous of the formed elements of the blood. In the normal adult male, they number about 5 million per cubic millimeter; in the adult female, about 4½ million. These figures represent averages, and actual normal counts may vary as much as a million, more or less, from the averages given. Prolonged residence at high altitude is accompanied by an increase in the number of erythrocytes. The figure for the total surface area of all of the red blood corpuscles in the human body is impressive. It amounts to about 3500 square meters. This enormous area is available for exchange between the corpuscles on the one hand and the plasma and air on the other.

In thin smears of freshly drawn blood, the erythrocyte is pale greenish-yellow. The characteristic red color becomes evident when the cells are crowded together. In a dried smear of peripheral blood, the erythrocytes stain red (i.e., are

**Figure 5–1.** *Scanning electron microscopic view of human erythrocytes.* Top: *Two erythrocytes in the lumen of a small capillary.* × *3600.* (Courtesy of Dr. H. Tung.) Bottom left: *The erythrocytes of human and most mammalian species are shown very clearly to be like biconcave discs.* × *5850.* Bottom right: *Irregular-shaped erythrocytes are characteristic of a form of anemia called spherocytosis. Platelets (P) are also present.* × *4645.* (Reproduced with permission from Fujita, T., et al.: SEM Atlas of Cells and Tissues. New York, Igaku-Shoin Medical Publishers, Inc., 1981.)

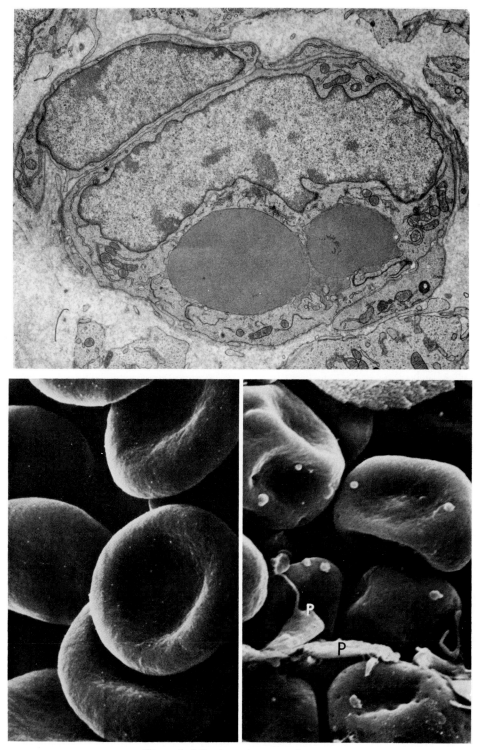

***Figure 5–1*** See legend on opposite page

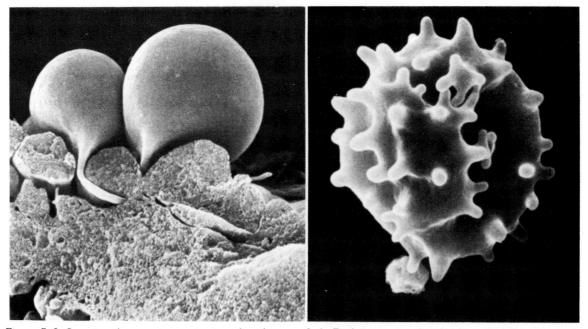

*Figure 5–2.* Scanning electron microscopic view of erythrocytes. Left: Erythrocytes are often fixed in a hanging state on the sinus wall. × 13,000. Right: Erythrocytes may transform into cells called echinocytes (prickly-husked cells) during preparation of blood smears. This deformation allows for a decrease in the resistance of the membrane and may occur in certain pathological conditions, including spherocytosis. × 9000. (Reproduced with permission from Fujita, T., et al.: SEM Atlas of Cells and Tissues. New York, Igaku-Shoin Medical Publishers, Inc., 1981.)

acidophil) with the Leishman and Giemsa stains. The cytoplasm appears homogeneous, and no nucleus is present. Each erythrocyte is bound by a delicate plasma membrane (i.e., a typical "unit" membrane) that consists of about 40 per cent lipid (e.g., phospholipid, cholesterol), 50 per cent protein, and 10 per cent carbohydrate. About 50 per cent of the proteins exist as integral membrane proteins. Several peripheral proteins are found within the plasma membrane and include *spectrin* and *actin*. These peripheral proteins form a cytoskeletal network composed of two layers: a vertical granular layer and a horizontal filamentous meshwork. The meshwork is mainly constructed of the contractile protein, spectrin. Both spectrin and actin are bound to the integral membrane proteins of the plasma membrane via other peripheral membrane proteins, called *ankyrin*. Spectrin maintains the biconcave shape and allows for efficient flow of oxygen and carbon dioxide within the interior. This flexibility of the membrane also permits the viscosity of the blood to remain low. While the shape of the mature

erythrocyte is affected by the subplasmalemmal network, membrane plasticity, which is necessary for survival, is dependent on the presence of membrane constituents in plasma membrane (e.g., cholesterol). Normally, about 1 per cent of the corpuscles encountered in peripheral blood are not fully mature. This percentage of immature erythrocytes (reticulocytes) reflects the rate at which erythrocytes are replaced daily by the bone marrow. Abnormal increases in the numbers of reticulocytes indicate an increased demand for oxygen-carrying capacity. The reticulocytes appear a little larger than the red blood cells and often contain ribosomal RNA that, in the presence of Romanovsky's stains, exhibits a slight bluish tinge. When stained supravitally with brilliant cresyl blue, this residual rRNA (ribosomal RNA) appears as a few granules or a delicate internal network, or reticulum.

Erythrocytes have a tendency to adhere to each other along their concave surfaces, thus forming columns or rows like piles of coins. This phenomenon is termed *rouleaux formation* and occurs spontaneously in a stagnant circulation or in blood removed from the circulation. Although the exact cause is not known, it is thought by many to be due to surface tension.

Chemically, the content of the erythrocyte consists of a lipid and protein colloidal complex that contains an approximately 33 per cent solution of *hemoglobin*. This is the oxygen-carrying protein that is responsible for the color of red blood corpuscles and partly determines the shape of the erythrocytes. The hemoglobin molecule represents a conjugated protein of four subunits, each of which contains a heme group, a porphyrin derivative plus ferrous iron, bound to a polypeptide. Variations in the polypeptide chain of a heme group result in various types of hemoglobin. Hemoglobin combines with oxygen (*oxyhemoglobin*) and carbon dioxide (*carbaminohemoglobin*) in a reversible chemical manner. Its combination with carbon monoxide (*carboxyhemoglobin*) is not reversible and could result in the death of the organism. Since erythrocytes lose their nucleus, mitochondria, ribosomes, and many cytoplasmic enzymes, they are unable to synthesize hemoglobin. The primary source of energy for this cell is the anaerobic degradation of glucose to lactate. A small portion of the glucose (10 per cent) is aerobically processed by means of the hexose monophosphate shunt. The enzymes for the aforementioned metabolic pathways are retained within the mature cell.

A slight structural change in a single amino acid in the Hb A, normal adult hemoglobin, results in a clinical syndrome called *sickle cell anemia*. This produces an altered form of hemoglobin (*Hb S*) and cells that are rod-like, very inflexible, and subject to rupture during their passage through splenic blood vessels.

The contents of the corpuscle normally are in osmotic equilibrium with the plasma. The plasma membrane of the erythrocyte contains an ATP-dependent active transport system that is specific for sodium and potassium. If plasma is concentrated by evaporation or if hypertonic solutions are added to the blood, *crenation* of the corpuscles occurs. This is the result of the passage of water from the corpuscles into the plasma, causing a shrinkage of the corpuscles and so producing protuberances on their surface or a scalloped contour. On the other hand, if the solution is diluted (hypotonic medium), water enters the corpuscles and they swell, becoming spherical, and lose hemoglobin to the surrounding plasma. This process is called *hemolysis*. The resulting form is called a *blood shadow* or *blood ghost* and virtually consists of a pure membrane preparation. Hemolysis is also accomplished by agents that damage the plasma membrane, and the substances that affect it are known as *hemolysins* or hemolytic agents.

*Agglutination*, or clumping of corpuscles, is induced by various agents. It may occur in the circulating blood in a variety of pathologic conditions. *Agglutinins* present in the plasma of some individuals may cause agglutination of erythrocytes in others. The agglutinins form the basis for the four main blood groups (ABO blood group). The factors that determine these blood groups are the terminal sugars of the glycocalyx on the plasma membrane, which are glycoproteins and glycolipids. The terminal amino acid composition and sequence of glycophorin on the external surface of the plasma membrane determine the MNS blood group.

In certain pathological conditions, not only the number but also the size, shape, and hemoglobin content of the erythrocytes may vary enormously. The presence of a high percentage of erythrocytes varying greatly in size is called *anisocytosis*. Cells smaller than 6 μm in diameter are termed *microcytes*, and cells larger than normal, found commonly in some types of anemia, are known as *macrocytes* or *megalocytes*. Cells with distortions in shape are termed *poikilocytes*. When the rate of red blood cell formation is greater than the rate of hemoglobin synthesis, red blood cells are produced that contain a concentration of hemoglobin less than normal. Such cells appear paler (*hypochromic*) than the normal erythrocytes (*normochromic*). There is a pathological condition that results in the retention of fragments of nuclear DNA during removal of the nucleus. Two or more granules are termed *Howell-Jolly bodies*.

## LEUKOCYTES

Leukocytes, or *white blood cells*, contain nuclei. There is an average of 5,000 to 9,000 leukocytes per cu mm in normal human blood. These cells do not present a constant form, owing to their capacity for ameboid movement. Unlike erythrocytes, leukocytes are functional only to a small extent in the blood stream. Their greatest activity is exhibited in the connective tissues. Their capacity for ameboid movement enables them to push the cells of the capillary walls (*endothelium*) apart and enter or leave these vessels (*diapedesis*). Leukocytes generally are involved in the cellular and humoral defenses of the organism against foreign materials. It is for this reason that they are found in considerable numbers in the connective tissue.

The leukocyte count in children is much higher, and marked variations from the normal number occur pathologically. If the number is increased above 12,000 per cu mm, the condition is referred to as *leukocytosis*; if decreased below 5,000, it is called *leukopenia*. It must be appreciated that leukocytes seen in the living state or in routine histological sections appear quite different from the same cells seen in dried smears. In sectioned material, the leukocytes appear rounded, as they do within the circulation, but their diameters are less than in the living condition owing to shrinkage. In smear preparations, cells flatten and appear larger than in life, and many structural details are altered or distorted; for instance, the nucleolus of granular leukocytes is obscured. Thus, the type of preparation must be borne in mind when consideration is given to the histological appearances of the various cells.

Leukocytes are of two main types, *agranular* and *granular* (Fig. 5–3). The agranular leukocytes are characterized by their clear, homogeneous, slightly basophilic cytoplasm. The nuclei are spherical to reniform in shape. The granular leukocytes have a cytoplasm that contains numerous characteristic granular bodies and possess nuclei that exhibit considerable variation in shape.

### Agranular Leukocytes

Two types of agranular leukocytes exist: *lymphocytes*, which are small cells with a scanty cytoplasm, and *monocytes*, which are slightly larger cells containing somewhat greater amounts of cytoplasm.

**Lymphocytes.** In human blood, the lymphocytes are spherical cells that vary from 6 to 8 μm in diameter, although a few may be larger. Most are only a little larger than erythrocytes. They make up from 20 to 35 per cent of the total white blood cells. In small lymphocytes, the nucleus is so large that it fills nearly the entire cell, leaving only a narrow rim of cytoplasm. The amount of cytoplasm is so small in quantity that in laboratory preparations the nucleus is the only part of a small lymphocyte that can be identified. The nucleus appears spherical and generally shows a small indentation to one side. This indentation is more obvious in the large lymphocyte. The densely packed chromatin of the nucleus stains intensely, and the nucleolus is invisible in stained dried smears. The cytoplasm stains basophil, owing to a concentration of ribosomes throughout the cytoplasm, as is seen on electron micrographs. Dry smears stained by the Romanovsky method show purplish, azurophil granules that may occasionally be seen within the cytoplasm, but unlike the specific granules of the granular leukocytes, they are variable in nature.

A few of the lymphocytes of normal circulating blood may be as large as 10 to 12 μm (measured in dried smears). In fresh blood, their size is somewhat smaller. The larger size is due chiefly to a greater amount of cytoplasm. These cells sometimes are referred to as *medium-sized lymphocytes*. Some of the larger cells may appear to be intermediate between lymphocytes and monocytes. None of these large cells should be confused with the *large lymphocytes* that reside in the lymph nodes and appear in the blood only in pathological conditions. The latter are distinguished by the presence of a vesicular nucleus with prominent nucleoli.

Although morphologically similar, lymphocytes of the blood constitute a heterogeneous cell population that may be classified on the basis of origin, fine structural appearance, surface markers, life cycle, and function. They also have the

---

**Figure 5–3.** *Human blood cells from a smear after Wright's stain. A and D, Neutrophil leukocytes. B and E, Eosinophil leukocytes. C, Basophil leukocyte. F, Plasma cell; this is not a normal constituent of the peripheral blood but it is included here for comparison with the nongranular leukocytes. G and H, Small lymphocytes. I, Medium lymphocytes. J, K, and L, Monocytes. (From Fawcett, D. W.: Bloom and Fawcett: A Textbook of Histology, 11th ed. Philadelphia, W. B. Saunders Co., 1986.)*

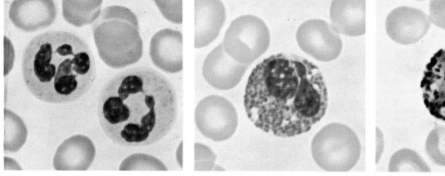

A
B
C

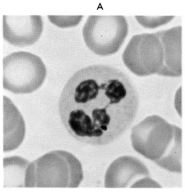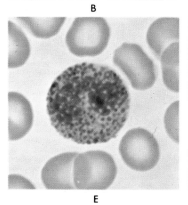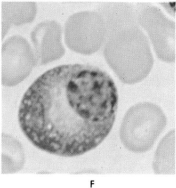

D
E
F

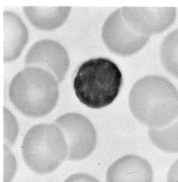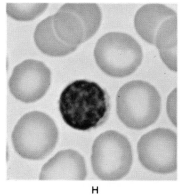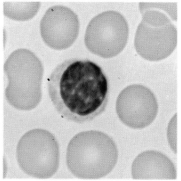

G
H
I

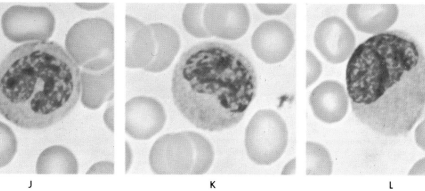

J
K
L

*Figure 5–3* See legend on opposite page

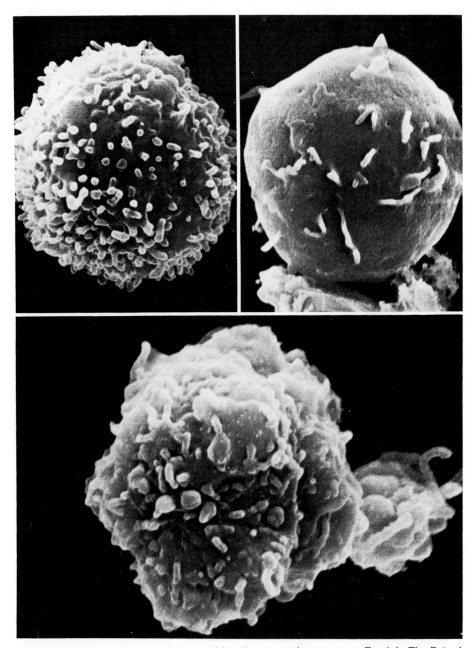

**Figure 5–4.** *Scanning electron microscope preparations of lymphocytes and a monocyte. Top left: The B (or bone marrow–derived) type of lymphocyte is generally characterized by fairly uniform microvilli, which densely cover the cell surface.* × *18,000. Top right: The T (or thymus-derived) type of lymphocyte is generally smooth, with only a few microprojections.* × *16,000. Bottom: Monocytes have a rather irregular surface structure possessing villous, lamellar, and granular microprojections. A pseudopodium is seen at the right, issuing long microvilli as the cell migrates along a glass surface.* × *19,000. (Reproduced with permission from Fujita, T., et al.: SEM Atlas of Cells and Tissues. New York, Igaku-Shoin Medical Publishers, Inc., 1981.)*

capacity to be transformed into other cell types. Large lymphocytes, with diameters of up to 18 μm, will differentiate into two major categories of effector cells, T or B lymphocytes, in response to specific antigens (Fig. 5–4). These are discussed in more detail in the latter part of this chapter.

**Monocytes.** Monocytes are large cells having an average diameter of 9 to 12 μm, but in dried smears, they may flatten out to achieve a diameter of 20 μm or more (Fig. 5–5). They constitute from 3 to 8 per cent of the leukocytes of the blood. The nucleus is located eccentrically in the cell and is ovoid or kidney-shaped. The nucleus may show a deep depression or a horseshoe shape in older cells. The nucleus does not stain as deeply as that of the lymphocyte, owing to the finely granular character of the chromatin that is disposed in a delicate network. The cytoplasm is relatively abundant and with Wright's stain is pale grayish-blue in dried smears. It often has a vac-

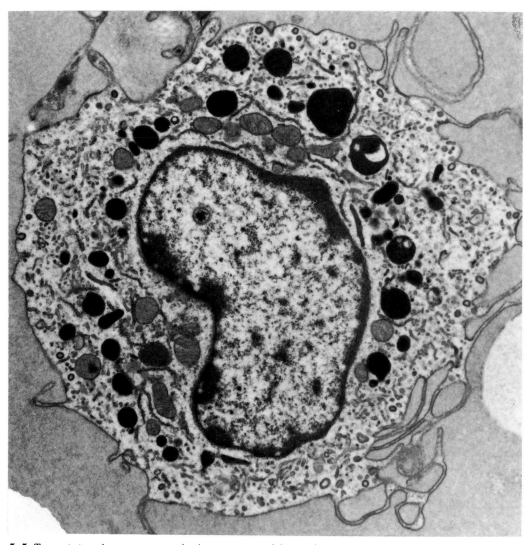

**Figure 5–5.** *Transmission electron micrograph of a monocyte exhibiting phagocytic microprojections along its marginal border. The nucleus is indented, and the cytoplasm contains electron-dense azurophil granules (primary lysosomes) and some granular endoplasmic reticulum.* × *15,300. (Courtesy of James Weber and H. N. Tung.)*

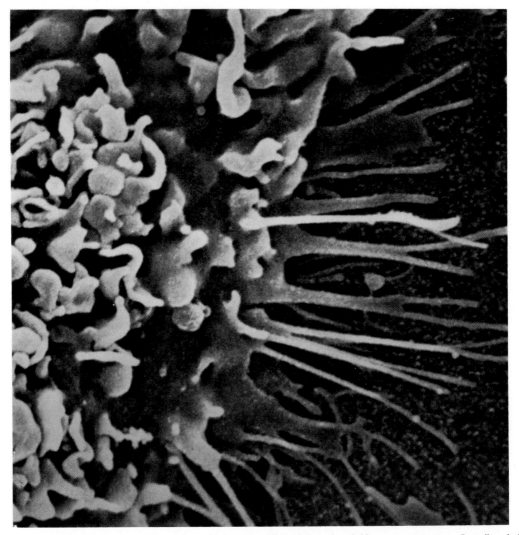

***Figure 5–6.*** *This SEM of a rat macrophage shows filamentous (*filopodia*) and web-like microprojections (*lamellipodia*) along the cell margin. The upper surface of the cell is covered by bulbous or twisted microprocesses (*microlamellae*). × 8700. (Reproduced with permission from Fujita, T., et al.: SEM Atlas of Cells and Tissues. New York, Igaku-Shoin Medical Publishers, Inc., 1981.)*

uolated or reticulated appearance and is seen to contain a population of azurophil granules. These granules are more numerous but smaller than those in lymphocytes. The granules are primary lysosomes. Electron microscopic examination reveals a well-developed Golgi apparatus, microfilaments and microtubules near the indentation of the nucleus, some granular endoplasmic reticulum but fewer free ribosomes than are found in lymphocytes, and one or two nucleoli in the nucleus.

The cell surface of the monocyte is richly supplied with microvilli and pinocytotic vesicles. Rarely, one may find intermediates between monocytes and medium-sized lymphocytes, and in such cases, positive identification is difficult.

Large monocytes show greater activity than small ones, and as they move, they send out many pseudopodia of varying sizes and shapes. After entering the connective tissues, monocytes are transformed into *macrophages*—phagocytic

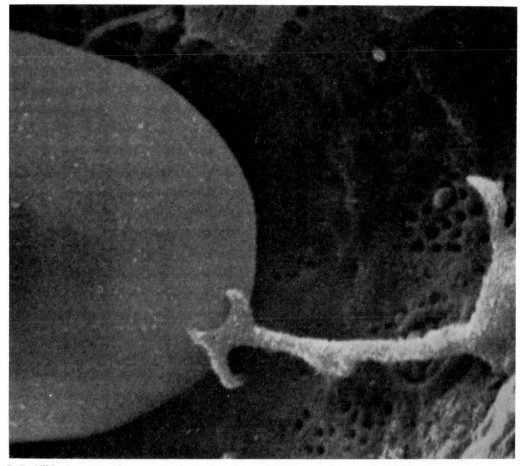

**Figure 5–7.** *SEM of a macrophage cortical filopodium in rat liver. A macrophage (Kupffer's cell) extends a filopodium in recognition of a damaged (previously fixed in glutaraldehyde for a few minutes) erythrocyte in the initial stage of phagocytosis. × 16,000. (Reproduced with permission from Fujita, T., et al.: SEM Atlas of Cells and Tissues. New York, Igaku-Shoin Medical Publishers, Inc., 1981.)*

cells (Fig. 5–6). These macrophages show filamentous microprojections called *filopodia* and web-like ones called *lamellipodia* along the cell margin (Fig. 5–7).

### Granular Leukocytes

The granular leukocytes are of three types: *neutrophil*, *basophil*, and *acidophil* (or *eosinophil*), distinguished by the affinity of their respective granules for neutral, basic, or acid components of the Romanovsky-type dye mixture.

These granules differ in size and in their refractive properties (which in life are semifluid droplets). In contrast with lymphocytes and monocytes, granular leukocytes always contain specific granules. Another characteristic of these cells is the form of their nucleus, which generally exhibits two or more lobes (polymorphous) held together by a delicate piece of nuclear material. For this reason, they are sometimes referred to as *polymorphonuclear leukocytes* (Fig. 5–8). These lobes may be separated in cells that presumably are undergoing degenerative changes.

**Neutrophils.** The neutrophil, polymorphonuclear leukocytes are large cells having a diameter

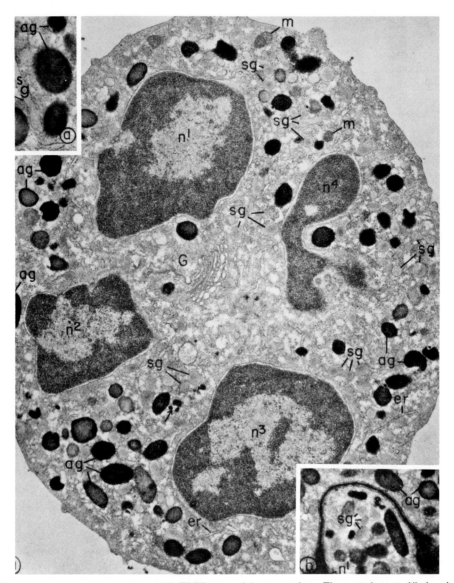

**Figure 5–8.** *Mature polymorphonuclear neutrophil (PMN) reacted for peroxidase. The cytoplasm is filled with granules; the smaller peroxidase-negative specifics (sg) are more numerous, azurophils (ag) having been reduced in number by cell divisions after the promyelocyte stage. Some small, irregularly shaped azurophil granule variants are also present (arrow). The nucleus is condensed and lobulated. The Golgi region (G) is small and lacks forming granules. Endoplasmic reticulum (er) is scanty, and mitochondria (m) are few. Note that the cytoplasm of this cell has a rather ragged, moth-eaten appearance, owing to the fact that glycogen, which is normally present, has been extracted in this preparation by staining in block with uranyl acetate. × 21,000. The insets depict portions of the cytoplasm of mature PMN reacted for peroxidase. Inset a demonstrates that the peroxidase-positive azurophils (ag) can be easily distinguished from the unreactive specifics (sg). Note that one of the specifics is quite elongated (1000 μm). Inset a, × 36,000; inset b, × 14,000 (From Bainton, D. F., et al.: The development of neutrophil polynuclear leukocytes in human bone marrow. J Exper Med 134:907–934, 1971, by copyright permission of the Rockefeller University Press.)*

of 7 to 9 μm in the fresh condition and 10 to 12 μm in dried smears. These cells are the most numerous of the white cells in human blood and constitute from 65 to 75 per cent of the total. The nucleus is highly polymorphous and shows a variety of forms. It usually consists of from three to five irregularly ovoid bodies connected by fine threads of chromatin. The number of lobes increases with age. The lobation of the nucleus has been the basis for the classification of these cells according to their age. There are no nucleoli present in the neutrophils of the peripheral circulation.

In dried smears of the peripheral blood of human females, one can see a small nuclear appendage attached to the remainder of the nucleus by a fine thread of chromatin in about 3 per cent of the neutrophils. This "drumstick," first noted by Davidson and Smith, represents the sex chromosome. Presumably, it is present in all the cells of females, but it is closely packed within one of the lobes of the nucleus in most cells and thus is obscured.

The neutrophils are very actively ameboid and phagocytic and have been estimated to move at an average rate of 35 mm per minute. Their abundant cytoplasm is homogeneous but is filled with fine granules, the majority of which are neutrophil (i.e., react to both acids and basic stains). The result is a characteristic purple or lilac color. In younger cells, the cytoplasm stains basophil, and the granules are bluish purple. With age, the cytoplasm stains faintly acidophil, and the granules are more reddish purple. In other mammals, the granules have variable sizes and staining reactions. In the rabbit and guinea pig, the granules accept the acid stain, and thus in these animals, the cells may be called *pseudoeosinophils*. Since the cells vary in their staining reactions in different species, sometimes they are called *heterophil* leukocytes rather than neutrophils. Most granules are called *specific granules*. These granules are salmon-pink and spherical or rod-shaped and contain alkaline phosphatase, collagenase, lactoferrin, and lysozyme. *Azurophil granules* represent a second type of granule that stains deep reddish-purple and are primary lysosomes that contain acid phosphatase, cathepsin, elastase, collagenase, cationic antibacterial proteins, and myeloperoxidase. These enzymes are principally hydrolytic enzymes and are liberated following ingestion by neutrophils of particles such as carbon, bacteria, and other microorganisms. Both specific and azurophil granules are formed within the Golgi apparatus, with approximately one third of the granules being azurophil in the fully differentiated neutrophil. There are very few mitochondria, a small rough endoplasmic reticulum, and a great amount of glycogen present in the cytoplasm. Since there are few mitochondria present, the Krebs's cycle is of little importance in the metabolic activities of neutrophils. Anaerobic metabolism (via hexose monophosphate shunt) is of great advantage to a cell that kills microorganisms mainly in unoxygenated environments.

**Eosinophils.** The eosinophil, or acidophil, leukocytes are somewhat larger than neutrophils and in the fresh condition are 9 to 10 μm in diameter (Fig. 5–9). They normally make up from 2 to 4 per cent of the white cell count in the adult, but in children, the percentage is somewhat higher, 6 per cent. In dried smears, the size of the flattened cells varies from 12 to 14 μm. The nucleus is usually bilobed (rarely three) and stains somewhat lighter than the nuclei of neutrophils. There are no nucleoli. The cytoplasm characteristically is filled with coarse, refractile granules of uniform size, which stain intensely with acid dyes. The specific granules, which number about 200 per cell, have a striking appearance in electron micrographs. They appear banded because of the presence within them of dense cylindrical crystals that lie parallel to the long axis of the granule. These specific granules are primary lysosomes, which contain acid phosphatase, β-glucuronidase, cathepsin, phospholipase, RNAase, myeloperoxidase, and basic protein (makes up about 50 per cent of granule protein and determines the staining reaction of the granule). The myeloperoxidase found here has far less antibacterial action than that present in neutrophils. These granules, like the azurophil granules of neutrophils, are lysosomal in nature.

**Basophils.** Basophils are difficult to find in human blood because they constitute only about 0.5 to 1.0 per cent of the total number of leukocytes in the blood (Fig. 5–10). They are about the same size as neutrophils, 7 to 9 μm in diameter in the fresh condition and 10 μm or a little more in dried smears. They are not actively

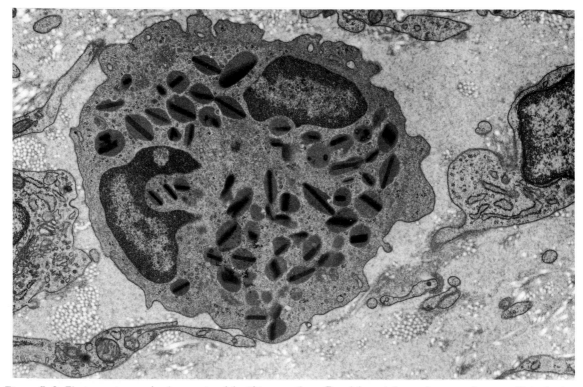

**Figure 5–9.** *Electron micrograph of an eosinophil within a capillary. Two lobes of the nucleus may be seen. Note the large specific granules, each containing a dark, angular mass.* × *12,000. (Courtesy of Dr. H. N. Tung.)*

ameboid but move about more slowly than either of the other granulocytes. The nucleus, less heterochromatic than that of other granulocytes, is irregular in outline and partially constricted into two lobes. It is usually obscured by the overlying specific granules. These cytoplasmic granules are spherical, coarse, and variable in size and stain metachromatically with basic dye owing to the presence of heparin. The granules are soluble in water and therefore are partly dissolved or absent in routine preparations. They are fewer in number and more irregular in size and shape than in the other granulocytes. These basophil, metachromatic granules also contain histamine and serotonin. Unlike the granules in the other types of granular leukocytes, they are not considered to be lysosomes.

Morphologically, there are two basophilic cell types: the basophil leukocytes of the blood and the basophil cells of tissues called *mast cells*. Both have granules that contain heparin and histamine.

But despite the similarities they present, in mammals the mast cell of the connective tissues may arise from several sources, but the basophil leukocyte is derived from the myeloid elements of the bone marrow. In addition, in some species, they have different appearances at the electron microscopic level of examination.

### Function of Leukocytes

Little is known about the functions of leukocytes while in the blood stream, where they appear to be largely inactive. They perform most of their functions outside the vascular system, where they show active movement, and some exhibit phagocytosis. The movement they show is a crawling or ameboid process on a substrate. Neutrophils are the most active, followed by monocytes and basophils. Lymphocytes generally

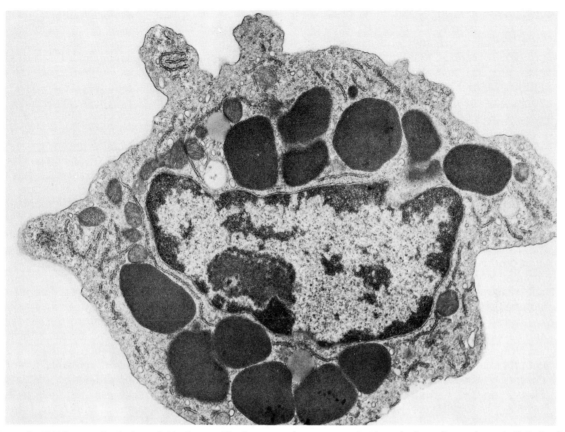

**Figure 5–10.** *Micrograph of a basophil leukocyte. The large granules are somewhat irregular in outline and vary in their density. (From Fawcett, D. W.: Bloom and Fawcett: A Textbook of Histology, 11th ed. Philadelphia, W. B. Saunders Co., 1986, p. 127.)*

appear the most sluggish but, under certain conditions, may become remarkably active. There is a constant migration of leukocytes out of the blood vessels (diapedesis) into the connective tissues. The number of leukocytes within connective tissue is so large that they are considered normal constituents of that tissue. Some of these cells may return into the blood or lymph vessels. Emigration is greatly increased toward the site of local injury or inflammation. This is a specific response to chemotactic stimulation, and cells are attracted by substances elaborated by the injured cells. The term *cytoclesis* is used to describe this attraction between cells. The first cells to respond to such a stimulus are granulocytes; later, monocytes respond. Lymphocytes accumulate in the tissue at sites of chronic inflammation.

Neutrophils constitute the first line of defense against invading organisms, especially bacteria. They are called *microphages* because they actively phagocytize small particles. They are spherical and inactive while circulating in the blood and change form to become active upon touching of a solid substrate. In the active state, they move via pseudopodia at a speed of about 30 μm per minute and spread in various directions. Their specific granules are lysosomal in character and contain hydrolytic enzymes that fuse with the phagosome to form secondary lysosomes. In addition to *lysozyme*, an enzyme that disrupts the glycosides in the cell wall of bacteria, they contain *lactoferrin*, a protein that not only is bacteriostatic to iron-requiring bacteria but also inhibits further neutrophil production. These granules can produce products such as chlorides and lecithins that may inhibit or kill microorganisms. Azurophil granules are another type of granule present in the cytoplasm. Lysosomal in character, they contain acid hydrolytic enzymes and a specific enzyme, *myeloperoxidase*, that combines with peroxide to produce activated oxygen, which is bactericidal. Neutrophils, especially during acute infections, may shed pseudoplatelets that can be readily distinguished from true platelets because they contain neutrophil myeloperoxidase. After this activity, neutrophils become depleted of all granules and eventually die.

Eosinophils, like neutrophils, possess granules that are lysosomal in nature, and they are thought to phagocytose antibody-antigen complexes formed as part of the allergic response in asthma and hay fever. These granules also can reduce inflammation by inactivating histamine and *leukotrienes* produced by basophils. The latter cause slow contraction of smooth muscles and, in this instance, may mediate an inflammatory response. The number of eosinophils is greatly increased in certain allergic diseases and parasitic infections. Eosinophils assist in killing helminths by digesting them with soluble hydrolases. Myeloperoxidase does not have the antibacterial activity of neutrophil enzyme. The eosinophils are attracted to the site of reaction by chemotactic factors that are produced by basophils and lymphocytes. Their number in the blood is decreased following the administration of adrenal corticosteroids. This hormone has no effect on bone marrow eosinophils.

Basophils increase in number in relatively few pathological conditions. The specific granules contain *heparin* (a powerful anticoagulant); *histamine* (increases permeability of blood vessels and thereby decreases the blood pressure); and *serotonin* (constricts blood vessels and assists in increasing blood pressure). These granules are capable of producing leukotrienes, which slow the contraction of smooth muscles. Recently, another substance that is lipid and possibly related to prostaglandins has been isolated. Unlike histamine, it produces a slow but sustained increase in vasodilation and vascular permeability. These materials are aggregated in the specific granules and are discharged at the cell surface by exocytosis. Such features indicate that basophils have a close relationship to mast cells, but despite the similarities, these cells originate from different

stem cells in the bone marrow. When the basophil is the major cell constituent at an inflammatory focus, the condition is termed *cutaneous basophil hypersensitivity*. The basophil, like the mast cell, can release its granular content in response to the action of certain antigens.

Monocytes migrate readily through blood vessel walls and are actively phagocytic. Once they leave the blood stream, they are indistinguishable from connective tissue macrophages (histiocytes), and it is generally considered that these two cell types are identical. In the tissues, they interact with the lymphocytes of the immune defense system.

In recent years, the functions of lymphocytes and the relationship of small, medium-sized, and large lymphocytes have received much attention. It is generally accepted that medium-sized lymphocytes represent either a step in the development of small lymphocytes from large lymphocytes or an intermediate stage in the differentiation of small lymphocytes into plasma cells. With regard to function, the majority of the evidence concerns small lymphocytes, which are known to play a major role in the initiation of the immune responses. It has been shown that small lymphocytes comprise at least two distinct populations of cells as determined by their site of formation, their life span, and their susceptibility to certain drugs. Some lymphocytes arise in bone marrow from a pluripotent or hemopoietic (or hematopoietic) stem cell and pass to the thymus, where they proliferate. These thymic-processed cells (T cells) then may re-enter the blood stream and return to the bone marrow or to peripheral lymphoid organs, where they may live for months or years. T cells are responsible for cell-mediated immune reactions and have surface receptors that are specific for foreign antigen recognition. Other lymphocytes, the B cells (so called because they require the *bursa of Fabricius*, a lymphoid organ in the cloaca of birds or its unidentified equivalent in mammals, for development) apparently do not pass through the thymus but move directly via the blood stream to the general lymphoid tissues. B cells are responsible for the production of antibodies (humoral antibody responses), which circulate in the blood stream and bind specifically to foreign antigens that induce them. Antibody-coated foreign antigen enhances phagocytosis, complement-mediated cell lysis, and killer (K) cell destruction of the invading organisms. T and B cells become morphologically distinguishable only when activated by antigen. Activated B cells have the plasma cell as their end stage of differentiation. Plasma cells have an extensive rough endoplasmic reticulum distended with antibody molecules. Activated T cells have little rough endoplasmic reticulum but are filled with free ribosomes. Both activated cell types migrate via the blood stream to separate areas lacking rigid boundaries within the peripheral lymphoid tissues. This ensures interaction between B and T cells in most antibody responses.

The immune system works by a clonal selection process whereby T or B cells are grouped into different clones or sets. Each set consists of cells committed, before ever being exposed to a particular antigen, to making a particular antibody. When activated by their specific antigen, these cells can differentiate into *effector cells* (cells actively engaged in making a response to an antigen) or into *memory cells* (cells that can readily be induced to become effector cells upon a subsequent antigen encounter). Memory cells may live for years without growing or dividing and are responsible for the secondary immune response. This explains why a second injection of antigen results in a greater and faster production of antibody than the first injection. T and B cells interact with one another in most antibody responses. These interactions are mediated by different T cell subpopulations. *Helper T cells* activate B cells, other T cells, and macrophages. *Suppressor T cells* inhibit B cells and other T cells. Occasionally, tolerance to self-molecules breaks down, causing T or B cells to react against their own cells—an *autoimmune reaction*. In the case of *myasthenia gravis*, antibodies are made against one's own acetylcholine receptors on the skeletal muscle membrane at the myoneural junction. This disrupts innervation of skeletal muscle cells.

Since lymphocytes play such an important role in both humoral antibody and cell-mediated immune responses, it is not surprising that they are particularly abundant ($2 \times 10^{12}$ in humans) in the connective tissues that underlie the epithelial lining of the respiratory and digestive tracts. Their cell mass is comparable to that of the liver or brain.

## BLOOD PLATELETS

Blood platelets are small protoplasmic discs that are colorless in circulating blood. They are 2 to 4 μm in diameter. Their number varies considerably, but usually it is given as 200,000 to 300,000 per cu mm of blood. Their number is extremely difficult to count, since they adhere to each other and to all surfaces as soon as blood is removed from a vessel (Fig. 5–11). Lower vertebrates lack platelets; instead, they possess small nucleated cells, the *thrombocytes*.

Platelets are round or ovoid on the flat; when seen in profile, they appear spindle- or rod-shaped. Blood stains demonstrate two regions of the platelet, a deeply basophil granular zone (the *granulomere*), usually centrally located, and a pale, homogeneous peripheral zone (the *hyalomere*). No nucleus is present. Electron micrographs of platelets reveal the presence of numerous bands of circumferential microtubules that give the platelet its shape. The plasma membrane has a heavy glycocalyx and is continuous with an open canalicular system. Platelets endocytose large particles by invagination of plasma membrane. Small particles and solute enter the system of canaliculi. Microfilaments, consisting of both actin and myosin, are present beneath the plasma membrane and are associated with the bundle of microtubules. Only after the platelets are activated by thermal or mechanical stimuli are the microfilaments assembled from amorphous precursors within the cytoplasm to form a striking network of interconnecting microfilaments.

Two types of granules are suspended within this interfilamentous network: *dense-core granules* and *alpha granules*. The dense-core granules (100 to 250 nm in diameter) contain serotonin, adenosine diphosphate (ADP), adenosine triphosphate (ATP), and calcium. Alpha granules, besides being lysosomal in character, contain various substances related to blood clotting—factors that neutralize heparin, increase vascular permeability, and are chemotactic for neutrophils. The activated platelet also exhibits lamellar bodies, which bear a striking resemblance to tertiary lysosomes (residual bodies). It could be surmised that lysosomal enzymes are being used in the manufacture of a secretory product. Microprojections, extending from the margin of the activated

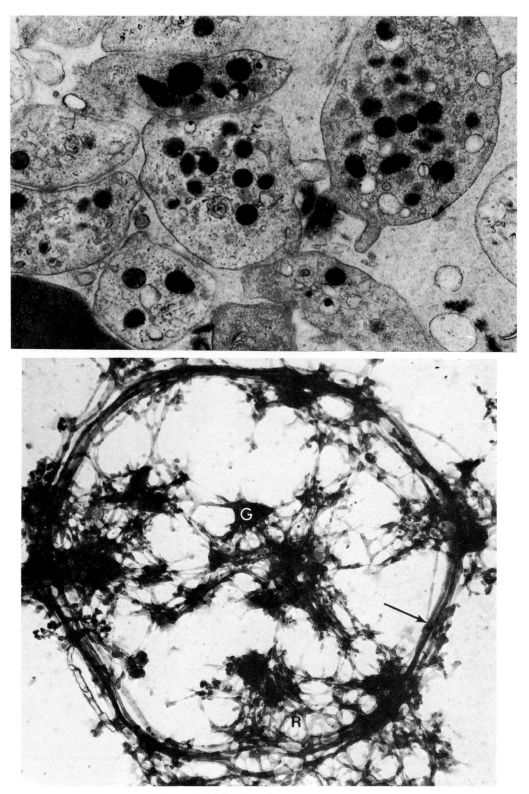

*Figure 5–11* See legend on opposite page

platelet, apparently play a principal role in platelet recognition of tissue damage and cause adhesion to damage sites. A dense tubular system that may be involved in sequestrating calcium and synthesizing prostaglandins is also present within the cytoplasm of platelets.

Platelets arise as detached portions of peculiar giant cells of bone marrow, the *megakaryoctes*. Platelets play several roles in hemostasis (Fig. 5–12). They adhere to injured regions of blood vessels, producing a *white thrombus*, which covers injured surfaces and plugs deficiencies within the vessel walls. They are presumed to produce an enzyme, *thromboplastin*, which is of importance in the clotting mechanism. Thromboplastin aids in the transformation of *prothrombin* into *thrombin*, and thrombin in turn transforms *fibrinogen* into *fibrin*. Serotonin, an agent that causes contraction of smooth muscle in small blood vessels, also is present in platelets, probably located in small cytoplasmic granules.

A decrease in the number of circulating platelets is seen clinically in a condition known as *thrombocytopenia*.

## PLASMA

Plasma is an aqueous solution that transports all nutritive materials. In it are found the nutritive substances derived from the digestive system, the waste substances produced in the tissues, and the hormones. A straw-colored fluid, plasma is homogeneous and slightly alkaline, having a "soapy" feel. It constitutes 55 per cent of a blood sample, with the cellular elements accounting for 45 per cent. Plasma also contains dissolved gases, inorganic salts, proteins, carbohydrates, lipids, and certain other organic substances. The plasma proteins account for about 7 per cent of the volume and consist of *albumin* (maintains the osmotic pressure of the blood and is the main constituent); *gamma globulins* (*immunoglobulins*

or antibodies), and *fibrinogen* (which is an important globulin necessary for the coagulation process). Suspended particles can be demonstrated within it by phase microscopy and dark-field microscopy. These are *chylomicrons*, minute fat globules that are more numerous after a fatty meal. As long as blood continues to flow normally through the blood vessels, the fibrinogen remains in a diffused or solvent condition. When the circulation ceases, or when blood is exposed to air, fibrinogen precipitates as a network of fine filaments, fibrin. The contraction of the clotted blood or plasma (*syneresis*) expresses a clear, yellowish fluid (*serum*) that lacks the formed elements of the blood.

## LYMPH

Lymph is the fluid that is collected from the tissues and returned to the blood stream. Its composition varies considerably. Lymph has a lighter specific gravity than that of blood. It contains no red corpuscles, platelets, or fibrinogen. However, it contains numerous lymphocytes and a few granulocytes. The cells are added to the lymph as it passes through the lymph nodes. The lymph nodes also add immunoglobulins to the lymph and, from there, to the blood stream. Lymph coagulates at a much slower rate than does blood, and the clot is soft. Unlike the blood, it does not carry oxygen but may contain carbon dioxide. Lymph draining from the walls of the small intestine is milky because of the fat globules that it contains and is referred to as *chyle*.

## LIFE SPAN AND DISPOSAL OF BLOOD CELLS

In contrast with many cells, red and white blood cells live for only a relatively short time. The life

---

**Figure 5–11.** Top: *Electron micrograph of a clump of platelets. Each contains a group of dense granules and microtubules, sectioned transversely within the finely granular cytoplasm. A portion of an erythrocyte is also present (lower left). × 8500. Bottom: Platelet on a polylysine-coated grid. This typical view shows a circumferential density that represents the microtubule coil (arrow). The coil appears to be developing angles at intervals. Note strands of the reticulum (R) and dense granules (G). × 32,000. (From Nachmias, V. T.: Cytoskeleton of human platelets at rest and after spreading. J. Cell Biol. 86:795–802, 1980, by copyright permission of the Rockefeller University Press.)*

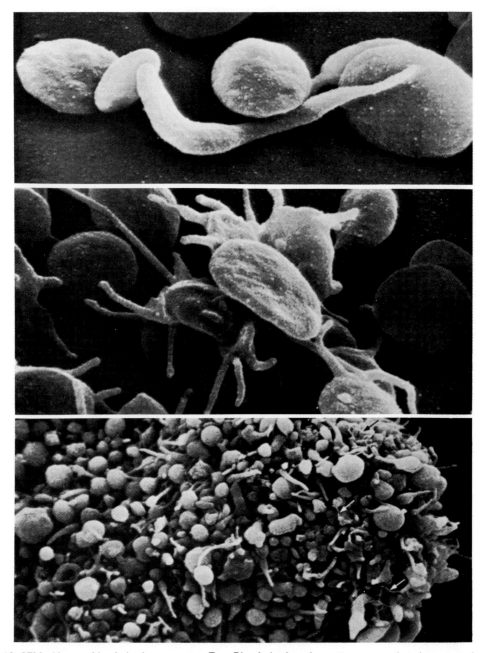

*Figure 5–12.* SEM of human blood platelet aggregates. Top: *Blood platelets play an important role in hemostasis by stimulating the process of blood clotting and thrombi formation. In the unstimulated condition in the blood, they are mostly lens-like discs 2–4 µm in diameter. A deviate form (club-shaped) is occasionally encountered in about 4 per cent of the platelets sampled.* × 15,500. Center: *Activated platelets are shown projecting filopodial microprocesses from the margin of the disc.* × 15,500. Bottom: *Fully activated platelets tend to form aggregates. The trapped cells become swollen and project filopodia that attach to fibrin fibers (arrows). The fiber formation is mediated by thromboplastin produced by the platelets.* × 4000. *(Reproduced with permission from Fujita, T., et al.: SEM Atlas of Cells and Tissues. New York, Igaku-Shoin Medical Publishers, Inc., 1981.)*

span of the human erythrocyte is approximately 120 days. This may be determined by several methods. Differential agglutination (which measures the length of time compatible donor cells survive in a recipient) is cumbersome and has been largely superseded by methods of tagging red blood cells with isotopes. Of the latter, chromium tagging, utilizing $^{51}$Cr, is now the most commonly used. A small quantity of washed red blood cells simply is mixed with a solution of $Na_2[^{51}Cr]O_7$, and this is injected into the subject from whom the blood is removed. The life span is estimated by the persistence of radioactivity.

It is believed that worn-out erythrocytes are removed from the circulation by the macrophages in the spleen, liver, and bone marrow. The worn-out erythrocyte seems to have a defect (removal of sialic acid) in the oligosaccharides on the surface of the plasma membrane. The timing mechanism involved in the "signal for removal" has not been elucidated. After destruction of the red blood cells by the phagocytic cells, hemoglobin is broken down into an iron-containing portion (*hematin*) and an iron-free portion (*globin*). The hematin is further broken down into iron, which is reutilized or stored, and into bilirubin, which is transported to the liver and excreted in the bile.

The life span of the various types of white blood cells is difficult to determine, since these cells leave the blood vascular system to enter the tissue spaces, but it appears to be quite variable. There is evidence that neutrophils have a half-life of about seven hours within the circulating blood but may live in the connective tissues for up to four days. Some lymphocytes may have a life span of only a few days, while others survive in the blood stream for many years (T cells). The half-life of a monocyte in the blood is believe to be from 12 to 100 hours. Many lymphocytes undoubtedly return to the lymphoid organs and recirculate. However, there is no strong evidence that monocytes recirculate in the blood after they enter the connective tissue and differentiate into phagocytic cells. Granulocytes appear to remain alive in the tissue spaces only a few days. Most appear to die whether or not they have taken part in phagocytosis. It is no wonder that neutrophils lack the protein-synthesizing machinery to produce additional granules. Senile and dead cells are thought to be removed by phagocytes within the liver and spleen and locally within the connective tissues. There is a considerable loss of white blood cells owing to migration through the lining epithelium of the mucous membranes, particularly into the lumina of the digestive and respiratory systems.

Platelets are believed to survive for four to six days in the circulating blood. They are thought to be removed from the circulation in a way similar to how erythrocytes are removed (i.e., by phagocytic activity of macrophages in the spleen and liver).

## HEMOPOIESIS

Formed elements of the blood, like the epithelial cells in the gut, are highly specialized cells that have a relatively short life span. The number of formed elements within the blood is kept at a constant number by the formation of new cells as worn-out ones are withdrawn from the blood stream. Specialized connective tissues, *hemopoietic* (or *hematopoietic*) tissues, which are derived from mesenchyme, make new blood cells. The process by which blood cells are formed is called hemopoiesis (hemo, blood; poiesis, making). The formed elements of the blood are divided into two groups according to the major sites of their development and differentiation in the adult. Lymphocytes and monocytes are developed chiefly in the lymphoid tissues and are termed *lymphoid elements*. Erythrocytes and granulocytes normally are produced within the red bone marrow (myeloid tissue) and are referred to as *myeloid elements*. This separation, however, is not absolute. Lymphocytes are produced not only in lymphatic tissue. While T cells are formed in the thymus (a lymphatic organ), B cells differentiate in myeloid tissue and secondarily take up residence in lymphatic tissue. There is now clear evidence, principally from radioautography and chromosome marker techniques, that monocytes also arise within the bone marrow from precursor cells. Additionally, the separation is not seen in the fetus, where hemopoiesis begins outside the embryo itself in different sites at different ages. Prenatal hemopoiesis appears successively in the yolk sac, mesenchyme and blood vessels, liver, spleen, and lymph nodes. Except for the thymus, the major hemopoietic organs in mammals are of mesenchymal origin. In the adult, in certain pathological conditions, myeloid elements may be formed again in the spleen, liver, and lymph nodes, a condition known as extramedullary hemopoiesis. Even the undifferentiated mesenchymal cells within the yellow bone marrow may proliferate, giving rise to myeloid cells in response to excessive hemorrhages (or excessive destruction of erythrocytes).

Hemopoiesis remains one of the greatest areas of controversy in the field of histology. Different interpretations regarding the origin and nature of the stem cell or cells have led to a confusion of ideas by which the subject remains still greatly obscured. One theory, the monophyletic (unitarian) theory of hemopoiesis, holds that all blood cells, red and white, rise from a common stem cell, the *hemocytoblast*, with polyvalent potentiates. The *dualistic* or *diphyletic* theory holds that lymphocytes and monocytes derive from one stem cell (called a *lymphoblast* by many investigators), and granular leukocytes and erythrocytes from a separate cell (the *myeloblast*). At the other extreme, the complete polyphyletic theory maintains that there is a primitive stem cell for each type of blood cell. There has been considerable misunderstanding in the past with regard to these theories, and much of this has been the result of the use of different terminologies by proponents of the different theories. Today, the unitarian theory appears to be accepted by the majority of hematologists. These polyvalent hemocytoblasts or stem cells have the following features: They are uncommitted and poorly differentiated and are capable of renewal and proliferation. Later, the pluripotential stem cells give rise to restricted populations of stem cells that contribute to the lymphoid or myeloid lines of differentiation. These cells are called *restricted progenitor cells*. Eventually, their progeny form the particular precursor that develops into the fully functional cell of a specific blood cell type.

The following account is based upon this interpretation, and it should be emphasized that the controversies do not affect the factual descriptions of the structural features of the blood cells of various developmental stages. The controversies essentially center around the relationships between cells of the earliest stages. These earliest stages contain progenitor cells that cannot be readily identified under the microscope. Experimentally, progenitor cells have been shown to be under the control of certain regulating substances (e.g., *erythropoietin*, which regulates erythrocyte production) and may even require special microenvironments (i.e., T cells) before maturing into fully functional blood cells. Even B cells need the splenic microenvironment to achieve final maturity before entering the circulation.

## DEVELOPMENT OF MYELOID ELEMENTS

Myeloid tissue, under normal conditions, is confined to the marrow cavities of bone, where it is termed *bone marrow* (Figs. 5–13 through 5–15). Bone marrow accounts for about 5 per cent of the total body weight and is the most important hemopoietic tissue in human beings from the fifth month of fetal life through adulthood. It provides a special hemopoietic microenvironment for multipotential stem cells and allows for their differentiation and release into the general circulation (Fig. 5–16). In the adult, there are two types of marrow, red and yellow, which may be interconvertible as a reflection of shifts in the hemopoietic demands. However, red bone marrow is normally actively hemopoietic, whereas in yellow bone marrow, most of the hemopoietic tissue has been replaced by fat. Under certain pathologic situations, the undifferentiated mesenchymal cells in yellow bone marrow may proliferate and form myeloid cells. In the adult, red bone marrow occurs principally in the sternum, ribs, vertebrae, skull, and proximal epiphyses of some of the long bones.

The myeloid tissue compartment provides special microenvironments that consist of a framework (or *stroma*), a vasculature (or blood vessels), and associated cells (or free cells) lying within the meshwork of the stroma (Fig. 5–17).

**Stroma.** The framework is a loose latticework of reticular (argyrophil) fibers in close association with primitive and phagocytic reticular cells. Some fat always occurs in the center of the red bone marrow around the venous sinuses. These fat cells are scattered singly within the stroma, unlike yellow bone marrow, in which the fat cells are so concentrated as to exclude nearly all other elements.

*Text continued on page 222*

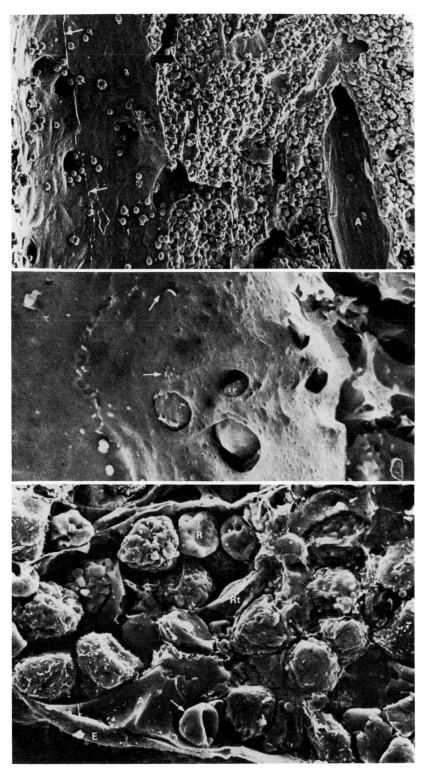

*Figure 5–13.* SEM of bone marrow parenchyme. Top: The longitudinal view of the bone marrow of the femur of a young rat is shown. The central vein is seen, on the left side, with numerous sinuses opening into it. Blood cells and a thread of forming blood platelets (arrows) are seen along the endothelium. Fenestrations in the endothelium are not seen at this magnification. The spaces outside are filled with bone marrow parenchyme (site of blood cell formation). A nutrient artery (A) is seen at the right. × 390. Center: The wall of a sinus shows two types of intracellular fenestrations: (a) large apertures (50–100 μm in diameter) occupied by migrating blood cells, and (b) small sieve-like pores (1–3 μm, arrows). × 8000. Bottom: Blood cell–forming tissue containing immature erythrocytes (R, identified by their smooth but indented surface), one (arrow) of which is seen migrating toward the sinus wall. The sinus wall consists of endothelial (E) and adventitial (A) cells. Reticular cell processes (Rt) divide the marrow tissue into compartments. × 31,000. (Courtesy of M. Muto, Tsuneo Fugita, Keiichi Tanaka, and Junichi Tokunaga. Reproduced by permission of Igaku-Shoin Medical Publishers, Inc.)

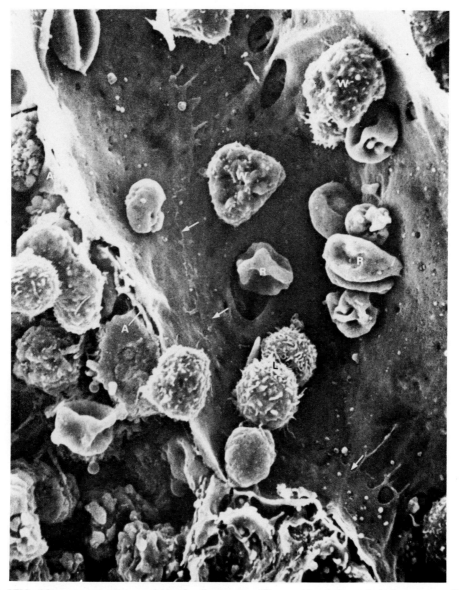

**Figure 5–14.** *SEM of bone marrow sinus and blood cell migration. The outside of the endothelium is partially covered by attenuated processes of adventitial cells (A). Boundaries of flat endothelial cells (arrows) show few microprojections. The apertures of the endothelial cells are occupied by white (W) and red (R) blood cells with some lymphocytes (L) just attached to the wall. × 4000. (Reproduced with permission from Fujita, T., et al.: SEM Atlas of Cells and Tissues. New York, Igaku-Shoin Medical Publishers, Inc., 1981.)*

**Figure 5–15.** *Development of myeloid elements. The double line in the illustration separates the cells that are found in the bone marrow from the mature cells below the line, seen normally in peripheral blood. Note that the myeloblast stage (between the hemocytoblast and the promyelocyte) has been omitted from this diagram. (Courtesy of J. H. Cutts.)*

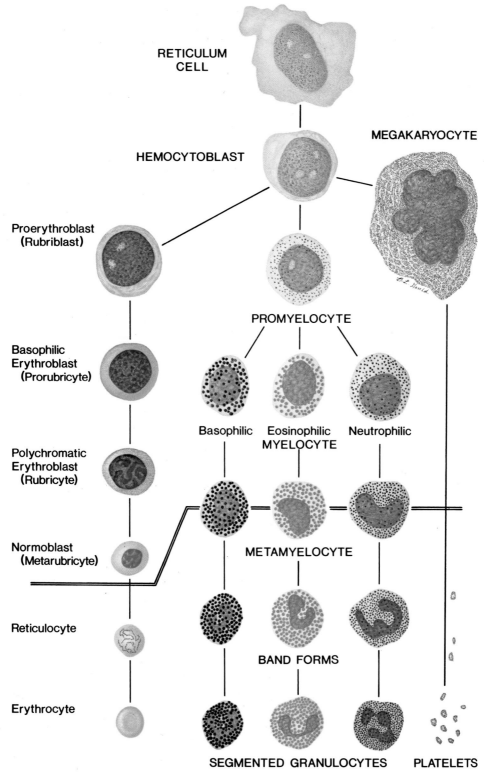

RETICULUM CELL

MEGAKARYOCYTE

HEMOCYTOBLAST

Proerythroblast
(Rubriblast)

PROMYELOCYTE

Basophilic
Erythroblast
(Prorubricyte)

Basophilic   Eosinophilic   Neutrophilic
MYELOCYTE

Polychromatic
Erythroblast
(Rubricyte)

Normoblast
(Metarubricyte)

METAMYELOCYTE

Reticulocyte

BAND FORMS

Erythrocyte

SEGMENTED GRANULOCYTES    PLATELETS

*Figure 5–15* See legend on opposite page

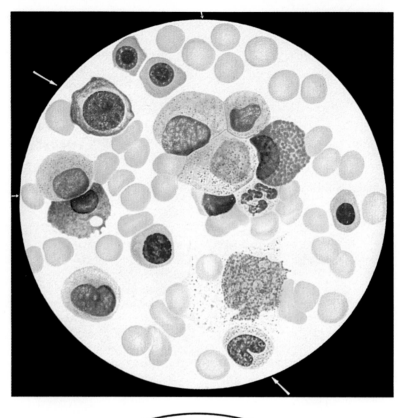

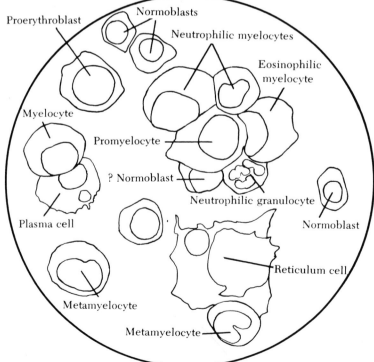

Proerythroblast

Normoblasts

Neutrophilic myelocytes

Eosinophilic myelocyte

Myelocyte

Promyelocyte

? Normoblast

Neutrophilic granulocyte

Normoblast

Plasma cell

Reticulum cell

Metamyelocyte

Metamyelocyte

A

*Figure 5–16.* See legend on opposite page

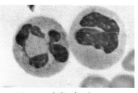

Neutrophilic leukocytes

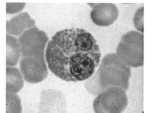

Eosinophilic leukocyte

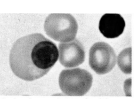

Orthochromatic erythroblast
(normoblast), extruded nucleus

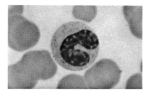

Neutrophilic metamyelocyte

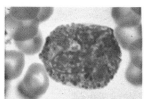

Eosinophilic metamyelocyte

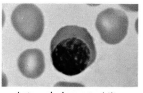

Late polychromatophilic
erythroblast

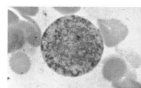

Neutrophilic myelocyte

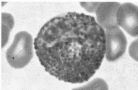

Eosinophilic metamyelocyte

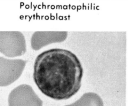

Polychromatophilic
erythroblast

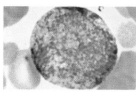

Early neutrophilic myelocyte

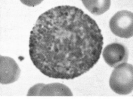

Eosinophilic myelocyte

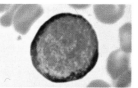

Early polychromatophilic
erythroblast

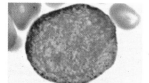

Very early myelocyte

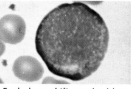

Basophilic erythroblast

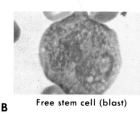

**B**   Free stem cell (blast)

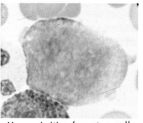

Very primitive free stem cell

Early basophilic erythroblast

*Figure 5–16.* A, *Normal marrow smear and diagram of a representative area. Leishman's stain. (From Heilmeyer, L., and Begemann, H.: Atlas der Klinischen Hämatologie und Cytologie. Berlin, Springer, 1955; reproduced with permission from Springer-Verlag, 1987.)* B, *Photomicrographs of developing blood cells in human bone marrow, showing steps in the transformation of stem cells into neutrophilic and eosinophilic leukocytes and into erythrocytes, as seen in dry smears stained with Wright's blood stain. (From Fawcett, D. W.: Bloom and Fawcett: A Textbook of Histology, 11th ed. Philadelphia, W. B. Saunders Co., 1986, p. 246.)*

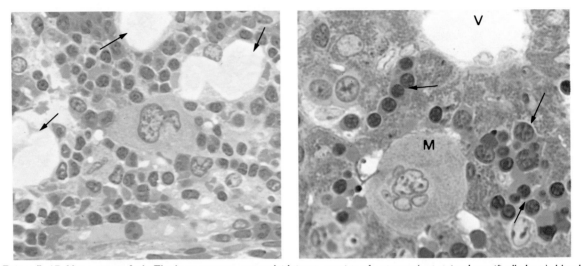

*Figure 5–17. Hemopoiesis.* Left: *The bone marrow, or myeloid tissue, consists of a stroma (not stained specifically here), blood vessels, and free cells. The free cells represent all stages in the maturation of red and white blood cells. Individual cell types generally cannot be recognized. The large cell in the center, with a large lobed nucleus, is a megakaryocyte. The large, clear areas within the stroma are fat cells (arrows). Plastic section. H and E. High power.* Right: *Blood cells are formed in different sites at different stages during development, and in the fetus, they appear successively in the yolk sac, mesenchyme, liver, spleen, and lymph nodes. Blood formation commences in the liver at about six weeks and gradually diminishes during the middle of fetal life. This section demonstrates active hemopoiesis within the liver. Hepatic cells are large and contain large vesicular nuclei. The cells are arranged in plates that radiate out from the central vein (V). Between the plates of liver cells are numerous hemopoietic elements (arrows), principally of the red cell series. A large megakaryocyte (M), with a complex lobed nucleus and finely granular cytoplasm, also is present. With the development of bone marrow (during the third fetal month), hemopoiesis wanes in the liver. Plastic section. Paragon. High power.*

**Blood Vessels.** The characteristic feature of the "closed" circulation of the myeloid tissue compartment is the presence of large, tortuous thin-walled sinusoids 50 to 75 μm in diameter consisting of an *endothelium* of simple squamous cells held together by zonulae adherens (probably associated with gap junctions); a variable *basement membrane*; and minimally phagocytic reticular cells associated with the outer surface of the *adventitia.* The walls of these vascular sinuses possess wide fenestrations with an incomplete basement membrane that permits blood cells to gain entry into the general circulation. Arterioles connect directly with the sinusoids, which themselves are drained by narrow, thin-walled veins that leave the bone marrow at numerous sites. Nerves are associated with this vasculature and appear to be vasomotor.

The adventitial reticular cell branches out into the cords of hemopoietic tissues to form supports for the cords consisting of hemopoietic cells. These reticular cells may play a role in the compartmentalization of hemopoietic cells in particular locations and, in that way, influence the maturation process of blood cells. The reticular cells may accumulate water and fatty substances and produce a white, gelatinous marrow that becomes yellow. In this way, they constitute a mechanism for increasing and decreasing the hemopoietic compartment as the need arises.

**Free Cells.** Cells lying free within the meshes of the stroma represent all stages in the maturation of red and white blood cells. Mature erythrocytes, the three types of granular leukocytes, and agranular leukocytes (lymphocytes, monocytes, and some plasma cells) are found between the immature elements.

## THE STEM CELL: THE HEMOCYTOBLAST

The hemocytoblast is an ameboid blood-forming cell of lymphoid nature. It is indistinguishable from most large lymphocytes and measures approximately 10 to 15 μm in diameter. The nucleus is relatively undifferentiated and contains one or two nucleoli. In dried smears, the nucleus shows dense accumulations of chromatin material. In sectioned material of bone marrow, the nucleus appears vesicular, with some peripheral condensation of heterochromatin, and nucleoli are distinct. Azurophil granules are seen occasionally within the rim of basophil cytoplasm.

Evidence for their capability of differentiating into a unipotent cell for each hemopoietic cell line comes from experimental data involving irradiated experimental animals. The evidence indicates that these multipotential stem cells are not fixed in the adult (as they are in the fetus) and that most stem cells are in the resting stage, since injections of ³H thymidine do not kill all these cells. Hemocytoblasts arise chiefly by mitotic divisions, with a very slow rate of proliferation. In the adult, they are sometimes referred to as *transitional cells*, or *transitional lymphocytes*. Although they occur in greatest numbers in the bone marrow, they do not represent a very high concentration—about 1 per 10,000 nucleated cells in the mouse marrow. These multipotent stem cells also occur in the blood—10 in each milliliter of mouse blood (1 per 100,000 nucleated blood cells). Most investigators believe that these circulating cells in the adult represent "old," although not dying, cells. These blood-borne cells in the fetus are believed to be responsible for the shift in the hemopoietic foci from liver to bone marrow (as indicated by the large numbers present at this particular time). In the adult, the hemocytoblast gives rise to all myeloid elements and, in addition, according to the unitarian theory of hemopoiesis, to lymphoid elements.

**Erythrocytes.** Although erythrocytes represent the majority of the formed elements of the blood, developing and mature erythrocytes constitute only a minority of the blood cells present within myeloid tissue. Two major reasons for this are that the development of a mature erythrocyte takes only about three days (whereas a granular leukocyte requires 14 days or more for development) and that the life span of the latter is short. It should be borne in mind that the principal processes involved in the differentiation of erythrocytes are reduction in size, condensation of the

nuclear chromatin and eventually loss of the nucleus and of cellular organelles, and acquisition of hemoglobin.

For descriptive purposes, erythrocyte development is divided into a number of stages, but it must be emphsized that the process is a continuous one (Fig. 5–18). The stages of erythrocyte development, in order of differentiation from the hemocytoblast, are *proerythroblast, basophil erythroblast, polychromatophil erythroblast, normoblast* (orthochromatic erythroblast), *reticulocyte*, and *erythrocyte*. The terminology used here has the advantage that it is descriptive of most of the stages, but the student should be aware of the fact that other terminologies do exist. A description of the stages follows, and the terms in parentheses represent those recommended by an International Committee on Nomenclature.

***Proerythroblast (Rubriblast).*** This is the earliest recognizable cell of the erythrocyte series and is believed to differentiate from the hemocytoblast, or pluripotential stem cell, by way of a committed erythroid progenitor cell. The proerythroblast is the largest of the precursor cells, about 15 to 20 μm in diameter. The nucleus has a uniform chromatin pattern, more distinct than that of the hemocytoblast, and one or more prominent nucleoli. The amount of cytoplasm is greater than that of the hemocytoblast, and it is moderately basophil. A small amount of hemoglobin can be detected within the cytoplasm by special techniques but is obscured by the basophilia of the cytoplasm in stained preparations at all subsequent stages of development. Submicroscopic membrane-limited structures, *siderosomes*, occur in the cytoplasm. They contain a protein that represents a storage form of iron called *ferritin*. It first appears as pinocytotic vesicles below the plasma membrane of the cell. This iron is brought to the cells in the bone marrow bound to a plasma globulin, *transferrin*.

After undergoing a number of mitotic divisions, the proerythroblast gives rise to the basophil erythroblast.

***Basophil Erythroblast (Prorubricyte).*** This cell is slightly smaller than the proerythroblast and averages 10 μm in diameter. The nucleus possesses a coarse network of dense heterochromatin, and the nucleolus usually is obscured. The sparse cytoplasm shows intense basophilia, indic-

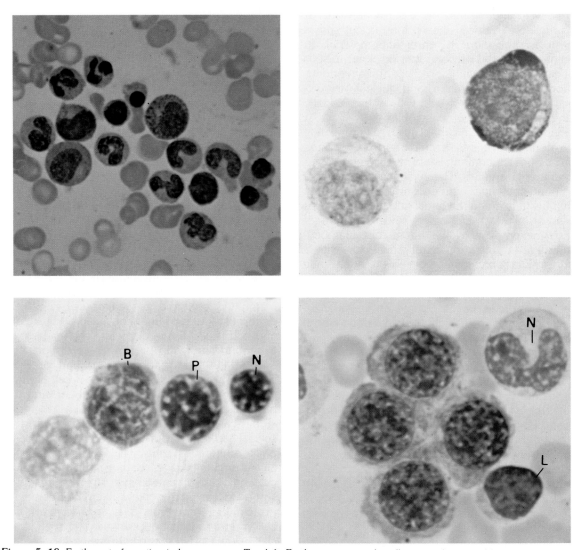

***Figure 5–18.*** *Erythrocyte formation in bone marrow.* Top left: *Erythrocytes are pale yellow, anucleate, and homogeneous. The nucleated cells are immature elements, principally of the white cell series. Wright's stain. High power.* Top right: *Reticular cell (left) and hemocytoblast (right). The reticular cell shows a large, pale nucleus and a faintly basophil, granular cytoplasm. The hemocytoblast possesses a large, ovoid nucleus with a fine pattern of chromatin material; a large, pale nucleolus; and a basophil cytoplasm. Wright's stain. Oil immersion.* Bottom left: *Basophil erythroblast (B), polychromatophil erythroblast (P), and normoblast (N). The basophil erythroblast is smaller than the hemocytoblast, and its nucleus possesses coarser chromatin granules. The cytoplasm is markedly basophil. The polychromatophil erythroblast, smaller than the basophil erythroblast, shows coarse clumping of nuclear chromatin and a cytoplasm that is gray owing to the presence of hemoglobin within the basophil cytoplasm. The normoblast, no larger than surrounding erythrocytes, contains a small, dense nucleus and a thin rim of pale cytoplasm, which later in development will be acidophil as a result of the accumulation of hemoglobin. Wright's stain. Oil immersion.* Bottom right: *The four polychromatophil erythroblasts exhibit large nuclei, with coarse chromatin clumps, and a polychromatophil cytoplasm owing to the presence of hemoglobin within the basophil cytoplasm. Also present are a juvenile (band) neutrophil (N) and a small lymphocyte (L). Wright's stain. Oil immersion.*

ative of a further increase in the numbers of free ribosomes and polyribosomes. Hemoglobin continues to be formed but is masked by the basophilia.

*Polychromatophil Erythroblast (Rubricyte).* Basophil erythroblasts undergo numerous mitotic divisions and produce cells that acquire sufficient hemoglobin for it to be observed in stained preparations. After staining with Leishman's or Giemsa's stain, the cytoplasm varies in color from a purplish-blue to a lilac or gray owing to the presence of varying amounts of pink-staining hemoglobin within the basophil cytoplasm of the erythroblasts. Thus, they are *polychromatophil.* The nucleus of the polychromatophil erythroblast has a denser chromatin network than that of the basophil erythroblast, and the cell is smaller.

*Normoblast (Metarubricyte).* The polychromatophil erythroblasts undergo a number of mitotic divisions. The basophilia of the cytoplasm decreases, and the amount of hemoglobin increases to such an extent that the cytoplasm stains approximately as acidophil as that of the mature erythrocyte. Cells that exhibit this degree of acidophilia within their cytoplasm are referred to as normoblasts. The normoblast is smaller than the polychromatophil erythroblast and contains a smaller nucleus that stains densely basophil. Gradually, the nucleus becomes pyknotic. There is no further mitotic activity. Finally, the nucleus is extruded from the cell together with a thin rim of cytoplasm. Extruded nuclei are ingested by macrophages associated with the stroma of the bone marrow.

*Reticulocyte.* The reticulocyte, or immature erythrocyte, has been described previously. It is thought that the majority of reticulocytes lose their reticular structure before leaving the bone marrow, since the reticulocyte count of peripheral blood normally is less than 1 per cent of the erythrocytes. The remaining organelles of the reticulocytes are broken down by *ubiquitin* (a nonlysosomal soluble ATP-dependent enzyme).

The stages just described in the process of *erythropoiesis* are, in the main, morphological manifestations of the synthesis of hemoglobin. The concentration of RNA in the ribosomal clusters (polyribosomes) that are synthesizing hemoglobin is responsible for the basophilia of the cytoplasm, most marked in the basophil erythroblast. The presence of RNA can be correlated with the active synthesis of nucleotides and hemoglobin.

The normal development of erythrocytes is dependent upon many different factors, including the presence of the parent substances (principally, globin, heme, and iron) of hemoglobin. Additional factors, such as ascorbic acid, vitamin $B_{12}$, and the *intrinsic factor* (normally present in gastric juice), that function as coenzymes or as precursors of coenzymes in the synthetic process are also necessary for the normal maturation of erythrocytes.

The most potent stimulus for development of erythrocytes is tissue hypoxia (oxygen deficiency), which induces formation of a humoral factor, *erythropoietin*, that travels in the plasma to the bone marrow, where it stimulates production of more erythrocytes. Erythropoietin is produced principally in the kidney and appears to act by stimulating committed erythroid progenitor cells to differentiate into proerythroblasts and erythroblasts. The rate of cell division also is increased, as is the rate of release of reticulocytes from the bone marrow. Thus, the synthesis and release of erythropoietin is directly related to the availability of oxygen in the tissue and to the number of circulating erythrocytes carrying oxygen.

**Granulocytes.** The stages of granulocyte development (*granulopoiesis*), in order of differentiation from the hemocytoblast, are *myeloblast, promyelocyte, myelocyte, metamyelocyte,* and *granular leukocyte* (Figs. 5–19 and 5–20). The transformation from myeloblast to the mature circulating neutrophil requires about 11 days, with a 70-kg man manufacturing about $7.5 \times 10^{10}$ neutrophils per day. The neutrophils spend a total of seven days within the *medullary formation* (*mitotic*) and *medullary storage* (*maturation*) compartments. The remainder of their time is spent in the *circulatory* (contains neutrophils circulating in the blood stream) and *marginating* (contains neutrophils in the blood stream but not circulating) *compartments.* The marginating compartment serves as a reserve pool of blood cells that can be mobilized as the need arises. The number of circulating blood cells remains relatively constant because, at any particular point in time, both the circulating and marginating compartments are in equilibrium.

Myelocytes of the three types (neutrophil, eosinophil, and basophil) contain their characteristic,

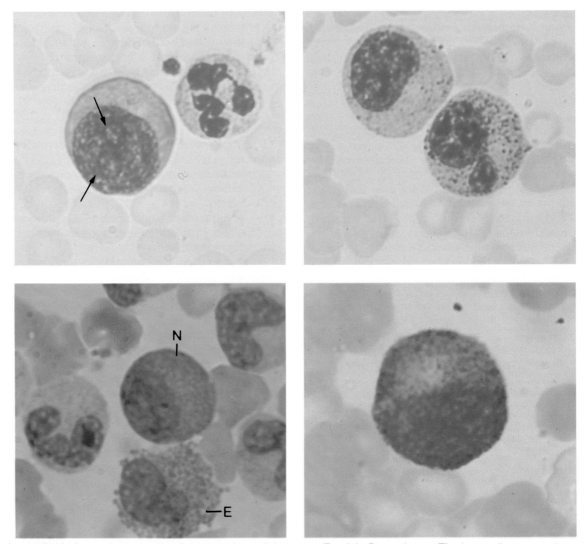

**Figure 5–19.** *Bone marrow smears illustrating white cell formation. Top left: Promyelocyte. The large cell, a promyelocyte, exhibits an ovoid nucleus with coarse chromatin strands and two nucleoli (arrows). The cytoplasm is basophil and contains a few nonspecific granules (pink). The other cell is a mature neutrophil granular leukocyte. Wright's stain. Oil immersion. Top right: Neutrophil myelocyte (left) and band neutrophil (right). The neutrophil myelocyte, somewhat smaller than a promyelocyte, shows more compact nuclear chromatin and fine cytoplasmic granules. The band neutrophil contains an irregular lobed nucleus and fine, specific cytoplasmic granules. Wright's stain. Oil immersion. Bottom left: Eosinophil (E) and neutrophil (N) myelocytes. The late eosinophil myelocyte shows an indented nucleus and large eosinophil granules. The early neutrophil myelocyte possesses a condensed ovoid nucleus and fine neutrophil granules. Also present are three neutrophil metamyelocytes with fine, specific granules and reniform nuclei. Wright's stain. Oil immersion. Bottom right: Basophil myelocyte. The outline of the nucleus appears indefinite, and the cytoplasm contains specific basophil granules. Wright's stain. Oil immersion.*

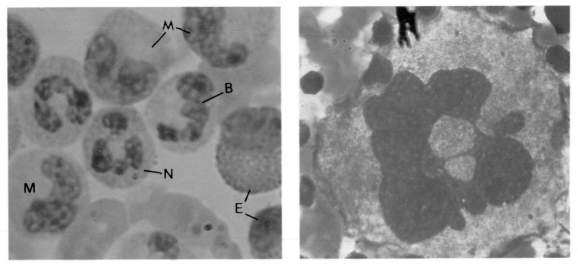

**Figure 5–20.** *Bone marrow smear. Left: Present in this field are eosinophil myelocytes (E), neutrophil metamyelocytes (M), band neutrophils (B), and a mature neutrophil granular leukocyte (N). Wright's stain. Oil immersion. Right: This giant cell (megakaryocyte), which occupies the majority of the field, has a large, irregular nucleus and a finely granular cytoplasm that exhibits a patchy basophilia. Wright's stain. Medium power.*

specific (peroxidase-negative) granules that are derived from the *cis* (immature) face of the Golgi apparatus. Further differentiation involves a progressive (but modest) reduction in size, an increasing darkening and lobation of the nucleus, and a further accumulation of specific granules. The azurophil (perioxidase-positive) granules appear first in the cytoplasm of the promyelocyte.

**Myeloblasts.** These are the most immature recognizable cells of the granulocyte series and are thought to arise from hemocytoblasts by way of an intermediate cell type. They are variable in size, ranging from 10 to 15 μm in diameter. The large spherical nucleus shows a delicate chromatin pattern and one or two nucleoli. Electron micrographs show that the cytoplasm, which is scanty and somewhat more basophil than that of the hemocytoblast, contains numerous mitochondria and free ribosomes but few elements of granular endoplasmic reticulum. No granules are present at this time.

**Promyelocytes.** Promyelocytes are somewhat larger than the myeloblasts. The nucleus is rounded or oval, with dense, peripheral heterochromatin and an indistinct nucleolus. Generally, the cytoplasm is basophil, but it may show localized acidophil areas. It is characterized by the presence of scattered, densely azurophil granules. These nonspecific, or primary, granules represent a special type of primary lysosome. These peroxidase-positive granules are synthesized at this stage of granulopoiesis, with subsequent stages exhibiting a decrease in the number of granules. Azurophil granules are derived from the *trans* (mature) face of the Golgi apparatus and have a homogeneous density. This granule is surrounded by a membrane and contains lysosomal enzymes. It is believed that the neutrophil-specific granules arise from the azurophil granules.

**Myelocytes.** These are derived from promyelocytes. In the process of differentiation, the essential change is the appearance of specific granules with the size, shape, and staining characteristics that allow one to recognize that they are neutrophils, eosinophils, or basophils. Since the primary, azurophil granules are produced only in the promyelocyte stage, their number in each cell is reduced with each myelocyte division. Myelocytes also show a reduction in size, averaging 10 μm in diameter, and decreased basophilia of the cytoplasm. There is an increased content of heterochromatin in the nucleus, and, in late myelocytes, the nucleus indents and begins to assume a horseshoe shape.

The specific granules first appear in the perinuclear region and later are dispersed throughout the cytoplasm. Neutrophil-specific granules (salmon-pink) are not visible at the light microscopic level, but the eosinophil-specific (orange) and basophil-specific (dark-purple) granules are not below visible resolution.

*Metamyelocytes.* Myelocytes undergo repeated divisions, become smaller, and cease dividing. The cells that are a product of the final division are *metamyelocytes.* They are juvenile forms of granular leukocytes and have a characteristic granular content. The nucleus, at first horseshoe-shaped, gradually indents further. At this stage, the late metamyelocyte is known as a *band cell.* As the cells age, the nucleus acquires its typical lobation, the number of lobes usually varying from three to five. The basophil metamyelocyte differs from the other two types of metamyelocytes in that its nucleus does not differentiate into distinct lobes. Thus, it is difficult to distinguish basophil metamyelocytes from mature basophil leukocytes. The mature cells (segmented granulocytes) enter the sinusoids and thus reach the blood stream.

In each of the aforementioned myelocyte stages, the neutrophils far outnumber the eosinophils and basophils. The granular leukocyte precursors greatly outnumber the progenitors of the erythrocytes. This preponderance of early leukocyte forms over erythrocyte progenitors is in contrast with the opposite relationship in blood. As explained earlier, the difference in the numerical relationship can be explained partly by the fact that erythrocytes survive for a much longer time in the circulation than do the leukocytes.

Loss of the leukocytes from circulating blood results in an increase in the rate of release of these cells from bone marrow, and a more severe loss induces an increased rate of differentiation of stem cells of the granulocyte series. This suggests that production of granulocytes is controlled by a humoral mechanism yet to be identified.

## MEGAKARYOCYTES AND PLATELET FORMATION

The megakaryocytes are giant cells (30 to 100 μm or more in diameter) that are thought to be derived from the hemocytoblast (Fig. 5–21). They are characteristic of all adult mammalian bone marrow, and they may be found also in the hemopoietic tissues (liver, spleen) during embryonic development. The nucleus is complexly lobed, and individual lobes may be closely packed or connected by fine strands of chromatin material. The cytoplasm contains numerous azurophil granules and exhibits a patchy basophilia. The cell outline often is indistinct, since pseudopodial cytoplasmic processes extend through the walls of the sinusoids.

Megakaryocytes are said to arise from hemocytoblasts via an intermediate stage, the *megakaryoblast.* The latter cell is distinguished from a hemocytoblast by its nuclear characteristics: the nucleus is large, and often indented, and the peripheral heterochromatin is dense. The cytoplasm is homogeneous and basophil. Megakaryoblasts differentiate into megakaryocytes by a peculiar form of nuclear division in which the nucleus undergoes multiple mitotic divisions without cytoplasmic division. The number of mitoses is not known. After their formation, megakaryocytes extend cytoplasmic processes, which become pinched off as platelets. Electron microscopic studies have revealed an extensive development of smooth-surfaced membranes within the cytoplasm, thus dividing it up into small compartments and delineating the extent of future platelets. The azurophil cytoplasmic granules form the chromomeres of the future platelets. Following formation of *demarcation channels* by the membranes, the compartments readily separate to become free platelets. Megakaryocytes are short-lived, and stages of degeneration are seen commonly. After the peripheral cytoplasm is shed as platelets, the megakaryocytes become shrunken and their nuclei fragment.

## DEVELOPMENT OF LYMPHOID ELEMENTS

The development of lymphocytes and monocytes occurs in the lymphoid tissues and, to some degree, in myeloid tissue as well. The process of differentiation of these cells, however, cannot be followed as readily as that of the myeloid elements. Morphological evidence of differentiation is not marked. The appearance of definitive characteristics such as nuclear disappearance or lobation, cytoplasmic granulation, and loss of cyto-

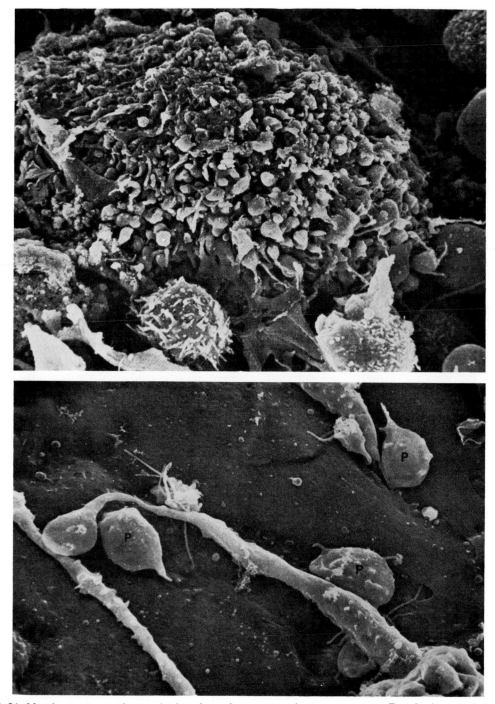

**Figure 5–21.** Megakaryocytes producing platelets shown by scanning electron microscopy. Top: In this megakaryocyte, the cytoplasm is entirely fragmented into blood platelets as seen in the mouse spleen. × 4875. (Courtesy of T. Ihzumi. Reproduced by permission of Igaku-Shoin Medical Publishers.) Bottom: In rat bone marrow, megakaryocytes may produce ribbon-like processes from which beaded and constricted shapes may be separated into platelets (P). × 3378. (Reproduced with permission from Fujita, T., et al.: SEM Atlas of Cells and Tissues. New York, Igaku-Shoin Medical Publishers, Inc., 1981.)

plasmic basophilia does not occur in lymphocytes and monocytes, which retain the cytoplasmic basophila and generally primitive nuclear shape of the stem cell.

The stroma of lymphoid tissue, like that of myeloid tissue, contains a framework of reticular fibers closely associated with primitive reticular cells and fixed macrophages. The sinuses present within lymphoid tissue are lined by *littoral cells* of the macrophage system. The meshes of the stroma contain the free cells, megakaryocytes, and some fat cells.

**Lymphocytes.** These cells are derived from the *lymphoblasts,* which are relatively large, spherical cells. The nucleus is large and contains relatively condensed chromatin and prominent nucleoli. The cytoplasm is homogeneous and basophil. These immature lymphocytes resemble the hemocytoblasts of bone marrow, and according to the unitarian theory of development, they are the same cells in a different location. (Proponents of the dualistic theory claim that the lymphoblasts differ slightly from the hemocytoblasts and can differentiate only into lymphoid elements.) As lymphoblasts undergo differentiation, the nuclear chromatin becomes more dense and compact, and azurophil granules appear within the cyto-

plasm. The cells are reduced in size and are termed *prolymphocytes* by some authors. These cells give rise directly to the circulating lymphocytes.

In postnatal mammals, most lymphocytes arise by proliferation of pre-existing lymphocytes within the lymphoid tissues, principally within lymph nodes and the spleen (Fig. 5–22). Only when such a production is unable to supply the demand for lymphocytes is it likely that there is any marked differentiation from the stem cells that enter the circulation from bone marrow.

The development of small lymphocytes, principally in the lymph nodes and the spleen, generally represents a reaction to an invasion by foreign-body proteins. A further reaction to such a stimulus is the formation of *plasma cells,* which are responsible for the synthesis of antibodies. These cells may arise directly from hemocytoblasts (lymphoblasts) or from immunologically competent lymphocytes. In the latter process, small lymphocytes (*B cells*) pass through intermediate stages that are indistinguishable from large and medium-sized lymphocytes.

**Monocytes.** Monocytes are developed from a stem cell within the bone marrow. It is not possible to distinguish this stem cell, the *monoblast,* from

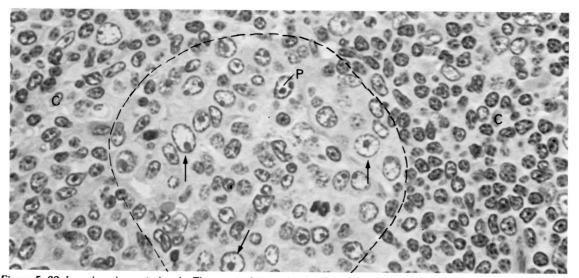

**Figure 5–22.** Lymph node, cortical node. The germinal center (outlined) contains principally medium-sized lymphocytes. A few cells (arrows) show large nuclei with distinct nucleoli. These are large lymphocytes and lymphoblasts. Occasional plasma cells (P) also occur in this zone. Small lymphocytes, produced within the germinal center, are pushed to the periphery and constitute the cortex of the nodule (C). Plastic section. H and E. Oil immersion.

the myeloblast. The monoblast gives rise to the *promonocyte*, which is about 15 μm in diameter. The nucleus is oval or indented and has a fine chromatin pattern with two or more nucleoli. The cytoplasm is basophil and contains a variable number of fine azurophil granules. This cell gives rise to the monocyte, which is present in both bone marrow and blood. It is slightly smaller than the promonocyte (10 to 12 μm), and nucleoli are indistinct within the nucleus. The cytoplasm contains an abundance of fine azurophil granules that give a positive peroxidase reaction, unlike those of lymphocytes that show a negative peroxidase reaction. Monocytes leave the blood to enter the tissues, where their life span as macrophages may be as long as 70 days.

## EMBRYONIC DEVELOPMENT OF BLOOD CELLS

There are three ill-defined phases of hemopoiesis during intrauterine development, and in all phases, the initiation of hemopoiesis is the same. It consists of a differentiation of mesenchymal cells into free cells whose cytoplasm acquires a definite basophil character. These cells, often termed hemocytoblasts, proliferate actively. Such a process occurs initially within the yolk sac during the third week of development. The hemocytoblasts become transformed into *primitive erythroblasts* by the elaboration and accumulation of hemoglobin within their cytoplasm. They differ from bone marrow—derived erythrocytes in that they are larger and retain their nuclei.

During the second phase, hemopoiesis occurs within the liver and spleen. It commences in the liver at about six weeks and continues actively until the middle of fetal life (Fig. 5–23). Hemocytoblasts proliferate and differentiate into nucleated and non-nucleated red blood cells, leukocytes, and megakaryocytes. The formation of nucleated red blood cells gradually diminishes prior to the middle of fetal life, and hemopoietic activity in the liver normally disappears at the time of birth. Hemopoiesis occurs within the spleen between the second and eighth months. Erythropoiesis here ceases at or just after birth, although lymphocytes continue to be produced within the spleen postnatally. Additionally, during

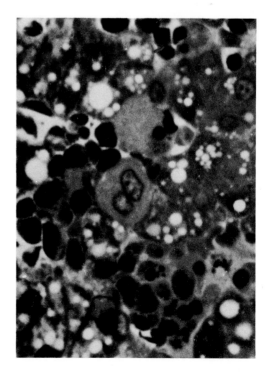

**Figure 5–23.** *Section of liver from a six-month-old human fetus. At this stage, liver cells contain large amounts of lipid material within their cytoplasm and appear vacuolated owing to loss of lipid during tissue preparation. Note the presence of extramedullary hemopoiesis. Numerous myeloid elements, principally of the erythrocyte series, lie between the liver cells. Note the megakaryocyte. High power.*

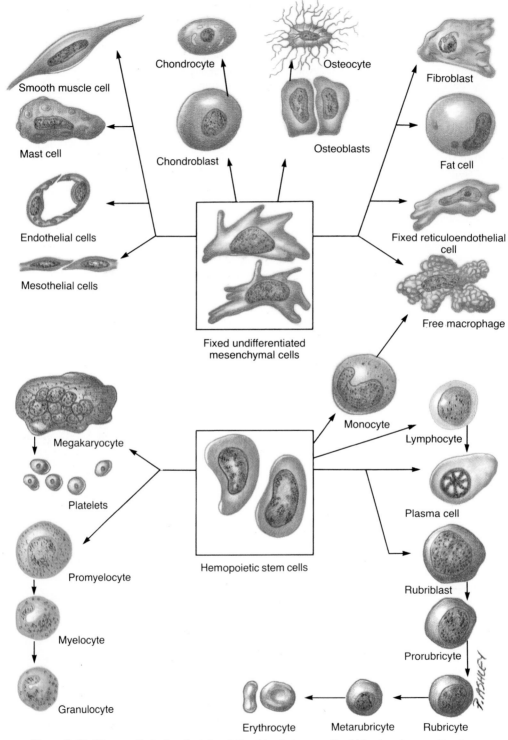

**Figure 5–24.** *Diagram illustrating the interrelationships between cells of blood and connective tissues.*

the second phase, the thymus commences to produce lymphocytes from the second month on.

The third phase involves the bone marrow and the lymph nodes. Myeloid tissue of bone marrow appears in the third fetal month when the cartilaginous primordia of the bones become invaded by mesenchyme during the process of ossification. Again mesenchymal cells round off and become hemocytoblasts, which give rise to erythroblasts, myelocytes, monocytes, lymphocytes, and megakaryocytes. With the appearance of bone marrow, production of nucleated red blood cells ceases. Lymph nodes develop relatively late during fetal life, and production of myeloid elements is never a marked feature within them. However, they continue to function throughout life, like the spleen, in the producion of lymphocytes.

### INTERRELATIONSHIPS BETWEEN CELLS OF BLOOD AND CONNECTIVE TISSUES: DEVELOPMENT POTENTIALITIES

Mesenchymal cells have great potentiality. They are able to differentiate along any one of several lines leading to the formation of many different kinds of cells in the connective tissues (Fig. 5–24). The process of cellular differentiation implies the acquisition of a property or properties not possessed previously and leads to specialization.

It is important to realize that complete differentiation is not achieved by all cells. Maximow originated the concept that, in the development of any kind of adult connective tissue from mesenchyme, some undifferentiated cells remain as a reservoir of multipotential cells. It should be appreciated that there is a tendency for the process of differentiation to be halted somewhere along the line of differentiation. Thus, in any connective tissue, there may be cells that are undifferentiated, cells that are partially differentiated, and cells that have achieved complete differentiation.

Two further concepts with regard to the process of cellular differentiation remain to be considered. In general, the more differentiated a cell becomes, the more restricted its developmental potencies. Once a cell has achieved a certain degree of differentiation along a particular line, further differentiation is possible only along the original line of differentiation. The second point is that once differentiation has been completed, cellular proliferation becomes markedly restricted. Many specialized cells are incapable of division.

*Metaplasia* is a process that illustrates well the concepts of cellular differentiation just described. It occurs under certain pathological conditions when one specialized type of connective tissue appears to transform into another. This, in fact, is not the case, since specialized cellular elements are unable to differentiate. Actually, metaplasia represents a replacement of one type of connective tissue by another from undifferentiated cells present within the tissue. It occurs in response to altered environmental factors.

Summary Table 5–1 appears on following page.

## Summary Table 5–1. Formed Elements of the Peripheral Circulation

| Formed Elements | Approx. Diameter in Dried Smears (μm) | Approx. Number (per ccl, or Percentage) | Nucleus | Cytoplasmic Background | Granules | Phagocytic Properties | Motility | Function |
|---|---|---|---|---|---|---|---|---|
| Erythrocytes | 7.0–7.6 | Newborn: 6 million; Female: 4 million; Male: 5 million | None | Pale greenish-yellow (fresh); red with Giemsa stain or when packed together | None | None | None | Transport of oxygen and carbon dioxide |
| Platelets | 2.0–4.0 | 250,000 | None | Pale blue | Delta (dense): serotonin; alpha: fibrinogen; lambda: lysosomal enzymes | None | None | Plugs (damaged tissues); blood coagulation; clot retraction and removal |
| Leukocytes | | | | | | | | |
| Granulocytes | | (differential WBC count) | | | | | | |
| Neutrophils | 10–12 | 65–75 per cent | Chromatin coarse (dark); segmented (2–5 lobes); no nucleoli | Unstained | Specific: salmon-pink; Azurophil: deep reddish-purple | Marked | Marked | Acute bacterial infections (coccal); acute hemorrhages; poisons (lead) |
| Eosinophils | 12–14 | 2–4 per cent (6 per cent in children) | Chromatin coarse (light); usually bilobed | Unstained | Specific: red (refractile) | Negligible | Negligible | Allergic and antiparasitic responses; dissolution of old blood clots |
| Basophils | 10–12 | 0.5–1 per cent | Chromatin coarse (light); usually trilobed; no nucleoli | Unstained | Specific: blue-black clusters (metachromatic, very soluble in water) | Negligible | Marked | Role in delayed hypersensitivity; eosinophil chemotactic factor; allergic responses; Hodgkin's disease |
| Agranulocytes | | | | | | | | |
| Monocytes | 20–25 | 3–8 per cent | Spherical, oval, or bean-shaped (light); no nucleoli | Faintly basophil | Azurophil: very light purple (few in number) | Marked | Marked | Transformed into macrophages, giant cells, and osteoclasts. Involved in inflammatory responses |
| Lymphocytes | 6–9 (small) 10–12 (medium) 13–18 (large) | 20–35 per cent (composite) | Oval or slightly indented in large cells (dark); nucleoli in some | Basophil | Azurophil: purplish | Negligible | Marked | Involved in both humoral and cell-mediated immunity |

# Muscle

## INTRODUCTION

The primary function of muscle cells is contraction, this resulting in movement of the body as a whole and of the many parts with respect to one another. Muscle cells lie in parallel arrays. They are elongated in the axis of contraction and, thus, usually are termed *muscle fibers*, not to be confused with connective tissue fibers (which are extracellular) or nerve fibers (which are elongated cell processes). Muscle tissue consists of three basic elements:

 1. The muscle fibers themselves, usually arranged in bundles or fasciculi, but occasionally occurring as single elements.

 2. A rich capillary network that provides oxygen and nutrients and eliminates toxic waste materials.

 3. Fibroconnective supporting tissue with fibroblasts and collagenous and elastic fibers. Blood vessels and nerves run in this connective tissue that also binds together the muscle fibers and provides a harness so that the pull resulting from contraction of the fibers may be exerted usefully.

6

A specific terminology is used in respect of muscle. The protoplasm is referred to as *sarcoplasm* (*sarcos,* muscle); mitochondria as *sarcosomes*; and endoplasmic reticulum as *sarcoplasmic reticulum*. The *sarcolemma* is the complex of the plasmalemma, its basal lamina, and associated collagen microfibrils. The bulk of the sarcoplasm is occupied by *myofibrils*, these contractile elements running in the long axis of the cells and responsible for the longitudinal striation seen in all muscle fibers. Each myofibril is a bundle of smaller *myofilaments*, the myofilaments being of two types: one composed primarily of actin and the other of myosin, the main contractile proteins. A *sarcomere* is a linear contractile unit (really a segment of a myofibril), resulting from the specific arrangement of myofilaments in a myofibril.

There are three types of muscle, classified on both a structural and a functional basis. Functionally, muscle either is under the control of the will (voluntary muscle) or is not (involuntary muscle). Structurally, it either shows regular transverse bands along the length of the fibers (striated muscle) or does not (smooth, or unstriated, muscle). On this basis, the three types of muscle are

1. Striated voluntary or skeletal muscle, attached to bones or fascia and constituting the flesh of the limbs and body wall.

2. Striated involuntary or cardiac muscle, forming the wall of the heart and also located in the walls of the adjacent major blood vessels.

3. Smooth involuntary muscle, present in the walls of the hollow viscera and most blood vessels.

## SKELETAL OR STRIATED MUSCLE

### Organization

The flesh or meat of animals is formed by skeletal muscle. In the fresh state, it has a pink color, resulting partly from a pigment present in the muscle fibers and partly from the rich vascularity of the tissue. Some variation in the color of individual muscle fibers does occur, and ''red'' and ''white'' fibers are recognized. Capillaries in muscle lie mainly parallel to the muscle fibers, with numerous cross anastomoses. Muscle also is

richly innervated. Striated muscle fibers are arranged in bundles or fascicles, are parallel, and are enveloped in connective tissue that contains the blood vessels and nerves. Each individual muscle fiber is long, cylindrical, and multinucleated, with the ends being rounded or tapering at the junction of muscle and tendon. In many muscles, individual fibers are shorter than the overall length of the muscle, one end attaching to tendon and the other to a connective tissue septum in the muscle. The power of a muscle depends not upon the length of the component fibers but upon the total number of fibers present in the muscle. With exercise, muscles increase in size because of an increase in the size of each individual fiber (*hypertrophy*) and not because of an increase in the number of fibers (*hyperplasia*).

Connective tissue associated with skeletal muscle is organized into three designated tunics (Fig. 6–1). First, each named muscle of gross anatomy is enveloped in a layer of relatively thick connective tissue called the *epimysium*, which appears as a white sheath to the naked eye. Within it are the muscle fibers arranged in bundles, or fasciculi, each bundle surrounded by a sheath of thinner connective tissue termed the *perimysium*. Within a fasciculus, finer connective tissue penetrates between and around individual muscle fibers as the *endomysium*, and it contains the capillary network and terminal nerve fibers. It is formed by a network of reticular and fine collagenous fibers and a few connective tissue cells with a varying content of elastic fibers (particularly prominent in the small muscles of the eye and face). The total amount of fibroconnective tissue varies with the muscle, from being abundant, coarse, and relatively tough (e.g., in the gluteus maximus) to being relatively sparse and thin (e.g., in the psoas major—the filet mignon). At the attachment of muscle to tendon, aponeurosis, raphe, dermis, or periosteum, the perimysium blends with the connective tissue of the attachment.

Striated muscle fibers show both longitudinal and transverse striation and vary from 1 to 40 mm or more in length and 10 to 100 μm in diameter (Figs. 6–2 through 6–7). Nuclei in each fiber are numerous (about 35 per mm of length) and ovoid and are situated peripherally, subjacent to the sarcolemma. The sarcolemma is a structureless, thin membrane, sometimes apparent

## MUSCLE

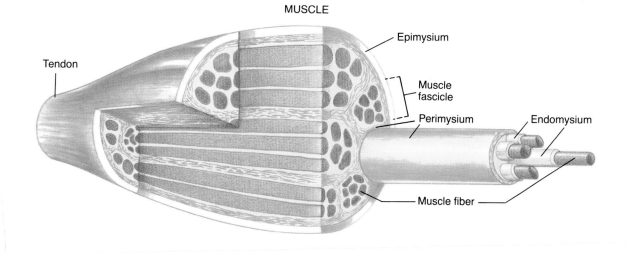

## MUSCLE FIBER

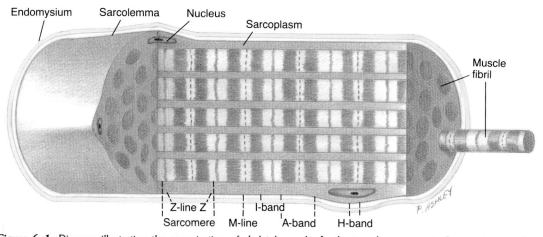

P. ASHLEY

*Figure 6–1.* Diagram illustrating the organization of skeletal muscle. In the top diagram, part of an entire muscle is shown ensheathed in its epimysium. Within the epimysium, bundles or fascicles of muscle fibers are surrounded by perimysium, and within the fascicle, individual muscle fibers are surrounded by endomysium. Perimysium and epimysium are continuous with the dense, regular connective tissue of the tendon (or aponeurosis). In the lower diagram, the structure of an individual muscle fiber, supported by endomysium, is illustrated. The fiber has multiple, peripheral nuclei located subjacent to the sarcolemma, and sarcoplasm is occupied mainly by myofibrils. Note the cross-banding of the myofibrils, with sarcomeres, and that this transverse striation is confined to the myofibrils, although the banding is in register across the entire fiber. Myofibrils sectioned through the I band (left) show only thin myofilaments but show both thick and thin myofilaments in the A band (right).

bounding the muscle fiber and usually seen clearly where a fiber has been crushed with subsequent retraction of sarcoplasm from the sarcolemma. The sarcoplasm is occupied largely by long, parallel, cylindrical filamentous bundles, the *myofi-*

*brils,* each 1 to 3 μm in diameter and showing a regular transverse striation. In transverse section, myofibrils appear as small dot-like profiles with clear, nonfibrillar sarcoplasm lying between and around them. Clear sarcoplasm also lies adjacent

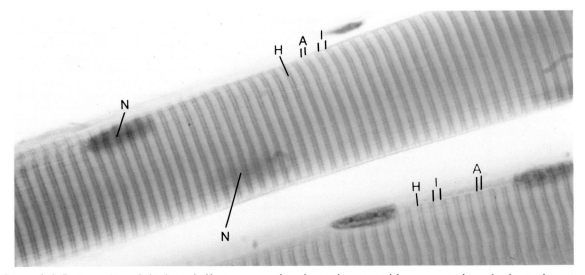

*Figure 6–2.* Portions of two skeletal muscle fibers are seen, these having been teased from a mass of muscle, that is, the entire thickness of the fibers is seen, and they have not been sectioned. The fibers are cylindrical and of considerable length and are multinucleated, with nuclei (N) located peripherally. Not all nuclei are in sharp focus owing to the thickness of the preparation. The sarcoplasm shows cross-striation with alternating dark (anisotropic-A) and light (isotropic-I) bands, with a central, light H band in the A band. The bands appear to cross the entire fiber, although they are confined to the myofibrils, which are not seen here as individual fibrils. Hematoxylin. Oil immersion.

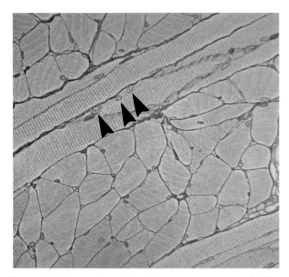

*Figure 6–3.* Striated muscle of the tongue is seen, with fibers cut in both longitudinal and transverse planes. The stain demonstrates endomysium (dark purple) surrounding individual muscle fibers, this network containing numerous blood capillaries (not seen here). In the muscle fibers in longitudinal section, transverse striations are seen, and nuclei are peripheral and multiple (arrowheads). Nuclei seen in transverse section are those either of muscle fibers or of fibroblasts (between fibers) of the endomysium, these being smaller and darker. Gridley's reticulum stain. Medium power.

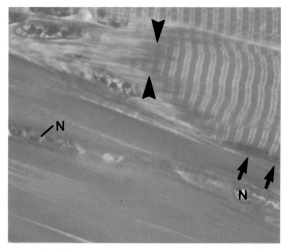

*Figure 6–4.* This section shows the junction of muscle fibers (above) with tendon (below). The fibers, in longitudinal section, show A, I, Z, and H bands with slender slips of nonfibrillar, clear sarcoplasm between myofibrils. The fibers are surrounded by endomysium, with fibroblast nuclei of the endomysium arrowed. At its extremity, the muscle fiber is rounded or tapered and shows grooves and ridges with slips of blue-staining connective tissue (arrowheads) of the endomysium passing from the sarcolemma to blend with the tendon (left). The tendon (below) is formed by dense, regular connective tissue with pink-staining collagen bundles and nuclei (N) of fibroblasts (tenocytes) between the bundles. Plastic section. Masson's trichrome. Oil immersion.

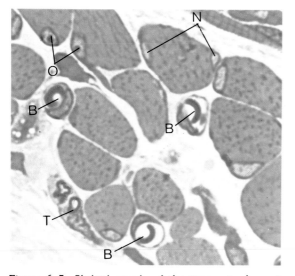

**Figure 6–5.** *Skeletal muscle of the tongue is shown in transverse section. Nuclei are peripheral in location and multiple (the fiber at top center with two nuclei labeled N) and often show prominent nucleoli (O). In the sarcoplasm, numerous sarcosomes (mitochondria) appear as darkly staining dots lying between the myofibrils. Between muscle fibers is supporting connective tissue with thin collagen fibrils staining pink, and this connective tissue contains numerous blood capillaries (B), also sectioned in transverse section and containing erythrocytes in their lumina. Also present is a small peripheral nerve (T) with two myelinated nerve fibers (black). Plastic section. Toluidine blue. Oil immersion.*

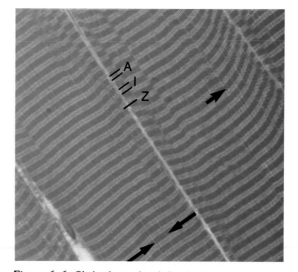

**Figure 6–6.** *Skeletal muscle of the diaphragm is sectioned longitudinally, and the fibers show A, I, and Z bands clearly. A sarcomere extends between two adjacent Z bands. The arrows indicate longitudinal, pale streaks of clear, nonfibrillar sarcoplasm between myofibrils, illustrating that banding is confined to the myofibrils. The nucleus (lower left) is of a fibroblast of the endomysium. Plastic section. Toluidine blue. Oil immersion.*

to nuclei, and these areas contain numerous sarcosomes (mitochondria), small Golgi apparatuses, glycogen, and some lipid droplets. More glycogen and sarcosomes arranged in linear chains lie between myofibrils, and here the sarcosomes are related to the cross striation of the myofibrils.

### Myofibrils

By light microscopy, the muscle fiber in longitudinal section shows alternating dark (A) and light (I) bands, so called because in polarized light the A band is birefringent, or anisotropic, while the I band appears dark or isotropic (Fig. 6–8). The A band stains more intensely than the I band and shows a central H band that stains less intensely and is less birefringent. In the center of

the H band, a slender, dark M line may be visible. Each I band is bisected by a distinct Z line or disc. While these bands may appear to cross the entire muscle fiber, they are, in fact, limited to the myofibrils, which are in register, and are not seen in interfibrillar sarcoplasm.

The segment between two adjacent Z lines, called a *sarcomere*, is about 2 to 3 μm long with the A band being 1.5 μm and the full I band (two halves at each end of the A band) about 0.8 μm (Fig. 6–9). The sarcomere is not only a structural unit but also the basic contractile unit. In relaxed muscle, the bands are distinct in longitudinal section. However, in contraction, they become less so, and the myofibrils become thicker and the sarcomeres shorter, the distance between Z bands progressively shortening. As I bands shorten, the ends of the A bands approach Z lines until, in full contraction, A and I bands are indistinguishable. During contraction, the length of the A band remains constant: The explanation for this is discussed below. In transverse section, the various bands are not seen.

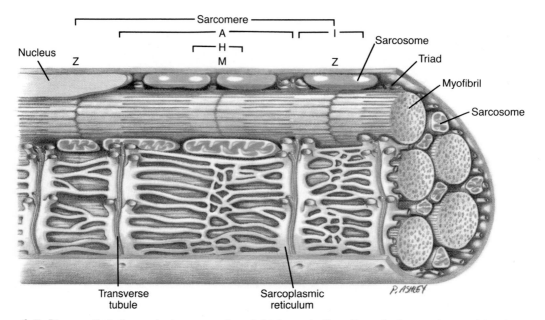

**Figure 6–7.** *Diagram illustrating part of a mammalian skeletal muscle fiber. Beneath the sarcolemma (above) is one the peripheral nuclei with sarcosomes in a row, with a second row of sarcosomes between myofibrils (center). One myofibril (top) shows thick and thin myofilaments, their arrangement in the sarcomere accounting for the banding. Below this lie two other myofibrils covered by sarcoplasmic reticulum, mainly in the form of longitudinal tubular elements with frequent cross anastomoses in the H-band region. At each A-I junction, these elements communicate with wider, terminal cisternae, each pair of cisternae separated by a slender T tubule to form a triad. The T tubules are invaginations of the surface plasmalemma (below). Two triads also are illustrated in transverse section (top right), again located at A-I junctions. Where the fiber is cut transversely through an A band (right), both thick and thin filaments are seen in regular array, the sarcoplasm between them containing elements of sarcoplasmic reticulum and sarcosomes.*

## Myofilaments and Striation

Myofibrils are composed of smaller units called myofilaments, and these are of two types, *thick* and *thin*, the former composed of myosin and the latter composed mostly of actin (Fig. 6–10). The thick and thin myofilaments are arranged in a regular manner, and the cross-banding seen on light microscopy is simply a reflection of their distribution in the sarcomere. The thick filaments are 12 to 15 nm in diameter and 1.5 μm in length, and they occupy the A band lying in the center of the sarcomere. The thin filaments are only 5 nm in diameter and 1.0 μm in length. They are attached to the Z bands and extend through the adjacent I bands and part of the way into A bands. They interdigitate there with the thick filaments, so that in a cross section of the peripheries of an A band, each thick filament is surrounded by six thin filaments in hexagonal array. The H band is simply the central area of the A band free of thin filaments, its width determined by the state of contraction. Thus, the banding pattern is accounted for by the presence or absence of overlap between the two types of filament, best seen in transverse section where the I band contains only thin filaments, the extremities of the A band contain both thick and thin, and the H band contains only thick. At the M line, in the center of the H band, thick filaments are interconnected by fine radial filaments, so that each is connected in the transverse plane with six adjacent thick filaments. The function of these cross filaments at the M line is to maintain the regular spacing and arrangement of thick filaments in the sarcomere. In the region of the overlap of thick and thin filaments, regularly spaced cross bridges extend radially from thick filaments toward the neighboring thin filaments. These bridges are absent in the H band.

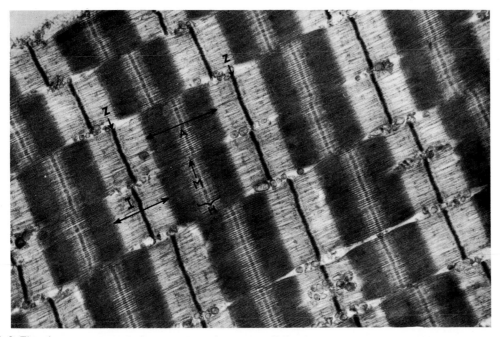

**Figure 6–8.** *This electron micrograph shows portions of seven myofibrils of a single muscle fiber of the rabbit psoas muscle. In this longitudinal section of noncontracted, relaxed muscle, cross-banding is seen clearly, with the dark A (anisotropic) bands bisected by the lighter H bands with a central thin, dark M line. The I (isotropic) bands are lighter-staining and are bisected by the very dark Z lines or discs, with sarcomeres extending between adjacent Z lines. Between myofibrils are slender slips of nonfibrillar sarcoplasm containing small sarcosomes and vesicular and tubular elements. ×13,000. (Courtesy of Dr. H. E. Huxley.)*

A *thick filament*, 1.5 μm long, has a smooth central region with short projections toward each end, these corresponding to the cross bridges. Each thick filament is formed by a bundle of myosin molecules, each a rod-like structure 200 nm long and about 2 nm in diameter, but in the form of a golf club with a shaft and a head. Two subunits are present in the molecule, light mero-myosin forming most of the shaft and heavy meromyosin forming the rest of the shaft and the head, the heads protruding from the bundle as the cross bridges. Centrally in the thick filament, the molecules lie in an overlapping antiparallel array, and only the shafts are present with no cross bridges, this corresponding to the H band. At each end, the heads of myosin molecules protrude in a spiral manner, the overlapping molecules being staggered, so that six longitudinal rows of heads connect with the six associated thin filaments, the heads being directed away from the midpoint (at the M line). The head of the myosin molecule is flexible on its shaft, and it is the heads,

or cross bridges, that possess the adenosine tri-phosphatase (ATPase) activity necessary for the actin-myosin interaction during contraction.

A *thin filament*, 1.0 μm in length, is formed mainly by F-actin, a filamentous protein that consists of two strands of globular subunits of G-actin, with the two strands arranged in a helix. All filaments inserting into one side of a Z disc are of the same polarity, whereas filaments of the opposite polarity insert into the other side of a Z disc (and to the Z disc at the other end of the same sarcomere). Associated with the double helix of actin is a long, slender filament of tropo-myosin that lies in the groove between the two strands of F-actin. It is formed by tropomyosin molecules lying end to end in the filament. Also present is troponin in the form of globular units attached to the tropomyosin at regular intervals.

The *Z disc* has a characteristic zigzag appearance because the attached thin filaments from the two sides are offset and not in register. As each thin filament reaches its attachment at the Z line,

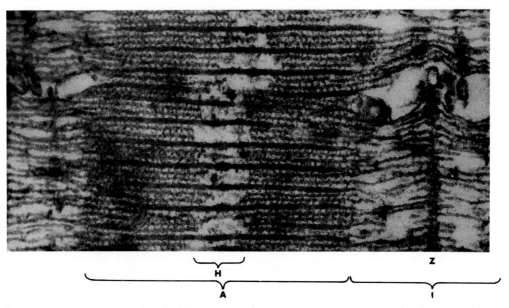

**Figure 6–9.** *In longitudinal section of relaxed rabbit psoas muscle, one sarcomere is seen extending between adjacent Z lines. The thick myosin filaments extend through the A band, while thin actin-containing filaments are located in the I band, extending into the outer parts of the A band. They are attached to Z discs, and two are seen between every two thick filaments. Cross-bridges are seen between thick and thin filaments. In the H band, only the central portions of thick filaments are present in this partially contracted muscle. ×74,000. (Courtesy of Dr. H. E. Huxley.)*

it attaches by four fine Z filaments to four thin filaments of the opposite sarcomere, the Z filaments forming a tetragonal pattern on transverse section. Associated with the Z filaments is a dense amorphous material (the Z disc matrix), mainly responsible for the density of the Z disc, and also the protein alpha-actinin, which helps to bind the thin actin filaments together and also contributes to the density of the Z disc.

Also present in muscle cells are filaments other than the thick and thin myofilaments. These are intermediate, 10-nm filaments of desmin and vimentin that surround and interconnect myofibrils, maintaining sarcomeres in register across the fiber. They play an important role in muscle fiber structure and mechanics.

### Membrane Systems

Each muscle fiber is bounded by a *sarcolemma*, too thin to be resolved clearly by light microscopy, and consisting of the muscle cell plasmalemma, its basal lamina, and a few associated collagen microfibrils. Within the muscle fiber is an extensive system of a special type of agranular (smooth) endoplasmic reticulum called the *sarcoplasmic reticulum*. This is a continuous system of membrane-limited tubules and cisternae forming cylindrical sheaths around each myofibril, the tubular elements mainly longitudinal with frequent cross connections in the region of the H band. At A-I junctions, tubules connect to channels of larger caliber called *terminal cisternae*, lying as rings around the myofibrils. A similar network of tubules surrounds I bands with another terminal cisterna at each A-I junction, so that pairs of cisternae lie at each A-I junction. The two cisternae of each pair are separated by a more slender *transverse* or *T tubule*, the entire complex being termed a *triad* (Fig. 6–11). Thus, there are two triads to each sarcomere in mammalian muscle. In amphibian muscle, the arrangement is similar, but triads are located at Z discs (i.e., triads lie between sarcomeres).

*Transverse* or *T tubules* are invaginations of the surface sarcolemma, their lumina continuous with the extracellular space (Fig. 6–12). At regular

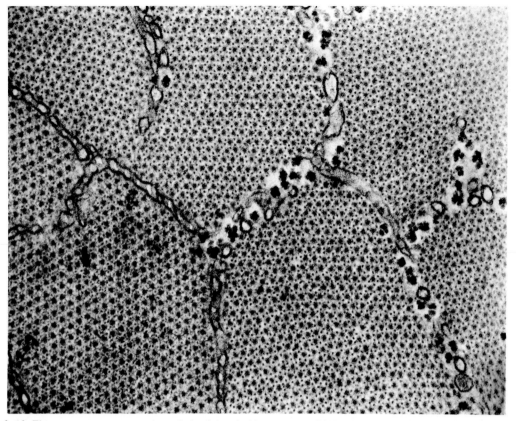

**Figure 6–10.** This, a transverse section through the A band of frog sartorius (skeletal) muscle, shows thick myosin myofilaments with thin myofilaments in a hexagonal arrangement around them. Note that myofibrils are delineated by thin slips of sarcoplasm containing elements of the sarcoplasmic reticulum and dark glycogen particles. ×50,000 (Courtesy of Dr. H. E. Huxley.)

intervals along the muscle fiber, they pass from the sarcolemma into the interior of the fiber, undergo branching, and lie between terminal cisternae of sarcoplasmic reticulum at the A-I junctions to form triads. Collectively, T tubules form the *T system* of the muscle fiber: They are slender and of relatively uniform diameter. Functionally, the T tubules provide for the rapid spread throughout the entire muscle fiber of surface membrane excitation/depolarization. In turn, at triads, the depolarization of T-tubules by an ATP-dependent mechanism causes release of calcium ions from the sarcoplasmic reticulum, this triggering contraction of the myofibrils. After stimulation ceases, calcium returns to the sarcoplasmic reticulum, where it is stored. This is discussed more fully later in respect of the mechanism of contraction.

## Mechanism of Contraction

As already mentioned, in contraction, a muscle fiber becomes shorter and thicker, and the A bands remain constant in length while both H and I bands decrease. Neither thick nor thin filaments change their length, and contraction occurs by a *"sliding filament mechanism"* that involves a change in relative position of the two sets of myofilaments (Fig. 6–13). The thin filaments slide past the thick filaments, the ends of the thin ones being drawn inward toward the M line, progressively shortening and then obliterating the H band. At the same time, the ends of the thick filaments approach the Z discs, shortening and obliterating the I bands. Thus, adjacent Z discs are brought closer, shortening the sarcomere with overall shortening of the myofibril. The

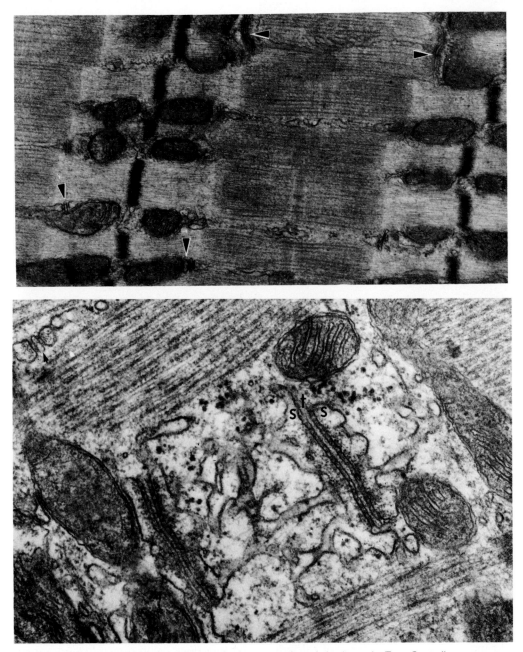

**Figure 6–11.** *Both electron micrographs are of longitudinal sections of rat skeletal muscle. Top: Centrally, a sarcomere extends between two Z discs, and all bands are visible. In this white muscle fiber, small sarcosomes lie in pairs on each side of the Z discs in intermyofibrillar sarcoplasm together with elements of sarcoplasmic reticulum, and triads (arrowheads) are present at A-I junctions, each with a small central transverse tubule bordered on each side by a terminal cisterna of sarcoplasmic reticulum. ×32,000. Bottom: In this partially contracted fiber, myofibrils lie above and below, with a triad in transverse section (top left). The T tubule is indicated by an arrowhead. Centrally is a meshwork of sarcoplasmic reticulum with the two triads of one sarcomere at A-I junctions, the right one labeled with a central T tubule (t) between terminal cisternae of sarcoplasmic reticulum (s). ×64,000.*

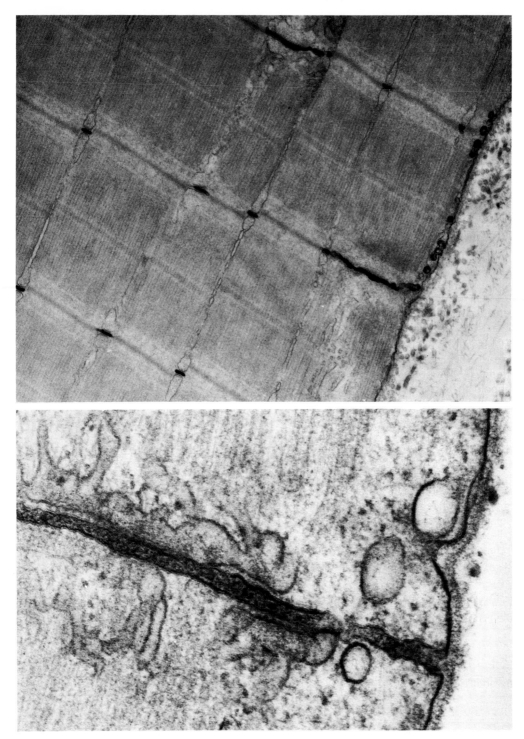

**Figure 6–12.** These electron micrographs of frog sartorius muscle demonstrate elements forming triads, here located at Z lines. Top: The T tubules stain densely, bordered on each side by terminal cisternae of sarcoplasmic reticulum. The sarcolemma (right) shows its basal lamina and associated collagen microfibrils (appearing as dots in transverse section), and subjacent to it are caveolae. ×22,000. Bottom: A T-tubule is seen to be in continuity with the plasmalemma and, within sarcoplasm, is bordered on each side, above and below, by terminal cisternae of sarcoplasmic reticulum. ×88,000.

SARCOMERE

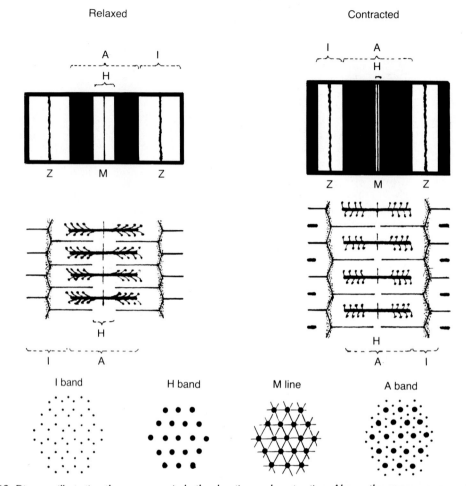

**Figure 6–13.** *Diagram illustrating the sarcomere in both relaxation and contraction. Above, the appearances are those seen by light microscopy. In contraction, note that both I and H bands become shorter, adjacent Z lines approach each other (in a shortened sarcomere), but the A-band length remains unaltered. The myofibril and the fiber become shorter and wider. In the central figures, the arrangement of thick and thin myofilaments is illustrated. In contraction, neither change length, but relative position is changed by the "sliding filament" mechanism, the cross bridges (heads of myosin molecules) of the thick filaments attaching to active actin sites on the thin filaments and sliding them toward the center of the sarcomere. Below, there are transverse sections of all regions of a sarcomere of a relaxed fiber showing the arrangement of thick and thin myofilaments.*

mechanism involves the heads of the myosin molecules moving toward globular actin subunits of thin filaments, engaging them, and then flexing at their points of junction with their shafts. By a cycle of attachment, flexion, detachment, and reattachment of the myosin heads, contractile force is generated, sliding the filaments past each other and drawing the thin filaments inward in the manner of an animated cogwheel. This process requires energy, the myosin heads acting as an ATPase to break down ATP to ADP. The store of ATP is limited and is replenished constantly by sarcosomes. In relaxation, myosin heads detach from thin filaments, permitting the two sets of filaments to slide back past each other to their original relaxed position of partial overlap.

Calcium ions are necessary for contraction. After stimulation of a muscle fiber, all myofibrils contract simultaneously and instantly, and contraction starts at A-I junctions, the site of triads. As explained, depolarization of the surface sarcolemma is carried to the interior of the fiber by T tubules, where, at triads, it causes release of calcium from sarcoplasmic reticulum (terminal cisternae). Calcium then binds with troponin of thin filaments, causing the troponin-tropomyosin complex to move deeper in the groove of the actin helix, thus exposing myosin-binding sites on the actin filament. Calcium thus "unlocks" the active myosin-binding sites on the thin filament, permitting the myosin heads to attach to them, swivel or flex, and thus displace the actin filaments a short distance. After stimulation, calcium returns to the sarcoplasmic reticulum, the troponin-tropomyosin complexes return to a more peripheral position along thin filaments, and the active actin sites thus are blocked. In effect, the troponin-tropomyosin complex forms a locking mechanism that prevents myosin-actin interaction: In contraction, calcium is the "key" that unlocks this mechanism.

It should be noted that a muscle fiber cannot contract other than to maximum capacity—the "all or none law"—and the power of contraction of a muscle is varied by the number of muscle units that contract.

### Types of Muscle Fiber

Muscles show some variation in color, and this is due to a variation in type of the component muscle fibers. Predominant in so-called "red" muscles are small, dark, granular or "red" fibers, while in "white" muscles, most fibers are larger and paler (Fig. 6–14). Red fibers are small in diameter, have a high myoglobin content, a large number of sarcosomes lying in rows at the periphery of the fiber and between myofibrils, a high succinic dehydrogenase reaction (due to mitochondrial enzymes), and a rich blood supply (Fig. 6–15). They have thick Z discs and a more complex sarcoplasmic reticulum. These red fibers are the *slow fibers* with a slow conduction rate,

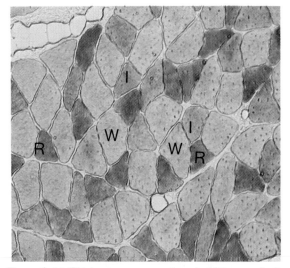

***Figure 6–14.*** *This is a transverse section of rabbit sacrospinalis muscle showing red (small, dark) (R) and white (larger, pale) (W) fibers. Fibers that are intermediate (in both color and size) (I) also are seen. Modified phosphatase reaction. High power. (Courtesy of Dr. K. D. McFadden.)*

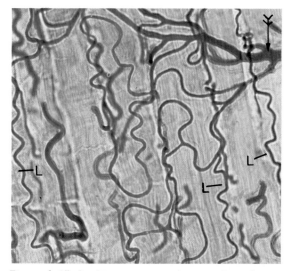

***Figure 6–15.*** *In this preparation, the arterial supply to a muscle was injected with red-colored gelatin, and the rich capillary plexus is demonstrated. Most capillaries run longitudinally (L), parallel to the muscle fibers, with numerous cross anastomoses. The coiling of the capillaries probably results from contraction of the muscle. The muscle fibers in the background are stained lightly, and a small arteriole (arrow) is seen supplying the plexus. Phosphotungstic acid. Medium power.*

are innervated by small axons, and fatigue relatively slowly. White fibers, the *fast fibers*, are of larger diameter and have fewer sarcosomes, a weak succinic dehydrogenase activity, and a less rich blood supply. They have thin Z discs, are innervated by large axons, have a fast conduction rate, and fatigue rapidly. Also found are fibers with characteristics intermediate between red and white fibers: These are called *intermediate fibers*. Most muscles contain a mix of both red and white fibers, although in red muscles, the red fibers predominate, and vice versa in white muscles.

### Nerve Supply

Each muscle has one or more nerves of supply, the nerve piercing the epimysium at the "motor point," which is fairly constant. In addition to motor fibers, the nerve also contains sensory fibers to muscle spindles and neurotendinous endings and autonomic fibers to blood vessels. Functionally, a muscle is composed of *motor units*, a unit being a single nerve fiber and the muscle fibers it supplies. Where delicate movement is required (e.g., in eye muscles), each muscle fiber may have its own nerve of supply, but in trunk muscles, for example, a single nerve may supply a hundred or more muscle fibers.

**Motor End-Plate.** The specialized junctional zone between a terminal motor nerve fiber and the muscle fiber it supplies is called a motor end-plate, or myoneural junction (Fig. 6–16). As the nerve fiber approaches its termination, it loses its myelin sheath but remains covered by a thin sheath of Schwann cell cytoplasm. The nerve then branches into either a plate-like mass or several terminal swellings that lie in gutters or depressions of the muscle surface, these being called the *primary synaptic clefts*. Beneath this is a specialization of the muscle fiber surface called the *subneural apparatus*.

By electron microscopy, the terminal nerve swellings are seen to contain mitochondria and numerous small synaptic vesicles 40–60 nm in diameter, these vesicles storing the neurotransmitter acetylcholine. On the muscle side, at the subneural apparatus, are numerous infoldings of the sarcolemma of primary synaptic clefts, these being the *secondary synaptic clefts*, and the adjacent sarcoplasm contains several nuclei and numerous sarcosomes. Between nerve and muscle and extending into primary and secondary synaptic clefts is a single basal lamina of glycoprotein material. The basal lamina of the secondary synaptic clefts contains acetylcholinesterase. On stimulation, acetylcholine is released into the synaptic clefts from synaptic vesicles of the nerve terminals by exocytosis and passes to receptor sites on the sarcolemma of the ridges and clefts, generating an action potential. This action potential passes over the sarcolemma and into the T tubules, causing release of calcium and triggering contraction. Acetylcholinesterase rapidly breaks down the acetylcholine, thus limiting the duration of contraction and permitting repetitive stimulation. In the disease *myasthenia gravis*, there is a pronounced reduction in the number of acetylcholine receptor sites, and the condition is characterized by profound muscular weakness and fatigability.

Thus, muscle contraction is controlled by motor end-plates but coordination of muscle activity involves sensory endings located in both muscle and tendon.

**Neuromuscular Spindles.** These are fusiform in shape with a connective tissue capsule and contain several small, modified muscle fibers called the *intrafusal fibers*, only 1 to 5 mm long and attached at their ends to tendon or endomysium (Fig. 6–17). Intrafusal fibers are of two types: One type, the *nuclear bag fibers*, is larger and less numerous with many nuclei contained in the centers of cells; the other type, the *nuclear chain fibers*, is smaller and more numerous with a single row of nuclei in the centers of cells. Afferent nerve fibers terminate on nuclear bag fibers in a spiral form (annulospiral endings) and as clusters (flower-spray endings) on nuclear chain fibers, and each type shows small, modified motor endings, or myoneural junctions. The sensory endings are proprioceptive and respond to tension or to stretch.

**Neurotendinous Endings.** These, also called tendon organs, are located in tendons near muscle-tendon junctions and consist of small bundles of encapsulated collagen fibers with sensory nerve fibers intertwined among them. They are stimulated by tension or stretching of the tendon during contraction. Other sensory endings simply ramify over the surface of collagen bundles of the tendon.

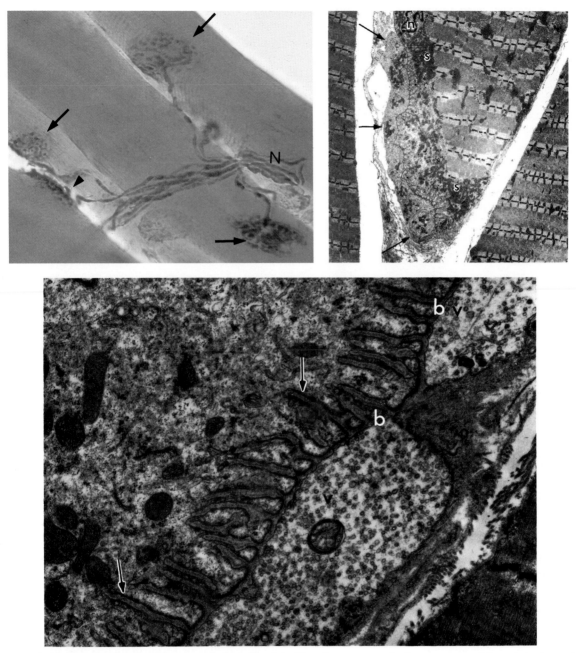

*Figure 6–16.* Myoneural junction (motor end-plate). Top left: This photomicrograph shows portions of four skeletal muscle fibers, each with a myoneural junction. A small nerve (N) shows several terminal branches. Three of the myoneural junctions are seen in surface view (arrows) as plate-like masses with terminal swellings of a nerve fiber. The fourth (arrowhead) appears as a disc on the surface of the muscle fiber. Medium power. Gold chloride. Top right: This electron micrograph of a white muscle fiber shows a myoneural junction (arrows), the subjacent sarcoplasm showing a nucleus (n) and numerous sarcosomes (s). ×3500. Bottom: At higher magnification, portions of two terminal nerve swellings show numerous synaptic vesicles (v) that contain the neurotransmitter acetylcholine. A basal lamina (b) lies in the primary synaptic cleft between nerve terminals and muscle sarcolemma, with numerous infoldings of the sarcolemma or secondary synaptic clefts (arrows), these also containing basal lamina material, the location of acetylcholinesterase. Numerous sarcosomes are seen in the sarcoplasm (left). ×26,000.

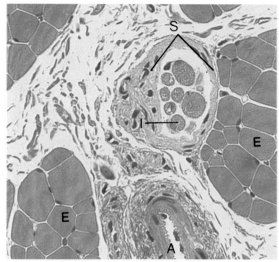

*Figure 6–17.* This section shows parts of several fasciculi, or bundles, of ordinary or extrafusal (E) muscle fibers in transverse section. Lying in perimysium between them (center) is a muscle spindle (S). This spindle shows seven intrafusal fibers (I), smaller than extrafusal fibers, enclosed in a connective tissue capsule. Afferent and efferent nerve fibers terminate on these intrafusal fibers, the sensory endings being proprioceptive, but no nerve fibers or endings are visible. A small artery (A) also is present. H and E. Medium power.

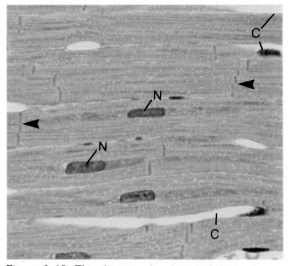

*Figure 6–18.* This shows cardiac (ventricular) muscle sectioned longitudinally. The muscle fibers, or trabeculae, are mainly parallel but show branching and cross bridges to give a pseudosyncytial arrangement. Between trabeculae are numerous blood capillaries (C) lined by endothelium with some endothelial nuclei seen. Nuclei (N) of muscle are large and are located centrally in the fibers with nonfibrillar sarcoplasm at their poles. The remainder of the sarcoplasm is occupied mainly by myofibrils. Intercalated discs (arrowheads) appear as dark lines crossing fibers either transversely (left) or in a staggered, zigzag manner (right). They are the sites of cell junctions. Plastic section. Weigert. Medium power.

## Regeneration

Muscle fibers have a limited capacity for regeneration, and gross damage is repaired by fibroconnective scar tissue. Similarly, if the nerve or blood supply is interrupted, muscle fibers degenerate and are replaced by fibrous tissue. However, adult muscle fibers contain *satellite cells*, which are small and uninucleated and are situated between sarcolemma and endomysium. These cells, which represent a reserve of embryonic myoblasts, can divide and play a role in repair and regeneration.

## CARDIAC MUSCLE

### Organization

Cardiac muscle is involuntary and striated and contracts rhythmically and automatically. It is found only in the myocardium (the muscle layer of the heart) and in the walls of large blood vessels joining the heart. By light microscopy, cardiac muscle has an overall appearance of long, mainly parallel fibers or trabeculae with numerous cross beams, giving the false impression of a syncytial network (Figs. 6–18 through 6–23). Each fiber is a linear unit composed of several cardiac muscle cells joined end to end at specialized junctional zones called *intercalated discs.* Each cell is about 100 μm long and 15 μm in diameter, often partially divided at one or both ends into two or more branches that meet adjacent cells, or parts of them, at intercalated discs. Each cell has a single, elongated nucleus, centrally located in sarcoplasm, and is bounded by a sarcolemma similar to that of skeletal muscle. Myofibrils are separated by abundant sarcoplasm containing numerous sarcosomes arranged in rows, with consequent obvious longitudinal striation. Myofibrils diverge around nuclei and show a pattern of cross striation identical to that of

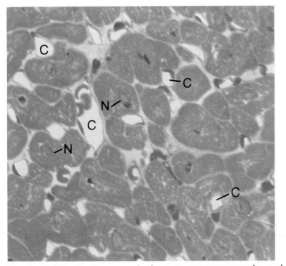

**Figure 6–19.** Cardiac muscle here is cut transversely and shows variation in size and shape of the fibers. Nuclei (N) are located centrally, and sarcoplasm appears reticular and pale-staining between darker-staining myofibrils. Numerous capillaries (C) are cut transversely also, lying in a delicate connective tissue endomysium. Methylene blue, basic fuchsin. Medium power.

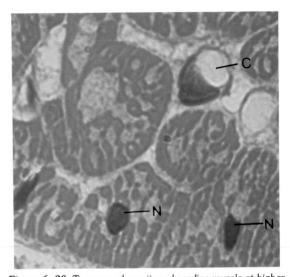

**Figure 6–20.** Transversely sectioned cardiac muscle at higher magnification shows variations in trabecular size and shape, central nuclei (N), and abundant sarcoplasm filled mainly by dark-staining (pink) myofibrils with pale-staining sarcoplasm between them. Between trabeculae is a delicate endomysium in which a capillary (C) is seen. Plastic section. H and E. Oil immersion.

skeletal muscle, with A, I, Z, H, and M bands. Around nuclei are fusiform areas of nonfibrillar sarcoplasm containing sarcosomes, a small Golgi apparatus, a few lipid droplets, and, with increasing age, some deposits of lipofuscin pigment (secondary lysosomes). This pigment may be so extensive as to give a brownish tinge to fresh myocardium ("brown atrophy" of the heart). Large deposits of glycogen are present throughout the sarcoplasm. Intercalated discs, areas of cell adhesion between adjacent cells, appear as dark lines crossing fibers at Z lines in an irregular, zigzag or step-like fashion. They function to maintain firm cohesion between adjacent muscle cells and to transmit tension of the myofibrils along the axis of an entire fiber.

Between the fibers, or trabeculae, is an endomysium of fine connective tissue containing small blood vessels and lymphatics.

## Fine Structure

Myofilaments containing actin and myosin are identical to those of skeletal muscle, but their grouping into myofibrils is not complete as it is in skeletal muscle. Transverse sections show that myofibrils are incompletely delineated by sarcoplasmic reticulum and sarcoplasm containing sarcosomes, and myofibrils do not appear as the discrete structures seen in skeletal muscle. Sarcosomes are large, up to 2.5 µm long (the length of a sarcomere), and show closely packed cristae, and frequently, lipid droplets lie between them. Glycogen occurs as 30- to 40-nm dense particles widely scattered not only throughout nonfibrillar cytoplasm but also in rows between myofilaments, particularly in relation to I bands.

The *T tubules* are invaginations of the sarcolemma, as they are in skeletal muscle, but differ in that they are of greater diameter and are located at Z discs and not A-I junctions. They contain extracellular basal lamina (glycoprotein) material continuous with that of the sarcolemma. The *sarcoplasmic reticulum* is less highly developed than that of skeletal muscle and consists of longitudinal, interconnected tubules that couple (i.e., form triads) with T tubules at Z discs by small, terminal expansions, but no large terminal cisternae are present. Also present are small,

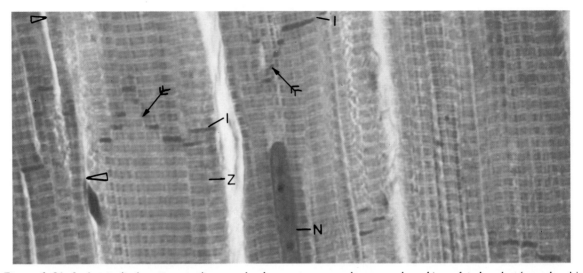

**Figure 6–21.** In longitudinal section, cardiac muscle shows some cross beams or branching of trabeculae (arrowheads), accounting for the pseudosyncytial appearance. A nucleus (N) shows several nucleoli and is centrally located in a trabecula. A, I, H, and Z bands are seen in the myofibrils with clear nonfibrillar sarcoplasm appearing as streaks between myofibrils. Intercalated discs (I) are dark-staining, located at Z discs, and often cross the fiber in a stepwise fashion (arrows). Azocarmine and thionin. Oil immersion.

flattened cisternae of sarcoplasmic reticulum located subjacent to the sarcolemma (subsarcolemmal cisternae) that function like triads by coupling with the sarcolemma and releasing the calcium necessary for contraction.

*Intercalated discs* are specialized cell junctions, located at Z lines (Figs. 6–23 and 6–24). Opposing cell surfaces at a disc show a complex pattern of blunt papillae and ridges with reciprocal pits and grooves. In that discs usually cross a trabecula or fiber in a stepwise pattern, they have transverse and longitudinal parts. In transverse regions are scattered *spot desmosomes* (maculae adherentes) for firm cell adhesion and extensive intermediate junctions, or *fasciae adherentes*. At a fascia adherens, the intercellular space is about 20 nm wide, with dense material on the cytoplasmic surfaces of each plasmalemma in which are anchored the thin myofilaments. These regions also function in firm cell adhesion, and calcium ions are necessary for this. In longitudinal regions, in particular, are extensive *gap junctions*, or *nexuses*, with a few less extensive gap junctions in transverse regions: Here the intercellular space is only 2 nm. These are areas of low electrical resistance and permit rapid impulse conduction between cells, enabling the myocardium to function as a syncytium.

### Contraction

Spontaneous myogenic contractions occur in cardiac muscle cells from early embryonic life, and the mechanism of contraction is identical to that of skeletal muscle (i.e., a sliding filament). In specific regions of the heart, cardiac muscle cells are modified to form the impulse-conducting system (see Chapter 8) that regulates the heart beat. Transmission of impulses occurs from cell to cell via gap junctions, or nexuses.

### Types of Cardiac Muscle

As indicated, in the impulse-conducting system, cardiac muscle is modified, but there also are differences between atrial and ventricular fibers. The preceding description applies to ventricular fibers.

*Atrial fibers* are smaller, their T system is poorly developed and even absent in the smallest fibers,

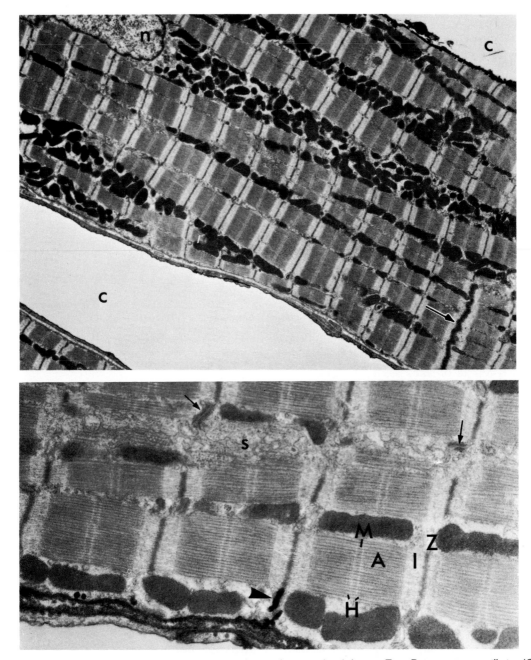

***Figure 6–22.*** *These electron micrographs are of ventricular, cardiac muscle of the rat. Top: Between two capillaries (C) is a single trabecula or fiber. A portion of a centrally located nucleus (n) has nonfibrillar sarcoplasm containing numerous sarcosomes at its (right) pole, with the remainder of the sarcoplasm occupied by myofibrils with rows of sarcosomes in the sarcoplasm between them. Banding of the myofibrils is identical to that of skeletal muscle with A, I, H, and Z lines, but myofibrils appear to branch and divide by interchange of myofilaments between adjacent myofibrils (i.e., they are not so clearly delineated or so discrete as in skeletal muscle). An intercalated disc (arrow) is located at a Z disc. ×4000. Bottom: A, I, Z, H, and M bands are seen in the myofibrils, with sarcosomes in rows between them and subjacent to the sarcolemma (bottom). Also seen is sarcoplasmic reticulum, triads located at Z discs (arrows), and a darkly staining T tubule (arrowhead) adjacent to (and would be continuous with) the sarcolemma, this located at a Z disc. ×22,000.*

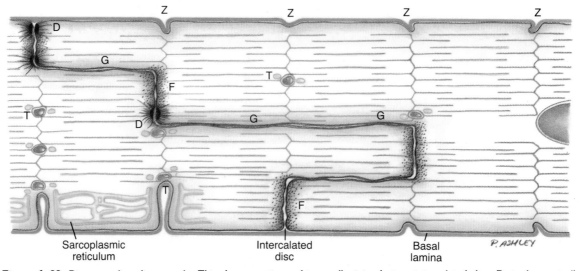

**Figure 6–23.** *Diagram of cardiac muscle. This shows portions of two cells, joined at an intercalated disc. Part of a centrally located nucleus (blue) is seen at right, with myofibrils formed by thick and thin filaments, their distribution in the sarcomere accounting for the banding as it is in skeletal muscle (see Figures 6–7 and 6–13). Note the branching of myofibrils that occurs by interchange of myofilaments (right). The intercalated disc shows transverse and longitudinal parts, the transverse parts located at Z discs with maculae adherentes (spot desmosomes, D) and fasciae adherentes (F) on transverse parts and gap junctions (G) on longitudinal parts. Also illustrated (lower left) is sarcoplasmic reticulum ensheathing myofibrils, and T tubules (T). T tubules are continuous with the sarcolemma, located at Z discs, of large diameter (compared with those of skeletal muscle); contain basal lamina material; and with sarcoplasmic reticulum, form triads at Z discs.*

and they contain homogeneous, electron-dense "atrial-specific granules," 0.3–0.4 μm in diameter. These lie adjacent to the Golgi apparatus and the nucleus and the granules contain two polypeptides called *cardionatrin*, which is a powerful diuretic, and *cardiodilatin*, which causes relaxation of vascular smooth muscle and consequent vasodilation.

*Purkinje's fibers* are specialized cardiac muscle cells, part of the impulse-conducting system, and are located just beneath the endocardium in relation mainly to the interventricular septum. As with ordinary cardiac muscle, they form a network composed of separate cellular units, but they are larger, thicker (up to 50 μm in diameter), and more palely staining. They have abundant central sarcoplasm, relatively few myofibrils located peripherally, and abundant quantities of glycogen. Intercalated discs are seen infrequently and are poorly developed. There are regions where a gradual transition occurs between Purkinje's and ordinary cardiac muscle cells, although many Purkinje's cells join directly to ordinary cells. In other portions of the conducting tissue (e.g., the

sinoatrial and atrioventricular nodes), the nodal cells are much smaller than ordinary cardiac muscle cells. These are described more fully in Chapter 8.

### Connective Tissue

Connective tissue is not prominent in cardiac muscle but extends between fibers as a delicate endomysium containing an extremely rich capillary network. Lymphatic capillaries also are prominent, and fine autonomic nerves are seen quite frequently (mostly sympathetic), terminating directly on cardiac muscle.

### Regeneration

Although cardiac muscle is more resistant to injury than other types of muscle, it shows little evidence of regeneration after injury. Damaged cardiac muscle is repaired by fibroconnective scar tissue.

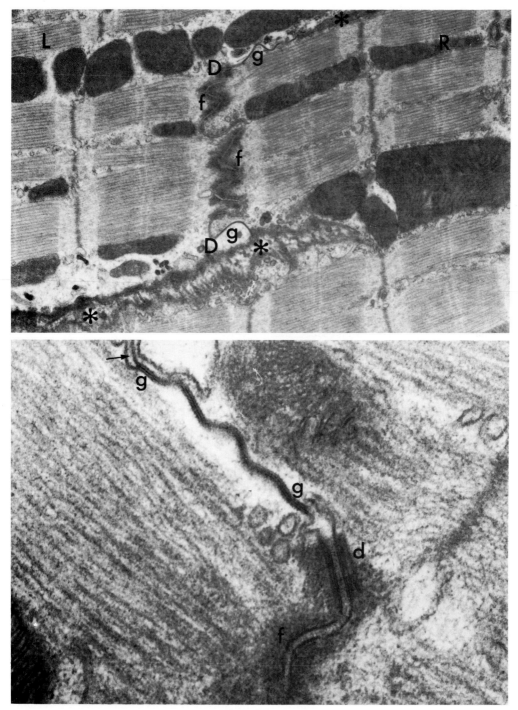

***Figure 6–24.*** *Electron micrographs of intercalated discs. Top: The extracellular (intercellular) space is indicated by asterisks, with parts of two cells (left L and right R) joining at an intercalated disc (D) located at a Z line. The disc shows gap junctions (g) on longitudinal parts and a fascia adherens (f) on the transverse part. ×24,000. Bottom: A higher magnification shows an extensive gap junction (g) on a longitudinal part of a disc (parallel to myofibrils), a macula adherens or spot desmosome (d), and a fascia adherens (f) on the transverse part. Intercellular space (arrow) appears above. ×84,000.*

## SMOOTH MUSCLE

Also called unstriped, nonstriated, or involuntary muscle, smooth muscle mainly is visceral in distribution, forming the contractile portion of the wall of the digestive tract from mid-esophagus to anus (Figs. 6–25 and 6–26). It also is found in the respiratory, urinary, and genital systems; in arteries, veins, and larger lymphatics; in the dermis; and in the iris and ciliary body of the eye. In these locations, it functions to moderate and maintain lumen diameter of the hollow viscera.

### Organization

Smooth muscle cells may occur singly or in small groups (e.g., in the dermis or in the cores of intestinal villi), intimately associated with fibroelastic connective tissue. In blood vessels, the muscle cells change lumen caliber and are oriented circumferentially or transversely around the vessels. Elsewhere, they usually lie in sheets with all fibers in the same orientation. Often, two sheets

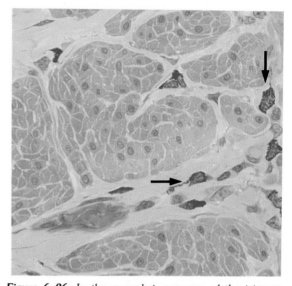

*Figure 6–26. In the muscularis mucosae of the jejunum, smooth muscle fibers are arranged in bundles and here sectioned transversely. Cell outlines vary in size, only the larger profiles showing centrally located nuclei, indicating elongation of the cells with the section cutting most at either end of the cell outside the nuclear area. Present in the surrounding connective tissue are blood vessels and numerous mast cells (arrow). Methylene blue, azure A. Medium power.*

form the wall of a duct or hollow viscus with fibers of the two sheets at right angles (e.g., in the intestine, an inner layer is circular, and an outer layer is longitudinal in orientation) (Fig. 6–27). In many cases, these orientations really are spiral in type, the "circular" being a closed and the "longitudinal" being an open helix. In other organs (e.g., the uterus and the bladder), layers are defined poorly, and muscle occurs as interlacing bundles oriented in all directions.

When lying in sheets and bundles, the cells usually are arranged with the nuclear (broad) region of one adjacent to the tapering (thin) ends of adjacent cells, with a slender intercellular space of only 50 to 80 nm. This space is occupied by reticular and fine elastic fibers, probably formed by the muscle cells themselves, as connective tissue cells are seen rarely in this location. More prominent connective tissue with fibroblasts, blood vessels, and nerves surrounds a large bundle or sheet of muscle. In such a sheet, the pull of a contracting cell first is transmitted to the fine reticular-elastic net that lies around it and then to

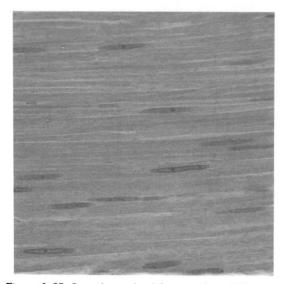

*Figure 6–25. Smooth muscle of the muscularis of the colon is cut longitudinally, the cells arranged in a layer, or coat. The cells are elongated and parallel, with little intercellular material. Nuclei are elongated, most show nucleoli, and they are staggered (i.e., nuclei of adjacent cells do not lie next to each other). Sarcoplasm is homogeneous. Methylene blue, azure A. Medium power.*

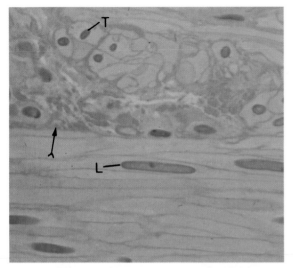

**Figure 6–27.** Smooth muscle cells here are cut both longitudinally (L) and transversely (T). In longitudinal section, cells are elongated with central, elongated nuclei and homogeneous cytoplasm, whereas only a few of the transverse profiles show nuclei. Muscle cells are closely apposed in the two layers, with slender pink-magenta fibrils between them. These are PAS-positive reticular fibers, with larger collagen fibrils (arrow) between the bundles of smooth muscle fibers of the wall of the gallbladder. H and E, PAS. Oil immersion.

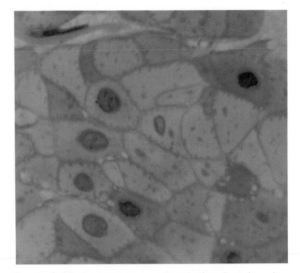

**Figure 6–28.** In transverse section, both cell and nuclear outlines vary in size in these smooth muscle fibers of the bladder wall, indicating elongation of the cells, confirmed by the fact that nuclei are seen only in a few cells. The cells are closely packed and show small dark bodies, both at the surface sarcolemma and within sarcoplasm. These are attachment plaques and dense bodies, are believed to be part of a skeletal network interconnected by intermediate (10-nm) filaments, and are similar to Z lines of striated muscle, serving as attachment regions for thin myofilaments. Toluidine blue. Oil immersion.

the stronger connective tissue of the bundle, giving a steady, general force to the enclosed or enveloped tissue (e.g., in constriction of a blood vessel).

When relaxed, smooth muscle fibers are elongated, spindle-shaped cells with tapering ends and a wider central nucleus-containing region. Size varies with location. In small blood vessels, they are only 20 μm long but can reach 0.5 mm in the pregnant uterus. Usually, they are 0.2 mm long and 6 μm in diameter at the nuclear region. Sarcoplasm usually appears acidophil and homogeneous, sometimes with small clear areas that may indicate the location of glycogen accumulations. Occasionally, a longitudinal striation can be demonstrated, a reflection of the presence of myofibrils running the full length of the fiber. No cross striation or banding is seen, which indicates a nonregular orientation of myofilaments. Small, darkly staining patches may be visible along the sarcolemma and in the sarcoplasm, particularly in thin plastic sections: These are termed *attachment plaques* and *dense bodies* (Fig. 6–28). Cyto-

plasmic organelles are few and located mainly at nuclear poles. In transverse section, only a few cells show the presence of nuclei because of the elongation of the cells, but when present, they are round and central in position. In longitudinal section, the nucleus is elongated and ovoid with rounded ends, stains lightly, and usually has a fine chromatin network. However, in cells fixed in contraction, the cell outline is irregular, and the nucleus characteristically shows a passive folded or pleated shape.

### Fine Structure

In the sarcoplasm around the nucleus, and particularly at its poles, are a few sarcosomes, a few elements of granular reticulum and some free ribosomes, a small Golgi apparatus, glycogen, and occasional lipid droplets (Figs. 6–29 through 6–32). Elsewhere, the sarcoplasm is occupied mainly by myofilaments of two sizes, generally

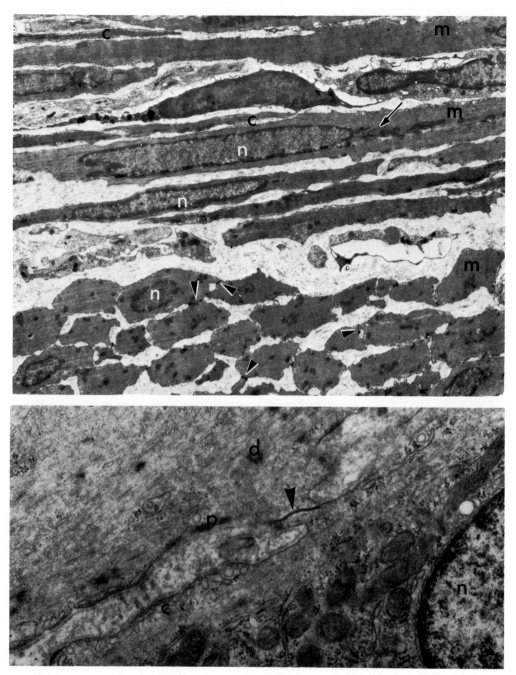

**Figure 6–29.** *Electron micrographs of smooth muscle. Top: This is a section of the duodenal muscularis with smooth muscle cells (m) of its two layers cut longitudinally (above) and transversely (below). Nuclei (n) are elongated, with organelles (arrow) at the nuclear pole and numerous subsarcolemmal caveolae (c). In transverse section, only a few cells are cut through the nuclear area. Cells lie closely apposed, with little intercellular material, and in those of the layer cut transversely, numerous gap junctions, or nexuses, are present (stained darkly, arrowheads). ×3000. Bottom: Parts of two cells of the muscularis trachealis are seen with a little intercellular material between them. Cut longitudinally, sarcoplasm shows myofilaments running longitudinally, most organelles (sarcosomes, granular endoplasmic reticulum seen here) in a paranuclear position (n, nucleus), attachment plaques (p) at the surface sarcolemma and dense bodies (d) in the sarcoplasm, and a nexus (arrowhead) between the two cells. ×36,000.*

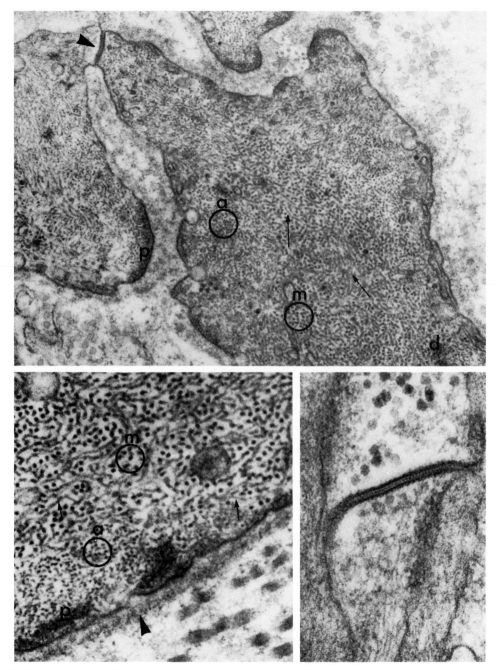

**Figure 6–30.** *Electron micrographs of smooth muscle (musculus trachealis). Top: Portions of three cells in transverse section are seen with a nexus (arrowhead) between two of them in the plane of section. Sarcoplasm contains filaments of three sizes: thick (myosin, m) myofilaments, thin (actin-containing, a) myofilaments arranged in bundles, and intermediate 10-nm filaments (arrows). The last interconnect dense bodies (d) and attachment plaques (p) and are believed to serve a cytoskeletal function. ×44,000. Bottom left: This higher magnification shows more clearly the filament types. Also seen is the basal lamina (arrowhead) and collagen microfibrils (below). ×180,000. Bottom right: A nexus, or gap junction, is seen between processes of two smooth muscle cells, this being a site of low electrical resistance for rapid passage between cells of electrical impulses and ions. ×68,000.*

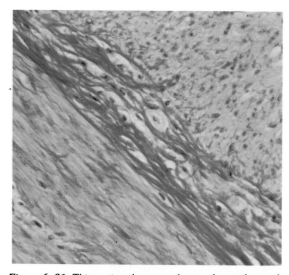

*Figure 6–31.* This section shows two layers of smooth muscle of the intestinal muscularis, one cut transversely (upper right) and one cut longitudinally (lower left). Sarcoplasm stains yellow, nuclei black, and extracellular collagen fibrils and fibers bright red. Between individual smooth muscle cells in both layers are thin, slender collagen fibrils (reticular fibers) only, with more dense connective tissue with larger collagen fibrils between the layers. Here, a few nuclei of fibroblasts are present between the collagen fibrils. A stain such as this (van Gieson's) clearly distinguishes between smooth muscle and connective tissue. Medium power.

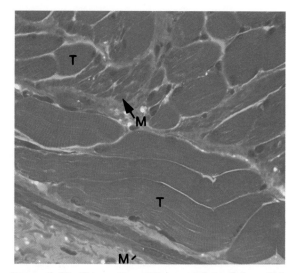

*Figure 6–32.* This section of the muscularis of the middle esophagus shows a mixture of smooth and skeletal muscle fibers in both layers of the muscularis cut transversely (above) and longitudinally (below). The skeletal muscle fibers (T) in transverse section are obviously of greater diameter and show peripheral, multiple nuclei and, in longitudinal section, show cross-banding. Smooth muscle fibers (M) are smaller, with single central nuclei, and do not show cross-banding. H and E. Medium power.

organized into parallel and longitudinal bundles or myofibrils, with a few sarcosomes and glycogen particles scattered between them. However, thick filaments vary in length and show cross bridges along their entire lengths. Thin filaments are similar to those of striated muscle but are more numerous with a ratio of twelve to one thick (instead of six to one in striated muscle). Both attachment plaques and dense bodies appear electron-dense, with thin myofilaments associated with them. They resemble Z discs in structure and also contain the protein alpha-actinin. Also present are intermediate 10-nm filaments, mainly interconnecting dense bodies and attachment plaques and believed to serve a skeletal function. No T system is present in smooth muscle, but there are elements of sarcoplasmic reticulum and *subsarcolemmal caveolae*, small pinocytotic-type vesicles beneath the sarcolemma. These vesicles are static, however, and have been shown to sequester calcium. They probably function in

calcium release and initiation of contraction comparable to the role of sarcoplasmic reticulum in striated muscle.

The sarcolemma is supported by a basal lamina and associated collagen microfibrils, and thus, a gap of about 50 to 80 mm usually separates adjacent smooth muscle cells. However, in regions, adjacent cells are separated by only 2 nm, these areas being gap junctions, or *nexuses*, sites of low electrical resistance where rapid passage of ions and electrical impulses can occur.

## Contraction

In smooth muscle, the contractile unit, in a sense, is the cell and not the sarcomere, which is not present. It is believed that contraction results from a sliding filament mechanism, similar to that of striated muscle, but the mechanism is not fully understood. It may be that the presence of bridges along the entire length of the thick filament permits actin-myosin interaction along the entire length of the thick filament, with force transmitted by the dense bodies and the intermediate filaments to decrease cell length. This process would require calcium ions for activation, with subsarcolemmal caveolae believed to be the reservoir for calcium.

In general, smooth muscle contracts slower than other types of muscle but can sustain contraction for long periods with little expenditure of energy.

## Nerve Supply

Smooth muscle contraction may follow nerve or hormonal stimulation. Generally, muscle is supplied by both sympathetic and parasympathetic nerve fibers, all being postganglionic and unmyelinated, with adrenergic and cholinergic transmitters involved, respectively. On the basis of innervation and function, two types of smooth muscle are recognized. The *multiunit* type has a rich nerve supply with all, or at least most, muscle cells receiving a nerve terminal. This type is found in the iris, larger arteries, and the ductus deferens, and contraction of muscle fibers occurs quickly and simultaneously. The *unitary* type of muscle contains fewer nerve terminals, and the stimulus spreads from cell to cell via nexuses. This gives a relatively slow contraction and is found in the viscera and smaller blood vessels. Intermediate types also are found. Uterine smooth muscle in late pregnancy responds to the hormone oxytocin, with other smooth muscle being unresponsive.

In visceral smooth muscle, two types of contraction are recognized and appear to be independent of each other. *Rhythmic* contractions occur as periodic waves of contraction after spontaneous generation of impulses. *Tonic* contraction is the continuous state of partial contraction re-

| Summary Table 6–1. Features of Muscle Types | | | |
| --- | --- | --- | --- |
| **Characteristics** | **Skeletal Muscle** | **Cardiac Muscle** | **Smooth Muscle** |
| Location | Flesh of limbs and trunk, attached to skeleton | Myocardium; major blood vessels | Hollow viscera, blood vessels, iris |
| Shape and arrangement | Elongated, parallel fibers; large | Parallel fibers or trabeculae with cross beams in pseudosyncytium | Elongated, fusiform; small |
| Transverse striations | Present | Present | Not present |
| Nucleus | Multinucleate, peripheral | Single, central | Single, central |
| Sarcoplasmic reticulum | Complex with terminal cisternae | Less well-developed, no cisternae | Poorly developed; subsarcolemmal caveolae |
| T system | At A-I junctions, slim | At Z discs, wider | Absent |
| Cell junctions | Absent | Intercalated discs with maculae adherentes, fasciae adherentes, and gap junctions | Nexuses (gap junctions) |
| Myofibrils, sarcomeres | Well-delineated | Less well delineated | Not clearly seen |
| Connective tissue | Epi-, peri-, and endomysium | Endomysium | Delicate fibroelastic around individual fibers. Stronger around bundles or sheets |
| Capillary plexus | Rich, mainly longitudinal and parallel, with cross connections | Extremely rich, plexiform | Less obvious, mainly parallel to fiber orientation |
| Nerve, specializations | Myoneural junctions, neuromuscular spindles, neurotendinous endings. Somatic | Fine terminals, autonomic | Fine terminals, autonomic |
| Contraction | Powerful: variation between white and red fibers in speed and fatigability. Voluntary | Powerful, constant, low fatigability. Involuntary | Slow, low fatigability. Involuntary. Rhythmic and tonic |

sulting in muscle tone. The physiology of these is poorly understood.

### Origin, Growth, and Regeneration

Most smooth muscle develops by differentiation of mesenchymal cells, although that of the iris is derived from ectoderm. Some glands and their ducts (e.g., salivary, sweat, and lacrimal) contain cells called *myoepithelial cells*, derived from ectoderm but with many of the characteristics of smooth muscle (*see* Chapter 2). Smooth muscle can respond to physiological (e.g., the uterus in pregnancy) and pathological (e.g., arterioles in hypertension) stimuli by increasing in size. While the increase in size of the uterus in pregnancy mainly is due to muscle cell hypertrophy, there may also be an increase in the number of cells (hyperplasia).

### Differentiation from Connective Tissue

A common difficulty in tissue identification is the distinction between smooth muscle and connective tissue when stained with hematoxylin and eosin. Muscle fibers are cellular and usually stain more intensely eosinophil than do collagen fibers, and nuclei are situated *within* cytoplasm and are larger than those of fibroblasts situated *between* collagen fibers. Additionally, muscle nuclei may be wrinkled when the cells are in contraction. Staining techniques such as Mallory and van Gieson readily distinguish between the two.

# Nervous Tissue

## INTRODUCTION

The nervous system is distributed widely through-out the body, and with a few minor exceptions, all organs include a nervous component. Basically, this is the communi-cation system of the body that collects stimuli, transforms or transduces these into electrical stimuli that pass into a large, highly organized reception and correlation area (the central nervous system, or CNS) where they are interpreted, and then, in turn, issues appropriate responses or sensations. These functions are performed by highly specialized cells called *neu-*

7

*rons,* in which the properties of irritability and conductivity are highly developed. The nervous system includes the neurons, their supporting cells, and a limited amount of connective tissue containing a rich vascular supply.

Anatomically, the nervous system is divided into a *central nervous system* (CNS) and a *peripheral nervous system* (PNS). The CNS consists of the brain and the spinal cord located in the cranium and the vertebral canal and thus protected by bone, while the PNS includes all other nervous tissue. In the CNS, neurons are supported by a variety of cells called *neuroglia,* while in the PNS, the supporting cells are *Schwann's cells* and other "satellite" cells. It is the CNS that functions as the integrating and communications center, receiving exterior stimuli from the body surface (*exteroceptive*), from internal organs (*interoceptive*), and from joints, muscles, and tendons (*proprioceptive*). The PNS interconnects all other tissues and organs with the CNS. Functionally, the nervous system is divided into *somatic* and *autonomic* parts. The somatic part (Gr. *soma,* body) is concerned with the receipt of sensation and the formation of appropriate motor responses that are voluntary (i.e., under the control of the will). The autonomic part (Gr. *autos,* self; *nomos,* control; i.e., automatic) regulates all other responses that are beyond voluntary control, and this includes the nervous supply of smooth and cardiac muscles, exocrine glands, and viscera. Additionally, there is a close coordination between nervous and endocrine systems, some neurons being secretory (e.g., in the hypothalamus and the neurohypophysis).

Although neurons vary greatly in size, shape, and the number and pattern of their branches, they show a basic similarity in form. Each has a *perikaryon,* or *soma,* consisting of the nucleus and surrounding cytoplasm, and one or more cell processes. These processes are of two types. *Dendrites,* usually branching and multiple, form, together with the perikaryon, the main area for receipt of impulses. *Axons* are more slender, and only one arises from each soma: They may give off branches or collaterals and terminally may show fine ramifications also. They conduct away from the soma, transmitting impulses to other nerve cells, glands, and muscle. Thus, neurons are polarized with dendrites and soma receiving

stimuli and the axon conducting the impulse to other cells, with transmission in one direction. Most, but not all, neurons conform to this pattern. The perikarya of most neurons lie in or near the CNS, while their processes may lie totally within the CNS, extend from it for some distance, or lie entirely outside the CNS. While neurons are separate, discrete cells, most are associated functionally with other neurons in chains to form pathways, the impulse from one neuron passing via its axon to the perikaryon or dendrite of

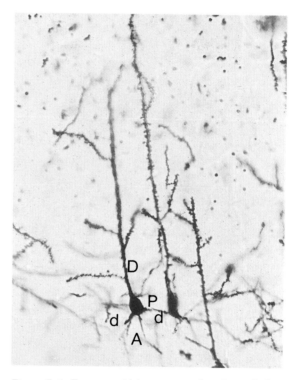

*Figure 7–1.* Two pyramidal neurons, and portions of others, from the cerebral cortex are seen. These are multipolar, Golgi type I and show the general features of all neurons, each with a perikaryon (P), or soma; a large apical branching dendrite (D) and several basal dendrites (d); and a single axon (A) leaving the base of the cell. The axon is long, and only its root is seen in the cell on the left. On the dendritic branches are small spines, areas of synaptic contact. As in most neurons, the perikaryon, or soma, and the dendrites receive impulses from other neurons (axosomatic and axodendritic synapses), and impulses pass via the axon to other neurons or effector organs. This is a silver impregnation specimen that demonstrates only the cell outline. Low power.

another, stimulating that neuron in turn to initiate its own impulse, which then passes along its axon. This specialized site of contact between neurons is called a *synapse*, where chemical or electrical signals pass from cell to cell.

Three main types of neurons are classified based on the number of processes (Fig. 7–1). Most neurons are *multipolar*, with one axon and, usually, two or more dendrites, and this type includes motor neurons and internuncial neurons (interneurons, that lie between sensory and motor neurons). *Bipolar* neurons have one axon and one dendrite, are not common, but are found in the retina and the vestibular and cochlear ganglia of the eighth (auditory) cranial nerve, and in olfactory epithelium. True *unipolar* neurons with a single process are rare but are found in embryonic stages and in the photoreceptors of the eye. Most of the neurons in which apparently only a single cell process leaves the perikaryon are originally bipolar, with the two processes later fusing into a single common stem that, at some distance from the soma, branches to form a Y or T shape. These are the *pseudounipolar* neurons, and all sensory neurons of craniospinal ganglia belong to this group.

In the CNS, nerve cell bodies (soma) are found only in the *gray matter,* while the *white matter* contains only their processes and supporting cells. Outside the CNS, perikarya lie in *ganglia* (simply, collections of nerve cell bodies) and in specialized sensory regions such as the retina and the olfactory mucosa.

(*Note on Terminology*: The perikaryon sometimes is referred to as the *nerve cell*, or nerve cell body, and both dendrites and axons may be termed *nerve fibers*.)

## THE REFLEX ARC

Functionally, as already indicated, neurons can be classified as *motor*, controlling effector organs such as muscle or glands; *sensory*, receiving exteroceptive, interoceptive, or proprioceptive stimuli; or *internuncial*, connecting other neurons to establish complex functional circuits or neural pathways.

Any nervous activity involves several neurons with potentially numerous interconnections via their synapses.

In humans, most actions involve reflex arcs, the simplest of which occurs with only two participating neurons (Fig. 7–2). In clinical examination, the *knee jerk* is used and is performed with the patient in a sitting, relaxed position and the knees crossed. The patellar tendon of the uppermost knee is tapped sharply, and, normally, the quadriceps muscle then contracts to kick the foot forward. This is a reflex action involving one afferent (sensory) and one efferent (motor) neuron. The pathway includes a peripheral dendritic process of the afferent neuron lying in the quadriceps tendon and sensing stretch of the tendon. Its cell body (soma) is located in a posterior (dorsal) root ganglion near the spinal cord, from whence its axon passes into the substance of the spinal cord where it synapses with an efferent nerve cell body. The axon of this second neuron then passes into a peripheral nerve to supply, and cause to contract, muscle fibers in the quadriceps muscle. This simple, two-neuron pathway can be made more complex by inserting a third internuncial (connector) neuron between the afferent and efferent neurons, establishing potentially numerous connections within the CNS. In fact, once a nervous impulse reaches the CNS, there is widespread activity. The simple reflex arc is an example of the basic principle that nervous activity involves neural pathways with inflow to the CNS by the afferent neuron, modification and integration by the internuncial neuron, and outflow by the efferent neuron to an effector organ.

## THE NEURON

The general features of neurons have already been described. Motor neurons and internuncial neurons are multipolar, with perikarya that are irregular and angular, the shape depending on the number of cell processes. Sensory neurons are pseudounipolar, with globular perikarya and only one cell process, while bipolar neurons are fusiform or spindle-shaped, with an axon and a single dendrite at opposite poles of the soma. In

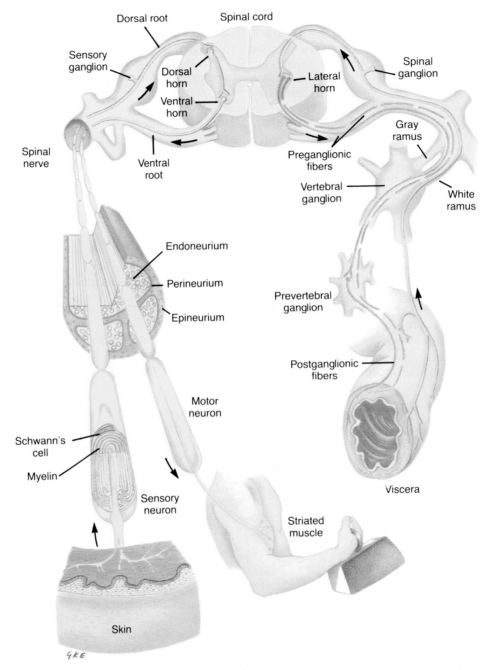

**Figure 7–2.** Diagram illustrating somatic (left) and sympathetic (right) reflex arcs. In the somatic arc, a sensory (pseudounipolar) neuron lies in the dorsal root or sensory ganglion with a peripheral process terminating in skin. The central process passes to the spinal cord, where it synapses with a connector or internuncial neuron (multipolar) in the dorsal horn of gray matter. In turn, the internuncial neuron synapses in the ventral horn of gray matter with a motor (multipolar) neuron, the axon of which passes to striated muscle, the effector organ. Thus, this is a three-neuron reflex arc. The simplest, a two-neuron reflex arc, is formed by a sensory and a motor neuron. In the sympathetic reflex arc, three neurons are involved, but the synapse between the sensory and the internuncial neurons occurs in the lateral horn (intermediolateral column), the internuncial neuron being the "preganglionic" neuron. The synapse between this and the motor, or "postganglionic," neuron occurs in a prevertebral ganglion.

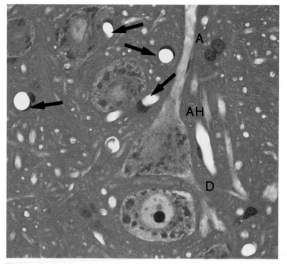

*Figure 7–3. Most features of a typical neuron are seen in this preparation showing motor neurons (anterior horn cells) of the spinal cord. These are multipolar, Golgi type I. The nerve cell bodies (somas, or perikarya) are large, and the lowest one shows a typical, large vesicular nucleus with a prominent nucleolus—the "owl's-eye" appearance. Perikarya contain clumps of blue-purple–staining material, the Nissl bodies, which extend into dendrites. The central cell shows a branching dendrite (D) and, at its upper extremity, a clear area of cytoplasm devoid of Nissl substance. This is the axon hillock (AH), and arising from the soma here is the axon (A). Smaller nuclei present are mainly of oligodendrocytes (a type of neuroglia), and numerous capillaries (arrows) also are seen. Methylene blue, basic fuchsin. High power.*

general, neurons are large cells, varying from 4 to 135 μm in diameter (Figs. 7–3 and 7–4).

## Perikaryon

The perikaryon (soma, or cell body), formed by the nucleus and surrounding cytoplasm, has a receptive function together with the dendrites, in most cases receiving stimuli generated in other nerve cells (Fig. 7–5). It is the trophic, or nourishing, center of the cell, supplying organelles and macromolecules to its processes. Usually, the perikaryon is large, up to 135 μm in diameter, with a large (up to 20 μm in diameter) euchromatic, spherical nucleus that is situated centrally. Chromatin is fine and dispersed, usually with a large prominent, single nucleolus. Sex chromatin (Barr's body) in the female may be visible as a

nucleolar satellite or at the periphery of the nucleus. The nuclear envelope is distinct and shows numerous pores. The large, pale vesicular nucleus with prominent nucleolus is often referred to as the "owl's-eye" appearance.

Contained in the perikaryon are organelles, usually arranged in a regular, even fashion around the nucleus. Mitochondria are small and rod-like, with cristae that lie both transversely and longitudinally. The Golgi apparatus is large and lies around the nucleus, often as several dictyosomes composed of closely apposed, flattened cisternae often with dilated ends, the cisternal stacks interconnected by smooth-surfaced tubular elements that may be continuous with granular endoplasmic reticulum. Centrioles rarely are seen (neurons are not capable of cell division). Primary lysosomes are common, and secondary lysosomes increase in number with age, some being lipofuscin granules, "inert" by-products of lysosomal activity (Fig. 7–6). Pigment granules of various types also are common and include melanin as dark-brown or black granules found in regions such as the substantia nigra of the midbrain, in spinal and sympathetic ganglia, and in the locus ceruleus near the fourth ventricle. Fat droplets may be present, representing either a normal reserve material or a product of pathological metabolism. Iron-containing granular deposits are found in regions such as the substantia nigra and the globus pallidus. Glycogen is not present in adult neurons. Two other components of the neuronal cytoplasm characteristically are well developed, as indicated below.

**Nissl Bodies.** These, the basophilic component, are stainable by basic aniline dyes, appearing as basophilic clumps throughout the cytoplasm and in dendrites, although they are absent in the axon and the *axon hillock*, a clear conical area at the origin of the axon from the soma (Fig. 7–7). In small neurons, instead of Nissl bodies, only a diffuse basophilia is seen. Nissl bodies consist of parallel arrays of cisternae of granular endoplasmic reticulum with associated polysomes and ribosomes, both free and attached. Nissl bodies react to injury or to prolonged stimulation in a characteristic manner by apparently breaking up and diffusing throughout the cytoplasm, a process called *chromatolysis*. The presence of extensive granular reticulum, prominent nucleoli, and numerous mitochondria is associated with

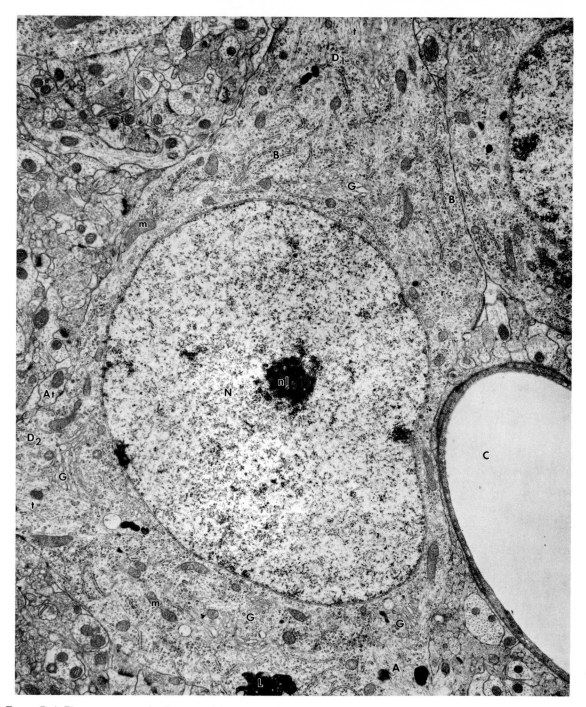

**Figure 7–4.** *Electron micrograph of a pyramidal neuron of rat cerebral cortex showing the root of an axon (A, lower right) and apical (D₁) and basal (D₂) dendrites. In the perikaryon is the nucleus (N) with its nucleolus (nl), cytoplasm with Nissl bodies (B), element of the Golgi apparatus (G), mitochondria (m), free ribosomes (r), lysosomes (L), and microtubules (t). Microtubules are more prominent and are arranged in parallel bundles in the cell processes. An axon terminal (At) forms a synapse with the neuron, and a capillary (C) also is seen. Approx. × 7000. (Reproduced with permission from Peters, A., Palay, S. L., and Webster, H. de F.: The Fine Structure of the Nervous System. Philadelphia, W. B. Saunders Co., 1976.)*

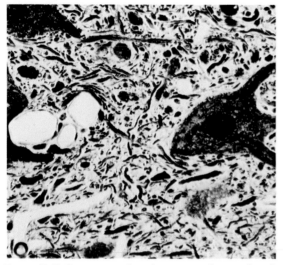

**Figure 7–5.** Demonstrated in this anterior horn cell is the shape of the perikaryon, which is multipolar, with the roots of three large dendrites. In both soma and dendrites, there are neurofibrils, appearing here as dark clumps and strands. Clear cytoplasmic areas between them probably represent Nissl bodies. The large, central nucleus appears black. Around the neuron, there is the neuropil formed by processes of other neurons and neuroglia, some small dark nuclei of neuroglia cells, and capillaries. Silver stain. High power.

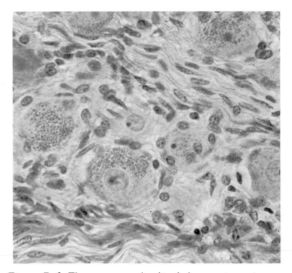

**Figure 7–6.** These neurons (multipolar) are autonomic ganglion cells of a sympathetic ganglion, showing large, vesicular nuclei with prominent nucleoli, and several contain in their cytoplasm yellowish-brown lipofuscin granules, by-products of lysosomal activity. The granules appear to increase in number with age. Each neuron has a "capsule" formed by small capsule or satellite cells, and between the neurons are nerve fibers. H and E. Medium power.

the synthesis of new protein that passes to all parts of the neuron, including the axon and the dendrites.

**Neurofilaments and Neurotubules.** Within neurons, there is a cytoskeletal network of *neurofibrils*, visible by light microscopy in silver preparations, lying between Nissl bodies and parts of the Golgi complex and extending into dendrites and the axon. These bundles are formed by neurofilaments, 10 nm in diameter and of indefinite length, and neurotubules, 25 nm in diameter and with a pale central core of 10 nm. The neurotubules appear to be identical to microtubules found in other cell types, but the neurofilaments differ from intermediate, 10-nm filaments of other cell types, including those of neuroglial cells (see later).

## Nerve Cell Processes

As explained previously, the processes are dendrites (usually multiple) and the axon (single),

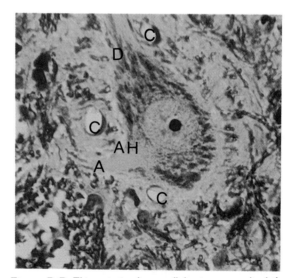

**Figure 7–7.** This anterior horn cell (motor neuron) of the spinal cord shows a large vesicular nucleus with prominent nucleolus and, in the cytoplasm, clumps of purple-staining Nissl bodies that (above) extend into the stem of a dendrite (D). They are absent in the axon hillock (AH) from which the axon (A) originates. Several capillaries (C) lie in gray matter adjacent to the neuron, while white matter is seen at left. Trypan blue and cresyl violet. Oil immersion.

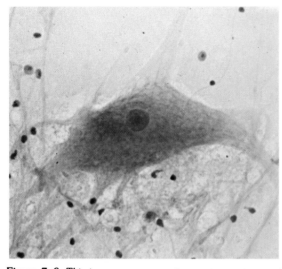

**Figure 7–8.** *This is a smear preparation, not a section, and shows an anterior horn (motor) cell of the spinal cord. This is a multipolar neuron with a large, central nucleus and a dense nucleolus, fibrillar cytoplasm, and numerous processes—all dendrites here, as the axon is not identifiable. Neurofibrils extend into these processes. The surrounding small, blue-staining nuclei are those mainly of oligodendrocytes. H and E. High power.*

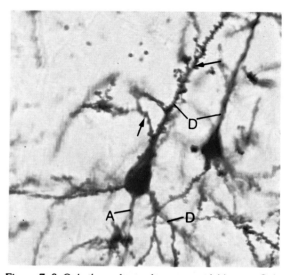

**Figure 7–9.** *Only the surfaces of two pyramidal (motor, Golgi type I) neurons of the cerebral cortex are seen in this preparation. Each shows an apical, branching dendrite and several basal dendrites (D), with the root of one axon (A). On the dendritic branches are small spines (arrows), the sites of synaptic contact. Silver impregnation. Medium power. (See also Figure 7–1.)*

with conduction along dendrites to the perikaryon and along the axon away from the cell body.

**Dendrites.** In most neurons, dendrites are multiple and comparatively short, located near the parent perikaryon. Most branch into primary, secondary, and higher orders of branching, and in larger dendrites, it is difficult to determine where a dendrite starts and the perikaryon ends (Fig. 7–8). The dendritic base usually is broad, narrowing toward the terminal branches. Main-stem dendrites contain Nissl bodies and ribosomes, and mitochondria and neurofibrils are found along their lengths, even into the finest ramifications. There is evidence that the neurotubules are involved in transport of protein and other material from the perikaryon to the terminations of the dendrites, as is also the case in axons (see following discussion on axonal transport).

Dendrites of many neurons appear to be beaded, covered by small, spine-like processes called *dendritic spines* that are specialized for synaptic contacts (Fig. 7–9). Generally, they have a short slender stem 0.5 to 1.0 μm long, with an expanded tip 0.5 to 2.0 μm in diameter. They may contain a few microtubules and a "spine apparatus" formed by one or more vesicular or sac-like membranous structures, between which are bands of electron-dense material. Spines are numerous on major dendrites, less so near the perikaryon and at dendrite tips, but are not present in many types of neurons. While they represent the main synaptic surface of dendrites, other synapses do occur along the dendritic tree. It should be noted that it is the dendrites that constitute much of the felt-like "neuropil" of the CNS.

**Axon.** The axon, or axis cylinder, is a single, cylindrical process usually thinner, straighter, and longer than the dendrites of the same neuron (Fig. 7–10). It often arises from the nerve cell body at a region called the *axon hillock* that contains no Nissl bodies but may arise from the base of a major dendrite. The so-called *initial segment* of the axon, lying between the axon hillock and the beginning of the myelin sheath (if present), shows a 20-nm electron-dense undercoat to the plasmalemma (axolemma), and here

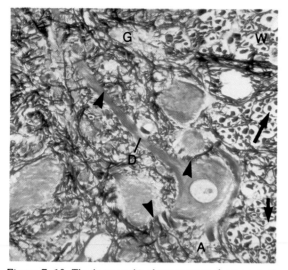

*Figure 7–10.* The large multipolar neuron in the gray matter (G) of the spinal cord (anterior horn) shows a large central vesicular nucleus, and both the cytoplasm and the cell processes contain faintly stained neurofibrils. The axon (A) is cut short. Small nerve fibers in the surrounding neuropil stain black. The long dendrite (D) and the soma show synapses at their surfaces (arrowheads). To the right is white matter (W) with axons stained black (as dots in transverse section) surrounded by clear, unstained myelin (arrows). Silver, aniline blue. High power.

in the axoplasm the microtubules (neurotubules) are arranged in parallel bundles with small cross bridges between adjacent microtubules.

Axons vary from less than a micrometer to several micrometers in diameter and from a fraction of a millimeter to more than a meter in length and generally have a smooth contour. Along its course, an axon may or may not show side-branches (*collaterals*) that leave the main axon at right angles and, often, more complex terminal arborizations (*telodendria*) in relation to the neuron on which it terminates. At their terminations, axonal twigs may show small swellings called *boutons terminaux;* similar swellings at synapses along the course of a terminal axon are called *boutons en passant.* In some cases, telodendria with their boutons are so extensive as to surround the neuron on which they terminate in a basket-like arrangement.

While there are no Nissl bodies in axoplasm, it does contain neurotubules, neurofilaments, and long slender mitochondria. Most axons are insu-

lated by a myelin sheath (see later) that distinguishes them from dendrites, but others are unmyelinated. Neurofilaments are more numerous in axons than in dendrites, but small dendrites and small unmyelinated axons are difficult to distinguish.

*Axonal Transport.* The long processes of neurons are maintained by the activity of the parent perikaryon, with constant movement of material from the perikaryon to the axon and dendrites, and, in some cases, back to the perikaryon. This transport is more necessary and more extensive in the axon in that dendrites contain organelles, including ribosomes.

Axonal transport is the transfer of materials to the terminal axon (*bouton*) (*anterograde* transport) and the return of material to the perikaryon (*retrograde* transport). There apparently are two components. A fast transport system goes in both directions at a speed of 2 to 40 cm per day and involves movement of organelles such as vesicles, elements of smooth reticulum, and mitochondria plus some metabolites. A slow transport system at a speed of 0.5 to 4 mm per day conveys cytoskeletal proteins associated with the neurofilaments and neurotubules and proteins of the cytoplasmic matrix. While the mechanism is poorly understood, it is known to involve the neurotubules. Involved also is the transport to the axon terminal of the materials necessary for reformation of transmitter substances and synaptic vesicles (see later).

## SYNAPSES

Synapses are the sites of transneuronal transmission of a nerve impulse. In relatively few instances, the electrical signal is passed directly from cell to cell by a low resistance gap junction. These are the *electrical synapses. Chemical synapses* are more common, and here the impulse is transmitted by a neurotransmitter substance. Usually the contact is between the axon of one neuron and a dendrite of another neuron (axodendritic) or its perikaryon (axosomatic), but occasionally between axons (axoaxonic) or between dendrites (dendrodendritic) (Figs. 7–11 and 7–12). Functionally, both excitatory and inhibitory

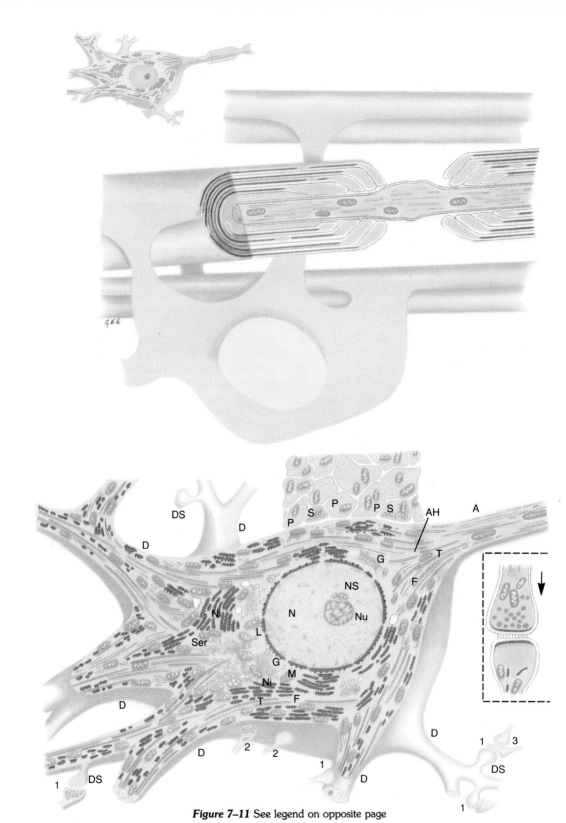

DS D D P S P P S AH A

P S G T

NS

F

N Nu

Ni

Ser L

G

M

Ni

T F

D D

D

DS

1 2 2

1 D

D

1 3

DS

1

*Figure 7–11* See legend on opposite page

synapses occur, and although there are morphological differences in various types, all have common features.

As already described, terminal axonal branches commonly show small swellings that contact another neuronal surface, as the axon lies adjacent to it (the *boutons en passant*) or at their tips (the *boutons terminaux*). Typically, a synapse consists of three elements: a presynaptic knob (the *bouton*); the synaptic cleft, a narrow extracellular space of 20 nm; and a postsynaptic element (usually a dendrite or soma). At a synapse, the pre- and postsynaptic membranes lie parallel to each other, separated by the synaptic cleft, which is crossed by fine filaments connecting the outer leaflets of the two membranes, sometimes with dense material bisecting the cleft. Lying in the presynaptic knob are collections of *synaptic vesicles*, 40 to 60 nm in diameter, filled by the neurotransmitter substance together with mitochondria, a few elements of smooth reticulum, and neurotubules and neurofilaments, with some dense material associated with the inner, cytoplasmic surface of the presynaptic membrane. The postsynaptic membrane also shows dense, fluffy material on its cytoplasmic surface. With the arrival of an action potential at the axon terminal and depolarization of the membrane, calcium enters the ending, which causes the vesicles to move to the presynaptic membrane, fuse with it, and discharge the transmitter into the synaptic cleft. The transmitter crosses the cleft and binds to receptors on the postsynaptic membrane, opening up channels in the membrane with consequent depolarization. After this cycle, the transmitter either is degraded by enzymes or is rapidly taken back into the presynaptic ending.

Variations in the appearance of synapses do occur. The preceding description is of a *symmetrical ending*. An *asymmetrical ending* has a wider synaptic cleft of 30 nm and shows pronounced thickening of the postsynaptic membrane. Some evidence suggests that the symmetrical type is inhibitory, whereas the asymmetrical is excitatory. However, intermediate types do occur, and morphology cannot be related directly to physiological function. A further type shows synaptic vesicles with a dense core, and in these, the neurotransmitter is catecholamine. Neurotransmitter substances include acetylcholine, norepinephrine, dopamine, serotonin, gamma-aminobutyric acid, glutamate, glycine, and a variety of peptides such as cholecystokinin and vasoactive intestinal peptide.

## TYPES OF NEURONS

As stated earlier, neurons are described as unipolar, pseudounipolar (Fig. 7–13), bipolar, or multipolar, depending on the number of processes. However, a great variety of neurons occur in the CNS, with differences in cell shape, size, and position; the number, length, and method of branching of processes; and synaptic relationships. Two main groups of multipolar cells are important. *Golgi type 1* neurons have a well-developed dendritic tree and a long axon that leaves gray matter and enters white matter to run in a major fiber tract of the CNS or contributes to a peripheral nerve. In contrast, *Golgi type 2* neurons have short axons that do not leave the area of their perikarya. Examples of Golgi type 1

*Figure 7–11. This composite summary diagram illustrates most features of a neuron in the CNS. Top left: As seen by light microscopy, there is a large vesicular nucleus and a prominent nucleolus, with a nucleolar satellite above. In the cytoplasm, Nissl bodies (blue) and neurofibrils (black) are seen. Both Nissl bodies and neurofibrils extend into dendrites, only neurofibrils into the axon (right, yellow), which becomes myelinated. Below it is the small nucleus of an oligodendrocyte. Center: This oligodendrocyte is shown forming myelin sheaths for several nerve fibers, with a node of Ranvier (see also Figure 7–30). Bottom: As seen by electron microscopy (see also Figure 7–4), the nucleus (N) is large and vesicular, with nucleolus (Nu) and nucleolar satellite (NS) containing the heterochromatic X chromosome. In the cytoplasm (pink) are Nissl bodies (Ni) (blue) of granular endoplasmic reticulum, Golgi apparatus (G) around the nucleus, smooth endoplasmic reticulum (Se), lysosomes (L), mitochondria (M) (green), and bundles of microtubules (neurotubules) (T) and neurofilaments (F). Six dendrites (D) are shown with dendritic spines (DS), and the axon (A) (yellow) leaves at the axon hillock (AH) (pink). In the bracket at top, the relation of the neuronal surface to synapses (S) (synaptic vesicles, red) and glial processes (P) (dark pink) is shown. Types of synapses seen are axodendritic (1), axosomatic (2), and axoaxonic (3). The dendrodendritic type is not illustrated. At right, in the bracket is an asymmetrical synapse, with the direction of conduction arrowed.*

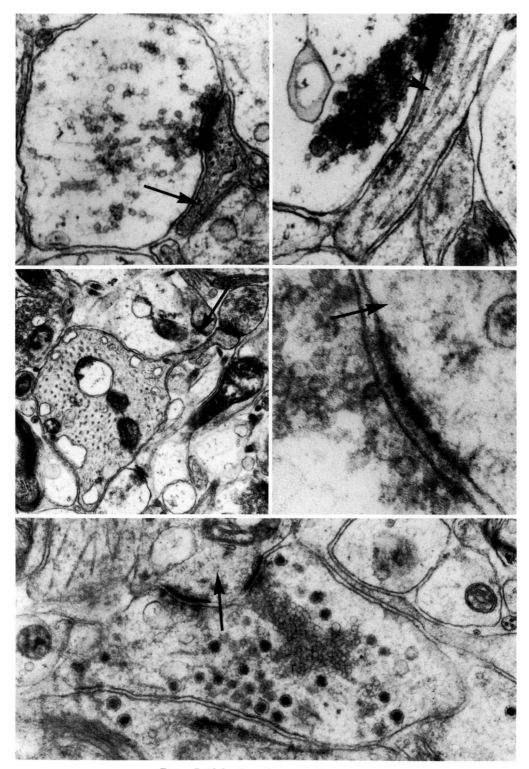

*Figure 7–12* See legend on opposite page

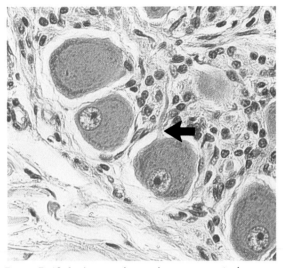

*Figure 7–13. In this pseudounipolar neuron, a single process (arrow) leaves the perikaryon and, at some distance from the soma, would divide in a T or Y fashion into a peripheral process (the functional dendrite) and a central process (the functional axon). In the soma is a large vesicular nucleus with prominent nucleolus and basophilic cytoplasm containing Nissl bodies (purple). The adjacent small nuclei are of supporting ("capsule") cells. H and E. Oil immersion.*

neurons are the anterior horn (motor) cells of the spinal cord, which are stellate, or star-shaped; pyramidal neurons of the cerebral cortex with an apical dendrite, four or more branching dendrites passing out from the base of the pyramid, and an axon leaving the cell base also; and Purkinje's cells of the cerebellar cortex. This cell has a flask-shaped cell body with a single dendrite arising from the pointed pole and branching extensively in one plane (in the manner of a pear tree branching against a wall), and a small axon leaving the opposite, broader pole of the perikaryon.

Examples of Golgi type 2 neurons are the cells of the cerebral and cerebellar cortices. This type includes the interneurons that connect or lie be-

tween two long links in a pathway. Many cells in the cortices are referred to as granule cells, with a few radiating, short dendrites and an axon that is confined to the immediate area or, if longer, never enters the white matter.

## NEUROGLIA

As the name suggests (*neuron*, nerve; *glia*, glue), this tissue binds together the nervous tissue of the CNS. In the PNS, the neurolemma (Schwann's), capsule, and satellite cells probably subserve similar functions (to be described later). Neuroglial cells are small, and only their nuclei are seen in routine preparations, the nuclei being 3 to 10 µm in diameter. They are studied best by silver and gold impregnation techniques that demonstrate the entire cell.

Neuroglia include two types of astrocytes and oligodendrocytes (the macroglia), microglia, and the ependyma. These cells provide a supporting framework for the neurons, form myelin, and are phagocytic. Some are mobile and, unlike neurons, retain the capacity to divide. Together, they form a dynamic system functioning in metabolic exchange between neurons of the CNS and their environment.

### Macroglia

**Astrocytes.** As the name suggests, these are small, star-shaped cells with branching cytoplasmic processes visible only after impregnation techniques. Nuclei are large and ovoid or spherical, and the cytoplasm contains a Golgi complex, few ribosomes and little granular reticulum, lysosomes, and glycogen. Characteristically, there are bundles of glial filaments, extending into the cell processes, 8 nm in diameter, and composed mainly of glial fibrillar acidic protein. The *proto-*

---

*Figure 7–12. Electron micrographs of synapses. In all figures, the arrow indicates the direction of conduction. Top left: Axodendritic, the dendrite in cross section at right. Presynaptic vesicles are seen at left. × 45,000. Top right: Axodendritic, the dendritic process containing neurotubules in longitudinal section. × 52,000. Center left: A dendrite in cross section shows a dendritic spine extending up and to the right to a synapse. × 22,500. Center right: Axodendritic at higher magnification. One presynaptic vesicle appears to be fusing with the axolemma at the synapse. Unit membrane structure is seen both in synaptic membranes and in presynaptic vesicles. × 98,000. Bottom: The axon terminal here contains small, spherical, clear synaptic vesicles and dense-cored vesicles of the neurosecretory type. × 37,000.*

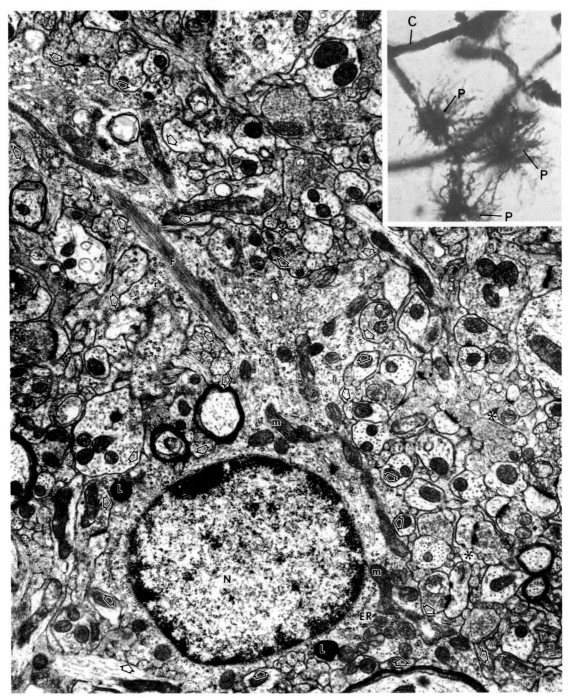

**Figure 7–14.** *Protoplasmic astrocytes. Top right (inset): Light photomicrograph showing three protoplasmic astrocytes (P) of the gray matter of the brain, in relation to capillaries (C) that they contact by perivascular feet. Note the numerous, branching processes. Protargol. Medium power. The electron micrograph shows a nucleus (N) of a protoplasmic astrocyte from rat cerebral cortex with a bundle of filaments (F), mitochondria (m), microtubules (t), free ribosomes (r) and granular reticulum (ER), and two lysosomes (L) in the cytoplasm. The cell outline is partially indicated by arrowheads, and in the surrounding neuropil are processes of other neuroglial cells (asterisks) of irregular outline and more regular dendrites and axons. Approx. × 14,000. (Reproduced with permission from Peters, A., Palay, S. L., and Webster, H. de F.: The Fine Structure of the Nervous System. Philadelphia, W. B. Saunders Co., 1976.)*

*plasmic* astrocyte has large, branching processes and is located in the gray matter of the CNS, with its processes attaching to the walls of blood vessels and the inner surface of the pia mater (that covers the CNS) by small pedicels, or feet (Figs. 7–14 and 7–15). Smaller protoplasmic astrocytes are one type of satellite cell, lying close to the surface of neurons. *Fibrous* astrocytes have long, slender processes with few or no branches, contain more prominent filament (glial) bundles, and are found in white matter (Fig. 7–16). Their processes also attach to blood vessels, and they lie mainly between fascicles of nerve fibers. Recent studies suggest that astrocytes regulate extracellular potassium levels. Potassium generated by neuronal activity perhaps is siphoned by astrocytes to the brain surface and, hence, to the cerebrospinal fluid and blood to maintain electrical neutrality.

**Oligodendrocytes.** Also known as *oligodendroglia,* they are smaller than astrocytes, with small heterochromatic, somewhat irregular nuclei, scanty cytoplasm that appears as a rim around the nucleus, and a few, short cell processes. The cytoplasm is more dense than that of astrocytes, with free and attached ribosomes, a large Golgi apparatus, many mitochondria, and numerous

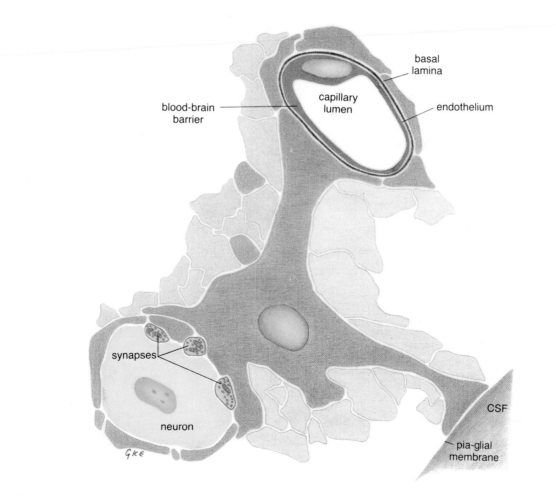

basal lamina

capillary lumen

blood-brain barrier

endothelium

synapses

neuron

CSF

pia-glial membrane

GKE

**Figure 7–15.** *Diagram of a protoplasmic astrocyte illustrates the relationships between it and other components of the gray matter. Note that by its cytoplasmic processes it contacts a capillary (top), a nerve cell (bottom left), and the pia-glial membrane (bottom right).*

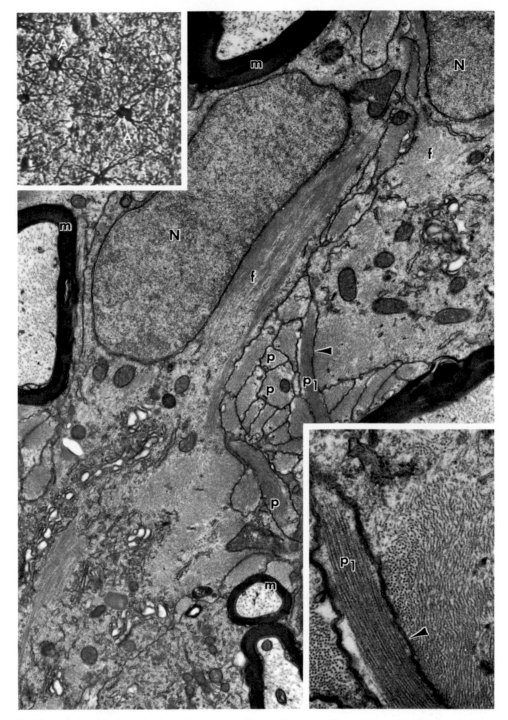

**Figure 7–16.** Fibrous astrocytes. Top left (inset): Light photomicrograph showing fibrous astrocytes with several slender processes in the white matter of the brain. Protargol. Medium power. The electron micrograph shows two fibrous astrocytes in cat optic nerve, with nuclei (N) and bundles of intermediate 10-nm filaments (f) in the cytoplasm. Note numerous processes (p) of other astrocytes and myelinated fibers (m). One region showing a gap junction (arrowhead) between one astrocyte and the cell processes ($P_1$) of another astrocyte is seen (below right, inset) at higher magnification and shows also cytoplasmic filaments in cross and longitudinal section. × 12,000. (Electron micrograph courtesy of Dr. P. T. Massa.)

microtubules that extend into the cytoplasmic processes. Oligodendrocytes occur mainly in two locations: (1) in the gray matter, around neurons, as perineuronal satellite cells, and (2) in the white matter, where they lie in rows between nerve fibers (interfascicular oligodendrocytes) (Fig. 7–17). Others lie in a perivascular position. They are responsible for myelin formation, leaf-like

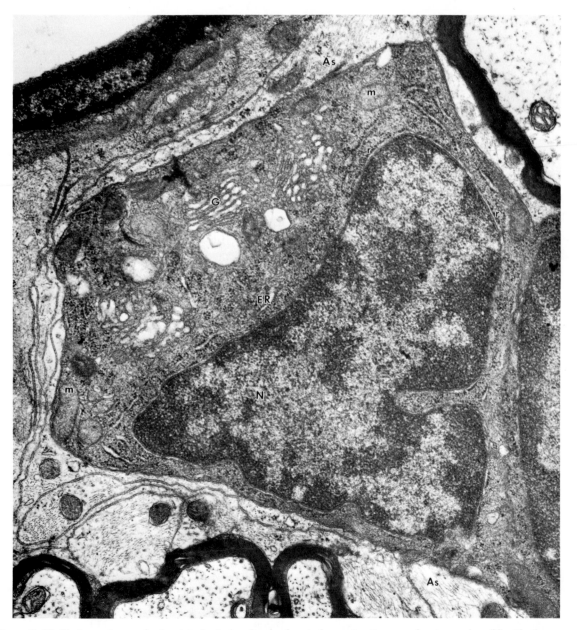

**Figure 7–17.** *Electron micrograph of an interfascicular oligodendrocyte from rat optic nerve showing nucleus (N) with ribosomes (r) attached to the nuclear envelope, granular reticulum (ER), Golgi apparatus (G), and mitochondria (m). Lighter processes of fibrous astrocytes (As) surround the dark oligodendrocyte. Approx. × 36,000. (Courtesy of Dr. A. Peters.)*

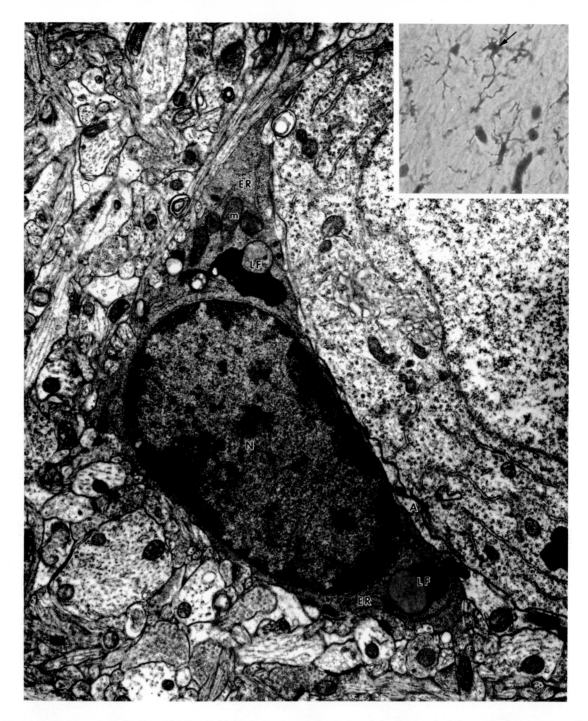

**Figure 7–18.** Microglial cells. Top right (inset): Light photomicrograph of microglial cell (arrow) of the cerebral cortex, a small cell with two or more short cytoplasmic processes. Protargol. High power. The electron micrograph shows part of a pyramidal neuron (right) separated from the microglial cell by a thin process of an astrocyte (A). In the microglial cell (nucleus, N) are mitochondria (m), endoplasmic reticulum (ER), and dense inclusions that appear to be lipofuscin (LF). Approx. × 13,000. (Reproduced with permission from Peters A., Palay, S. L., and Webster, H. de F.: The Fine Structure of the Nervous System. Philadelphia, W. B. Saunders Co., 1976.)

cytoplasmic processes of the cells wrapping around nerve fibers, serving the same function as Schwann's cells in the PNS. Unlike Schwann's cells, however, each oligodendrocyte has several processes and forms myelin sheaths around several adjacent nerve fibers (see later).

### Microglia

Microglia are small cells with small deeply stained nuclei, scanty cytoplasm, and a few, short, spiny processes (Fig. 7–18). They lie throughout the CNS, often adjacent to blood vessels. They contain lysosomes, inclusions, and generally sparse organelles and are capable of migration and phagocytosis.

Developmentally, astrocytes and oligodendroglia—the macroglia—are derived from *spongioblasts*, a primitive ectodermal cell. This cell, intermediate in structure between an astrocyte and an oligodendrocyte, may be present normally in the CNS of the adult and, when stimulated, may proliferate to form phagocytes. Generally, it is believed that microglia are of mesodermal origin, perhaps from blood monocytes, but they may be derived from primitive spongioblasts that persist in the adult. Functionally, neuroglia are involved in a communication function and in normal metabolism of CNS neurons. It appears that neurons virtually are wrapped in glial cells and their processes, except at the sites of synaptic contact. Neuroglia also play an important role in disease, forming many of the tumors of the CNS and being involved in degenerative disorders and infectious diseases.

### Ependyma

The CNS develops as a hollow cylinder—the neural tube—and in the adult, cavities remain as the brain ventricles and the central canal of the spinal cord. These cavities are lined by ependyma that retains its epithelial character present in the early embryo (Figs. 7–19 and 7–20). In the embryo, ependymal cells are ciliated, and some cells of the adult retain cilia. Most ependymal cells show numerous apical microvilli and are cuboidal.

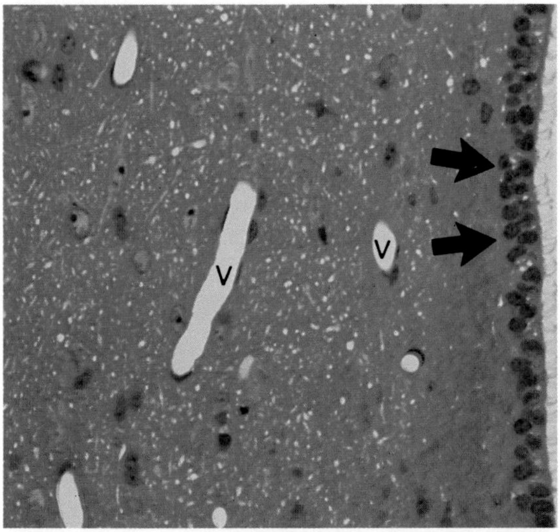

*Figure 7–19. To the right is the lumen of the third ventricle of the brain lined by ependyma (arrows), a simple cuboidal epithelium that lines the entire ventricular system of the CNS. In this location, the ependyma retains apical cilia. The remainder of the field shows thalamic (diencephalic) substance in which are numerous capillaries (v) and many small nuclei, some with thin cytoplasmic rims. The larger, vesicular, ovoid nuclei probably are those of astrocytes. The darker, smaller, more irregular ones are of oligodendrocytes. Methylene blue, basic fuchsin. High power.*

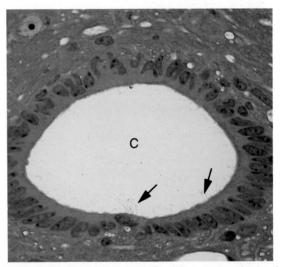

*Figure 7–20. The central canal (C) of the spinal cord is lined by ependyma, here appearing as a simple, low columnar epithelium. The luminal (apical) border of the cells appears irregular owing to the presence of microvilli, and a few cells show cilia (arrows). Methylene blue, basic fuchsin. High power.*

All have basal processes that extend into surrounding nervous tissue, and in several locations, the ependyma is modified as the choroid plexuses to secrete cerebrospinal fluid (see later).

### GANGLIA

A collection of nerve cell bodies located in the CNS is called a *nucleus*. A similar collection lying outside the CNS is called a ganglion (although not all ganglia lie outside the CNS). Ganglia of the PNS are of two main types: (1) sensory ganglia of the *craniospinal group* and (2) visceral, motor *autonomic* ganglia.

Ganglia vary greatly in size, ranging from large ones with 50,000 or more cells to very small ones containing only a few nerve cell bodies. All also contain nerve fibers (axons and dendrites) with their supporting sheaths, and usually, each ganglion (nerve) cell has a capsule of small cuboidal cells called *capsule*, or *satellite*, cells (Fig. 7–21).

Around ganglia is a connective tissue capsule, which may be quite dense around large ganglia, continuous with which is a network of fine collagenous and reticular fibers extending into the ganglion. Blood vessels run in the connective tissue, between the mesh of which are situated the nervous elements.

### Craniospinal Ganglia

Spinal, or dorsal root, ganglia are fusiform or globular swellings of the posterior (dorsal) roots of all spinal nerves; similar swellings of some cranial nerves are the cranial ganglia (Figs. 7–22 and 7–23). Nerve cell bodies lie peripherally in the ganglia in groups, separated by bundles of nerve fibers, while the central, medullary zone contains mainly nerve fibers with few perikarya. Ganglion cells are pseudounipolar, globular, with a single process, the axon, that may coil around the perikaryon before (at some distance from its origin) splitting in a T or Y fashion (Fig. 7–24). A long peripheral process, the functional dendrite, passes to the periphery, where it originates in a

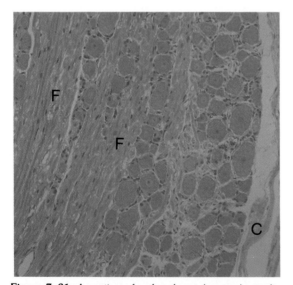

**Figure 7–21.** A portion of a dorsal root (sensory) ganglion shows capsule (C) to the right and, within the ganglion, groups of nerve cell bodies located mainly at the periphery, while in the central, or medullary, zone are bundles of nerve fibers (F) with smaller groups of perikarya between them. The pseudounipolar ganglion cells have a "capsule" formed by small satellite cells with small dark nuclei. H and E. Low power.

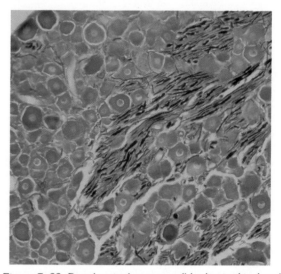

**Figure 7–22.** Pseudounipolar nerve cell bodies in this dorsal (spinal) root ganglion show pale-staining nuclei, the perikarya located mainly in the cortical zone (top and left) and varying in size, the smaller with unmyelinated fibers, the larger with myelinated fibers. The fibers are darkly stained, in groups, and located mainly in the medullary zone. Silver, aniline blue. Low power.

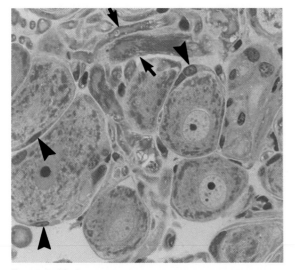

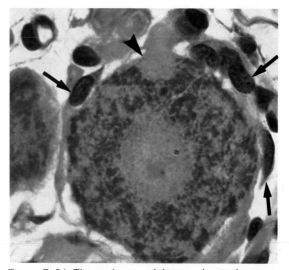

**Figure 7–23.** Several perikarya of pseudounipolar neurons of a dorsal root (sensory) ganglion are seen. They vary in size and some show a large vesicular nucleus with a prominent nucleolus (the "owl's-eye" appearance). In the cytoplasm, blue-staining Nissl bodies are seen, and around the ganglion cells are small satellite cells (arrowheads), with nerve fibers in small groups (arrows) between the cells. Methylene blue, basic fuchsin. High power.

**Figure 7–24.** The perikaryon of this pseudounipolar sensory (dorsal root) ganglion cell is globular with a large vesicular nucleus and cytoplasm filled with blue-staining Nissl bodies. At the top, a single cell process leaves the soma at the axon hillock devoid of Nissl substance (arrowhead), the process later dividing into central and peripheral fibers (not seen here). Around the soma are small satellite cells (arrows). Toluidine blue. Oil immersion.

receptor organ, while a shorter, usually thinner, process passes centrally to the CNS. Both branches are similar in structure and part of the axon. Perikarya show the usual features of neurons, with large central nuclei and prominent nucleoli and prominent Nissl bodies in the cytoplasm and lipofuscin pigment. Smaller cells of 15 to 25 μm in diameter have unmyelinated axons; larger ones up to 100 μm have myelinated axons. Each perikaryon has a "capsule" formed by a layer of small, low cuboidal cells, the satellite cells (*amphicytes*), analogous to neuroglial cells of the CNS.

Impulse transmission in the ganglion cells is directly from the peripheral to the central process, bypassing the soma, which receives no synapses from other neurons and has an exclusively trophic function.

### Autonomic Ganglia

These appear as swellings along the sympathetic (thoracolumbar) chain and its ramifications

and in the walls of organs supplied by the autonomic system (parasympathetic, craniosacral) (Figs. 7–25 and 7–26). Peripheral ganglia may be very small, and unlike sensory ganglia, the perikarya and nerve fibers are intermingled and show no tendency to group. Ganglion cells are multipolar, usually with several dendrites and a single unmyelinated axon, and 15 to 45 μm in diameter. Capsule cells are seen but are relatively few in number and discontinuous around perikarya, lying between cell processes.

### NERVE FIBERS

A nerve fiber is composed of an axon and its associated sheaths. All axons of the PNS have a *sheath of Schwann* (neurolemma, or neurilemma) extending from near their origins to close to their terminations, and the larger axons, within the sheath of Schwann, have an inner sheath of *myelin*. Thus, nerve fibers are either *myelinated*

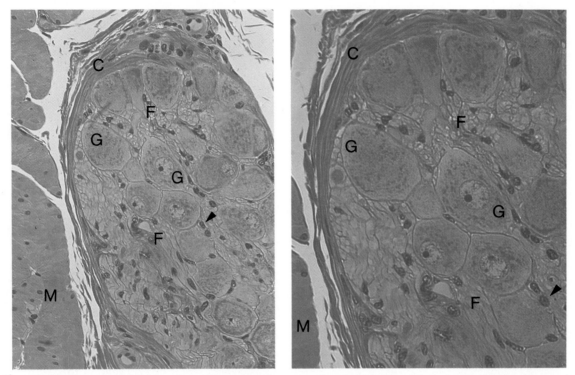

**Figure 7–25.** *These micrographs are of a small autonomic (parasympathetic) ganglion from the wall of the bladder. The ganglion shows a capsule (C) of fibroconnective tissue and contains multipolar ganglion cells (G), some showing large vesicular nuclei with prominent nucleoli and blue-staining Nissl bodies in the cytoplasm, intermingled with nerve fibers (F). A few capsule cells (arrowheads) lie in relation to perikarya. Smooth muscle (M) of the bladder wall is present at left. H and E. Left: low power; right: Medium power.*

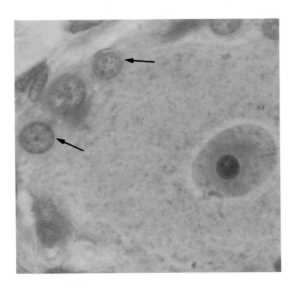

**Figure 7–26.** *This photomicrograph shows a portion of a large ganglion (multipolar) cell of a sympathetic ganglion. The cytoplasm is granular, the nucleus is vesicular with a prominent nucleolus, and satellite cells (arrows) form a partial capsule around the soma of the ganglion cell. H and E. Oil immersion.*

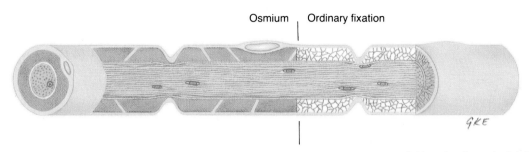

**Figure 7–27.** Diagram of a single myelinated nerve fiber as it would appear after osmium (left) and ordinary (right) fixation. Note the clefts of Schmidt-Lantermann seen in the osmium-fixed material (myelin, black; axon, yellow) and the neurokeratin network seen after ordinary fixation.

or *unmyelinated* (Figs. 7–27 through 7–29). In the CNS, nerve fibers may be partially covered by glial cells (unmyelinated) or may have a myelin sheath formed by oligodendrocytes (myelinated).

Myelin appears as homogeneous, white, refractile material in fresh preparations and is responsible for the white color of peripheral nerves and of fiber tracts in the CNS. In fixed preparations, myelin is darkened by osmium tetroxide or Weigert's method, the axon remaining unstained. Being a lipoprotein complex, myelin is dissolved by fat solvents. Silver impregnation and methylene blue vital staining methods demonstrate axons, the myelin being unstained, and are of particular value in demonstrating unmyelinated fibers, which are not easily seen in routine preparations.

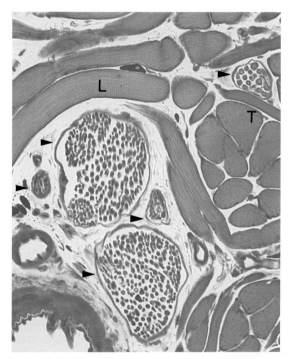

**Figure 7–28.** This is a section of the tongue. Skeletal muscle fibers are seen in both longitudinal (L) and transverse (T) sections with five small peripheral nerves in transverse section, of varying size. All show a perineurium (arrowheads) within which are nerve fibers, axons staining lightly, myelin staining pink. Most of the nerves present contain both myelinated and unmyelinated fibers, but the small nerve at top right contains only myelinated fibers. H and E. Low power.

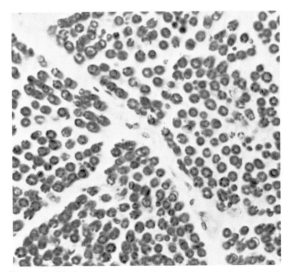

**Figure 7–29.** In this transverse section of a spinal nerve, only myelin is stained, surrounding unstained nerve fibers, and it appears as ring shapes. The myelinated nerve fibers are collected into fascicles. Methylene blue. Medium power.

**285**

## Sheath of Schwann

This sheath is formed by a chain of flattened cells with elongated, flattened, heterochromatic nuclei and cytoplasm that shows a small Golgi apparatus and a few mitochondria, but generally organelles are sparse. Externally is a basal lamina of glycoprotein material. Between adjacent cells in the chain, the axon is partially uncovered, although some cytoplasmic interdigitation occurs between the Schwann's cells. These sites where the sheath of Schwann and the myelin are interrupted are called the *nodes of Ranvier*. In myelinated fibers, an individual Schwann's cell and its myelin, thus, cover an *internodal segment*. Internodal segments vary in length, but generally, the segments are of greater length in longer, large-diameter fibers. If an axon has collateral branches, the branching occurs at a node of Ranvier. In unmyelinated fibers, the relationship of Schwann's cells to the axons is not clearly seen by light microscopy, but electron microscopy shows that axons lie singly or in groups in deep, longitudinal gutters, or invaginations, of a Schwann's cell with the original line of invagination being the *mesaxon*. At the mesaxon, a double fold of the Schwann's cell plasma membrane extends deeply to surround the nerve fiber or fibers, with a gap of only 15 to 20 nm (the periaxonal space) separating Schwann's cell plasma membrane and the axolemma. There is a similar gap between the two folds of plasmalemma at their point of invagination.

## Myelin Sheath

As indicated, myelin is white and highly refractile in the fresh state. Being largely composed of lipid, it is dissolved after routine fixation, leaving a network of protein material called *neurokeratin*. Electron microscopy demonstrates that myelin is neither structureless nor extracellular but is formed by fused, spiral laminae of Schwann's cell plasmalemma. Developmentally, an axon indents the Schwann's cell longitudinally, and then the flap of Schwann's cell cytoplasm along the side of the axon spirals around the axon probably as a result of growth at the site of invagination of the mesaxon. After forming several, often very many, spiral layers of the Schwann's cell plasma membrane, cytoplasm between the layers is forced back into the outer part of the Schwann's cell, allowing the apposed surfaces of the plasma membrane to become closely apposed, and eventually, they fuse. Mature myelin shows a repeating pattern of dark and light lines. The 3-nm dark lines are the *major dense lines* formed by fusion of inner cytoplasmic surfaces, while less dense lines that bisect the spaces between them are the *intraperiod lines*, formed by apposition of the outer leaflets of the Schwann's cell plasma membrane.

While this hypothesis, often termed the "jelly roll," explains the formation of myelin as seen in cross section, it is necessary also to visualize the process in longitudinal section, particularly in respect of the nodes of Ranvier. In longitudinal section, lamellae of myelin are seen to be progressively of shorter length from external to internal lamellae, the juxta-axonal lamella being the shortest. As each lamella bends toward the axon, the major period line splits to enclose a small area of Schwann's cell cytoplasm that contacts the axolemma near a node of Ranvier. In transverse section, a periaxonal space of 15 to 20 nm is continuous with the deepest lamella of myelin by the *internal mesaxon,* while an *external mesaxon* connects the outermost lamella with the surface of the plasma membrane.

Visible by light microscopy are small radial clefts or fissures extending through the thickness of the myelin called *Schmidt-Lantermann clefts*. These are really discontinuities in the close packing of myelin lamellae and are composed of slips of Schwann's cell cytoplasm formed by failure of fusion of cytoplasmic surfaces of the Schwann's cell plasma membrane, so that a major dense line appears to split, enclosing a small amount of cytoplasm. They may provide channels for conduction of metabolites into the deeper layers of the myelin sheath and to the axon.

In myelinated fibers of the CNS, myelin is formed by oligodendrocytes. However, while Schwann's cells of the PNS wrap a single axon in myelin, in the CNS an oligodendrocyte can form myelin sheaths around several axons, each axon wrapped by a cytoplasmic process of the glial cell, so that the cell body of the oligodendrocyte is not directly apposed to the myelin sheath(s), as is the case with a Schwann's cell in the PNS (Figs. 7–30 through 7–32).

## PERIPHERAL NERVES

Peripheral nerves include spinal nerves connected to the spinal cord and cranial nerves connected to the brain. All are composed of bundles of nerve fibers held together by connective tissue, and most appear white owing to their content of myelinated fibers, although nearly all also contain unmyelinated fibers. Most nerves are mixed, containing both sensory (afferent) and motor (efferent) fibers; a few are sensory or motor only.

A large nerve is enveloped in a sheath of relatively strong connective tissue termed the *epineurium,* composed of fibroblasts and collagenous fibers, mainly longitudinal in orientation, and a few elastic fibers (Fig. 7–33). Within the epineurium, nerve fibers lie in *bundles,* or *fascicles*, each surrounded by *perineurium* (Figs. 7–34 through 7–37). This perineurial sheath is formed by concentric layers or sheaths of flattened, fibroblast-like cells with basal laminae between the cellular sheaths (Fig. 7–38). The number of sleeves decreases as the nerve branches, with the last sleeve terminating just before the nerve ending. The perineurium is continuous with the pia arachnoid membrane of the CNS when traced centrally, and it provides a barrier to the passage of material into or out of the nerve fascicle. Within the perineurium, delicate collagenous and reticular fibers with flattened, elongated fibroblasts lie longitudinally between and around individual nerve fibers in relation to their neurilemma, although separated by the basal lamina that surrounds neurilemma cells. This is the *endoneurium* (Figs. 7–39 and 7–40).

A peripheral nerve has a rich blood supply with branches from adjacent arteries entering the epineurium, anastomosing and branching, with smaller vessels passing from them to run longitudinally in the perineurium. These vessels then form an extensive capillary plexus in the endoneurium.

## MEMBRANES AND VESSELS OF THE CENTRAL NERVOUS SYSTEM

The tissue of the CNS is soft and delicate and requires both adequate protection and nourishment. Externally, and providing protection, is the bone of the cranium and the vertebral column, and within the bony case are three membranous, connective tissue investments called the *meninges* (Fig. 7–41).

## Dura Mater

This, the outermost of the meninges, is a fibrous, tough relatively inelastic coat, usually described in two layers over the brain. The outer or *endosteal layer* adheres to bone of the cranium, contains a relatively rich vascular plexus, and functions as the periosteum of the cranium. The inner, *fibrous layer* is less vascular, with its internal surface covered by a layer of squamous cells of mesodermal origin. In specific regions, it is separated from the outer layer to form the large venous sinuses of the brain and also is reflected inward to form partitions in the large fissures of the brain, that is, as the sagittally oriented *falx cerebri* between the two cerebral hemispheres and *falx cerebelli* between the two cerebellar hemispheres, as the horizontal *tentorium* between the occipital lobes of the cerebrum above and the cerebellum below, and as an extension forming the roof of the hypophyseal fossa called the *diaphragma sella.*

The vertebral column has its own periosteum, and the spinal dura corresponds to the fibrous layer of the cranial dura, with which it is continuous at the foramen magnum. The spinal dura covers the spinal cord loosely as a cylindrical membrane but is connected to the spinal cord on both sides by a series of denticulate ligaments. Like the fibrous layer of the cranial dura, the inner surface of the spinal dura is covered by squamous cells. Externally, it is separated from vertebral periosteum by the *epidural space*, in which are anastomosing venous plexuses lying in fatty, areolar tissue.

## Arachnoid

This central layer of the meninges is separated from the dura by a slender capillary interval, the *subdural space*, containing lymph-like fluid. The arachnoid consists of a thin, delicate, nonvascular membrane lining the dura with, from its inner

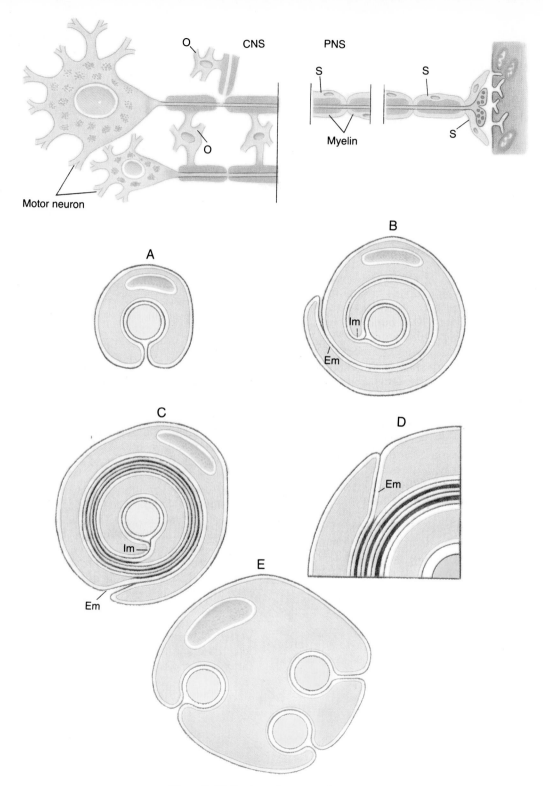

*Figure 7–30* See legend on opposite page

Illustration continued on opposite page

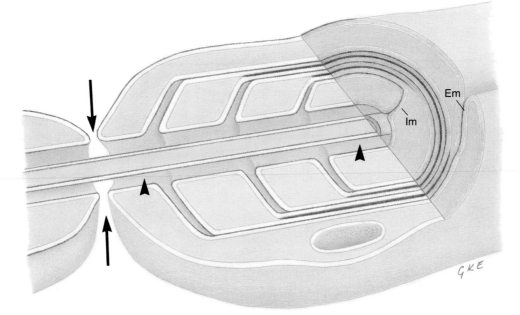

**Figure 7–30.** Diagrams of myelination. Top left: *Two motor neurons (anterior horn cells of the spinal cord) with perikarya and dendrites (left) lie in gray matter with Nissl bodies (dark blue) in cytoplasm but absent from the axon hillock (right). From the axon hillocks, the axons in white matter of the CNS are myelinated by oligodendrites (O). Note that an individual oligodendrocyte can myelinate nodal segments of more than one axon. In the PNS (right), Schwann's cells (S) provide the myelin. One axon is shown terminating at a myoneural junction (effector organ). Bottom left: A, B, and C illustrate successive stages in myelination by a Schwann's cell in the PNS. In A, the axon (yellow) lies in a groove, or longitudinal depression, in the Schwann's cell. In B, both internal and external mesaxons (Im and Em) are defined with one turn of the fused plasmalemma, the fused central lamina being a future intraperiod line. At C, myelin is formed with basically three turns, the cytoplasmic surfaces of the plasmalemma fusing to form major dense lines, intraperiod lines formed by fusion of external surfaces. At D, a portion of a myelinated axon is shown to illustrate major dense and intraperiod lines and the external mesaxon (Em). In E, three unmyelinated axons are seen invaginated into a Schwann's cell. Above, A node of Ranvier (arrows) of a myelinated axon is shown, the nerve fiber in both transverse and longitudinal section. Note that myelin lamellae vary in length from external to internal, the juxta-axonal being the shortest. Between the axon and the myelin of the Schwann's cell is the periaxonal space (arrowheads). External (Em) and internal (Im) mesaxons are seen. (See also Figure 7–11.)*

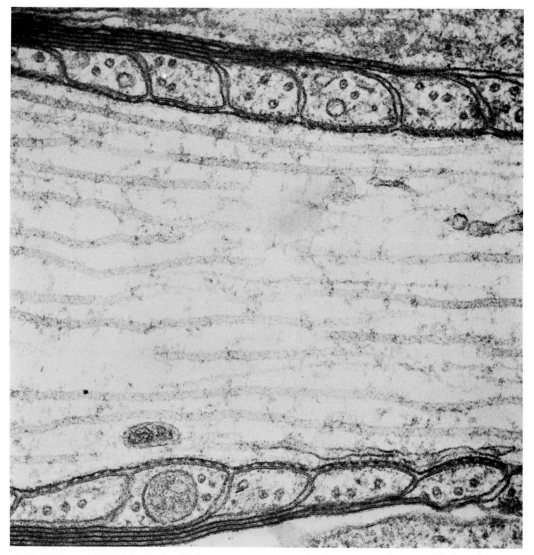

**Figure 7–31.** *Electron micrograph of a longitudinal section of a myelinated axon near a node of Ranvier from a rat brain. × 100,000. (Courtesy of Dr. A. Hirano. Reproduced by permission from the Editors, The Journal of Cell Biology, 34:561, 1967.)*

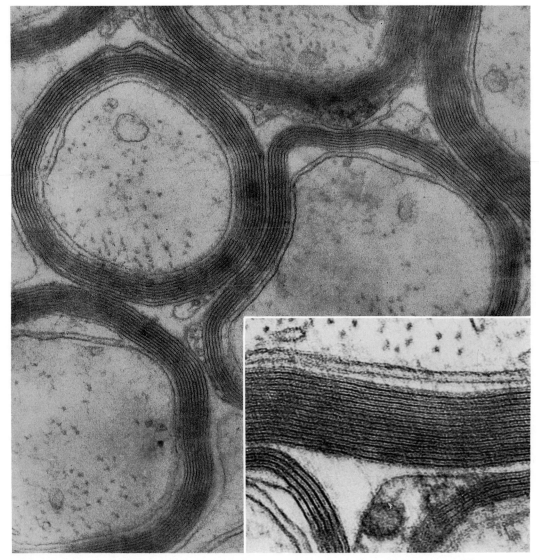

**Figure 7–32.** Electron micrograph of myelinated nerve fibers in a cross section of the rat optic nerve. × 70,000. Inset, bottom right: Higher magnification shows major dense and intraperiod lines. × 125,000. (Preparation by A. Peters.)

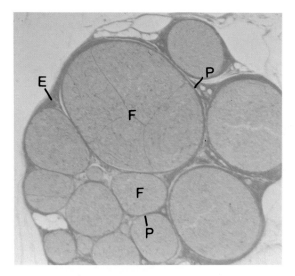

*Figure 7–33.* In this transverse section of a peripheral nerve, the associated connective tissue is demonstrated. The entire nerve is enveloped by relatively strong epineurium (E) within which are bundles, or fascicles, of nerve fibers (F), each ensheathed by perineurium (P). Within the fascicle, endoneurium lies around and between individual nerve fibers. (See Figures 7–34 and 7–40.) H and E. Low power.

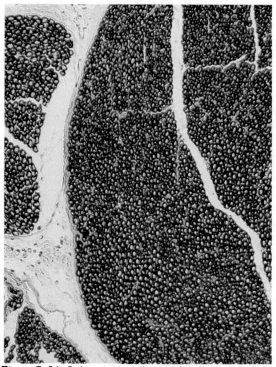

*Figure 7–34.* Only a portion of a peripheral nerve is seen in transverse section, with portions of three fascicles of nerve fibers. Each fascicle is enveloped in perineurium (arrowheads). The myelin stains black, the axons appear unstained. Osmium tetroxide. Low power.

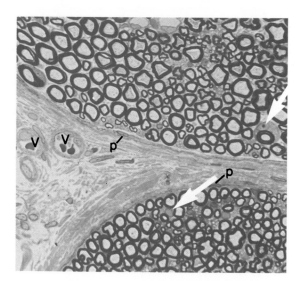

*Figure 7–35.* Portions of two fascicles of peripheral nerve are seen, each enveloped in perineurium (p). Myelin appears as dark-blue rings around unstained nerve fibers. Myelin varies in thickness, and nerve fibers vary in size. In some fibers, Schwann's cells are seen clearly in relation to the myelin (arrows). In the connective tissue between nerve fascicles are blood vessels (V). Toluidine blue. Medium power.

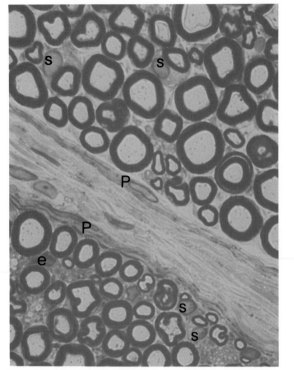

**Figure 7–36.** In transverse section, myelinated nerve fibers lie in two fascicles, each enveloped in perineurium (P). Nerve fibers are unstained and vary in size. Myelin appears as dark-blue–staining rings around them and varies in thickness, and in some, a clear relationship to Schwann's cells and their nuclei (s) is seen. Endoneurial nuclei (e) also are seen. Toluidine blue. Oil immersion.

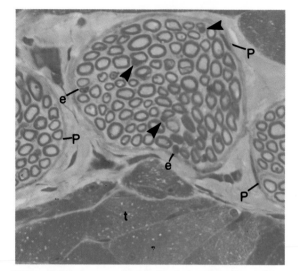

**Figure 7–37.** A nerve fascicle (center) and portions of two others are seen in transverse section. Each is enveloped by perineurium (P), and within the fascicle are nuclei of endoneurial cells (e). Other nuclei are of Schwann's cells (arrowheads), forming myelin (purple) around the unstained axons. This nerve lies in striated muscle (below [t] and top right). Methylene blue, basic fuchsin. High power.

surface, many thin trabeculae, or ribbon-like strands, attached to the underlying pia. The membrane and its trabeculae are composed of thin collagenous and elastic fibers, and all surfaces are covered by a simple squamous epithelium. The spaces between the trabeculae and the membranous roof constitute the *subarachnoid space*, filled with cerebrospinal fluid. Over the spinal cord, the trabeculae are few. Here, the subarachnoid space is continuous, and the arachnoid is separated more clearly from the pia.

In some areas, arachnoid penetrates dura as *arachnoid villi* that lie within the venous sinuses of the dura and function to transfer cerebrospinal fluid to the venous sinuses.

Pia and arachnoid have a similar structure and are regarded by some as a single layer called the *leptomeninx* or *leptomeninges*.

## Pia Mater

This delicate membrane closely invests the brain and spinal cord and, unlike the arachnoid, extends into the depths of cerebral sulci. The more superficial layer (the epipial tissue) is composed of a network of collagenous fibers closely apposed to the arachnoid and is more obvious over the spinal cord where it contains the spinal blood vessels. The deeper inner layer (the intima pia) is a close meshwork of fine reticular and elastic fibers adherent to neural tissue but separated by a layer of neuroglial cell processes. As blood vessels pass from the pia into nervous tissue, they take with them a covering of intima pia; in the case of larger vessels, there is an intervening perivascular space containing cerebrospinal fluid. The outer surface of the pia is covered by simple squamous epithelium.

Pia contains branches of the internal carotid and vertebral arteries that pass into and supply the CNS, the vessels losing their investment of pial tissue as they form capillary networks. The capillaries are ensheathed in neuroglial cell proc-

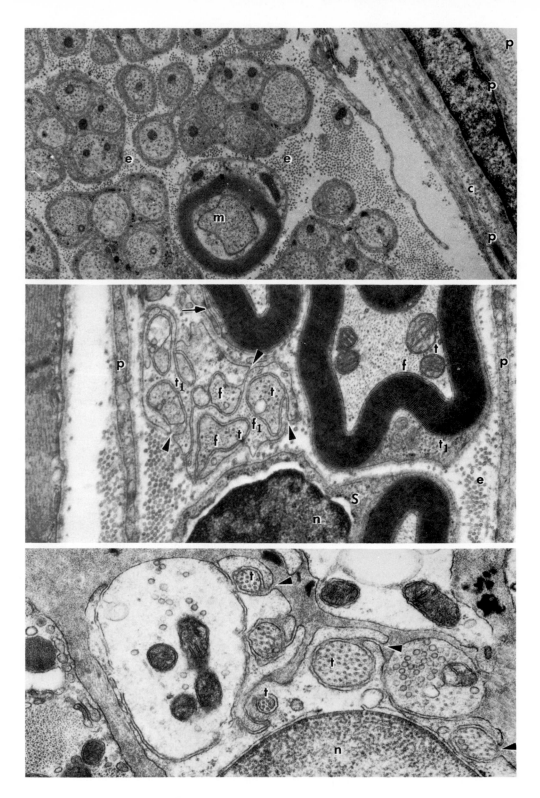

*Figure 7–38* See legend on opposite page

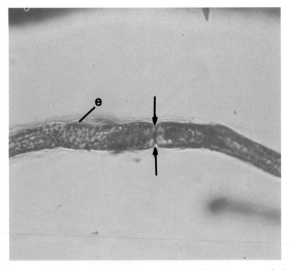

**Figure 7–39.** This single myelinated nerve fiber is surrounded by strands of endoneurium (e) and shows the neurokeratin network and a node of Ranvier (arrows). Iron hematoxylin. High power.

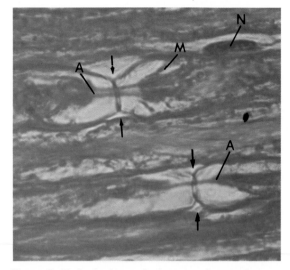

**Figure 7–40.** In this longitudinal section of a spinal nerve, a few myelinated nerve fibers are seen, two of which show axons (A) traversing nodes of Ranvier (arrows), the axons ensheathed in myelin (M). The nucleus (N) of an endoneurial cell also is seen. Iron hematoxylin, phosphotungstic acid. Oil immersion.

esses and are more numerous in gray matter than in white. Venous return from nervous tissue is to the pia and hence to dural sinuses. Both dura and pia contain a rich plexus of nerve fibers, mainly of the autonomic system to the blood vessels, but some sensory fibers also are present. There are no lymphatic capillaries in the CNS.

### Choroid Plexus

The choroid plexuses are responsible for the secretion of cerebrospinal fluid and are located in the roof of the third and fourth ventricles and in the medial walls of the lateral ventricles (Fig. 7–

42). In these regions, ependyma retains its embryonic character as a non-nervous epithelium with associated highly vascular pia mater invaginating into the ventricular space as a collection of villus-like processes, covered by the ependyma. The ependyma here is a cuboidal, regular layer with apical bulbous microvilli, the cells showing spherical nuclei and numbers of rod-shaped mitochondria (Fig. 7–43). Junctional complexes near the luminal border close off the intercellular spaces, and the cells are supported by a basal lamina beneath which is pial tissue consisting of loose connective tissue with numerous capillaries lined by thin, attenuated and fenestrated (type II)

**Figure 7–38.** Electron micrographs of peripheral nerves of three sizes all in cross section. Top: Part of one fascicle of a larger nerve with perineurium (top right) formed by concentric layers of flattened cells (p) with basal laminae and collagen fibrils (c). The fascicle contains one myelinated nerve fiber (m) and many unmyelinated fibers, in singles and in small groups lying in Schwann's cell cytoplasm, with collagen fibrils of the endoneurium (e). × 5500. Center: An autonomic nerve of myocardium with perineurial sheath (p) contains parts of three myelinated fibers, one (below) enveloped by a Schwann's cell (S) with its nucleus (n). One fiber shows the mesaxon (arrow), also seen in unmyelinated fibers (arrowheads). Neurotubules (t) and neurofilaments (f) are present in both myelinated and unmyelinated fibers, with microtubules ($t_1$) and microfilaments ($f_1$) in Schwann's cell cytoplasm. × 28,000. Bottom: A small unmyelinated nerve of myocardium with Schwann's cell nucleus (n) and nerve fibers, some very small, with neurotubules (t). × 35,000.

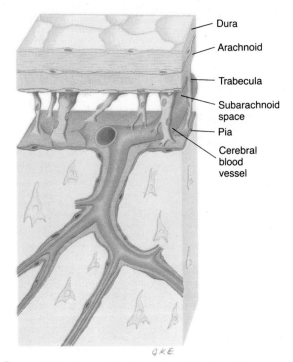

**Figure 7–41.** *Diagram illustrates the relationship of the meninges to the brain.*

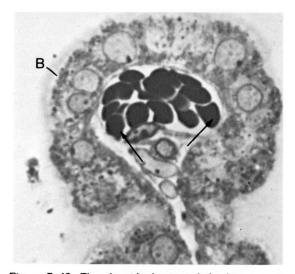

**Figure 7–42.** *The choroid plexuses of the brain secrete cerebrospinal fluid and are formed by ependyma (in the roof of the third and fourth ventricles and in the medial walls of the lateral ventricles) protruding into ventricular spaces in association with blood capillaries of the pia mater. Here, the ependymal epithelium is cuboidal, with central spherical nuclei and numerous mitochondria (blue-staining dots and rods) in the cytoplasm, with an apical border (B) composed of bulbous microvilli. Beneath the epithelium are numerous, thin-walled capillary blood vessels containing erythrocytes (black). Toluidine blue. Oil immersion.*

endothelium. These choroidal capillaries are highly permeable.

### Cerebrospinal Fluid

*Cerebrospinal fluid* is produced actively in the choroid plexus at a rate of up to 150 ml per day, and formation normally is balanced by absorption back to the venous system. The circulation is as follows: From the ventricles, fluid passes through three foramina in the roof of the fourth ventricle (a median foramen of Magendie and two lateral foramina of Luschka) into the subarachnoid space, where it circulates freely. It is absorbed mainly into cranial venous sinuses through arachnoid villi, which are tufts of pia arachnoid that penetrate dura to lie in the sinuses.

Cerebrospinal fluid is a clear, colorless liquid with a low specific gravity (1.004 to 1.007), containing inorganic salts, glucose, small amounts of protein, and, usually, a few lymphocytes. In that it fills the ventricles (and central canal of the spinal cord) and the subarachnoid space, it acts as a water cushion to protect the CNS from concussion and trauma, in general, and is important in CNS metabolism.

### BLOOD-BRAIN BARRIER

Many substances are exchanged rapidly between blood and the CNS, others are not, and capillaries do show reduced permeability to certain macromolecules. This *blood-brain barrier* is located in the endothelium of the blood vessels where zonulae occludentes between endothelial cells block intercellular transport. Additionally, capillaries of the CNS have a close investment of neuroglial cells and their processes (mainly astro-

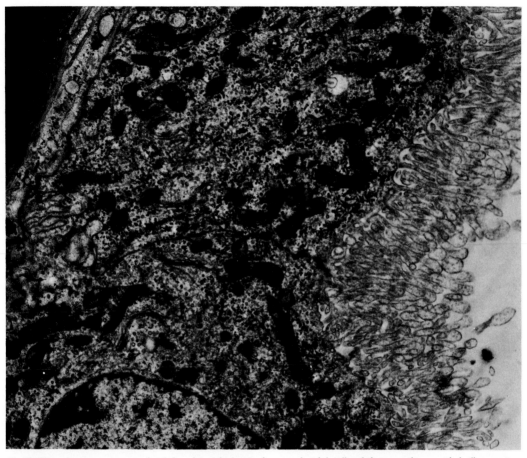

**Figure 7–43.** This electron micrograph of the choroid plexus shows cuboidal cells of the ependyma with bulbous microvilli on the apical surface (right) and some basal infoldings of the basal plasmalemma (left center). At top left is a portion of a capillary of the associated pia mater containing an erythrocyte. × 8500.

cytes), although this represents no barrier, as fluid passes freely via channels between astrocytic processes.

## CYTOARCHITECTURE OF THE CENTRAL NERVOUS SYSTEM

This subject is described fully in textbooks of neuroanatomy, but a brief outline follows of the arrangement of nerve cells and their processes in the more important parts of the CNS.

### Spinal Cord

In transverse section, the spinal cord is oval and partially divided into right and left halves by a posterior median septum and an anterior cleft called the anterior median fissure (Figs. 7–44 through 7–46). The entire cord is surrounded by pia mater, which extends into this fissure. There are variations in shape and structure at different levels of the cord (cervical, thoracic, lumbar, and sacral), although a basic pattern is seen throughout. Centrally lies gray matter, containing nerve cells, in the form of an H, each side with anterior

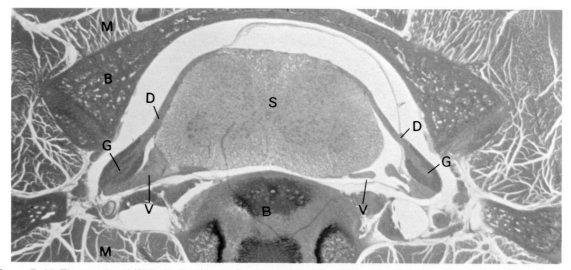

**Figure 7–44.** *The spinal cord (S) lies within the vertebral canal (bone, B), with muscle fibers (M) around the vertebra. Attached to the spinal cord are anterior (ventral) motor (V) and posterior (dorsal) sensory roots (D) of spinal nerves with dorsal root ganglia (G). White matter of the cord is stained palely, and in the central gray matter are dark-pink profiles of neurons. H and E. Low power.*

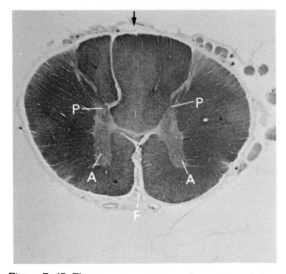

**Figure 7–45.** *This transverse section of the spinal cord shows peripheral white matter (formed by nerve fibers in tracts) stained dark gray. The central gray matter stains lighter and is in the form of an H, with anterior (A) and posterior (P) horns, large motor neurons lying in the anterior horns. The cord is divided into right and left halves by the anterior median fissure (F) and the posterior median septum (arrow). Weigert's stain. Low power.*

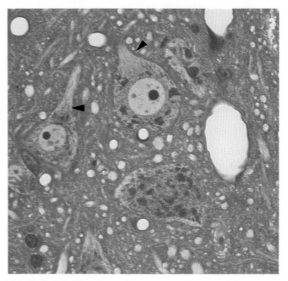

**Figure 7–46.** *This shows large motor neurons of the anterior horn of gray matter of the spinal cord. These are multipolar cells with large vesicular nuclei and prominent nucleoli, dark-staining Nissl bodies in the cytoplasm, and two neurons show the roots of their axons (arrowheads) from axon hillocks devoid of Nissl substance. Methylene blue, azure A, basic fuchsin. High power.*

and posterior horns connected by a cross bridge or commissure containing the central canal, lined by ependyma. Additionally, in the thoracolumbar region (T1 to L2), there is a lateral horn of gray matter on each side. Nerve cell bodies lie in groups in the gray matter with the large motor neurons (multipolar) lying in the anterior horn.

White matter formed by nerve fibers surrounds the gray matter and is divided into longitudinal columns, or *funiculi*. The posterior funiculus lies between the posterior horn of gray matter and the posterior median septum; the lateral funiculus is between the posterior horn and the anterior horn and the nerve (motor) roots passing from it to the surface; and the ventral funiculus lies between the anterior horn and the anterior median fissure. Between the tip of the posterior horn and the surface is a small area containing fine nerve fibers called the *zone of Lissauer*. Generally, the white matter contains no perikarya or dendrites and is formed by myelinated and unmyelinated fibers. At the surface of the cord is a narrow marginal area composed only of neuroglia.

Large, Golgi type 1 neurons lie in the anterior horn, with their axons passing as ventral (anterior) root fibers to spinal nerves; others send their axons into white matter of ipsilateral and contralateral sides. Golgi type 2 neurons have short axons that terminate on other adjacent neurons, being confined to gray matter.

## Cerebellum

The cerebellum consists of right and left *hemispheres* with a central *vermis* showing transverse fissures, so that a lobule comprises a part of the vermis with two lateral, wing-like extensions into the hemispheres. The surface of the hemispheres has numerous folds, or folia, lying parallel to the main fissures, so that in sagittal section, there is the appearance of a central stem or trunk with numerous branches—the *arbor vitae*. Gray matter is found as a thin cortex overlying the centrally placed white matter and as collections of nerve cells (nuclei) in the central white matter.

On section, the *cerebellar cortex* shows three layers (Fig. 7–47). The innermost or *granular* layer contains many small cells, each with three to six short dendrites and a nonmyelinated axon that ascends toward the surface where it divides into two lateral branches that run along the length of a folium. The central layer is formed by a single row of *Purkinje's* cells (Fig. 7–48). These are large and flask-shaped, with a main apical dendrite or dendrites that expand into a fan-shaped network of branches lying at right angles to a folium and thus at right angles to the terminal axonal branches of the granular cells (Fig. 7–49). Axons of Purkinje's cells arise at the cell bases, acquire myelin sheaths, and give off collaterals.

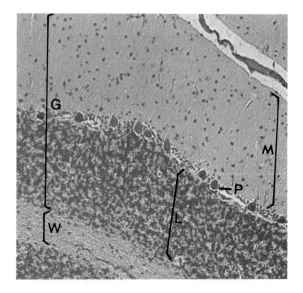

***Figure 7–47.*** *A portion of one folium of the cerebellar cortex is seen with peripheral gray matter (G) and central white matter (W). The three layers of the cortex are (1) an outer, thick, molecular layer (M) with a few small nerve cell bodies and many unmyelinated fibers; (2) a thin layer of scattered large Purkinje's cells (P); and (3) an inner granular layer (L) of small, closely packed cells. H and E. Medium power.*

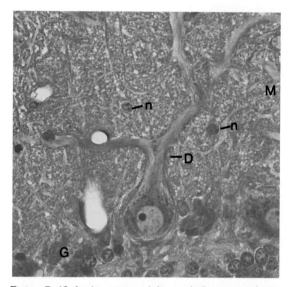

*Figure 7–48. In this section of the cerebellar cortex, there is the large flask-shaped perikaryon of a Purkinje's cell with a large vesicular nucleus, a prominent nucleolus, and Nissl bodies (blue) in the cytoplasm. Its single, large, branching dendrite (D) passes upward into the molecular layer (M), and below are a few small granule (G) cells. Seen in the molecular layer are nuclei (n) of neuroglial cells. Methylene blue, basic fuchsin. High power.*

Then the main axon traverses the deeper granular layer either to terminate in one of the deep cerebellar nuclei or to pass to another region of the cortex. The surface *molecular* layer contains a few small nerve cells and many unmyelinated fibers. These are stellate cells. Those near the surface have short dendrites and axons, but the deeper ones have longer axons showing collaterals in relation to several Purkinje's cells.

The cortex also contains fibers passing to it from the brain stem and spinal cord. "Mossy" fibers are thick and synapse on cells of the granular layer, while "climbing" fibers pass through the granular layer to terminate on Purkinje's cells.

Functionally, the cerebellum is related to movements of striated muscle, being concerned with coordination, posture, and equilibrium.

## Cerebrum

Gray matter of the cerebral hemispheres forms the *cerebral cortex* on the surface and also lies in ganglia or nuclei in the centrally placed white matter. There are right and left *hemispheres*.

The cerebral surface is convoluted, with projecting folds called *gyri* and intervening depressions, or *sulci*. The cortex is 1.5 to 4 mm thick and contains nerve cells, fibers, neuroglia, and blood vessels. In shape, the cells vary from pyramidal to stellate (granule) to fusiform, arranged in a laminated manner with six layers seen (Fig. 7–50). The following lists these layers, from superficial to deep

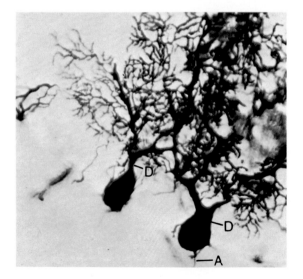

*Figure 7–49. In this preparation, only surface features are seen. The Purkinje's cells of the cerebellar cortex have large, flask-shaped perikarya with a single large dendrite (D) that enters the molecular layer and branches into a flat, fan-shaped network with numerous dendritic spines. A single axon (A) passes from the base of the cell into the granular layer and terminates either in a deep central nucleus or in another part of the cerebellar cortex. Golgi. High power.*

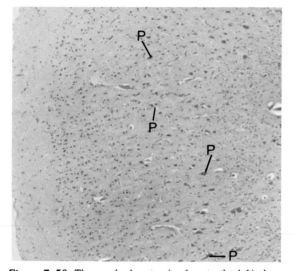

**Figure 7–50.** *The cerebral cortex (surface to the left) shows six layers in the gray matter, not seen clearly here, with large pyramidal neurons (P) in layers 3 and 5, and white matter deeply (to the right). H and E. Low power.*

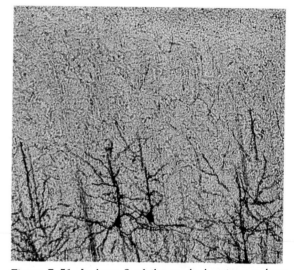

**Figure 7–51.** *In layer 3 of the cerebral cortex are large pyramidal (motor) cells with a large, branching apical dendrite, and several more dendrites and a single axon from the base. Only surface features are seen in this Golgi preparation. Low power.*

1. Molecular layer, largely formed by fibers running parallel to the surface and originating in deeper layers, with a few small perikarya.

2. External granular layer, with small triangular nerve cell bodies.

3. Pyramidal cell layer, with small pyramidal cells and many small granule cells (Fig. 7–51).

4. Internal granular layer of small, stellate granule cells.

5. Internal pyramidal (ganglionic) layer of large and medium-sized pyramidal cells.

6. Multiform (polymorphic) cell layer, the cells here varying in shape.

The layers blend one with another, and all contain neuroglia, the nerve cells lying in the *neuropil* (a feltwork of naked nerve fibers and neuroglial cell processes). There is variation in thickness (and prominence) of layers in different regions of the cortex, this being related to function.

Beneath the gray cortex, the white matter is formed by bundles of myelinated fibers, supported by neuroglia. Some of these fibers interconnect different regions of one cortical hemisphere and are called *association fibers*. Others connect regions of one cortex with other areas of the opposite hemisphere and are termed *commissural fibers*. *Projection fibers* leave the cortex and pass to lower centers.

## AUTONOMIC NERVOUS SYSTEM

The autonomic nervous system (ANS, visceral system) regulates the activities of smooth and cardiac muscle and glandular epithelium. Visceral afferent (sensory) neurons convey impulses to the CNS in a manner identical to other sensory neurons, with perikarya in sensory ganglia and long peripheral and central branches of their axons; however, these, while forming the afferent side of visceral reflex arcs, are not considered part of the ANS (which thus is entirely motor).

The ANS differs from the somatic motor system (in which a single neuron conveys impulses from the CNS to the effector organ), in that a chain of two neurons, with a synapse between them, is involved. Thus, there are *presynaptic* and *postsynaptic* neurons.

The ANS is divided into two divisions, the *sympathetic* and *parasympathetic*. Both include numerous small ganglia, as already described, these being, respectively, the thoracolumbar and craniosacral ganglia with associated nerve fibers. Presynaptic neurons of the sympathetic division lie in the lateral horn of gray matter of the spinal cord (T1 to L2), and their axons synapse in the

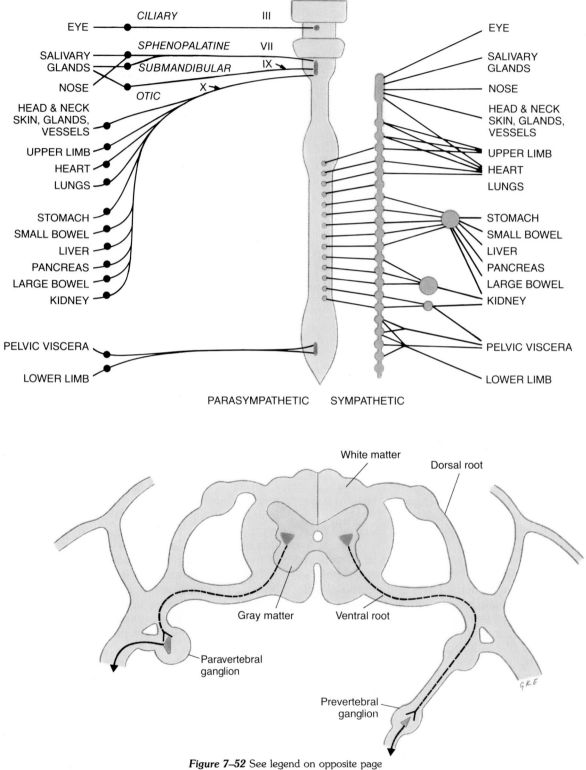

*Figure 7–52* See legend on opposite page

thoracolumbar (vertebral) chain of ganglia and in prevertebral ganglia (Fig. 7–52). Axons of presynaptic neurons of the parasympathetic system leave the brain as components of cranial nerves III, VII, IX, and X and also leave the spinal cord in the sacral region, synapsing in small cranial ganglia and in peripheral ganglia located in or near the organs they supply. In many cases, an organ receives nerve supply from both sympathetic and parasympathetic systems, and often, the two are antagonistic.

Histologically, preganglionic neurons (sympathetic) located in the lateral horn of gray matter (intermediolateral column) are small and spindle-shaped. They have very few terminal *boutons* or synapses compared with somatic motor neurons, with the majority of their axons terminating in the sympathetic chain. These preganglionic fibers are thinly myelinated. Sympathetic ganglion cells in the sympathetic chain are small, mostly multipolar, but of varying shapes, usually with some associated satellite or capsule cells. Their axons, the postganglionic fibers, are mostly unmyelinated and relatively long, passing to effector organs. Preganglionic neurons of the parasympathetic system lie in the brain and spinal cord and are usually small, and postganglionic neurons generally lie adjacent to, or in, the viscera supplied. Thus, preganglionic fibers (the axons of preganglionic neurons) are relatively long, and postganglionic fibers (the axons of postganglionic neurons) are relatively short. Preganglionic fibers are lightly myelinated, and postganglionic fibers are unmyelinated, as they are in the sympathetic system.

## NERVE ENDINGS

Peripheral nerve fibers, both motor and sensory, terminate in a peripheral organ, some as free nerve endings among non-nervous cells, others by specialized endings. Those fibers ending in *sensory receptors* are dendrites, those with *motor* or *secretory* endings are axons. The structure of the endings varies greatly but generally increases the area of contact between nerve terminal and non-nervous element. Sensory endings are discussed more fully in Chapter 17, and somatic motor endings (myoneural junctions) and the sensory endings associated with muscle have already been described.

Autonomic nerve endings generally are quite simple. The terminal nerve fiber generally shows swellings associated closely with the effector cell but separated from it by a synaptic cleft. Numerous synaptic vesicles are present in these swellings, with norepinephrine generally being the neurotransmitter at sympathetic endings and acetylcholine at parasympathetic endings.

## DIFFERENTIATION

Details of development of the nervous system are given in textbooks of embryology and neurology. The *neural tube* develops as an infolding of ectoderm along the dorsum of the embryo, from which cells detach on each side to form the *neural crests*. From neural crests are developed craniospinal and sympathetic ganglia, the adrenal medulla, and other cells. The wall of the neural tube at first is a single layer of epithelium, but this undergoes rapid division and differentiation to form neuroblasts, later forming neurons, and spongioblasts, later forming neuroglia (except perhaps microglia) (Fig. 7–53). Ependyma develops from the primitive lining of the neural tube. Neurons, satellite cells, and neurolemma develop from cells of the neural crest.

Throughout life, neuroglia, neurolemma, and capsule cells are capable of proliferation, but

---

**Figure 7–52.** Top: *Diagram of the peripheral distribution of components of the autonomic system; parasympathetic division on the left, sympathetic division on the right. The three peripheral or prevertebral ganglia represented by circles on the right are the celiac, superior mesenteric, and inferior mesenteric.* Bottom: *Diagram of a cross section of the spinal cord showing two possible courses taken by preganglionic (dashed lines) and postganglionic (dotted lines) fibers of the sympathetic nervous system.*

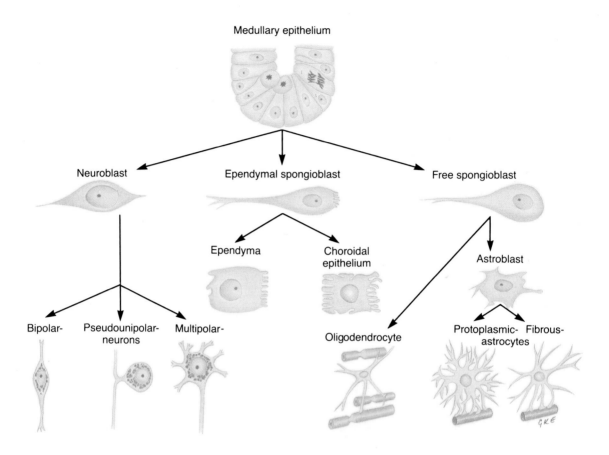

**Figure 7–53.** *Diagram illustrates the histogenesis of cells in the central nervous system, all derived from medullary epithelium of the neural tube. Microglial cells are not illustrated. The relation of an oligodendrocyte to myelinated nerve fibers and of astrocytes to blood vessels is seen.*

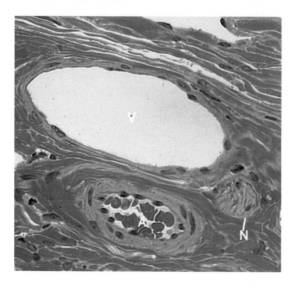

**Figure 7–54.** *This "neurovascular bundle" illustrates that peripheral nerves of all sizes often are associated with arteries and veins of comparable size. Here, a small nerve (N), a small arteriole (A), and a small venule (V) lie in connective tissue. H and E. High power.*

neurons do not reproduce after about the time of birth and cannot be replaced after destruction.

## DEGENERATION AND REGENERATION

Although neurons cannot reproduce after birth, they do have the capacity to withstand and recover from a certain degree of injury. After a nerve fiber is crushed or severed, both central and peripheral portions show changes. As described previously, the soma undergoes chromatolysis, with dispersion of Nissl substance and, later, re-formation, which may occur rapidly or may be prolonged over months. The axis cylinder beyond the damaged area degenerates, and fragmented material from it and the myelin are removed by phagocytosis of macrophages. Later, neurolemma cells proliferate to form a band or cord of cells.

After a period of about a week, from its central end, the divided axon starts to grow peripherally at a rate of 1 to 2 mm per day. Numerous sprouts

## Summary Table 7–1. The Nervous System

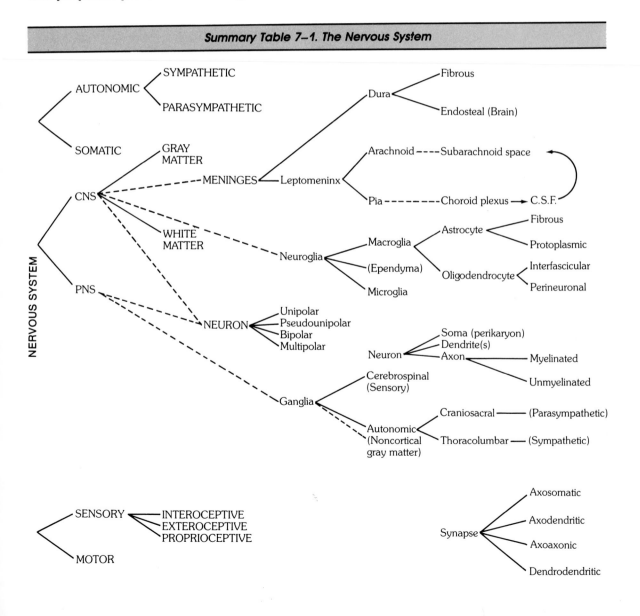

or branches grow across scar tissue at the injury site, enter the cords of neurolemma, and follow them to reach the original site of termination. However, because usually many axons are divided, any axon obviously may reach a termination that is inappropriate, and others are lost in scar tissue. Myelin is re-formed slowly. In the CNS, where a neurolemma sheath is lacking, regeneration is not possible.

## NEUROVASCULAR BUNDLE

Peripheral nerves frequently are associated with arteries and veins in so-called *neurovascular bundles* (Fig. 7–54). This occurs at all levels, the bundles branching and becoming smaller, so that near their terminations, small nerves travel with blood vessels of the order of arterioles and venules, as illustrated in Figure 7–54.

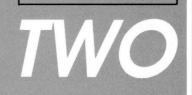

# TWO

# HISTOLOGY OF THE ORGAN SYSTEMS

# The Circulatory System

## GENERAL ORGANIZATION

The circulatory system consists of two major components: the *blood vascular system* and the *lymph vascular system*.

The blood vascular system is composed of the following structures:

1. The *heart*, a modified blood vessel that is specialized as a double pump for propulsion of blood. Blood from the body enters the right side of the heart and is pumped to the lungs. The left side of the heart receives the blood from the lungs and distributes it to all other organs and tissues of the body. The heart and the blood vessels thus form two circulations: the *systemic circulation*, from the heart to the tissues and organs of the body and back, and the *pulmonary circulation*, from the heart to the lungs and back.

2. The *arteries*, a series of efferent vessels, which become smaller as they branch. They distribute nutrients, oxygen, and hormones to all parts of the body.

3. The *capillaries*, a network of small, thin-walled vessels, through whose walls the interchange between blood and tissue occurs.

4. The *veins*, the afferent vessels to the heart, which converge into a system of larger vessels that convey the cellular products of metabolism.

The lymph vascular system, which commences in the tissues as blind tubules, consists of lymphatic capillaries and various-sized lymphatic vessels that return colorless fluid (lymph) from tissue spaces to the blood stream via the large veins in the neck.

8

Lymph nodes are interspersed along the course of lymphatic vessels and add lymphocytes to the lymph passing through them.

## THE BLOOD VASCULAR SYSTEM

The blood vascular system has a continuous lining that consists of a single layer of endothelial cells. In the capillaries, this single layer of cells forms the primary structural component of the wall. Thereafter, accessory coats are added progressively to the larger vessels.

### Capillaries

The capillaries are simple, endothelium-lined tubes that connect the arterial and venous sides of the circulation (Figs. 8–1 and 8–2). They have an average diameter of about 7 to 9 micrometers (μm). They form a network of narrow canals. The intensity of metabolism in a region determines the closeness of the mesh: a close network in lung, liver, kidney, glands, and skeletal muscle, and an open network in tendon, nerve, smooth muscle, and serous membranes.

The wall of a capillary consists of a single layer of flat endothelial cells supported by a basal lamina. Each endothelial cell is a curving, thin plate, with an ovoid or elongated nucleus. The cell borders, which can be made visible readily by the injection of silver nitrate, are serrated or wavy. Two or three cells, and occasionally only one, line the circumference of a capillary at any level of section. The endothelial cells are held together by tight junctions (zonulae occludentes).

Capillaries are surrounded by a thin sheath of delicate collagenous and reticular fibers and are accompanied by occasional perivascular cells, or

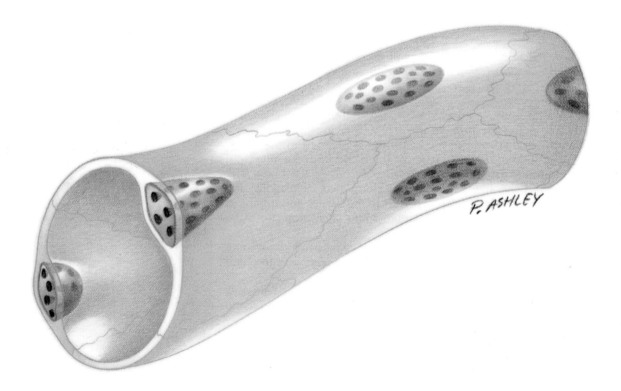

**Figure 8–1.** *Diagram illustrating the arrangement of endothelial cells comprising the wall of a capillary. The circumference of the capillary, sectioned at the left, is lined by two endothelial cells. A basal lamina, not shown here, surrounds the endothelium.*

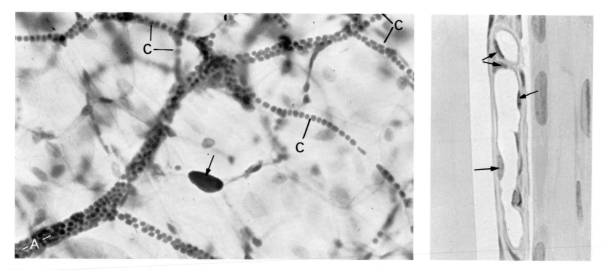

*Figure 8–2.* Capillaries. Left: *In this spread preparation of mesentery, stained with nuclear fast red, there is an open network of small blood vessels that contain packed erythrocytes within their lumina. A small arteriole (A) branches into numerous capillaries (C). The walls of the blood vessels are not stained. The background connective tissue, which is adipose, is indistinct and contains a mast cell (arrow). Medium power.* Right: *Section of a tendon (dense, regularly arranged connective tissue), with a portion of peritendineum present between two fiber bundles. The peritendineum contains a capillary, sectioned both transversely (above) and longitudinally (below). Endothelial nuclei (arrows) project into the lumen, and the cytoplasm of these cells is attenuated. The capillary is embedded within delicate connective tissue (pink). Plastic section. H and E. High power.*

*pericytes.* These slender, elongated cells generally appear similar to fibroblasts and are invested by a basal lamina that occasionally is deficient where the cell membrane of the pericyte is closely apposed to that of the endothelial cells. The pericytes are relatively undifferentiated cells that may transform into other cell types, including smooth muscle. In the past, it was suggested that they may be contractile and capable of altering the luminal diameter of capillaries. Recent evidence, however, indicates that endothelial cells themselves can contract and are able to reduce the diameter of the capillary lumen.

Variations in the structure of the endothelial cell wall form the basis of a classification of capillaries into three major types: *continuous, fenestrated,* and *sinusoidal.*

**Continuous.** Continuous (type I) capillaries are found in many tissues, including lung, muscle, skin, and the central nervous system (Fig. 8–3). The endothelial cytoplasm, which is relatively thick opposite the nucleus but which becomes attenuated elsewhere, lacks pores. Characteristically, it contains fine filaments and numerous small vesicles (*pinocytotic vesicles* or *caveolae intracellulares*) along both the luminal and basal surfaces. The vesicles are thought to form on one surface by invagination of the cell membrane, to detach, to cross the cytoplasm, and to fuse with the opposite surface, thus discharging their contents. Functionally, they are involved in the two-way transport of fluid across the capillary wall, and they represent the site of the so-called large-pore system of capillary permeability.

**Fenestrated.** Fenestrated (type II) capillaries, found in the intestinal mucosa, many endocrine glands, and the renal glomerulus are characterized by the presence of pores (*fenestrae*) within the attenuated endothelial cytoplasm (Figs. 8–4 and 8–5). The pores range in diameter from 30 to 80 nm and are closed by a thin diaphragm, except in capillaries of renal glomeruli. Macromolecules injected into the blood stream cross the capillary wall through these pores to enter the tissue space.

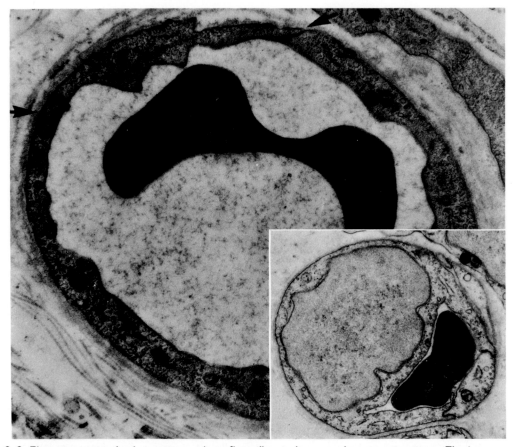

**Figure 8–3.** Electron micrograph of a continuous (type I) capillary in loose areolar connective tissue. The lumen contains a portion of an erythrocyte. Note the numerous pinocytotic vesicles in relation to the cell membrane of the endothelium and the two interfaces between endothelial cells (arrows). A basal lamina (at the tips of the arrows) surrounds the endothelium. × 18,500. Inset: A continuous capillary, the wall of which is composed of two endothelial cells, one showing a prominent nuclear area. An erythrocyte is present in the lumen. × 7500.

**Sinusoidal.** Sinusoidal capillaries, or *sinusoids*, have a luminal diameter much greater than that of normal capillaries. They may be 30 μm or more in diameter, and they have irregular tortuous walls. The walls show wide gaps between endothelial cells. Macrophages are closely associated with the endothelial cells. The basal lamina is incomplete, and the endothelial cells are separated from the parenchyma of organs only by a fine network of reticular fibers. These structural characteristics indicate that the interchange of fluids and macromolecules between blood and tissues is greatly facilitated through the sinusoidal capillaries. Such capillaries are found in the liver and in hemopoietic organs such as the bone marrow and spleen.

### Arterial and Venous Capillaries

*Arterial (pre-)* and *venous (post-) capillaries* are vessels intermediate between arteries and capillaries, and capillaries and veins, respectively. Arterial capillaries (or *metarterioles*) generally possess a wider lumen than that of capillaries and contain a discontinuous layer of smooth muscle

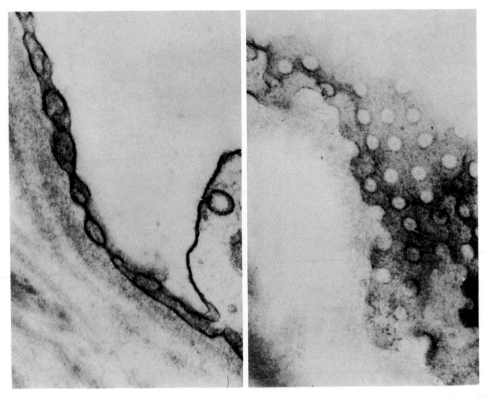

*Figure 8–4.* Electron micrographs of segments of two fenestrated capillaries from the choroid plexus. Left: The circular fenestrations (pores), each covered by a thin diaphragm, are cut transversely. Right: The endothelium has been sectioned obliquely, and the fenestrations are seen in surface view. Left: × 50,000; right: × 40,000.

cells in their walls. The vessels are surrounded by a sparse perivascular connective tissue that merges with the surrounding connective tissue of the organ. *Precapillary sphincters* are situated at the site where capillaries arise from metarterioles or arterioles proper, and these by intrinsic contraction control the amount of blood flowing through the capillary bed.

Venous capillaries, or *postcapillary venules*, may be up to 30 μm or more in diameter. The wall consists of an endothelial lining, a basal lamina, and a thin connective tissue coat containing pericytes, the latter occurring in greater numbers than in the general capillary network. Functionally, venous capillaries are closely related to the true capillaries in that they allow considerable exchange of metabolites and fluid between the blood and the fluid of the intercellular spaces.

### General Structure of Blood Vessels

All blood vessels with lumina greater than the diameter of capillaries exhibit a common pattern of organization (Fig. 8–6). The wall of each such vessel contains three concentric coats, or tunics:

1. The innermost coat, the *tunica intima*, consists of the inner *endothelial lining*, its underlying *basal lamina*, a *subendothelial layer* of delicate fibroelastic connective tissue, and an external band of elastic fibers, the *internal elastic membrane*, which is absent in many smaller vessels.

2. The middle coat, the *tunica media*, consists chiefly of smooth muscle cells, circularly arranged. Interspersed between the muscle cells are varying amounts of elastic and collagenous fibers and proteoglycans.

3. The outermost coat, the *tunica adventitia*,

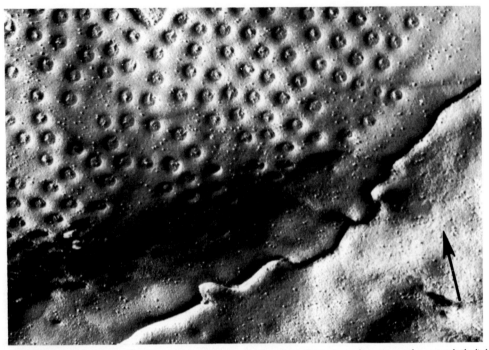

**Figure 8–5.** *Freeze-etch preparation of a fenestrated capillary, showing a surface view of portions of two endothelial cells. The interface between the two cells runs obliquely across the figure, and in the upper cell, circular fenestrations, each closed by a diaphragm, are frequent. The arrow indicates the direction of shadowing during preparation. Compare with Figure 8–4 (right). × 38,000.*

is composed principally of fibroelastic connective tissue, with most of the collagenous fibers running parallel to the long axis of the vessel. Closest to the media, there may be a definite concentration of elastic fibers to form the *external elastic membrane*. Externally, the tunica adventitia merges into the enveloping connective tissue of the organ through which the vessel is passing. In larger blood vessels, smaller blood vessels (the *vasa vasorum*) lie within the adventitia and supply it and the media with nutritive substances, since the tunics are too thick to be nourished by diffusion from the lumen.

Frequently, large blood vessels are bound together with peripheral nerves in so-called *neurovascular bundles*. As the bundles pass peripherally to the various tissues, they branch and become smaller, so that near their terminations small nerves are associated with smaller arteries (arterioles) and veins (venules).

## Arteries

There is a continuous and gradual transition in size and in structural components of the vessel wall from the largest arteries down to metarterioles supplying the capillary bed. It is thus customary to classify arteries into three groups:

1. Large elastic arteries.
2. Muscular arteries of small to medium size.
3. Arterioles, the smallest arterial branches.

**Large Elastic Arteries.** This group includes the aorta and its largest main branches, the brachiocephalic, the common carotid, the subclavian, and the common iliac (Fig. 8–7). The wall is relatively thin for the size of the vessel, and the amount of elastic tissue present is sufficient to impart a yellow color to the freshly cut wall.

The endothelial cells of the intima are polygonal in shape, not elongate as in smaller vessels. The subendothelial layer is thick and consists of col-

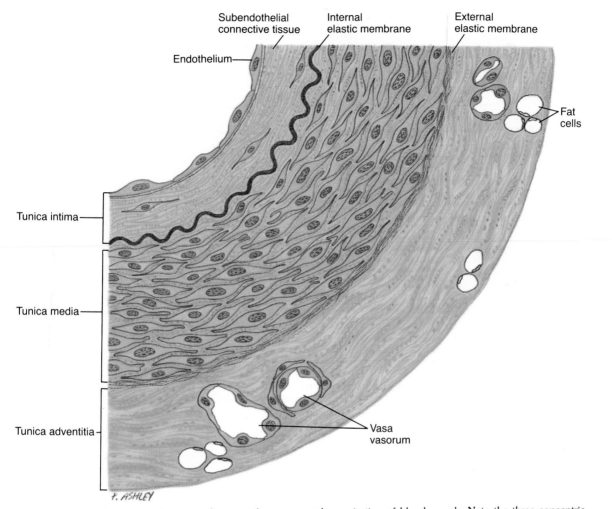

*Figure 8–6.* Schematic diagram illustrating the general structure and organization of blood vessels. Note the three concentric tunics surrounding the lumen.

lagenous and elastic fibers, which show a longitudinal orientation, some fibroblasts, and, in the deeper portion of the intima, small bundles of smooth muscle cells. The internal elastic membrane that marks the periphery of the intima is difficult to distinguish, since it is confused with the elastic membranes of the media. The media is characterized by numerous fenestrated elastic membranes, which are arranged concentrically. Their number, 40 to 60, increases with age. Interspaces between the membranes contain fi-

broblasts, an amorphous ground substance, and smooth muscle cells that pursue a spiral course. The adventitia is a thin coat. It consists largely of elastic and collagenous fibers and cannot be separated sharply from the surrounding connective tissue. There is no distinctive external elastic membrane. The adventitia contains both vasa vasorum and lymphatic vessels.

The elastic arteries absorb some of the pulse beat by the distention of the elastic tissue within their walls and make the blood flow less intermit-

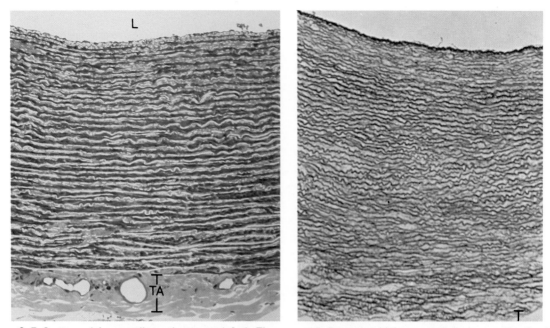

**Figure 8–7.** *Sections of the aorta (large elastic artery). Left: The concentrically arranged laminae of elastic tissue within the thick tunica media are unstained and appear wavy in this preparation. The stained material between the laminae contains fibroblasts, an amorphous ground substance, collagenous fibers, and scattered smooth muscle cells. The tunica adventitia (TA) contains numerous small blood vessels, the vasa vasorum. The thin tunica intima in relation to the lumen (L) cannot be defined at this magnification. Plastic section. Methylene blue. Low power. Right: The elastic laminae of the thick tunica media have been stained specifically. The thin tunica intima is represented by the densely stained, irregular strand immediately in relation to the lumen (above). A small portion of the tunica adventitia (T) is present, lower right. Verhoeff's elastic stain. Low power.*

tent than it would be if the vessels were rigid tubes. Often, they are termed *conducting arteries*, emphasizing their function of conducting blood to the smaller ramifications of the vascular system.

**Muscular Arteries.** This group includes all arteries of small and medium size (Figs. 8–8 and 8–9). The walls of the muscular arteries are relatively thick, owing principally to the large amount of muscle in the media. They also are called *distributing arteries*, since they distribute blood to the various organs and regulate the volume of blood in response to varying functional demands.

The tunica intima has three definite layers: an endothelium that lies upon a thin basal lamina, a subendothelial layer of delicate collagenous and elastic fibers, and an internal elastic membrane that is prominent and composed of closely interwoven elastic fibers (Fig. 8–10). The internal elastic membrane, in histological sections, typi-

cally is thrown into folds because of post-mortem contraction of the muscular elements within the media. The media consists almost exclusively of circularly disposed smooth muscle cells. Between the layers of muscle (up to 40 in number), there are small amounts of connective tissue, including collagenous, reticular, and elastic fibers. In the larger muscular arteries, elastic fibers are prominent between the muscle layers, where they form close networks. The adventitia is variable in thickness but often is as thick as the media. It contains collagenous and elastic fibers, mostly longitudinally arranged. Elastic fibers are concentrated internally, where they commonly form a definite external elastic membrane.

**Arterioles.** These vessels, with a diameter of 100 μm or less, have a tunica intima that consists of only endothelium and an internal elastic membrane (Figs. 8–11 and 8–12). The latter is really a network of fibers that by light microscopy

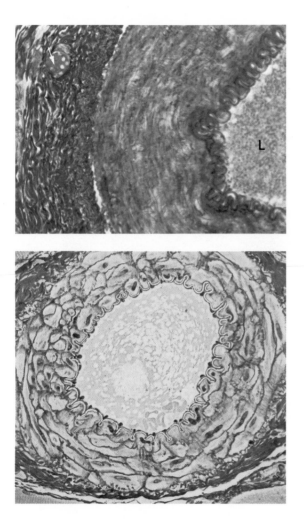

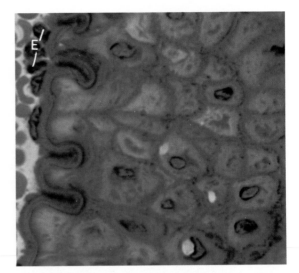

*Figure 8–9. Small muscular artery sectioned longitudinally. The tunica intima is composed principally of endothelium (E) and a distinct internal elastic membrane (red). Muscle cells, circularly arranged and here sectioned transversely, compose the tunica media. Plastic section. Toluidine blue, safranin. High power.*

*Figure 8–8. Muscular arteries. Top: Medium-sized muscular artery. The artery is sectioned transversely and shows a lumen (L) full of erythrocytes. The endothelium cannot be discerned at this magnification. A thin subendothelial layer of delicate connective tissue (blue) lies internal to the prominent internal elastic membrane (red), which shows a wavy outline. The thick tunica media (light blue) is composed of numerous layers of circularly disposed smooth muscle cells, between which are a few elastic fibers (red). The tunica adventitia (dark blue), composed principally of collagenous fibers, is almost as thick as the tunica media. It contains a small blood vessel (arrow), one of the vasa vasorum. Mallory stain. Low power. Bottom: Small muscular artery. The thick tunica media is bounded internally by the internal elastic membrane (unstained) and externally by a concentration of reticular fibers (specifically stained) in the tunica adventitia. Smooth muscle cells within the tunica media are outlined by staining of the delicate reticular fibers that surround them. Gridley's reticulin stain. Medium power.*

appears as a thin, bright line immediately beneath endothelium. The media is composed of one to five complete layers of smooth muscle cells and scattered elastic fibrils. The number of layers of muscle cells decreases as the caliber of the vessel decreases, and, at a diameter of about 20 μm, the muscle coat becomes a single layer. The thin adventitia is a layer of loose connective tissue with longitudinally oriented collagenous and elastic fibers. No definite external elastic membrane is present.

The arterioles have relatively thick walls and they control the distribution of blood to capillary beds by vasodilation and vasoconstriction. They are the prime controllers of systemic blood pressure. Most of the fall in blood pressure occurs within the arterioles, so that only a gentle stream passes into the delicate capillary beds.

## SPECIALIZED ARTERIES AND AGE CHANGES IN ARTERIES

Certain arteries show pronounced structural deviations from the generalized plan. These variations reflect adaptations to special locations and

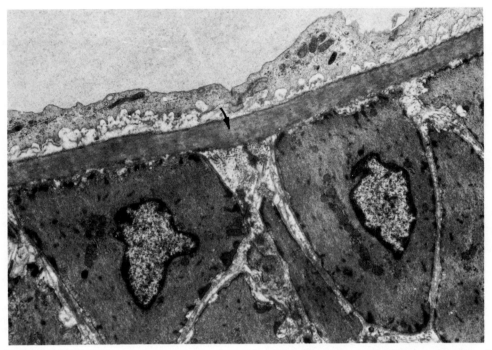

***Figure 8–10.*** *Electron micrograph of the tunica intima and a small portion of the tunica media of a muscular artery. A complete internal elastic membrane (arrow) is interposed between the endothelium and the transversely sectioned smooth muscle cells. × 20,000.*

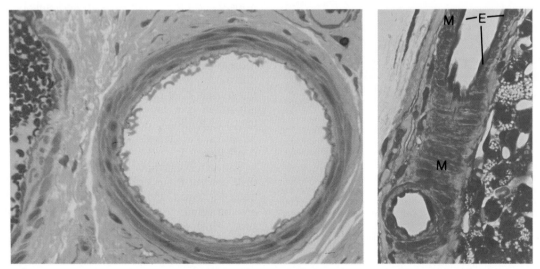

***Figure 8–11.*** *Sections of small arterioles. Left: The arteriole, embedded in loose connective tissue, shows a tunica intima, consisting of endothelium and a narrow internal elastic membrane (pale orange), and a tunica media composed of three to four layers of smooth muscle cells. The tunica adventitia is narrow and ill-defined and blends with the surrounding connective tissue. The accompanying venule (left) has a much thinner wall than the arteriole, and the tunica media shows one to two layers of smooth muscle cells widely spaced and separated by connective tissue. Plastic section. Methylene blue, azure A. High power. Right: This arteriole, within the capsule of the suprarenal gland, is sectioned both transversely (below) and longitudinally (above). In the intermediate portion, the section passes through the wall and demonstrates the circular arrangement of smooth muscle cells. Nuclei of endothelial cells (E) appear elongated, and the tunica media consists of a single layer of smooth muscle cells (M). Plastic section. H and E. High power.*

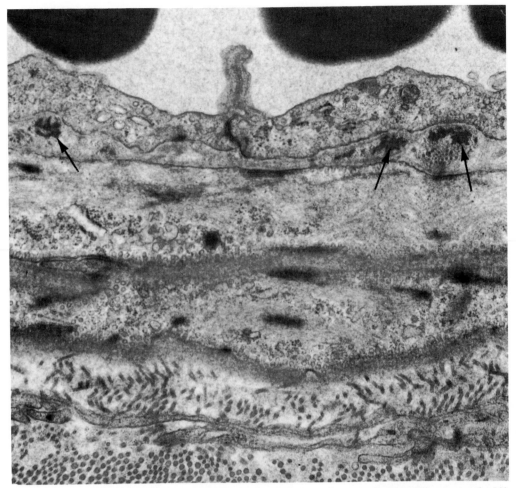

**Figure 8–12.** *Electron micrograph of a small arteriole. The internal elastic membrane is represented by a network of fibers, here sectioned transversely (arrows). The tunica media, composed of two layers of smooth muscle cells, is covered externally (below) by the connective tissue, principally collagenous fibrils, of the tunica adventitia.* × *22,000.*

functional demands. Arteries of the lung have thin walls owing to a reduction in both muscle and elastic tissue. This reduces their resistance and thus is correlated with a lower blood pressure in the pulmonary circulation. Arteries protected within the skull have a thin wall and a well-developed internal elastic membrane. The umbilical arteries possess a media composed of two thick muscular layers, an inner longitudinal layer and an outer circular layer. In the penile arteries, the intima is greatly thickened and contains many longitudinal muscle fibers. These groups of smooth muscle cells form the cores of *intimal cushions* that serve functionally as valves. Cardiac muscle extends into the media of the roots of the aorta and pulmonary artery.

Arteries tend to undergo regressive changes in adult life, especially in senescence. Arteries of the elastic type show greater changes with age than do arteries of the muscular type. Elastic tissue shows irregular thickenings; individual elastic fibers fragment; and fat infiltrates the interstitial substance. Later, calcification may occur within the media.

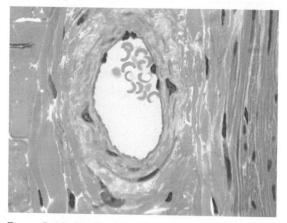

*Figure 8–13. Small venule. The wall consists of endothelial cells, nuclei of which project into the lumen, and a thin outer sheath (adventitia) of scattered fibroblasts and collagenous fibers that merge with those of the surrounding connective tissue. Plastic section. H and E. High power.*

## Veins

Venous blood vessels usually are classified into three groups:

1. Venules, the smallest venous branches.
2. Small to medium-sized veins.
3. Large veins.

Since blood within the veins is under much less pressure because of frictional losses than that within the arteries, veins must accommodate a greater volume of blood. Hence, veins generally are larger in diameter than their corresponding arteries, and their walls are thinner, chiefly owing to a reduction in muscular and elastic components.

**Venules.** The transition from capillary or venous capillary to venule is a very gradual one and involves the acquisition of connective tissue elements first and smooth muscle fibers later. The smallest venules possess an intima consisting of endothelium only and an outer sheath of collagenous fibers (Figs. 8–13 and 8–14). These venules participate in the interchange of metabolites between blood and tissues. When the vessel attains a diameter of about 50 μm, elastic fibers appear in the tunica intima and smooth muscle fibers are present between the intima and the outer fibrous sheath (adventitia). In venules of 200 μm or more, the circular muscle fibers form a continuous layer (media), one to three cells thick. The muscle fibers are more widely spaced than in an arteriole of similar size and are separated by bundles of collagenous and elastic fibers. The adventitia is thick in comparison with the overall thinness of the wall and consists of longi-

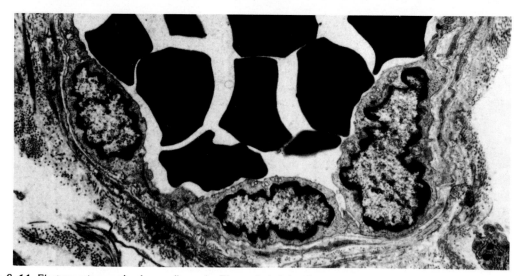

*Figure 8–14. Electron micrograph of a small venule. The endothelial cells surrounding the lumen, which contains numerous erythrocytes, are bounded externally by a delicate sheath of collagenous fibrils. × 8000.*

tudinally oriented collagenous fibers and scattered elastic fibers and fibroblasts.

**Small and Medium-Sized Veins.** These include practically all the anatomically named veins and their principal branches, except the main trunks (Fig. 8–15). The tunica intima is thin and consists of endothelium and a subendothelial layer that is inconspicuous and may be bounded externally by a network of fine elastic fibers, which does not form a distinct internal elastic membrane. The media is thin also and is composed of small bundles of circularly arranged muscle fibers separated by collagenous and elastic fibers. The adventitia is well developed and forms the bulk of the wall. It consists principally of thick, longitudinal collagenous bundles and frequently a few smooth muscle fibers arranged in small, longitudinal fascicles.

**Large Veins.** This group includes the superior and inferior venae cavae, the portal vein, and the main tributaries leading into these trunks (Fig. 8–16). The intima has the same structure as that of smaller veins, but it may be a little thicker. The media is poorly developed, and smooth muscle elements within it are much reduced or absent. The adventitia is the thickest of the three coats and contains many longitudinal muscle fibers, separated by collagenous fibers.

**Special Features of Certain Veins.** Some veins lack smooth muscle and thus are without a definite media. This group includes cerebral and meningeal veins, dural sinuses, and veins of the retina, bones, penile erectile tissue, and the maternal components of the placenta. Veins that are rich in smooth muscle include those of the gravid uterus and limbs, the umbilical vein, and some mesenteric veins. Cardiac muscle extends for a short distance into the adventitia of the venae cavae and pulmonary veins near their entrance into the heart.

**Venous Valves.** Many small and medium-sized veins, particularly those of the lower limbs, possess valves that prevent retrograde blood flow. The valves are paired, semilunar folds of the intima that project into the lumen with their free margins directed toward the heart. Both surfaces of the valves are covered by endothelium. In these veins, blood flow against gravity and toward

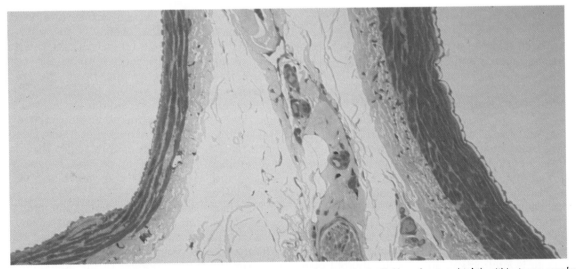

*Figure 8–15.* Medium-sized vein and muscular artery. Comparison between vein (left) and artery (right) within loose areolar connective tissue. The vein is identified by the overall thinness of its wall; a thin tunica intima; a tunica media composed of small bundles of smooth muscle cells separated by connective tissue, principally collagenous fibers; and a well-developed tunica adventitia. The artery has a much thicker wall than does the vein and exhibits a thick tunica media and a prominent internal elastic membrane (unstained). Plastic section. Methylene blue, azure A. Low power.

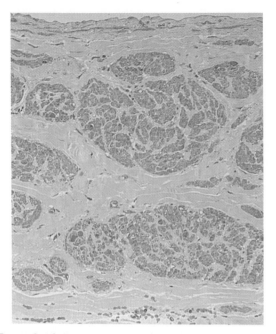

**Figure 8–16.** *Large vein. The inferior vena cava, here sectioned transversely, exhibits a thin tunica media within which are scattered smooth muscle cells, circularly arranged. The tunica adventitia is thick and contains numerous large bundles of longitudinally arranged smooth muscle cells, here sectioned transversely, that are separated by collagenous fibers. Plastic section. H and E. Low power.*

the heart is aided by contraction of neighboring skeletal muscles and the system of valves.

### Arteriovenous Anastomoses

In addition to capillary and sinusoidal connections between arteries and veins, in certain regions arteries are connected directly to veins by *arteriovenous anastomoses*. In the anastomoses, most commonly between arterioles and venules, endothelium lies directly upon a specialized tunica media comprising a sphincter. These vascular shunts are particularly numerous in the skin of exposed parts and in tissues where metabolic activity is intermittent, such as the thyroid gland and the digestive system. When the shunt is closed, arterial blood passes into the regular capillary bed. When the shunt is open, much of the blood bypasses the capillary bed and passes directly into the vein.

### The Heart

The heart is a highly specialized portion of the vascular system that propels blood through the blood vessels. The wall of the heart consists of three layers:

1. The inner layer, or *endocardium.*
2. The middle layer, or *myocardium.*
3. The outer layer, or *epicardium.*

**Endocardium.** The endocardium is analogous to the tunica intima of blood vessels and is lined by endothelium continuous with that of blood vessels entering and leaving the heart. Beneath the endothelium there is a *subendothelial layer* of fine collagenous fibers, a layer of relatively dense connective tissue, and an outer *subendocardial layer* of loose connective tissue that binds the endocardium to the myocardium. The subendocardial layer contains blood vessels, nerves, and branches of the impulse-conducting system.

**Myocardium.** The myocardium, which corresponds to the tunica media, is composed of cardiac muscle, which in the ventricles is arranged in two layers, superficial and deep. The superficial fibers run a spiral course, and the deep fibers generally follow a circular course around each ventricle. The muscle sheets of the atria and ventricles are attached by way of their interstitial connective tissue (endomysium) to the central supporting structure of the heart, the *cardiac skeleton.*

**Epicardium.** The epicardium (or *visceral pericardium*) is a serous membrane covered externally by a single layer of mesothelial cells. Beneath the mesothelium, there is a relatively thick layer of areolar or adipose tissue, the *subepicardial layer*, that contains the coronary blood vessels and nerves.

**Cardiac Skeleton.** The central supporting tissue of the heart is dense fibrous connective tissue on which cardiac muscle inserts and valves attach. Its main components are the *septum membranaceum*, or fibrous portion of the interventricular septum; the *annuli fibrosi*, or fibrous rings that surround the origins of the aorta and pulmonary artery and the atrioventricular canals; and the *trigona fibrosa,* masses of fibrous tissue between the arterial foramina and the atrioventricular canals. In certain larger animals, the dense connective tissue of the cardiac skeleton may become chondroid in nature and give rise to either cartilage or bone (the *os cordis*).

**Cardiac Valves.** The *atrioventricular valves* (*tricuspid* and *mitral*) between atria and ventricles and the *semilunar valves* between the ventricles and the aorta and pulmonary artery are reduplications of endocardium containing a core of dense connective tissue continuous with that of the annuli fibrosi. The atrioventricular valves are connected to papillary muscles of the ventricles by fibrous cords, the *chordae tendineae,* which serve to restrain the valves and prevent eversion of the valves when the ventricles contract. The semilunar valves each have three cusps, and the central fibrous plate of each cusp forms a thickening (the *nodule of Arantius*) at the free border.

**Impulse-Conducting System of the Heart.** A system of specialized cardiac muscle fibers, *Purkinje's fibers,* conducts the heart beat that has originated in the right atrium in the sinoatrial node, the rhythmic pacemaker of the heart (Figs. 8–17 and 8–18). Purkinje's fibers have a larger diameter than ordinary cardiac muscle fibers and contain relatively more sarcoplasm. Myofibrils are reduced in number and usually are limited to the periphery of the fibers.

An impulse begins at the *sinoatrial node,* which consists of a dense network of small Purkinje's fibers that peripherally are in continuity with atrial cardiac muscle fibers. The impulse spreads via the specialized conduction fibers to the *atrioventricular node,* a dense mass of fibers located in the median wall of the right atrium. The node continues into a common stem, the *atrioventricular bundle* (or *bundle of His*), which divides into two trunks that lie beneath the endocardium on either side of the interventricular septum. These trunks terminate in a system of Purkinje's fibers that connects with ordinary cardiac muscle fibers of the two ventricles.

The parasympathetic (vagus) and the sympathetic divisions of the autonomic nervous system extrinsically innervate the heart. The vagus and sympathetic fibers are complementary, the vagus fibers inhibiting and the sympathetic fibers accelerating the heart action. These fibers form exten-

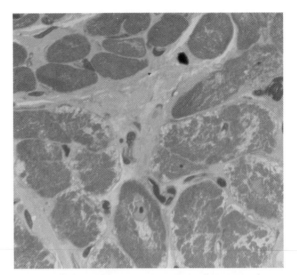

*Figure 8–17.* Purkinje's fibers, sectioned transversely, are present within the subendocardial layer of the right ventricle. The fibers have a larger diameter than that of ordinary cardiac muscle fibers and exhibit a clear sarcoplasm centrally that contains an occasional nucleus and peripheral concentrations of myofibrils. The Purkinje's fibers may be identified readily from the regular cardiac muscle fibers of the myocardium (above). Plastic section. Methylene blue, azure A. High power.

sive plexuses and terminate principally in relation to the sinoatrial and atrioventricular nodes and along the atrioventricular bundle. The vagus is the principal regulator of the sinoatrial pacemaker. Its fibers do not appear to reach the ventricular muscle.

### THE LYMPH VASCULAR SYSTEM

The lymph vascular system, the second component of the circulatory system, is unidirectional and functions to drain off excess tissue fluid as *lymph,* filter this through the lymph nodes, and return it to the blood stream. The smallest lymphatic vessels, *lymph capillaries,* end blindly. They form plexuses that drain into *lymphatic vessels,* which centrally converge into one of two *main lymphatic trunks,* which empty into veins at the root of the neck (Figs. 8–19 through 8–22).

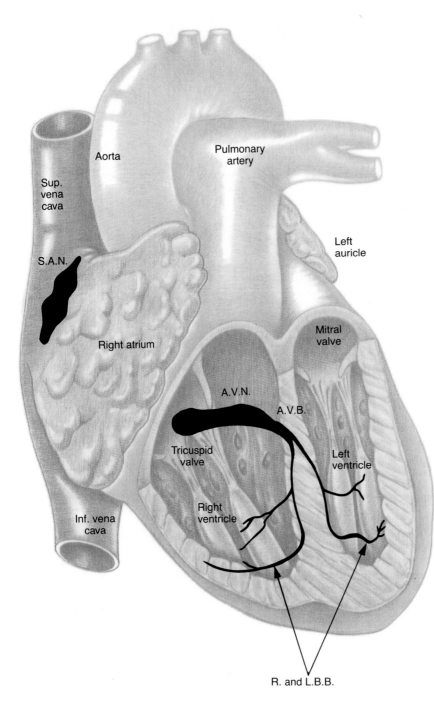

Aorta

Pulmonary artery

Sup. vena cava

Left auricle

S.A.N.

Right atrium

Mitral valve

A.V.N.

A.V.B.

Tricuspid valve

Left ventricle

Right ventricle

Inf. vena cava

R. and L.B.B.

*Figure 8–18.* Diagram of the heart, with the interior of the ventricles exposed, showing the principal components of the impulse-conducting system. S.A.N., sinoatrial node; A.V.N., atrioventricular node; A.V.B., atrioventricular bundle (of His); R. and L.B.B., right and left branches of the bundle.

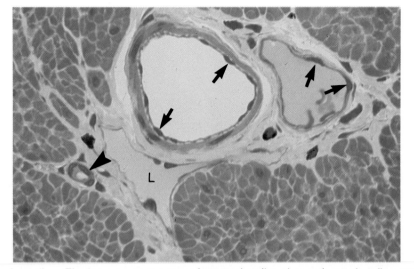

**Figure 8–19.** *Lymph capillary. The loose connective tissue between bundles of smooth muscle cells, sectioned transversely, contains a lymph capillary (L), which appears as an irregular cleft within the connective tissue lined by endothelial cells. Nuclei of these cells project into the lumen. The thin wall of the lymph capillary is in contrast to that of the venule (below), which has a wall that consists of endothelium (arrows) and a definite outer sheath (adventitia) of collagenous fibers that merge with those of the surrounding connective tissue. Also present are a small arterial (above) and an arterial capillary (arrowhead, upper left). The arteriole shows a tunica intima, consisting of endothelium (arrows) and a narrow internal elastic membrane (unstained), and a tunica media composed of a single layer of smooth muscle cells. The tunica adventitia is narrow and ill-defined and blends with the surrounding connective tissue. The small arterial capillary has an endothelial lining and a discontinuous layer of smooth muscle cells. Plastic section. Methylene blue, azure A. High power.*

**Lymph Capillaries.** Lymph capillaries, like blood capillaries, are simple, endothelium-lined tubes, but they are somewhat larger than blood capillaries and are not uniform in caliber. The wall is composed of a continuous endothelium that exhibits numerous small pinocytotic vesicles. The capillaries lack a complete basal lamina and are surrounded by a thin layer of collagenous and

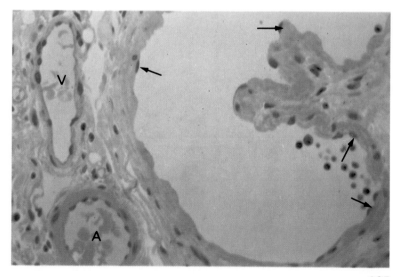

**Figure 8–20.** *Lymphatic vessel. The vessel, sectioned obliquely, lies within the connective tissue at the hilum of a lymph node. The section has passed through the roots of two valve leaflets. The wall of the vessel consists of endothelial cells, a few nuclei of which are apparent (arrows), and a thin outer sheath (adventitia) of collagenous fibers. Also present are a venule (V) and an arteriole (A). Plastic section. H and E. Medium power.*

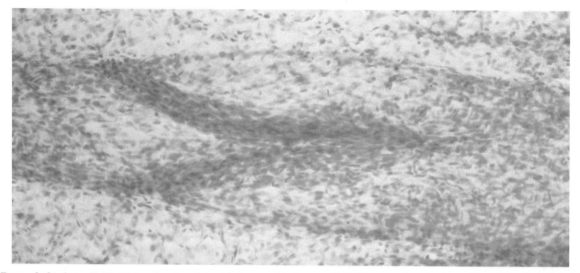

*Figure 8–21. Lymphatic vessel with valve. A lymphatic vessel is shown within this spread preparation of connective tissue. Only nuclei, both within the vessel wall and within the surrounding connective tissue, are stained. A pair of valves within the lumen of the vessel is seen clearly, with the free ends of tne valves directed centrally (to the right). The vessel expands in diameter beyond the attachment of the valves. Nuclear fast red. Medium power.*

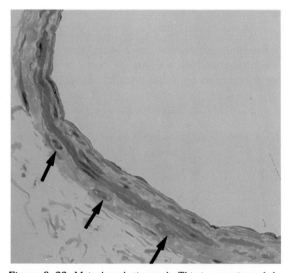

*Figure 8–22. Main lymphatic trunk. This is a section of the thoracic duct. The thin tunica intima consists of an endothelial lining, a delicate subendothelial layer, and a thin, inconstant elastic membrane; however, only the endothelial lining can be defined at this magnification. The tunica media consists of smooth muscle cells, mostly arranged concentrically. The tunica adventitia, which consists principally of coarse collagenous fibers, contains a few small blood vessels (vasa vasorum, arrows). Plastic section. Methylene blue, azure A. Medium power.*

reticular fibers that extend into the surrounding connective tissues as *anchoring filaments.*

**Lymphatic Vessels.** Lymph passes from lymph capillaries into larger vessels that have thicker walls and valves. These vessels resemble veins in structure, but their walls tend to be thinner. The endothelium is surrounded by collagenous and elastic fibers and a few smooth muscle cells. In larger vessels, three coats—intima, media, and adventitia—may be distinguished, but usually they are poorly demarcated. The vessels contain numerous valves that are more closely spaced than those found in veins. Between the valves, the vessels are swollen; thus, they have a beaded appearance.

**Main Lymphatic Trunks.** These are the thoracic and right lymphatic ducts. In structure, they are much like a vein of equal size, except for a greater concentration of smooth muscle fibers within the media. The intima consists of an endothelial lining, a delicate subendothelial layer that may contain some longitudinal muscle fibers, and a thin, inconstant, elastic membrane. The media contains longitudinal and circular smooth muscle bundles separated by abundant connective tissue. The adventitia consists of coarse collagenous fibers and a few longitudinal muscle fibers.

## Summary Table 8–1. The Circulatory System

| Component | Tunica Intima | Tunica Media | Tunica Adventitia | Total Wall Thickness | Principal Functions |
|---|---|---|---|---|---|
| **BLOOD VASCULAR SYSTEM** | | | | | |
| Continuous capillary | Thin. Endothelium and basal lamina (and pericytes) | Absent | Extremely thin. Traces of connective tissue | Thin | Site of interchange between blood and tissue fluid |
| Fenestrated capillary | Thin. Endothelium with pores | Absent | Extremely thin. Traces of connective tissue | Thin | Site of increased interchange between blood and tissue fluid |
| Sinusoidal capillary | Thin. Wide gaps between endothelial cells | Absent | Extremely thin. Delicate connective tissue fibers | Thin | Site of major interchange between blood and tissue fluid |
| Elastic artery | Relatively thick. Endothelium and subendothelial layer with smooth muscle | Extremely thick and with elastic laminae | Thin. No definite external elastic lamina | Thick | Conducts blood from heart under high pressure |
| Muscular artery | Thin. Endothelium and subendothelial layer and prominent internal elastic membrane | Thick. Many layers of muscle and interspersed elastic fibers | Thick. Collagenous and elastic fibers. Definite external elastic membrane | Thick | Distributes blood to various organs and tissues |
| Arteriole | Thin. Endothelium and internal elastic membrane | Relatively thick. One to five layers of muscle | Thin. Collagenous and elastic fibers | Relatively thick | Lowers blood pressure prior to entry to capillary bed |
| Venule | Thin. Endothelium | Absent in small venules. Thin in large venules | Thin. Collagenous fibers | Thin | Collects blood from capillary bed + site of interchange between blood and tissue fluid |
| Small and medium-sized veins | Thin. Endothelium, delicate subendothelial connective tissue, and valves present | Thin. Muscle + collagenous and elastic fibers | Thick. Connective tissue and muscle fibers | Relatively thick | Conduct blood toward heart. Under low pressure |
| Large vein | Thin. As in medium-sized vein | Thin. Muscle fibers reduced | Thick. Connective tissue + longitudinal bundles of collagenous and muscle fibers | Thick | Returns blood to heart |
| Heart | = Endocardium. Endothelium + supporting connective tissue + Purkinje's fibers + valves | = Myocardium. Thick. Cardiac muscle | = Epicardium. Mesothelium + supporting connective tissue | Thick | Pumps blood into systemic and pulmonary circulations |
| **LYMPH VASCULAR SYSTEM** | | | | | |
| Lymph capillary | Very thin. Endothelium lacks complete basal lamina | Absent | Extremely thin. Traces of connective tissue with anchoring filaments | Thin | Collects surplus tissue fluid |
| Lymphatic vessel | Thin. Endothelium + few connective tissue fibers. Valves present | Thin. Few muscle fibers | Relatively thick. May contain smooth muscle | Relatively thick | Conveys lymph to main trunks |
| Main lymphatic trunk | Thin. Endothelium + subendothelial connective tissue. Thin internal elastic membrane | Thin. Longitudinal and circular muscle fibers | Relatively thick. Longitudinal muscle fibers | Relatively thick | Returns lymph to blood stream |

# Lymph Organs

**9**

## INTRODUCTION

Several organs and structures within the body consist largely of *lymphoid (lymphatic) tissue* (Fig. 9–1). Lymphoid tissue is not one of the primary tissue types but is merely a variety of connective tissue. It has two principal components: *reticular tissue,* comprising a framework of reticular cells and reticular fibers, and *free cells,* chiefly lymphocytes, which lie within the interstices of the reticular tissue. In many regions of the body, the lymphoid tissue is not sharply delineated from the surrounding connective tissue; this is known as *diffuse lymphoid tissue,* in contrast with the more dense form (*lymph nodules*) in which the component cells are densely aggregated. Numerous gradations between the two varieties of lymphoid tissue are found.

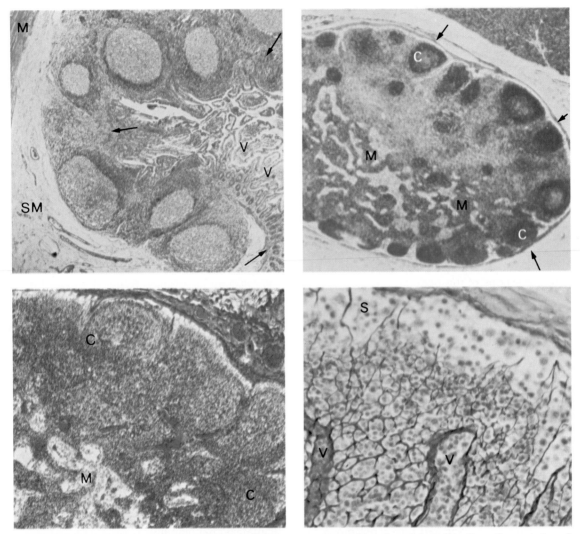

**Figure 9–1.** Lymphoid tissues. Top left: *Peyer's patches are aggregations of lymph nodules within the antimesenteric wall of the ileum. Here, each nodule shows a pale germinal center and a darker periphery. Over the patch, villi (V) are present in reduced numbers and appear somewhat irregular in outline. The muscularis mucosae (arrows) is interrupted by the nodules, which extend into the submucosa (SM). The muscularis externa (M) limits the submucosa externally. H and E. Low power.* Top right: *The lymph node is surrounded by a definite capsule (arrows), composed principally of densely packed collagenous fibers. The parenchyma of the node is specialized into two regions, an outer cortex (C) and an inner medulla (M). The cortex consists of lymph nodules, most of which show pale germinal centers. The nodules are separated from the capsule by a narrow space, the subcapsular sinus, through which lymph circulates. The medulla appears pale, and the lymphoid tissue within it is arranged in dense, irregular anastomosing strands or medullary cords. The cords are surrounded by medullary lymph sinuses. H and E. Low power.* Bottom left: *Lymph node. The capsule (blue) contains numerous blood vessels, and from its inner aspect, small bundles of fibers extend as trabeculae into the interior of the node. The cortex (C) contains lymphocytes closely packed into nodules, some of which show pale germinal centers. The lymph spaces between the cortex and the capsule constitute the subcapsular sinus. The medulla (M) contains irregular lymph (medullary) cords that are surrounded by wide medullary lymph sinuses. A few blood vessels (red) are present in both cortex and medulla. Azan. Medium power.* Bottom right: *Lymph node. The capsule (top) contains collagenous fibers (yellow-brown) and scattered delicate reticular fibers (black). Small lymphocytes are present within the subcapsular sinus (S), which is bridged by a few reticular fibers. Below this, there is a portion of a cortical lymph nodule in which there is a delicate meshwork of reticular fibers between the massed lymphocytes. Concentrations of reticular fibers also are present around small blood vessels (V), sectioned obliquely. Bielschowsky's method. High power.*

*Diffuse lymphoid tissue* is the simplest form of lymphoid tissue. It occurs principally as an infiltration of the lamina propria of mucous membranes. The chief locations are the alimentary and respiratory tracts. The lymphocytes that infiltrate the lamina propria are not packed closely together and do not show any special organization. The reticular cells are arranged in an apparent syncytium in close relation with the reticular (argyrophil) fibers. The manner in which lymphocytes are assembled varies with the locality and the amount of reticulum present. There are cells present within the reticulum that possess little cytoplasm and are relatively undifferentiated. Others have more cytoplasm and have acquired phagocytic properties. These are fixed macrophages that, on detachment from the reticular network, become free macrophages. These cells play an important part in the defense reactions of the body and in the general metabolism. In the defense reactions, their role is destruction of invading bacteria. In the general metabolism of the body, these cells dispose of disintegrating cellular material. Small lymphocytes are the most common of the free cells present. In addition, hemocytoblasts (lymphoblasts), monocytes, and plasma cells occupy spaces between the reticular cells and fibers.

*Lymph*, or *primary*, *nodules* are nonencapsulated aggregations of lymphocytes arranged in spherical masses. These aggregations, which present a more or less definite or circumscribed outline, have been called the structural units of lymphoid tissue. Encapsulated aggregations of lymph nodules form the so-called lymph organs. Nodules vary in diameter from a few hundred microns, or micrometers ($\mu$m), to a millimeter or more, and the periphery of each nodule is poorly defined and is not separated from the surrounding tissues by a connective tissue capsule. A diffuse border of small lymphocytes circumscribes these irregular masses and separates the nodule from the surrounding connective tissue. Each nodule may be homogeneous, or it may have an outer peripheral darker zone (*cortex*), containing closely packed small lymphocytes, and an inner pale *germinal center* (or *secondary nodule*). The presence of a germinal center is not constant but is correlated with the functional activity of the nodule. The central area develops in response to an antigenic stimulation and contains lymphoblasts

and large- and medium-sized lymphocytes in addition to small lymphocytes. In the germinal center, the lymphocytes are not as closely crowded as in the darker area by which it is surrounded. The meshes of the supporting reticular network are wider in the germinal center than in adjacent parts and permit the lymphocytes to separate from one another. It is a zone of rapid proliferation, and the size of the center is an indication of the level of the immunological response. Active proliferation is indicated by the presence of mitotic figures in the centers. A germinal center is lighter than the surrounding lymphatic tissue because its cells have more cytoplasm than do mature lymphocytes, and their nuclei are less chromatic. Generally, many more lymphocytes are produced in the center than are released, and these are phagocytosed by the macrophages present within the supporting reticular tissue. It should be emphasized that lymph nodules are not constant features, either in structure or in position. Involution may be associated with cessation of mitotic activity in the germinal center, which stains lightly when its stem cells disappear, leaving only reticular cells and a few macrophages. In this manner, they appear, remain for a time, and then disappear. Nodules are rare in the newborn and in animals maintained in an aseptic environment, since their formation is dependent upon antigenic stimuli. Similarly, new nodules may arise in diffuse lymphatic tissue at any time as an expression of the cytogenetic and defense functions of the lymphatic tissue. Thus, lymphatic nodules may exhibit a germinal center that contains activated B lymphocytes in the process of dividing and ultimately changing into plasma cells.

These nonencapsulated structures may be *solitary* or may occur as *aggregate nodules* in specific lymphoid organs such as lymph nodes, tonsils, and the spleen. The solitary nodules or *follicles* present in the mucosa of the intestinal tract are isolated nodules. Nodules may also be closely grouped into structures less highly organized than lymph nodes, forming nonencapsulated masses called *Peyer's patches* that are located in the small intestine, especially the ileum, and in the appendix.

The lymph nodes, encapsulated kidney-shaped structures, are the only lymphoid organs interposed along the course of the larger lymphatics

(Fig. 9–2). Thus, they possess both afferent and efferent lymphatic vessels. The tonsils, spleen, and thymus have efferent vessels draining from them, but they are not associated with afferent lymphatic vessels.

### THE LYMPH NODES

Lymph nodes are variable in number but occur in certain areas of the body such as the prevertebral region and the axillary and inguinal regions,

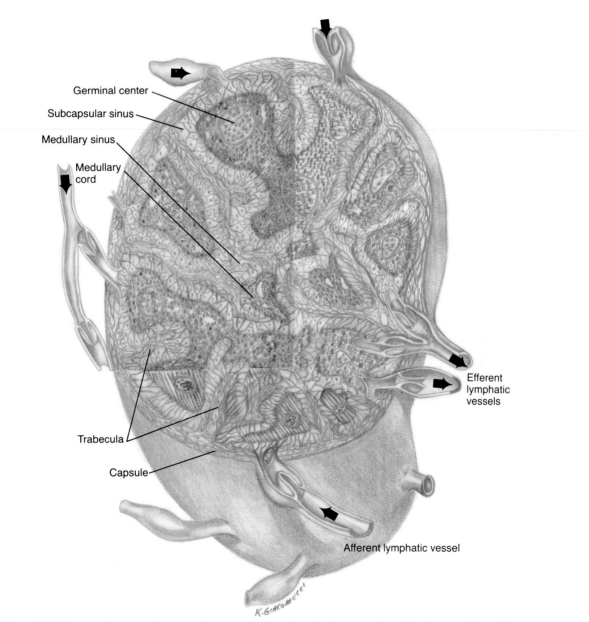

Germinal center

Subcapsular sinus

Medullary sinus

Medullary cord

Trabecula

Capsule

Efferent lymphatic vessels

Afferent lymphatic vessel

K·GIACOMUCCI

***Figure 9–2.*** *Diagram illustrating the general structure of a lymph node. Arrows indicate the direction of lymph flow.*

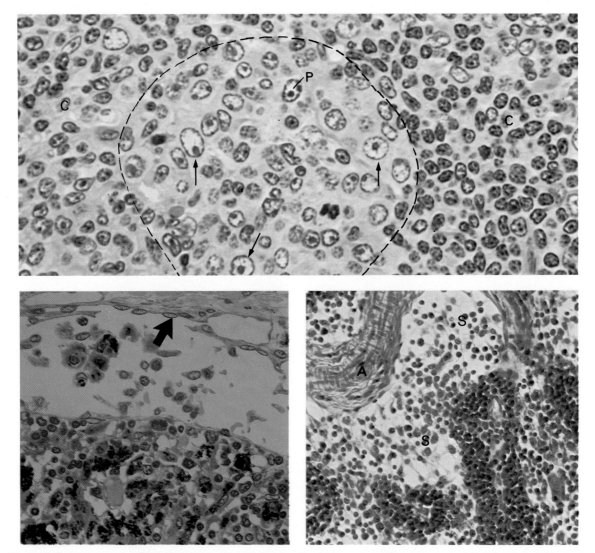

**Figure 9–3.** Lymph nodes. Top: The germinal center (outlined) contains principally medium-sized lymphocytes. A few cells (arrows) show large nuclei with distinct nucleoli. These are large lymphocytes and lymphoblasts. Occasional plasma cells (P) also occur in this zone. Small lymphocytes, produced within the germinal center, are pushed to the periphery and constitute the cortex of the nodule (C). Plastic section. H and E. Oil immersion. Bottom left: A portion of the capsule is present at the top. Immediately beneath it is the subcapsular sinus, lined by endothelium (arrow) and containing a few cells, principally small lymphocytes. Below this, there is a portion of the cortex of a lymph nodule. The collections of black material are carbon particles that have been taken up by the actively phagocytic cells associated with the reticulum. The carbon particles were inhaled and passed via the pulmonary lymphatic vessels to the node. Plastic section. H and E. High power. Bottom right: Portions of several medullary cords occupy the lower half of the field. They appear densely stained owing to the concentrations of lymphocytes within them. A small arteriole (A) shows elongated nuclei of the endothelium lining the narrow lumen and nuclei of smooth muscle cells circularly arranged. The vessel lies within connective tissue of a trabecula. Medullary sinuses (S) occupy the interval between the medullary cords and the trabeculae. They are incompletely lined by fixed macrophages and reticular cells and contain numerous free cells, principally small lymphocytes. H and E. Medium power.

where they exist in groups. Lymph nodes are especially numerous in the mesentery, in connection with the mesenteric lymph vessels. Each node is a somewhat flattened, bean-shaped body, ranging from 1 to 25 mm in diameter (Fig. 9–3). It has a convex contour except at an indented region, the *hilum* (or *hilus*), on one of its borders, where the blood vessels enter and leave the node. A number of afferent lymphatic vessels penetrate the capsule at multiple points on the convex surface of the node. Efferent vessels leave only at the hilum.

Lymph nodes are covered by a definite *capsule* of connective tissue that does not lie directly on the parenchyma but is separated from it by a space, the *marginal sinus*. The capsular material is continuous with a number of *septa* or *trabeculae* that extend into the substance of the organ. Reticular fibers may be seen crossing the sinus from the capsule, and trabeculae, to the parenchyma. The parenchyma of each node is specialized into two regions, an outer, or *cortical, portion,* characterized by the presence of lymph nodules,

and an inner, or *medullary, portion,* in which the trabeculae branch and anastomose to form irregular, anastomosing cords (Fig. 9–4). The connective tissue of the capsule also penetrates the gland at the hilum.

### Framework

The capsule consists of compactly arranged collagenous fibers with scattered elastic fibers. The latter form a loose network of fibers, particularly on the inner surface of the capsule, where they become more plentiful. At the hilum, the capsule is somewhat thicker. Trabeculae of dense collagenous fibers arise from the inner aspect of the capsule (at right angles), extend into the cortical portion of the gland, and incompletely divide it into compartments. In the medullary portion, the trabeculae become highly branched and finally fuse with the connective tissue of the hilum. A few smooth muscle fibers occur in the capsule, particularly at sites where lymphatic vessels enter

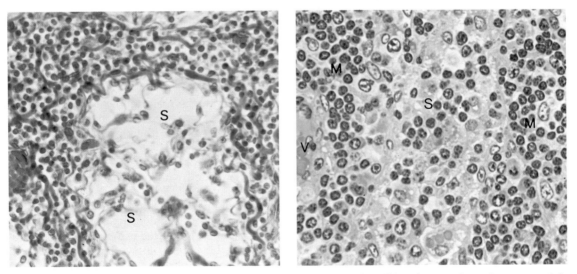

***Figure 9–4.*** *Lymph nodes. Left: Lymph node. The dark, irregular masses of small lymphocytes shown here are medullary cords. In addition to lymphocytes, the cords contain a few collagenous fibers (blue) and small blood vessels (red). The wide, irregular spaces are medullary lymph sinuses (S), which contain a few small lymphocytes. The sinuses are lined by reticular cells and fixed macrophages, which are irregular in shape and have long cytoplasmic extensions that appear to join with those of neighboring cells. The supporting reticular network has not been stained specifically. Azan. High power. Right: Lymph node, medulla. Portions of two medullary cords (M), composed mainly of small lymphocytes, are shown. Between them, there is a medullary sinus (S) containing numerous small lymphocytes. A small blood vessel (V) is associated with one medullary cord. Plastic section. H and E. High power.*

the node, and in the trabeculae. Their functional significance is unknown. The capsule, hilum, and trabeculae constitute the collagenous framework. Within the framework, there is a delicate meshwork of reticular connective tissue, comprising reticular fibers, reticular cells, and fixed macrophages. The spaces within this reticulum form the *lymph sinuses*, through which lymph percolates, and these sinuses contain free cells. The fibers of the reticulum blend with the fibers of the trabeculae and capsule. The reticulum extends as a delicate network and can be visualized readily in silver-impregnated histological preparations.

### Cortex

The degree of development of the trabeculae and the separation of the cortex into compartments vary in nodes of different animals and in nodes taken from different regions of the body. In humans, the compartments are not as definite as in many lower mammals. Within the cortical compartments, the lymphocytes are closely packed into nodules that are attached indirectly by reticulum to the nearby capsule and trabeculae (Fig. 9–5). The nodules are separated from the capsule and trabeculae by spaces, the lymph sinuses, through which the lymph circulates. Although the cortex usually is found surrounding the medulla except at the hilum, it shows considerable variation in thickness.

The cortical nodules often contain germinal centers; as in solitary nodules, however, these are inconstant features. Component cells of each germinal center are larger and possess more cytoplasm and paler nuclei than do the small lymphocytes. Hence, the whole central area appears lighter in stained sections. Most of the cells are medium-sized lymphocytes. A few are large, undifferentiated lymphocytes (lymphoblasts) and plasma cells. During an active phase, small lymphocytes are produced by the cells of the germinal center and are pushed outward into a peripheral zone, which becomes the *cortex of the nodule*. After a time, mitotic activity diminishes, the former growth pressure subsides, and the sharp boundary between the germinal center and the cortex disappears. The center becomes inactive, and the nodule returns to its homogeneous, resting appearance. Under certain pathological conditions,

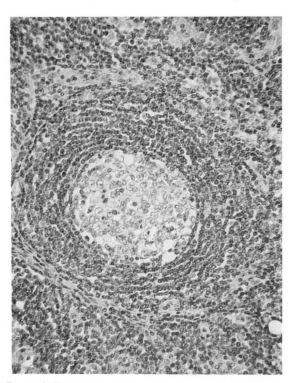

*Figure 9–5.* A cortical nodule. Component cells of the germinal center are large with pale nuclei and are surrounded by closely packed small lymphocytes. H and E. Medium power.

some of the pale centers contain numerous free macrophages. These areas have been called *reaction centers*.

Internal to the major cortical zone, there is an intermediate zone, called the *paracortex*, which separates the cortex (the more peripheral portion) from the medulla. The cortex is recognized by the presence of lymphatic nodules. The paracortex is provided with numerous specialized postcapillary venules lined with a simple cuboidal endothelium (venules in other parts of the body are lined by a simple squamous endothelium) and many lymphocytes within their walls. Experimental studies have shown that the lymphocytes of this zone, unlike those of the cortex proper, are of thymic origin (*T* lymphocytes) and are concerned with the cell-mediated immune response. T lymphocytes in the general circulation seem to be attracted to the cuboidal cells of the endothelium, adhere, and then squeeze between them to penetrate the paracortex, or *thymus-*

*dependent zone.* The postcapillary venules represent sites of exchange from blood to lymph of T lymphocytes. The latter may leave the lymph node via the efferent lymph vessels at the hilus.

On the other hand, the cortex proper, and particularly its nodules, is a region where *B* lymphocytes are concentrated and where stimulation by an antigen leads to the proliferation of small lymphocytes and plasma cells concerned with the production of specific humoral antibodies. The latter cells develop from the activated B lymphocytes and are primarily found in the medullary cords (tail regions of lymphatic nodules that enter the medulla) as nonmotile cells whose secreted immunoglobulin may be found in peripheral blood. Plasma cells are rarely seen in lymph or in the general blood circulation as fully differentiated cells. Activated B lymphocytes are seen in the germinal centers of the lymph nodules as intense basophil cells owing to increased RNA content. The germinal centers of lymph nodes, unlike those present in unencapsulated lymphatic nodules, have a specialized kind of reticular cell called a *dendritic reticular cell.* The long cytoplasmic processes of these cells offer an extensive surface area for the binding of newly formed immunoglobulin. If they are exposed again to the same antigen, these cells can bind it and make it readily available to the B lymphocytes. The germinal centers, in addition to containing the aforementioned cells, have many macrophages and some T lymphocytes. With age, nodules involute, and lymphatic activity is markedly reduced, with subsequent replacement of parenchymal cells by adipose cells.

## Medulla

The cellular components of the medulla and cortex are similar, but there is a difference in arrangement. The medulla consists of diffuse lymphoid tissue in the form of branching lymphoid strands, or *lymph cords,* that enclose a number of open lymph spaces. These cords contain B lymphocytes and descendants of activated B lymphocytes (plasma cells) and are seen coursing between the irregular branching and anastomosing trabeculae in the middle of the gland. Some lymph (medullary) cords are continuous with the deep surface of the cortical tissue and appear as extensions of it into the underlying medulla. They are surrounded by medullary lymph sinuses. Reticular fibers may be seen crossing the sinus and attaching the cords to adjacent trabeculae. This arrangement of dense lymph tissue, sinuses, and trabeculae is similar to that found in the cortex. The medulla is surrounded on all sides by the cortex, except at the hilum.

## Lymphatic Vessels and Sinuses

The circulation of lymph through a lymph node involves afferent lymphatic vessels, a system of lymph sinuses within the node, and efferent lymphatic vessels. Several afferent vessels pierce the capsule on the convex side of the node and open into the system of lymph sinuses. The afferent vessels are provided with valves that open toward the node. Each node contains a tortuous system of irregular channels, the *sinuses,* within the lymphoid tissue (Fig. 9–6). Unlike the endothelium-lined blood vascular and lymphatic vessels, the sinuses generally have walls that are not continuous. They are incompletely lined by reticular cells and fixed macrophages (*littoral cells*), supported by reticular fibers. The sinuses are bridged by further reticular cells that are interconnected by delicate cytoplasmic processes to form a network that is three-dimensional. The walls allow the free movement of lymphocytes from the nodules and medullary cords into the sinuses and thus into the efferent lymphatic vessels. The sinus system comprises three parts. Afferent vessels enter the *marginal,* or *subcapsular,* sinus, which separates the capsule from the cortical parenchyma. From the marginal sinus, lymph flows into the *cortical sinuses,* which lie between the cortical nodules and the trabeculae. Some electron microscopic studies indicate that the outer wall of the marginal sinus and the trabecular side of cortical sinuses possess an intact, continuous endothelium with a basal lamina. Thus, sinus walls adjacent to connective tissue limit movement of lymphocytes, whereas those adjacent to lymphoid tissue have gaps that permit free movement of cells. Cortical sinuses are continuous with *medullary sinuses,* which are interposed between medullary trabeculae and medullary cords. The medullary sinuses pierce the thickened portion of the capsule at the hilum and continue into the

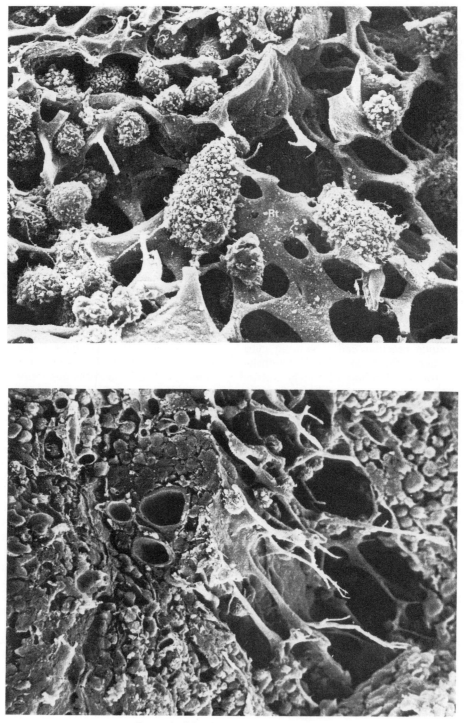

***Figure 9–6*** See legend on opposite page

efferent lymphatic vessels. The efferent vessels are fewer and wider than the afferent vessels and contain valves that open away from the nodes. The arrangement of valves in the afferent and efferent vessels allows a flow of lymph in only one direction through the node.

### Blood Vessels and Nerves

Arteries enter the lymph node at the hilum and give branches to the medullary cords and to the trabeculae. The branches to the cords continue into the cortex to supply the cortical nodules. Branches to the trabeculae supply the connective tissue of the trabeculae and ultimately reach the capsule. Dense capillary plexuses are present within the medullary cords and the cortical nodules. From the capillaries, blood is collected into postcapillary venules that, in the deep (paracortical) cortex, are lined by cuboidal endothelial cells. Lymphocytes of the recirculating type, principally T lymphocytes, apparently recognize the cuboidal endothelium as a site for migration. The migration may occur either by an intercellular or intracellular (transcellular) route, but more recent evidence favors the latter. Lymphocytes that leave the venules penetrate the paracortical zone and medullary sinuses and leave the node by the efferent vessels to return via the thoracic duct to the blood vascular system. By this route, most T lymphocytes recirculate many times. The postcapillary venules then drain into veins that follow the same general route taken by the arteries and leave the node at the hilum.

Nerves, which are mostly vasomotor, enter the hilum with the blood vessels and follow them into the interior of the node.

### Functions of Lymph Nodes

One of the primary functions of lymph nodes is the production of lymphocytes, which enter the sinuses partly by ameboid activity and partly by crowding pressure. Lymph is not markedly cellular until it has passed through a lymph node. The development of new lymphocytes from undifferentiated cells has been described previously (see Chapter 5). The actual stimuli for lymphopoiesis both in physiological and in pathological conditions are unknown. In certain pathological conditions, extramedullary hemopoiesis occurs, and the lymph nodes produce myeloid elements. The fact that lymph in efferent vessels is more cellular than that in afferent vessels is not due principally to production of lymphocytes in lymph nodes, however. Studies using transfused labeled cells have shown that the majority of lymphocytes leaving a lymph node are of the recirculating type.

Lymph nodes filter lymph by means of the phagocytic activity of the fixed and detached reticular cells. They remove degenerating cells, including erythrocytes, and particulate matter from the lymph. A good example of the latter is provided by the bronchial lymph nodes. Inhaled carbon particles eventually reach the bronchial lymph nodes, where they are taken up by the macrophages, often in such quantity that the nodes appear entirely black.

The lymph nodes also play a role in the formation of antibodies and engage in cellular immunity responses to regional antigens. The antigens engulfed in the venous sinuses and medullary regions are able to interact with recirculating T cells and B cells. Activated T cells in the paracortical areas and activated B cells in the

**Figure 9–6.** *Sinus and pulp in closer view. Top: Axillary node of the guinea pig. Reticular cells (Rt) in the sinus are smooth-surfaced, though in this micrograph they are contaminated by a small amount of coagulated lymph plasm. Macrophages (M) in the guinea pig are especially large and, as in other species, characteristically rough-surfaced. The pulp, upper right in the micrograph, is bounded by a lining cell layer next to the sinus. The pulp consists of round cells and reticular cells that are smaller in size than the sinal reticular cells. × 1900. Bottom: Trabeculae of lymph node. Mesenteric node of the dog. The lymph node tissue is supported by the capsule and trabeculae composed of thick collagen fibers. This micrograph shows a trabecula revealing its blood vessels and collagen bundles transversely cut. The latter fan out into fine fibrils supporting the parenchyma of the node. Facing the sinus, the surfaces of the trabecula and its branches are covered by a thin layer of lining and reticular cells. × 780. (Reproduced with permission from Fujita, T., et al.: SEM Atlas of Cells and Tissues. New York, Igaku-Shoin, 1981.)*

lymphoid follicles proliferate into cell groups (*clones*) having the same antigen specificity. Later, the T cells move into the lymphoid follicles and interact with B cells and macrophages. These latter cells proliferate to form the *germinal centers*, which push the smaller lymphocytes to the periphery, or *mantle*. The resulting mantle plus germinal center is called a *secondary nodule*. Within the germinal center, the activated B cells are transformed into plasma cells, which produce large quantities of antibody. Both T and B cells may differentiate into *memory cells*; these do not make a response but are readily induced to become activated cells by a later encounter with the same antigen. In this manner, lymph nodes provide a pool of stem cells capable of changing into antibody-producing cells and mounting an immune response that is both humoral and cellular. Additionally, lymphocytes return from the blood stream to the lymphatic channels via the lymph nodes.

Thus, the lymph node exhibits a filtering function by the removal of foreign substance from lymph via macrophagic action. This may lead to additional lymphocyte formation through activated clonal expansion of its resident lymphocyte population. The latter could take the form of increased numbers of plasma cells or *killer cells* (a cytotoxic T lymphocyte produced in immune responses). The waxing and waning of germinal centers is a good predictor of the antigenic responses and demonstrates the continuous functional changes that occur within the parenchyma of the lymph node.

### Development of Lymph Nodes

Lymph nodes develop after the formation of the primary lymphatic vascular system. These lymphatic vessels develop from the vessels of the circulatory system. Through a process of budding and fusion of isolated groups of mesenchymal cells, a one-way primitive lymphatic system is formed that empties into the venous system. In the connective tissue associated with the developing lymphatic plexuses, peripherally located mesenchymal cells form the lymph nodes as interposed periodic lymphatic beads produced by infiltration of the lymphatic plexuses. Lymphocytes form *in situ* from the mesenchymal cells.

Lymph sinuses develop as isolated lymph spaces within mesenchyme. The spaces fuse to form a system of anastomosing sinuses throughout the developing node. Later this system comes into contact with the afferent and efferent lymphatic vessels. Connective tissue fibers aggregate against the flattened ends of the lymphatic buds, forming the capsule around the developing lymph node. The buds continue to proliferate around the nodes which eventually fuse to form the marginal sinus under the connective tissue capsule. The capsule extends into the node as the trabeculae, which always remain separated from the concentrations of lymphoid tissue by sinuses. The medullary region differentiates in advance of the cortex, and germinal centers within the latter usually do not appear until after birth. Thus, the basic pattern of the adult lymph node is formed.

### Hemal (Hemolymph) Nodes

In certain animals, there are structures that are very similar to lymph nodes, except that they contain large numbers of erythrocytes. These structures, the *hemal nodes*, are common in ruminants, such as sheep, but they probably do not occur in humans. The general organization is similar to that of a lymph node, in that the hemal node consists of a mass of lymphatic tissue covered by a connective tissue capsule. The sinuses, however, are purely blood sinuses. In the hog, there are structures that are intermediate between a lymph node and a hemal node. Both blood vessels and lymphatics connect with the sinuses. Both afferent and efferent lymph vessels are wanting. Thus both sinuses and lymph spaces are filled with erythrocytes. In this instance, the term *hemolymph node* is most appropriate. The presence of macrophages containing pigmented cytoplasm indicates that the worn-out erythrocytes are dispatched in the hemolymph nodes. Hemal nodes are lymphopoietic and also filter blood.

### THE TONSILS

The *tonsils* are aggregates of unencapsulated lymphoid tissue that lie in close association with a wet epithelial membrane. There are three tonsillar groups, the *palatine tonsils*, the *lingual tonsil*, and the *pharyngeal tonsil*, forming a ring of lymphoid tissue surrounding the pharynx, where nasal and oral passages unite. Small accumulations of lymphoid tissue about the pharyngeal orifice of the *Eustachian* (auditory) tubes are called the *tubal tonsils*. The latter is sometimes considered as the fourth tonsillar group. The tonsils are characterized by depressions of the surface epithelium around which aggregates of lymph nodules are grouped. The extension of the overlying epithelium down into the lymphatic tissue forms deep pits called *crypts*. Lymphocytes can pass through this epithelium, and mucus-secreting glands, in the peritonsillar tissue, can cleanse the crypts. The incomplete ring of lymphoid tissue consisting of pharyngeal, palatine, and lingual tonsils is known as the *pharyngeal lymphoid ring of Waldeyer*.

### Palatine Tonsils

The palatine, or *faucial*, tonsils are paired, ovoid masses of lymphoid tissue that occupy the inter-vals between the glossopalatine and pharyngo-palatine arches (Figs. 9–7 and 9–8). They lie in the connective tissue of the mucosa and are covered on their free surface by a stratified squamous epithelium that is continuous with the lining of the mouth and pharynx. The epithelium rests upon a basal lamina, under which there is a thin layer of fibrous connective tissue. At various places on the surface of the tonsil, deep indentations, ten to twenty in number, occur. These indentations, or *tonsillar crypts*, penetrate into the interior of the tonsil and are lined by a continuation of the surface epithelium. Frequently, secondary crypts, also lined by epithelium, extend from the bases and sides of the main, or primary, crypts. Lymphoid tissue surrounds the crypts as a diffuse mass in which are embedded lymph nodules. The nodules, like those of lymph nodes, may contain germinal centers. In the deeper parts of the crypts, there is no clear delineation between epithelium and lymphoid tissue because of an intense infiltration of the epithelium with lymphocytes.

Adjacent to the deepest portions of the tonsil, the fibrous tissue is condensed to form a thin

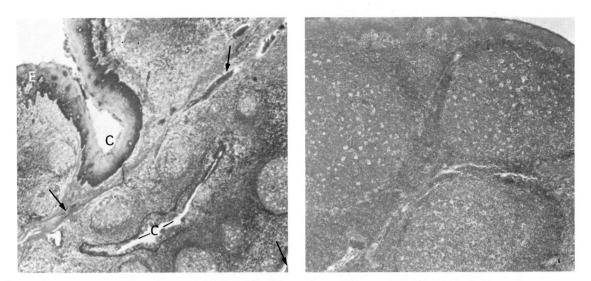

***Figure 9–7.*** *Tonsils. Left: Palatine tonsils are masses of lymphoid tissue within the mucosa and are covered by nonkeratinizing stratified squamous epithelium. Here, the surface epithelium (E) invaginates into the underlying lymphoid tissue to form an irregular crypt (C). Lymphoid tissue surrounds the crypt as a diffuse mass in which are embedded lymph nodules, some with germinal centers. Connective tissue septa (arrows) surround the lymphoid tissue associated with the crypt. Masson. Low power. Right: Palatine tonsil. The tonsillar tissue consists of a diffuse mass of lymphoid tissue that contains circumscribed lymph nodules with large germinal centers. At the top, the tissue is covered by stratified squamous epithelium. H and E. Medium power.*

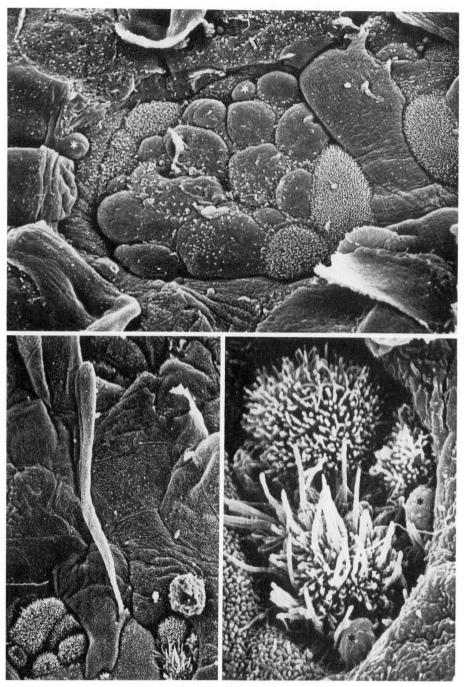

***Figure 9–8*** See legend on opposite page

capsule that covers the base and sides of the tonsil. Connective tissue septa extend into the interior of the tonsil and separate the various crypts, with their surrounding zones of lymphatic tissue, from one another. Small mucous glands lie in the connective tissue beneath the tonsil and its capsule. Their ducts open, for the most part, onto the free surface; occasionally, they may open into the tonsillar crypts.

### Lingual Tonsil

The *lingual tonsil* is located in the root of the tongue, behind the circumvallate papillae. It consists of an aggregation of wide-mouthed epithelial pits, each surrounded by lymphoid tissue. Each simple pit, or crypt, is lined by a continuation of the surface stratified squamous epithelium. The lymphoid tissue comprises a layer of lymph nodules, often with germinal centers. In most crypts there is marked infiltration of the epithelium with lymphocytes. Ducts of underlying mucous glands open onto the surface or into the crypts.

### Pharyngeal Tonsil

The *pharyngeal tonsil* is an accumulation of lymphoid tissue in the median posterior wall of the nasopharynx (Fig. 9–9). The lymphatic tissue is similar to that of the palatine tonsils. The epithelium over the free surface is folded, but no true crypts occur. In general, the epithelium is pseudostratified with cilia and goblet cells, but in the adult, there may be islands of stratified squamous epithelium. The epithelium is extensively

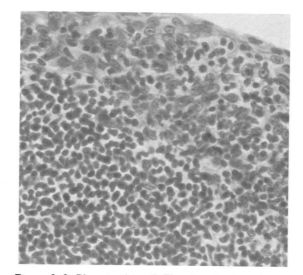

**Figure 9–9.** *Pharyngeal tonsil. The pharyngeal tonsil is an accumulation of lymphoid tissue within the posterior wall of the nasopharynx. The epithelium over the free surface generally is pseudostratified with cilia and goblet cells, but in the adult, there often are extensive islands of stratified squamous epithelium, as shown here. The boundary between the epithelium and the underlying lymphoid tissue is indistinct because of the extensive invasion of epithelium by lymphocytes. H and E. High power.*

infiltrated with lymphocytes. A thin capsule surrounds the pharyngeal tonsil and sends septa into the cores of epithelial folds. Mixed seromucous glands occur in the connective tissue beneath the capsule, and their ducts open onto the free surface or into the furrows between the folds. Hypertrophy of the pharyngeal tonsil, with consequent obstruction of the nasal openings, is common and is known clinically as *adenoids*.

---

**Figure 9–8.** *Human palatine tonsil. Top: An overview of a fungiform cell patch. Careful observation of this picture suggests that there may be transitional forms between the fungiform cells and the cells forming the stratified epithelium. Some of the fungiform cells are covered by microvilli. A few small round cells (*) may be lymphocytes passing through the epithelium. × 5900. It seems an attractive hypothesis that the fungiform cell patch represents a pass through which antigenic and invasive information from the oral cavity is introduced into the lymphoid tissue and through which antibodies, lymphocytes, and other protective elements may come out. Bottom left: Shows another part of the cryptal epithelium. The squamous epithelial cells are noteworthily polymorphous. The microplicae conspicuously differ in density from cell to cell; a few cells are covered by microvilli. A peculiar, long projection of an apparently waste cell is shown in the middle. At the bottom are two fungiform cell patches. × 2100. Bottom right: A closer view of one of the patches. Besides fungiform cells covered by microvilli, a cell possessing cilia in addition to microvilli is demonstrated. Bodies labeled with an asterisk possibly represent the heads of migrating lymphocytes. × 10,000. (Reproduced with permission from Fujita, T., et al.: SEM Atlas of Cells and Tissues. New York, Igaku-Shoin, 1981.)*

### Tubal Tonsils

The *tubal tonsils* sometimes are considered a separate tonsillar group. Each tubal tonsil lies around the pharyngeal orifice of the pharyngotympanic (auditory) tube and constitutes a lateral extension of the pharyngeal tonsil. The tubal tonsil is covered with ciliated columnar epithelium.

### Functions and Development of Tonsils

Blood vessels course in the capsule and septa of the tonsils and supply the lymphoid tissue. The tonsils possess no afferent lymphatic vessels. Plexuses of lymph capillaries occur around the lymphoid tissue and drain into efferent lymphatic vessels. The tonsils, which reach their maximum development in childhood and thereafter decline, constitute a discontinuous ring of lymphoid tissue around the pharynx. They participate in lymphocyte production and aid in the protection of the body against invading bacteria, viruses, and other foreign proteins. As in other lymphoid tissue, the foreign proteins (antigens) stimulate the production of antibodies in plasma cells, which themselves are derived from lymphocytes. On the other hand, epithelial erosion would seem to enhance an invasion by microorganisms, and the tonsils are known to be frequent portals of infection.

### THE THYMUS

The thymus, a lymphoepithelial organ, is the only lobulated lymphoid organ (Fig. 9–10). The thymus varies in size and development with the age of the individual. It attains its maximum development around puberty, after which it becomes inconspicuous.

It has neither lymph nodules nor sinuses, consists of two large lobes closely applied and united by connective tissue, and extends from the root of the neck into the upper part of the thorax, where it is located behind the sternum. A lobe is composed of thousands of *lobules*, each containing a peripheral *cortical* and a central *medullary* component. The lobules are incompletely isolated

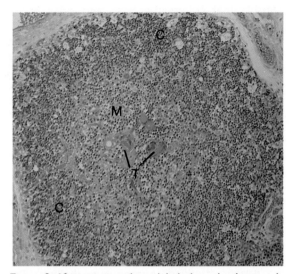

**Figure 9–10.** *A portion of one lobule from the thymus of a child is shown. It is surrounded by a delicate capsule composed of collagenous fibers. Lymphocytes (thymocytes) are densely packed within the cortex (C) and are less numerous in the medulla (M). The pale-staining bodies within the medulla are thymic corpuscles (T). Plastic section. H and E. Low power.*

units separated from one another only along their lateral margins, since the medulla constitutes a central core to each lobe and sends prolongations into each lobule. A capsule encloses each lobe and is composed mainly of collagenous fibers and some elastic fibers. It is not highly organized, and it merges with the surrounding areolar connective tissue. The inward extensions from the capsule (*septa*) delineate the lobules. Interlobular septa extend from the capsule as far as the medulla and thus partially separate the lobules from each other. In addition, intralobular *trabeculae* arise from the fibroelastic capsule and pass into the cortex of the lobules. The reticular connective tissue of the thymus differs in some respects from that of the other lymphoid organs. The reticular cells, which support the parenchyma, arise from entoderm rather than from mesoderm. These reticular cells are not phagocytic and do not have associated reticular fibers. True mesodermal reticulum is confined to the area around the blood vessels. In tissue culture, these cells have been shown to possess epithelioid characteristics reflecting their origin as tubular diverticula from the epithelium of the third pharyngeal pouch. As a result of the growth of these cells, the lobation of the thymus becomes more definitely established.

These *epithelial reticular cells* are stellate and possess ovoid, pale-staining nuclei with distinct nucleoli. The cells form an interconnecting meshwork by opposition of their branching cytoplasmic processes. The junctions between processes of neighboring cells show typical desmosomes with associated tonofibrillae. The cytoplasm is characterized by the presence of lysosomes, vacuoles, and electron-dense granules, possibly secretory in nature. The arrangement of the meshwork varies with location; in the cortex, it is open and has large interstices, and in the medulla it forms a system of incomplete anastomosing sheets. Additionally, the meshwork occurs as incomplete sheets over the connective tissue of the capsule and the trabeculae and ensheathes the major blood vessels of the cortex and the medulla. Many investigators believe that the latter arrangement constitutes a *blood-thymic barrier*, similar to the blood-brain barrier in the central nervous system formed by the glial cells, and that it limits access of certain circulating materials, particularly proteins, into the thymic parenchyma. The epithelial reticular cells, unlike true reticular cells of mes-

enchymal origin, do not phagocytose colloidal dyes and generally are not associated with reticular fibers.

The thymus appears to be the only part of the human body with reticular cells derived from endoderm. The epithelial reticular cells of the cortex appear to be responsible for the secretion of *thymic hormone* (or thymosin). This hormone influences the differentiation of T lymphocytes. The differentiated progeny can be visualized as dark-staining small lymphocytes that obscure the cellular reticulum. The blood-thymic barrier is believed to shield the small lymphocytes from antigenic substances within the cortex.

### Cortex and Medulla

The small lymphocytes, mentioned above, are present in the cortex and sometimes are called *thymocytes* (Fig. 9–11). The latter are densely and uniformly packed dark-staining cells that are found only in the cortex, the medulla appearing pale in comparison. The thymocytes appear similar in structure to lymphocytes elsewhere, although their origin differs. They arise by division of stem cells that originally migrated to the thymus

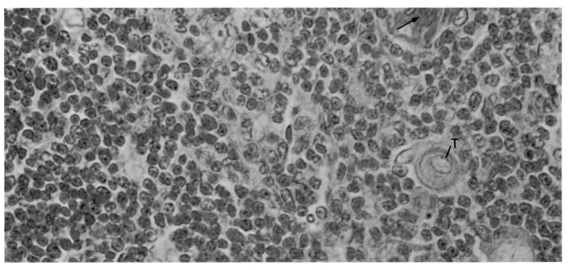

*Figure 9–11.* The cortex of the thymus, which occupies the left half of the field, contains densely packed lymphocytes within a meshwork of delicate connective tissue (pale blue). In the medulla (right half of field), lymphocytes are less densely packed and a thymic corpuscle of Hassall (T) is present. A portion of a trabecula (arrow) also is shown. Azan. High power.

from the bone marrow. The thymocytes occupy the interstices of the sparse reticular meshwork and obscure the epithelial reticular cells. The lymphatic tissue, unlike that of lymph nodes, is not arranged in nodules. The medulla stains more lightly and is less compact than the cortex. The thymocytes are less numerous in the medulla, and consequently, the epithelial reticular cells are prominent. In addition to thymocytes, lymphocytes of medium and large size are present, particularly in the medulla. Myoid cells also have been described in the medulla of some species.

True macrophages vary in number but are most common in the cortex in perivascular regions and in relation to the capsule and to the trabeculae. They are similar in structure to macrophages elsewhere and are concerned with the phagocytosis of thymocytes. It has been estimated that the majority of thymocytes produced in the cortex are destroyed and that only a small minority of cells is released.

The most characteristic feature of the thymus is the presence of *thymic corpuscles* (of Hassall) (Fig. 9–12). They are spherical or ovoid structures composed of concentrically arranged epithelial reticular cells and are localized principally in the medulla. The thymic corpuscle results from the growth and transformation of epithelial reticular cells. The corpuscle is acidophil and varies in diameter from 20 to more than 100 micrometers ($\mu$m). The central cells are large and often show evidence of hyalinization and degeneration into a formless mass that may even undergo calcification. The surrounding cells are flattened, crescentic elements concentrically arranged about the central cells. It is by the initial enlargement of the central cells that crescentic transformations of the surrounding cells are brought about. The surrounding cells may retain connections with the nearby typical epithelial reticular cells. The corpuscles become increasingly prominent during periods of intense destruction of thymocytes and during involution. Their significance is as yet unknown.

### Blood Vessels

The arteries supplying the thymus are derived from the internal thoracic and the inferior thyroid arteries. They branch and pass along the trabeculae before giving off arterioles, ensheathed by epithelial reticular cells, that enter the lobules at the junction between cortex and medulla. Nu-

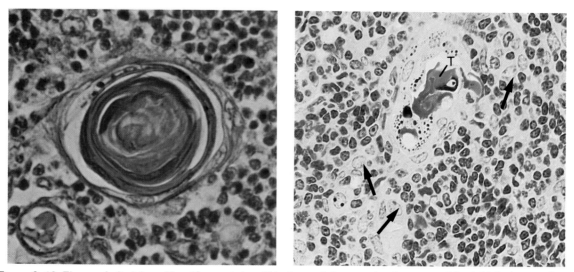

*Figure 9–12.* Thymus. Left: A large Hassall's corpuscle, within the medulla, occupies the center of the field. It shows a dense, hyalinized core surrounded by concentrically arranged, flattened epithelial cells. H and E. High power. Right: Scattered between the small lymphocytes are epithelial reticular cells (arrows) that possess pale, vesicular nuclei. Also present is a small thymic corpuscle (T) with a hyalinized core surrounded by flattened epithelial cells. H and E. High power.

merous capillary branches pass from the arterioles into the cortex, and less regular branches into the medulla. Epithelial reticular cells surround all smaller vessels in the thymus, and although incomplete, they constitute a layer that separates blood from the thymocytes, particularly in the cortex. From the capillary bed, blood passes through postcapillary venules that, unlike those of lymph nodes, do not show a thickened endothelium. Thymocytes (lymphocytes) that proliferate in the cortex enter the blood vascular system through the walls of these vessels. Returning venules pass mainly into the medulla and from there to veins in the interlobular trabeculae. The latter drain into the left brachiocephalic and thyroid veins.

## Lymphatics

There are no afferent vessels and no lymph sinuses in the thymus. Efferent lymphatics run mainly in the interlobular connective tissue trabeculae to the anterior mediastinal lymph nodes.

## Nerves

A few branches of the vagus and cervical sympathetic nerves reach the thymus. They run along the walls of the blood vessels. Only vasomotor endings for the sympathetic nerves have been observed.

## Involution

The thymus reaches its maximum size at puberty and then begins to involute, a process that continues into old age. This age involution first involves a gradual loss of thymocytes from the cortex, with the result that the boundary between cortex and medulla becomes indistinct. The medulla also begins to atrophy at puberty. Adipose tissue replaces the thymocytes and epithelial reticular cells. The last elements to be replaced are the thymic corpuscles, which may be recognizable even in old age.

The thymus may show accidental involution (severe atrophy) as a result of a serious infection or increased secretion of adrenocorticoids.

## Functions of the Thymus

Lymphopoiesis is a known thymic activity and occurs principally during fetal and early postnatal life. Plasma cells and myelocytes also are formed in small numbers. In mice, removal of the thymus shortly after birth results in lymphocyte deficiency and in some form of diminished immunity. The mice grow for several months and then die, presumably owing to an inability to produce antibodies. In the meantime, the mice do not resist bacterial infections and will not reject skin grafts from other strains of mice. These phenomena do not occur if thymectomy is delayed until a few days after birth—when the extralymphatic lymphoid tissues and circulation are already stocked with T cells. Thus, it is postulated that the thymus is responsible for the production of a pool of circulating lymphocytes, or T cells. Most T cells, through their association with epithelial-reticular cells, recognize foreign antigens when these antigens are associated on the cell surface with membrane glycoproteins encoded in the major histocompatibility complex (*MHC*). The *MHC* glycoproteins are thought to serve as antigen-binding receptors that activate the appropriate T cell response to a specific foreign antigen. T cells migrate to other lymphoid organs, principally lymph nodes and spleen. Here they settle down in so-called *thymus-dependent* zones, including the paracortical zones of lymph nodes, the periarterial sheaths in the white pulp of the spleen, and the lymphoid tissue of Peyer's patches in the small intestine. They give rise to immunologically competent cells.

The cortical portion of the thymus has the function of producing T lymphocytes and, for this reason, is referred to as a *primary lymphoid center*. Lymphoid organs and tissues that harbor T lymphocytes (and are sites for antibody production) are called *secondary lymphoid centers*. Since lymphoid nodules do not occur in the thymus, antibodies are not produced in this organ. The primary lymphoid center in mammals for the maturation of B lymphocytes is probably the bone marrow.

In the adult, the thymus continues to be an important source of small lymphocytes, particularly if the individual has suffered depletion of the lymphoid organs by irradiation. There is evidence that, in addition, the thymus exerts a humoral effect upon other lymphoid tissues, particularly with regard to the stimulation of lymphocyte production and development of immunological competence. These substances appear to diffuse through a cell-tight filter and substitute for the thymus. The best known of these substances is *thymosin*. It is believed to be synthesized by the epithelial-reticular cells and can be separated into two low-molecular-weight glycoprotein fractions. Thymosin relieves T cell deficiencies in thymectomized mice. *Thymoprotein* is a substance that induces T cell maturation. *Thymic humoral factor* enhances the graft-versus-host reaction and *serum thymic factor* induces the development of markers in T cells.

The thymus contains stem cells for mast cell differentiation. Eosinophilopoiesis requires the presence of the thymus. The thymus is influenced by the gonads, adrenals, and thyroid gland. Gonadal hormones induce involution, and thyroidectomy hastens it.

There appears to be some relation between the thymus and *myasthenia gravis*, a clinical condition characterized by muscle weakness. Many individuals suffering from this disease have either a thymic tumor or an enlarged thymus, but the significance of the relationship remains obscure.

## Development of the Thymus

In humans, the thymus arises as a paired ventral outgrowth from the third branchial pouch. Each outgrowth has a narrow lumen at first, but this quickly is obliterated by proliferation of the lining epithelial cells. The epithelial cells differentiate, and some transform into epithelial reticular cells at about the end of the second month of development. Thymocytes (or lymphocytes) appear at this time also. It is thought that they arise from mesenchymal cells that invade the developing thymus. The lymphocytes proliferate rapidly, and the epithelium is converted into a reticular cell mass. Lobules form at this time, and connective tissue invades the lobes to form septa and trabeculae. Hassall's corpuscles first appear during fetal life and continue to form until involution is initiated. They are thought to arise from hypertrophied and degenerating epithelial cells.

## THE SPLEEN

The spleen is the largest of the lymphoid organs, and, with the possible exception of the hemal nodes, it is the only organ specialized for filtering blood (Fig. 9–13). It has no afferent lymphatic vessels, and its sinuses, as in the hemal nodes, are filled with blood instead of lymph.

The spleen, like the lymph nodes, has a collagenous framework within which is suspended a reticular network. It is surrounded by a capsule that itself is covered by a serous membrane, the *peritoneum* (Fig. 9–14). Many trabeculae pass from the capsule into the interior of the organ. At one point on the surface of the spleen, there is a deep indentation, the *hilum*, where blood vessels enter and leave. The parenchyma (*splenic pulp*) is of two distinct types:

1. *White pulp* is typical lymphatic tissue that surrounds and follows the arteries. At intervals, it is thickened into ovoid masses, the *splenic nodules* (or *Malpighian bodies*).

2. The *red pulp* is more abundant, often forms plates, the *pulp cords*, and is associated with numerous erythrocytes.

The structure of the spleen and the relations between the red and white pulp depend upon the arrangement and distribution of blood vessels. Arteries are connected closely with the white pulp, and the terminal blood vessels (sinuses and veins) with the red pulp.

The trabeculae delineate many compartments, or *lobules*, within the spleen (Fig. 9–15). A lobule is about 1 mm in diameter and is bounded by several trabeculae. Each lobule is supplied by a central artery and is drained by veins that run in trabeculae to leave the lobule (Fig. 9–16). The lobules are not distinct, since they are not outlined completely by trabeculae.

## Framework

The capsule and trabeculae of the spleen consist of dense collagenous connective tissue with some elastic fibers and some smooth muscle fibers. The capsule is thickest at the hilum, where it surrounds the major blood vessels. The external surface of the capsule is covered by a layer of

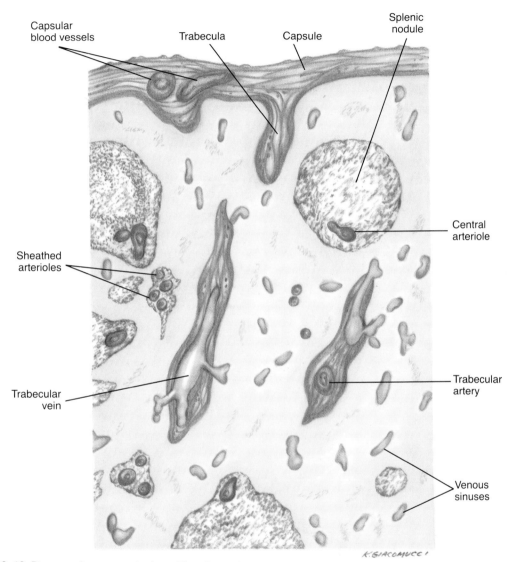

**Figure 9–13.** *Diagram of a section of spleen. The white pulp consists of nodules and aggregations of lymphocytes, and the red pulp is an open mesh with sinusoids.*

flattened mesothelial cells, a component of the peritoneum. Trabeculae radiate inward from the hilum and from the internal surface of the capsule. They branch and anastomose repeatedly to form a fairly complex framework throughout the interior. Smooth muscle elements within the capsule and trabeculae are responsible for the slow, rhythmical changes in volume of the spleen. The splenic pulp is supported by a fine meshwork of reticular fibers that blends with the capsule, trabeculae, and walls of the blood vessels. The cells in relation to the reticulum are, as in other lymphoid organs, primitive reticular cells and fixed macrophages.

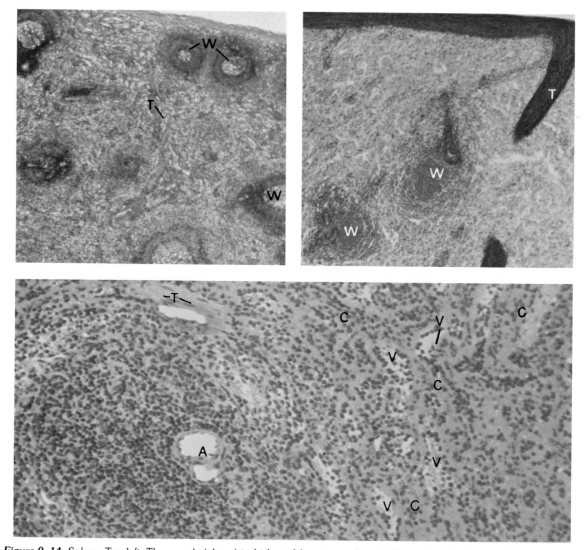

**Figure 9–14.** *Spleen. Top left: The capsule (above) is thick, and from it, a trabecula (T) runs into the interior of the organ. Red pulp forms the bulk of the parenchyma, and within it are accumulations of lymphoid tissue, the white pulp, forming splenic nodules or Malpighian bodies (W), many with germinal centers. H and E. Low power. Top right: The capsule, covered by a layer of mesothelial cells (not visible), and a trabecula (T) passing into the interior consist principally of collagenous fibers (blue). The majority of the parenchyma is red pulp, consisting of cellular cords and numerous venous sinuses. Two splenic nodules (W) of white pulp are dense accumulations of lymphocytes, each associated with a small artery (blue). Azan. Low power. Bottom: A central arteriole (A) is surrounded by densely packed lymphocytes that constitute a splenic nodule. The arteriole is somewhat eccentric in position with regard to the nodule. Above the nodule, there is a trabecula (T) associated with a small vein. The right half of the field is occupied by red pulp, consisting of loose lymphatic tissue in the form of irregular, anastomosing cords (C) separated by venous sinuses (V). Nuclei of the specialized reticular cells that line the sinuses project into the lumina. Plastic section. H and E. Medium power.*

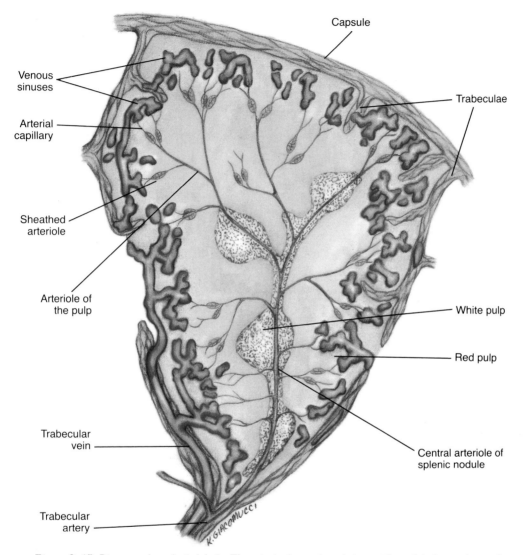

**Figure 9–15.** *Diagram of a splenic lobule. The principal vascular relations within a lobule are depicted.*

## Splenic Pulp

The parenchyma, or pulp, of the spleen consists of two distinct types: *white pulp* and *red pulp*. The former surrounds and follows arteries, and the latter is present as pulp cords.

**White Pulp.** This pulp appears on a cut surface as scattered gray areas of compact pulpal tissue.

It forms a *periarterial sheath* of lymphocytes about the arteries, the adventitia of which is largely replaced by reticular tissue. The reticular tissue is infiltrated with lymphocytes, which form areas of diffuse and nodular lymphatic tissue. The cells present within this tissue are predominantly small lymphocytes, but in addition, there are medium-sized and large lymphocytes, monocytes, and

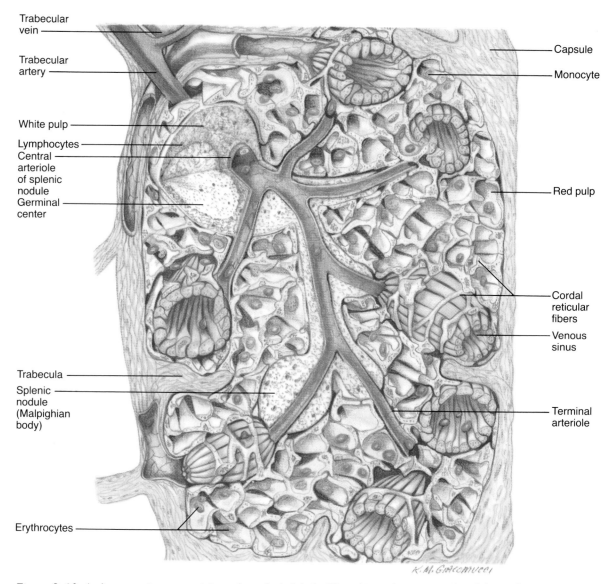

Trabecular vein

Trabecular artery

White pulp

Lymphocytes

Central arteriole of splenic nodule

Germinal center

Trabecula

Splenic nodule (Malpighian body)

Erythrocytes

Capsule

Monocyte

Red pulp

Cordal reticular fibers

Venous sinus

Terminal arteriole

K. M. Giacomucci

**Figure 9–16.** *A diagrammatic representation of a splenic lobule. The white pulp consists of nodules and aggregations of lymphocytes that surround and follow the arterial blood vessels, and the red pulp is an open mesh with sinusoids.*

plasma cells. The amount of lymphoid tissue is not constant but varies, as it does in all lymphatic tissue, in response to certain stimuli. *Splenic nodules* are denser accumulations of lymphocytes along the strands of white pulp. They are typical lymph nodules that may show germinal centers. In the spleen, the nodules are arranged around a

blood vessel, the so-called *central artery*, which in most instances is an arteriole and is eccentric in position, since it avoids the germinal center.

Between the white and red pulp are poorly delineated *marginal zones* of diffuse lymphatic tissue containing few lymphocytes and numerous macrophages. These zones trap circulating antigens and are important in the immunological activity of the spleen. In the white pulp, T and B lymphocytes generally are segregated into two different sites. T lymphocytes populate the periarterial sheath, and B lymphocytes are concentrated in the marginal zones and in the nodules. From birth to early adulthood, the white pulp forms the greater volume of the spleen, but with increasing age, it regresses, the number of splenic nodules decreases, and the red pulp becomes increasingly prominent.

**Red Pulp.** This pulp is a paste-like, red mass that can be scraped from a freshly cut surface (Fig. 9–17). It is looser in texture than white pulp and is infiltrated with all elements of circulating blood. It occupies all space not utilized by trabeculae and white pulp and contains numerous venous sinuses. Between the sinuses, the pulp appears as cellular cords (*splenic,* or *Billroth's, cords*), which form a spongy network of modified lymphatic tissue that merges gradually into the white pulp.

The support of the pulp is a typical reticulum with its associated reticular cells, both primitive and phagocytic. Within the meshes of this framework are lymphocytes, free macrophages, and all the elements of circulating blood. Lymphocytes of large, medium, and small sizes are numerous in the white pulp but are less numerous and more loosely arranged in the red pulp. The various types of lymphocytes arise in the white pulp and spread to the red pulp by amebism. Monocytes also are fairly numerous. Some are brought by the blood stream; others arise within the spleen by proliferation of existing cells or by differentiation from hemocytoblasts. The red pulp also contains numerous plasma cells, granular leukocytes, and erythrocytes.

In many mammals and mammalian embryos, the red pulp of the spleen contains megakaryocytes, myelocytes, and erythroblasts. These myeloid elements are absent from the spleen in adult humans, except in certain pathological conditions when the spleen undergoes *myeloid metaplasia.*

**Blood Vessels.** The distribution and organization of the red and white pulp depend upon the vascular arrangement. An appreciation of this arrangement is necessary also to an understanding of the structure of the spleen as a whole.

The arteries enter the spleen at the hilum and divide into branches that are typical muscular arteries, which pass along the trabeculae as *trabecular* or *interlobular arteries.* As the trabeculae branch, the arteries subdivide also. When reduced to a diameter of approximately 0.2 mm, they leave the trabeculae to enter the splenic parenchyma. As they do so, the tunica adventitia of the arteries loosens, takes on the character of reticular tissue, and becomes infiltrated with lymphocytes. At various points along the course of the vessels, the lymphatic sheath is increased in amount to form the splenic nodules. These vessels, called "central arteries or arterioles," although they are eccentric with reference to the corpuscles, give off capillaries that supply the white pulp and continue into the red pulp. After numerous divisions, the arterioles become reduced in size, lose their investment of white pulp, and enter the red pulp. Here, each arteriole subdivides into several small branches that lie close together like a brush, or a *penicillus.* The *penicilli vessels* show three successive segments (Fig. 9–18). The first portion, the longest segment, is the *pulp arteriole (artery of the pulp),* which possesses a thin tunica of smooth muscle. This vessel becomes narrow and divides into the *sheathed arterioles,* or *ellipsoids,* which have markedly thickened walls, the *Schweigger-Seidel sheath.* The thickened sheath, which is not as well developed in humans as in many lower mammals, is spindle-shaped and is composed of a mass of concentrically arranged cells and fibers continuous peripherally with the reticulum of the red pulp. Each sheathed arteriole divides into two or more *terminal arterial capillaries,* lined by a continuous endothelium. The terminations of the arterial capillaries are the subject of considerable controversy. Some authors claim that the arterial capillaries open directly into the pulp reticulum and that the blood gradually filters back into the venous sinuses (the "open" or slow, circulation theory). Other investigators consider that the arterial capillaries empty directly into the venous sinuses (the "closed" or rapid, circulation theory). There is considerable evidence for both theories, and it is possible that structurally and functionally both systems exist in the spleen. The exact routing of the blood is, in a sense, a detail of academic interest only, since there is an interchange of cells between the red pulp and the sinuses.

The *venous sinuses* constitute a system of

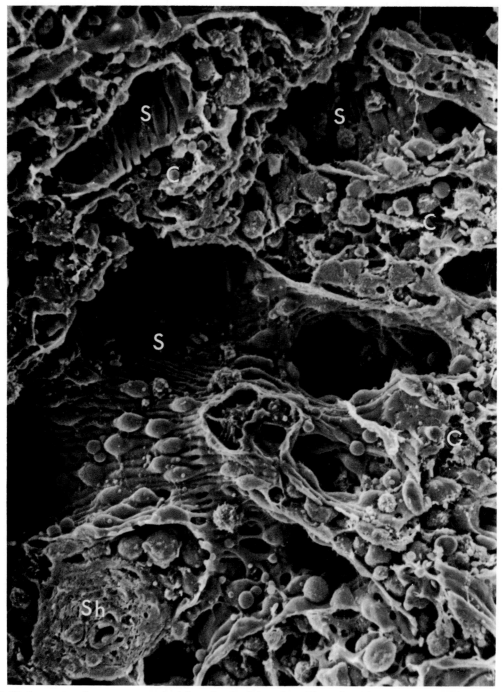

**Figure 9–17.** *A scanning electron micrograph of the red pulp of the spleen. The walls of the venous sinuses (S) are seen mainly in surface view. Also shown are splenic cords (C) and a sheathed arteriole (Sh). × 700. (Courtesy of Dr. T. Fujita.)*

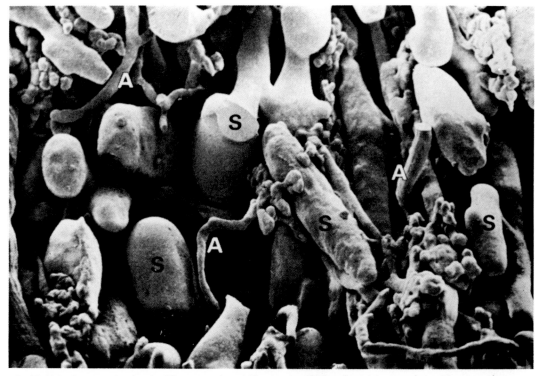

**Figure 9–18.** *Vascular cast of red pulp. The twigs of penicillar arteries (A) break up into granular resin masses that correspond to the spaces in the splenic cords. The granular masses, in turn, are attached by sausage-like casts of sinuses (S). This resin vascular cast of human red pulp gives support to the open theory of splenic circulation. × 230. (Courtesy of T. Murakami, T. Fujita, K. Tanaka, and J. Tokunaga and IGAKU-SHOIN Medical Publishers.)*

irregular, anastomosing tunnels throughout the red pulp (Fig. 9–19). They occupy more space than that occupied by the splenic cords that lie between them. These vessels are called *sinuses,* since they have an irregular lumen and are highly distensible. The sinus wall is composed of specialized endothelial cells that are rod-shaped and run longitudinally in the vessel wall. The cell bodies bulge into the lumen of the sinus (Figs. 9–20 and 9–21). This bulging is most pronounced in the region of the nucleus. The lining cells, termed *littoral, rod,* or *stave cells,* are connected by short transverse processes, and large gaps, or oval clefts, are present between them (Fig. 9–22). These deficiencies are large enough to allow formed element of blood to cross the sinusoidal wall. The cells rest upon an incomplete basal lamina, and the wall of the sinus is supported by thick, anastomosing reticular fibers circularly arranged.

The venous sinuses empty into the *pulp veins,* large thin-walled vessels lined by endothelium (Fig. 9–23). These veins leave the pulp and unite to form larger veins that pass into the trabeculae as *trabecular* or *interlobular* veins. The trabecular veins, which consist only of endothelium supported by the fibromuscular tissue of the trabeculae, travel to the hilum, where they drain into the splenic vein.

## Lymphatics

Efferent vessels are present in the capsule and in the larger trabeculae. A few deep efferent

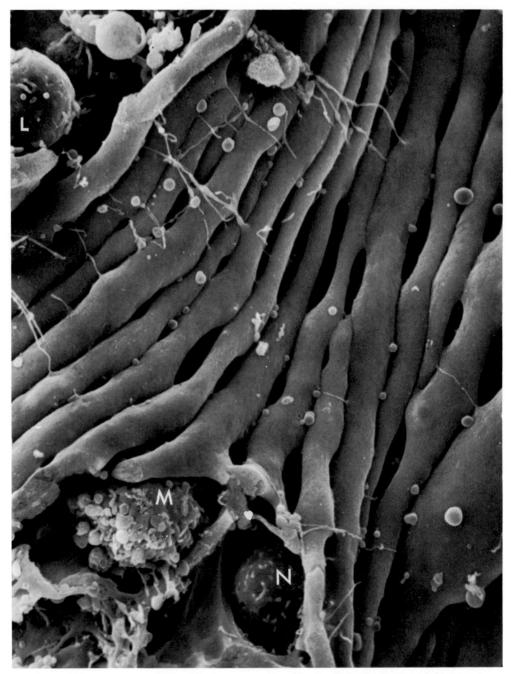

*Figure 9–19.* Spleen, scanning electron micrograph of a venous sinus. The littoral (rod) cells show deficiencies between them. Also present are a lymphocyte (L), a macrophage (M), and a neutrophil leukocyte (N). × 3700. (Courtesy of Dr. T. Fujita.)

*Figure 9–20.* Spleen, scanning electron micrograph of the cordal (outside) aspect of a sinus wall. The littoral (rod) cells at each level are bound by the cytoplasmic processes of reticular cells (Rt). On the left, a juxtaterminal portion of a penicillar artery is shown with perforations in its endothelium (arrows). Also present are red blood cells (R), macrophages (M) and their processes (m), and blood platelets (P). × 4400. (Courtesy of Dr. T. Fujita and IGAKU-SHOIN Medical Publishers.)

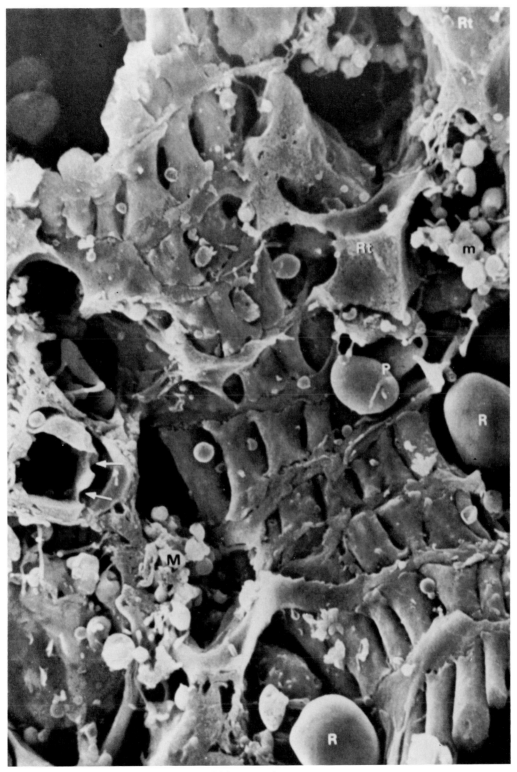

*Figure 9–20* See legend on opposite page

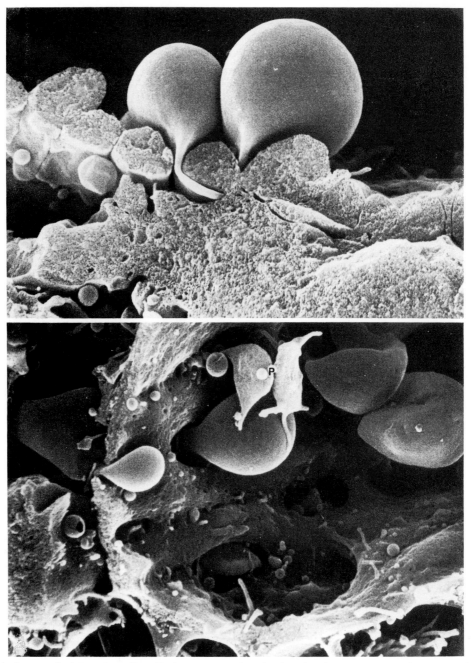

**Figure 9–21.** Sinus wall of the spleen. Top: Erythrocytes are often fixed in their hanging state on the sinus wall. × 13,000. Bottom: Erythrocytes are seen passing through the perforations in the sinus wall along with blood platelets (P). × 9300. (Reproduced with permission from Fujita, T., et al.: SEM Atlas of Cells and Tissues. New York, Igaku-Shoin, 1981.)

lymphatic vessels, which follow the arteries, may be present also in the white pulp.

### Nerves

Unmyelinated nerve fibers follow the arteries and terminate in the smooth muscle of their walls. Nerves also terminate in the capsule and in the trabeculae in species that possess smooth muscle cells in these sites. A few branches enter both the red and white pulp, but their endings here are unknown. Occasional myelinated fibers, which probably are sensory in function, are seen also.

### Functions of the Spleen

Splenic functions are not understood completely. The spleen is said not to be essential for life. However, although in some cases, it can be removed without harm to the individual, in others, morbidity may follow the operation. Often the morbidity is related to an increase in the number of lymphocytes in the blood as a result of excessive compensation by the lymph nodes. After extirpation, the functions of the spleen are taken over by various organs, principally other lymphoid organs and the bone marrow.

The spleen is an important hemopoietic organ, producing lymphocytes, which are formed chiefly in the white pulp, in particular in its nodules. From the white pulp, they pass to the red pulp and so into the sinuses and splenic vein. In the embryo, the spleen also produces myeloid elements. In certain pathological conditions, it may undergo myeloid metaplasia, as mentioned previously, and may produce all types of blood cells. Also, platelets may be trapped in the spleen with such zeal that too few are present in the general circulation; this may result in excessive bleeding. Similarly, the spleen may remove red blood cells with such avidity that an anemic crisis may ensue.

The spleen separates plasma from the blood cells, so that the blood cells are highly concentrated in the red pulp, thus enhancing the storage function of this organ. This elastic, controllable reservoir is capable of rapidly reintroducing blood cells into the circulation and adjusting the volume of the circulating blood. The spleen monitors red blood cells and is capable of detaining or modifying and phagocytizing these cells in the venous sinuses of red pulp. In the latter instance, the spleen functions as an organ of blood destruction. Red blood cells are engulfed by phagocytic cells, and iron recovered from the hemoglobin is stored in the cells. The iron is given up as needed and is utilized in the formation of new hemoglobin. From time to time, large numbers of red blood cells are expelled, when needed, into the general circulation by contraction of smooth muscle fibers and stretched elastic fibers in the trabeculae and capsule. Monocytes are sequestered in the white pulp, marginal zone, and red pulp and there transformed into macrophages. The latter cells contribute to the spleen's great phagocytic capacity. The spleen may release a humoral factor that induces bone marrow to produce and release monocytes and thereby augment the rate of the conversion process from monocyte to macrophage. Eosinophils are released to the spleen from the bone marrow for the final step in their maturational process prior to their entrance into the general circulation. B cells and T cells of the recirculating lymphocyte pool enter the spleen and follow specific pathways. After coursing through the red pulp and the marginal zone, they migrate through the reticular meshwork into the white pulp. T cells enter the periarterial lymphatic sheaths and may remain there for several hours. B cells enter the lymphatic nodules and stay there for a longer period of time. T cells and B cells may either engage in antibody production or rejoin the recirculating lymphocyte pool. Even in the absence of a capsule, the human spleen is capable of exhibiting a reservoir function for approximately one third of the platelets of the body. Labeling experiments with radioactive isotopes have demonstrated that the spleen's clearance rate per gram of tissue far exceeds that of lung, liver, bone marrow, and other components of the mononuclear phagocytic system.

The production of antibodies is another important function of the spleen. Foreign particles that are circulating in the blood can stimulate a strong immune response in the spleen. The antigen is trapped by the reticular network of the red and white pulp, thus allowing it to come in contact

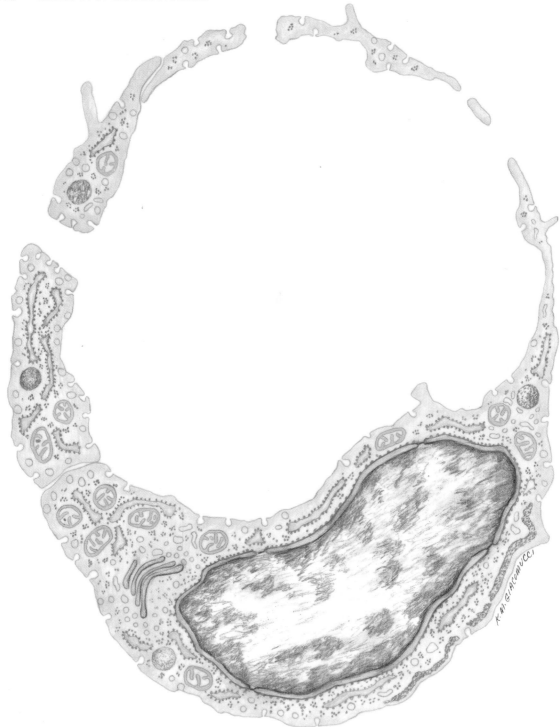

*Figure 9–22* See legend on opposite page

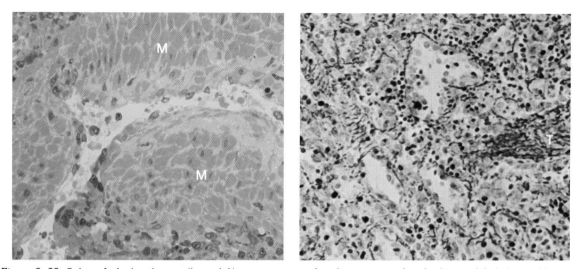

*Figure 9–23.* Spleen. Left: *A pulp vein (lower left) passes into a trabecula to join a trabecular (or interlobular) vein. Note the numerous smooth muscle fibers (M), here sectioned transversely, within the trabecula. Plastic section. H and E. High power. Right: In this section of red pulp, reticular fibers have been stained specifically (black), outlining clearly the venous sinuses within the parenchyma. The walls of the sinuses are supported by reticular fibers that are circularly arranged; thus, in sections that pass obliquely through the sinus walls, the reticular fibers appear as short dark profiles. Nuclei of reticular cells lining the sinuses are interposed between the fibers and the lumen. The remainder of the red pulp between the sinuses is composed of irregular cords of lymphatic tissue. A trabecula (T) contains delicate reticular fibers and collagenous fibers (brown). Bielschowsky's method. High power.*

with the T cells and B cells. T cells are located close to the central artery of the lymphatic sheaths, while B cells are situated in the periphery of the white pulp. Thus, the spleen traps antigen from the blood and permits T and B cells to interact and produce antibody. The trapped antigen is first phagocytized by macrophages in the marginal zone and red pulp. Then, it migrates into white pulp and surrounds the lymphatic nodules at the level of the junction of T cell and

B cell populations. The antigen can then be retained on the surface of the antigen-presenting cells (*APCs*) and macrophages. The *APCs* originate in the bone marrow and may migrate to lie within the white pulp of the spleen in both the B and T cell zones. The *APCs* in the T cell zones are called *interdigitating cells*. These latter cells have a specific *MHC* antigen on their cell surface that causes T cells to cluster. Clustering seems to elicit a rapid immune response and appears to

*Figure 9–22.* Littoral cells form the lining of the vascular sinusoids of the spleen, bone marrow, liver, and lymph nodes. They are components of the reticuloendothelial system and are phagocytic or potentially phagocytic. The sinuses formed by the littoral cells differ from vessels lined by endothelium. The cells are not always thin and attenuated but may be much thicker than those of endothelium. Gaps exist in the wall of the sinusoid. These may be large, and they could represent channels through the cell or spaces between adjacent cells. Fenestrations can also occur in thin regions of the lining, but these do not seem to be bridged by a diaphragm. There are also junctions between adjacent cells, and there may be small areas of membrane fusion. In contrast to endothelia, the basement lamina is discontinuous or entirely lacking in these sinuses. The littoral cells are irregular in shape and, as already indicated, vary greatly in thickness. They are functionally similar to other components of the reticuloendothelial system in that they are capable of phagocytosis. The cytoplasm is rich in mitochondria and contains cisternae of rough-surfaced endoplasmic reticulum, lysosomes, free ribosomes, and a Golgi complex. Pinocytotic vesicles are abundant in littoral cells, especially near the cell surfaces. A band of dense material (lower right) is often seen in these cells, usually near the surface of the cell facing the subsinusoidal space. The space contains the collagenous fibers and ground substance comprising the extracellular reticulum. (From Lentz, T. L.: Cell Fine Structure. Philadelphia, W. B. Saunders Co., 1971, p. 115.)

contribute to the development of T cell zones and to sorting of these cells. The antigens of the *MHC* are overwhelmingly preferred as target antigens by T cells, even though a large number of other antigens on the cell surfaces are recognized by T cells. *APCs* also may be present in the skin (*Langerhans's cells*) and in the cortex of lymph nodes.

In primary immune response, antibody-producing cells appear first within the periarterial lymphatic sheaths and simultaneously proliferate and secrete antibody as they move to the outer limits of the sheaths. Later, they appear in the red pulp as mature *plasma cells*. The latter cells are the most mature antibody-secreting cells that develop from activated B cells. The plasma cells are filled with an extensive rough endoplasmic reticulum and have a characteristic morphology. In contrast, activated T cells contain very little endoplasmic reticulum and do not secrete antibody. However, resting T cells and B cells look very much alike. Under the electron microscope, both cell types are small and only slightly bigger than red blood cells, with a nucleus occupying most of the cytoplasm. Fortunately, one means of distinguishing the two cell types has been found, *Thy-1 glycoprotein* (a plasma membrane protein). The use of a cell-surface antigenic marker (anti-Thy-1 glycoprotein) has revolutionized cellular immunology by functionally distinguishing even subpopulations of T and B cells. During a secondary immune response, or prolonged primary encounter, germinal centers are the predominant histological feature. These centers add antibody to the system and increase the number of memory cells.

Antibodies appear in the plasma as immunoglobulins (also called gamma globulins) and are secreted by plasma cells. By immunofluorescence, it has been shown that plasma cells, at any given time, produce a type of immunoglobulin. There are five groups of immunoglobulins in humans:

1. *IgG* (immunoglobulin G) occurs in the largest amounts (75 per cent of the total serum immunoglobulins) and has a molecular weight of 150,000. It can pass the placental barrier and forms the first passive protective mechanism for the newborn.

2. *IgE* has a molecular weight of 190,000 (monomeric form). It can adhere to the receptors on the plasma membranes of mast cells and basophil leukocytes and bring about the release of heparin, histamine, and leukotrienes (e.g., eosinophil chemotactic factors of anaphylaxis).

3. *IgA* has a molecular weight of 160,000 (monomeric form) and is found in tears, saliva, and vaginal secretions. This antibody can aid in the defense against proliferation of microbes in body fluids.

4. *IgD* (molecular weight of 180,000) makes up 0.2 per cent of the total immunoglobulins and functions in the morphogenic process of B lymphocytes.

5. *IgM* exists in a complex form with a molecular weight of about 900,000. Together with IgD, they are involved in the early immune responses via their interaction in the differentiation process of B lymphocytes. This results in the production of antibody-secreting plasma cells.

The spleen, which is interposed in the blood stream, produces antibodies that are derived from plasma cells and react mainly to antigenic stimuli from the blood during the immunological process.

## Development of the Spleen

The primordium of the spleen in human embryos appears as a thickening of the mesenchyme in the dorsal mesentery of the stomach during the fifth week of embryonic development. At this time, it consists of a mass of mesenchymal cells that later divide actively. The mass of the primordium is added to by apposition of cells from the covering mesothelium of the body cavity. The mesenchymal cells differentiate into cells of the reticulum and into primitive free cells resembling lymphocytes. Later, the tissue becomes myeloid in type, containing all stages in the development of megakaryocytes, granulocytes, and erythrocytes. The development of lymphocytes and monocytes continues throughout life, but myeloid elements disappear shortly after birth.

In the early stages of development, the spleen is supplied by a rich capillary plexus, but as a characteristic distribution of vessels is established, lymphocytes become compactly arranged around the arteries to form the white pulp. Definite nodules do not appear until later in fetal life, and germinal centers are not present until after birth. The venous sinuses develop as irregular spaces that later become connected with the established blood vessels.

## Summary Table 9–1. Lymphoid Organs

| Organ | Capsule | Separate Lobes | Cortex | Medulla | Epithelium | Lymphatic Nodules | Lymphatic Vessels | Function | Age of Maximum Development |
|-------|---------|----------------|--------|---------|------------|-------------------|-------------------|----------|----------------------------|
| Lymph nodes | Convex, well-developed, mostly collagenous, with trabeculae penetrating cortex at right angles | Absent | Present | Present | Absent | Present in cortex and surrounded by diffuse lymph tissue | Afferent and efferent | Filtration and phagocytosis; follicular dendritic cells bind and expose antigen; B lymphocytes differentiate into plasma cells (produce immunoglobulins) and memory cells (responsible for secondary immune response); paracortical T lymphocytes regulate response by producing T-helper factor, T-suppressor factor, and memory cells | Puberty |
| Tonsils Pharyngeal | Poorly defined, with trabeculae | Absent | Absent | Absent | Pseudostratified | Present as clusters about crypts | Efferent | Marked phagocytic capacity; lymphopoiesis | Puberty |
| Palatine | Well-defined, with trabeculae | Absent | Absent | Absent | Stratified squamous | Present beneath epithelium and around crypts | Efferent | Marked phagocytic capacity; lymphopoiesis | Puberty |
| Lingual | Not definite, with no trabeculae | Absent | Absent | Absent | Stratified squamous | Present as clusters about a single crypt | Efferent | Marked phagocytic capacity; lymphopoiesis | Puberty |
| Thymus | Mostly connective tissue with septa and trabeculae | Present | Present | Present | As scattered epithelial reticular cells and in thymic corpuscles | Absent | Efferent (small) | Production of T lymphocytes for cell-mediated immune reactions; thymosin to stimulate T production and maturation; stem cells for mast cell differentiation; eosinophilopoiesis; thymic hormone that enhances graft-versus-host reaction; minimal phagocytic activity | Before puberty |
| Spleen | Fibrous and muscular, with peritoneum cover. Incomplete trabeculae containing smooth muscle | Absent | Absent | Absent | Absent | Present in relation to central arteries of white pulp | Efferent; limited to capsule and trabeculae | Blood storage and release; presence of both B and T lymphocytes; phagocytic for blood cells and platelets; main source of circulating antibody in body; removal of lipid droplets in blood; extramedullary myelopoiesis under stress conditions | After puberty |

# The Skin and Its Appendages (The Integument)

## INTRODUCTION

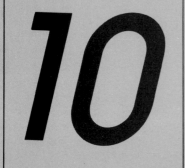

The integument comprises the skin that covers the surface of the body together with certain specialized derivatives of the skin. These include nails, hair, and several kinds of glands.

The skin protects the organism from injurious substances and influences; provides a barrier to invasion by microorganisms; helps to regulate the temperature of the body; and, by sweating, excretes water and various waste products of catabolism. It is the most extensive sense organ of the body for the reception of tactile, thermal, and painful stimuli. In addition, the epidermal cells can form enzymes (carboxylase, phosphatase, and sulfatase) and immune complexes in response to a viral invasion.

## THE SKIN

The skin is composed of two layers: the *epidermis*, a specialized epithelium derived from the ectoderm, and, beneath this, the *dermis* (or *corium*), of vascular dense connective tissue, a derivative of mesoderm. The dermis corresponds to the lamina propria of a mucous membrane (Fig. 10–1). These two layers are firmly adherent to each other and form a membrane that varies in thickness from about 0.5 to 4 mm or more in different parts of the body. Beneath the dermis is a layer of loose connective tissue that varies from areolar to adipose in character. This is the superficial fascia of gross anatomy, sometimes referred to as the *hypodermis*, but it is not considered to be part of the skin. The dermis is connected to the underlying hypodermis by connective tissue fibers that pass from one layer to the other. The superficial fascia permits great mobility of skin over most regions of the body. It is only in local areas such as the palm and the sole, where there

is considerable interlocking of fibers between dermis and hypodermis, that mobility is limited.

The free surface of the skin exhibits numerous ridges that can be seen with the naked eye. They run in various directions and are most apparent on the palms of the hands and the soles of the feet. The patterns, which consist of loops, whorls, and arches, are determined in the main by hereditary factors and correspond to similar patterns on the surface of the dermis, the *dermal ridges*. Thus, in sections, the boundary between epidermis and dermis appears uneven. However, variations in the degree of development of ridges do occur, and ridges are absent on the forehead, external ear, perineum, and scrotum. The ridges seen on the skin of the palmar surface of the fingers constitute the basis for the prints used in personal identification, since they are subject to marked individual variation and never change (apart from enlargement) after they are formed during the third and fourth months of fetal life.

Skin is classified commonly as *thick* or *thin*.

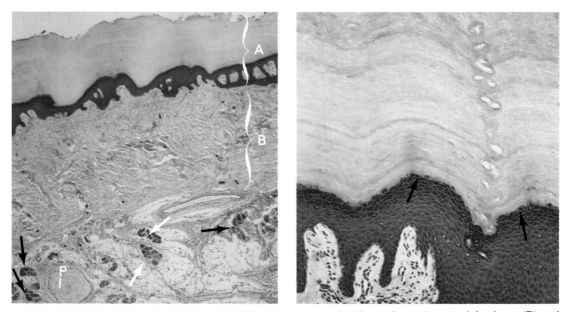

**Figure 10–1.** *Thick skin of the sole of the foot. Left: The skin is composed of the epidermis (A) and of the dermis (B), with an uneven boundary between the two. Note that the epidermis consists chiefly of keratin (stratum corneum). Beneath the dermis is the hypodermis, here adipose in character and containing sweat glands (arrows) and a Vater-Pacini corpuscle (P). H and E. Low power. Right: The epidermis shows the Malpighian layer (strata germinativum and spinosum), the stratum granulosum (arrows), and the stratum corneum, traversed by the duct of a sweat gland. The stratum lucidum is not apparent on this section. A small portion of the papillary layer of the dermis is present at lower left. H and E. Medium power.*

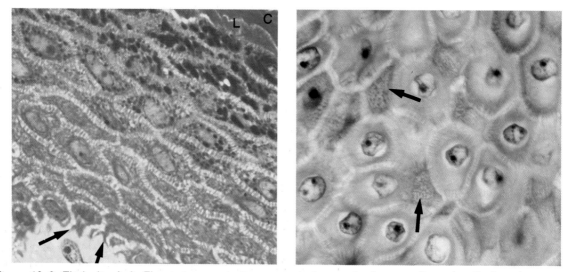

**Figure 10–2.** Thick skin. Left: The stratum germinativum is a single row of columnar cells, each cell of which has short cytoplasmic processes on its basal surface (arrows). The stratum spinosum, several layers thick, is composed of irregular, polyhedral cells, slightly separated from each other. The surface of the cells is covered with short cytoplasmic spines that meet with similar projections of adjacent cells to form intercellular bridges. The stratum granulosum consists of four to five layers of flattened cells that contain basophil keratohyalin granules. Small portions of the stratum lucidum (L) and the stratum corneum (C) are present at upper right. Plastic section. H and E. High power. Right: Epidermis, stratum spinosum. The prickle cells have large nuclei with distinct nucleoli and show intercellular cytoplasmic bridges. In two regions (arrows), the cytoplasmic processes are shown in cross section. Masson. Oil immersion.

Thick skin is found on the palms of the hands and soles of the feet; moderately thick skin over the back of the neck and the shoulders (Fig. 10–2). Thin skin covers the remainder of the body except for the eyelids and parts of the external genitalia where it is very thin (Fig. 10–3). It should be emphasized that these terms, thick and thin, do not refer to the thickness of the skin as a

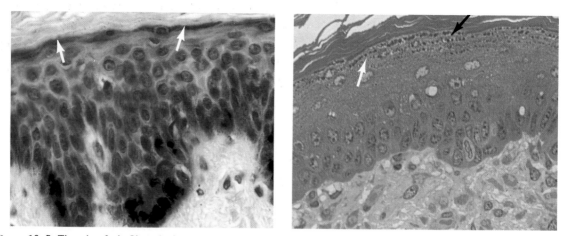

**Figure 10–3.** Thin skin. Left: Skin of a black person. Note the scattered cells representative of the stratum granulosum (arrows) and the thinness of the stratum corneum. There is marked deposition of pigment (melanin) in the Malpighian layer, particularly in the stratum germinativum. H and E. Medium power. Right: Keratohyalin granules (arrows) are seen clearly in cells of the stratum granulosum. Plastic section. H and E. High power.

whole, only to the epidermis. Thin skin itself varies greatly in thickness in different parts of the body, and these variations are due, in actual fact, almost entirely to variations in the thickness of the dermis. The dermis of extensor surfaces is usually thicker than that of flexor surfaces. Both regions, however, have an epidermal component that is classified as thin.

### The Epidermis

The epidermis, a stratified squamous keratinized epithelium, consists of four distinct cell types (Figs. 10–4 and 10–5):

1. Keratinocyte.
2. Melanocyte.
3. Langerhans's cell.
4. Merkel's cell.

The predominant cell type is the *keratinocyte*, an epithelial cell that differentiates to produce keratin. This results in the formation of the dead superficial layers of skin. These superficial keratinized cells are lost continuously from the surface and must be replaced by cells that arise as a result of mitotic activity of cells of the basal layers of the epidermis. Cells resulting from this proliferation are displaced to higher levels, and as they move upward, they elaborate keratin. Keratin eventually replaces the majority of the cytoplasm; the cell dies and finally is shed. Thus, it should be appreciated that the structural organization of the epidermis into layers reflects stages in the life of a keratinocyte, involving cellular proliferation and growth, outward displacement and differentiation, and death and desquamation.

The epidermis of the palms and the soles is particularly thick and exhibits maximal layering and cellular differentiation. It consists of five layers, or strata:

1. The *stratum germinativum*, or *stratum basale*, resting upon the dermis.

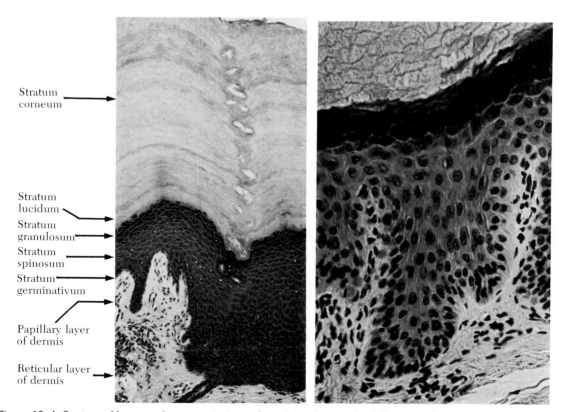

Stratum corneum

Stratum lucidum
Stratum granulosum
Stratum spinosum
Stratum germinativum

Papillary layer of dermis

Reticular layer of dermis

*Figure 10–4.* Sections of human sole, perpendicular to the surface, illustrate the different layers of the skin. Left: *Low power.* Right: *Medium power.*

2. The *stratum spinosum*, or *prickle cell layer*.
3. The *stratum granulosum*.
4. The *stratum lucidum*.
5. The *stratum corneum*, the outermost horny layer.

**Stratum Germinativum.** The stratum germinativum consists of a single layer of columnar or cuboidal cells. These primitive cells contain indented nuclei that are circumscribed by a thin rim of heterochromatin with one or two prominent nucleoli. Clusters of free ribosomes predominate in the cytoplasm. Each cell has short, thin cytoplasmic processes on its basal surface. These tooth-like processes fit into pockets of the basal lamina and appear to anchor the epithelium to the underlying dermis. The plasma membrane in relation to the basal lamina exhibits numerous hemidesmosomes. Desmosomes occur frequently at the lateral and upper surfaces of the cells and serve to bind the cells together. Electron microscopy shows that the cells contain bundles of fine filaments about 10 nm in diameter, randomly distributed throughout the cytoplasm. Aggregates of these filaments are visible on light microscopy as *tonofibrils*. Some of these aggregates are associated with the desmosomes, and the remainder are found throughout the cytoplasm forming the cytoskeleton. Mitotic figures occur in this layer, thus producing new cells that are displaced into the layer above.

**Stratum Spinosum.** The stratum spinosum is several layers thick and is composed of irregular, polyhedral cells, slightly separated from each other (Fig. 10–6). Toward the surface the cells become flattened. The surface of the cells (*prickle cells*) is covered with short cytoplasmic spines, or projections, that meet with similar projections of adjacent cells to form "intercellular bridges." It should be emphasized that these do not indicate cytoplasmic continuity between cells. Electron micrographs demonstrate that the short processes constituting a "bridge" make intimate contact at a desmosome. Hence, the keratinocytes are independent entities. The cytoplasm of these cells is basophil, indicating a considerable content of ribonucleic acid (RNA), in this case associated with protein synthesis for growth and division of cells. The cytoplasm also contains numerous bundles of filaments that form the tonofibrils. Many of these pass into cytoplasmic processes and terminate in the desmosomes. They do not extend across cell membranes. It appears that the filaments, particularly those in relation to desmosomes, help to maintain cohesion between cells and to resist the effects of abrasion.

It should be mentioned at this point that the two layers just described, the stratum germinativum and the stratum spinosum, are grouped together as the *malpighian layer—stratum (or rete) malpighii*—by many authors (Fig. 10–7). This layer is responsible for proliferation and for initiation of the keratinization process. The malpighian layer also contains *melanocytes*, which produce the pigment melanin, described later in the discussion on pigmentation. Additionally, scattered in this layer are Langerhans's and Merkel's cells.

Under normal conditions, the frequency of mitoses is far greater in the stratum spinosum than in the stratum germinativum. An increase in

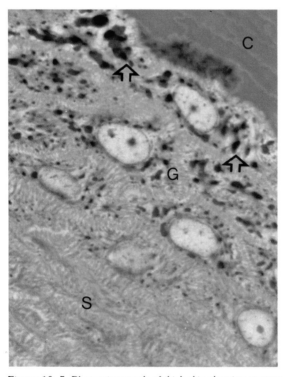

*Figure 10–5. Photomicrograph of thick skin showing stratum corneum (C), stratum granulosum (G) with irregular granules of keratohyalin (arrows), and stratum spinosum (S). H and E. High power.*

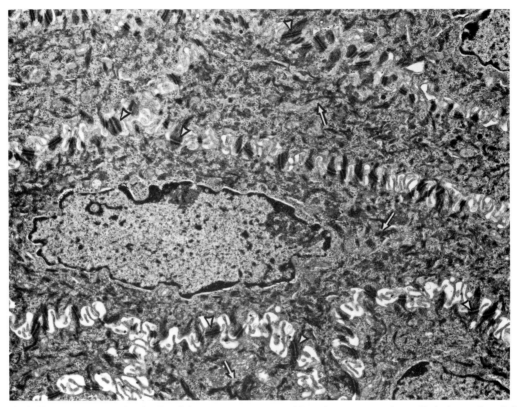

**Figure 10–6.** Electron micrograph of cells of the stratum spinosum. Note the presence of tonofibrils (arrows) and the wide intercellular spaces crossed by cytoplasmic processes. The areas of contact between the latter are marked by desmosomes (arrowheads). × 7500.

the mitotic index (*hyperplasia*) in the latter may lead to a carcinoma.

**Stratum Granulosum.** The next layer, the stratum granulosum, consists of three to five layers of flattened cells whose long axis is parallel to the skin surface. The flattened polyhedral cells have vesicular nuclei lacking nucleoli—morphological evidence for diminished cell activity. The cytoplasm of these cells contains granules of *keratohyalin*, which stain with some acid dyes and with certain basic dyes (Figs. 10–8 and 10–9). On electron microscopy, the granules appear as irregularly shaped masses of electron-dense material in association with bundles of filaments. The origin of these granules is obscure, but they appear to be involved in the process of formation of soft keratin. With increases in the size and number of these granules, the nuclei become pale and indis-

tinct and show degenerative changes. The granules later become intimately associated with tonofibrils, and cell contacts become indistinct. It is in this layer that the cells of the epidermis die. It should be noted that, as keratinization proceeds, increasing numbers of autophagosomes appear within the cytoplasm of keratinocytes. Digestion of cellular organelles by lysosomal enzymes within the autophagosomes results in the loss of cell structure. Keratinocytes in the granular layer also contain small *membrane-coating granules*, or *keratinosomes* (histidine-rich and cystine-containing protein having many phosphate groups). One of the functions of these granules seems to be to bind the tonofilaments and thus bring about a compartmentalization of these intermediate filaments within the cytoplasm. These granules, which are formed in association with the Golgi

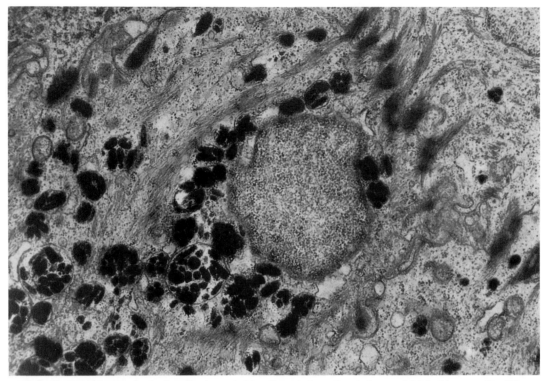

*Figure 10–7. Electron micrograph of a heavily pigmented keratinocyte from the stratum malpighii of human skin. Whereas the melanosomes of melanocytes occur singly, those of keratinocytes are found in clusters of varying size enclosed by a membrane. (Courtesy of G. Szabo and D. W. Fawcett, from Fawcett, D. W.: Bloom and Fawcett: A Textbook of Histology, 11th ed. Philadelphia, W. B. Saunders Co., 1986.)*

apparatus, later move to the cell periphery and eventually discharge their contents into the intercellular space. This extruded material is thought to function as a barrier to penetration by foreign materials, particularly water, since the epidermis is permeable to water in both the deeper and more superficial layers but not in the central region of the stratum granulosum.

**Stratum Lucidum.** The stratum lucidum is a clear translucent layer, three to five cells deep. Cells are not distinguishable clearly as separate entities. They are flattened and closely packed. Nuclei are indistinct or absent, and the cytoplasm lacks mitochondria, endoplasmic reticulum, ribosomes, and Golgi complexes. The cytoplasm contains a semifluid substance, keratohyalin, which is presumed to be a product of the granules noted in subjacent layers. The keratohyalin is distributed among the tonofibrils, which generally now are arranged parallel to the surface of the skin. Occurring at random throughout the cell are granules of *eleiden*, which are responsible for the acidophilia and refractility of this rather thin homogeneous layer. Nothing is known about the function of this substance.

**Stratum Corneum.** The fifth and outermost layer, the stratum corneum, is composed of clear, dead, scale-like cells that become progressively flattened and fused. These horny cells possess a thickened plasmalemma (15–20 nm) with many folds interdigitating with those of neighboring cells (Fig. 10–10). The nucleus is absent, and the cytoplasm is replaced with keratin, thought to be derived principally from the tonofibrils of the deeper layers of the epidermis (see Fig. 10–9). This is "soft keratin," low in sulfur content, as distinct from "hard keratin," found in nails and the cortex of hairs. The most superficial layers of

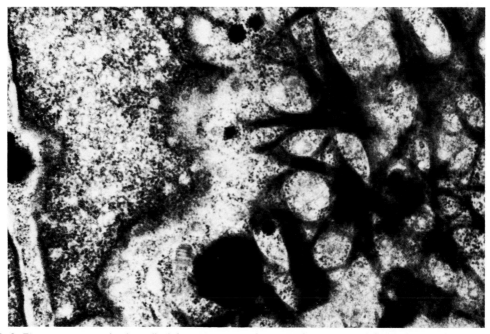

**Figure 10–8.** Electron micrograph of a cell of the stratum granulosum, with a portion of the nucleus (left). Note the irregular granules of keratohyalin. × 35,000.

the stratum corneum (sometimes called *stratum disjunctum*) are flat horny plates that are desquamated constantly. The stratum corneum stains pink with eosin and often is shredded during specimen preparation. Thus, from the surface of the epidermis, there is a constant loss of dead cells; these cells are replaced by new cells formed as a result of mitoses in the deeper layers, principally in the stratum germinativum and the stratum spinosum, and are pushed toward the surface during the process of keratinization.

### Epidermis of the General Body Surface

The epidermis of the rest of the body is both thinner and simpler than that of the palms and soles. All layers of the epidermis are reduced, and the stratum lucidum is usually absent. The stratum germinativum is similar to that of thick skin, but the stratum spinosum is not so extensive. The granular layer may be present as one or two rows of cells or may be represented by scattered cells along the line where this layer might be expected.

The reduction in thickness of the epidermis of thin skin is due probably to the fact that keratinization here is less marked and is not a continuous process.

### Pigmentation

The color of the skin is dependent upon three factors. The color of skin itself is yellow, owing to the presence of *carotene*, a plant pigment that is deposited in the stratum corneum and in the fat cells of the dermis and hypodermis. *Blood*, showing through from the underlying vascular dermis, imparts a reddish hue. Finally, the presence of varying amounts of *melanin* pigment is responsible for shades of brown. Melanin is present mainly in the stratum germinativum and in the deeper layers of the stratum spinosum.

Melanin is produced by specialized cells of the epidermis, the melanocytes, which are found scattered between keratinocytes of the stratum germinativum and stratum spinosum, as well as within hair follicles and dermal connective tissue

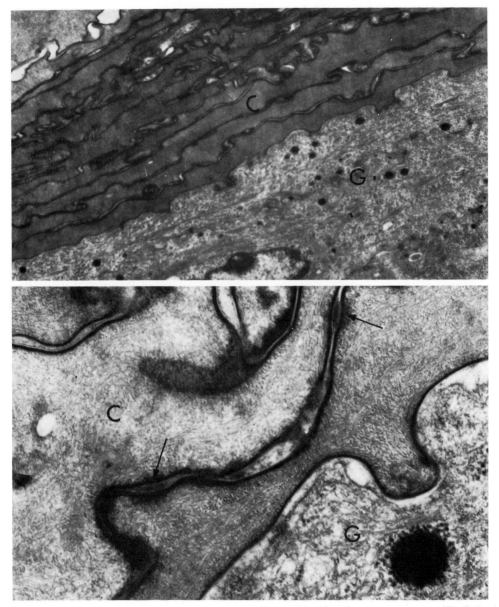

*Figure 10–9.* Electron micrograph of portions of the stratum granulosum (G) and of the stratum corneum (C). Cells of the latter are filled with keratin, which, at low magnification, appears amorphous. Desmosomes (arrows) between the cells are relatively well preserved. Top: × 20,000; bottom: × 70,000.

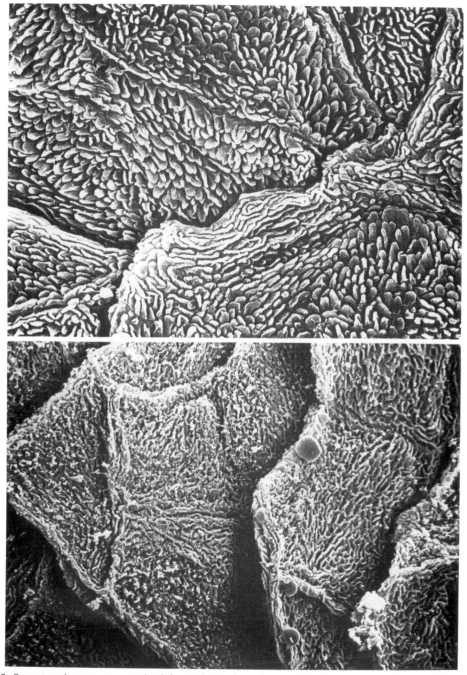

*Figure 10–10.* Scanning electron micrograph of the epidermis from the sole. Top: Long, tongue-like microfolia are shown on the deeper side of the epidermal cells. The microfolia tend to fuse into long ridges near the cell margins. × 4700. Bottom: Reticular microridges are demonstrated on the opposite (superficial) side of the stratum corneal cells. × 3700. (Reproduced with permission from Fujita, T., et al.: SEM Atlas of Cells and Tissues. New York, Igaku-Shoin, 1981.)

(Fig. 10–11). Developmentally, melanocytes are derived from neural crest ectoderm. The cells possess a small, spherical nucleus and numerous dendritic processes that extend between adjacent keratinocytes. Melanin formation occurs within *melanosomes*, membrane-bound granules present within the cytoplasm of melanocytes. These granules contain tyrosinase, an enzyme that is synthesized in ribosomes and transferred by the endoplasmic reticulum to the Golgi zone. Here, the enzyme is packaged into vesicles that fuse with premelanosomes. The latter mature through four defined stages into the melanin-packed melanosomes. These migrate through the dendritic processes of the melanocyte and are transferred to keratinocytes of the stratum germinativum and stratum spinosum. In a hematoxylin and eosin preparation, the melanocyte is not seen as a pigmented cell, since the dendritic processes are not visualized. The mechanism of dendritic transfer is not certain; either keratinocytes phagocytize the melanosome-containing processes of the melanocytes or melanocytes inject their pigment into neighboring keratinocytes. The process whereby the melanin granules are injected into keratinocytes is called *cytocrine secretion*. Within keratinocytes, the melanosomes generally accumulate above the nucleus and are closely associated with lysosomes and their contained enzymes. This is thought to be the reason that melanin disappears from keratinocytes of the more superficial epidermal layers.

Melanocytes are difficult to identify in routine histological preparations. However, they can be made visible by incubating wholemount preparations of the epidermis in *dopa*. This compound is oxidized by tyrosinase to produce in melanocytes a deposit of dark-brown melanin. The use of such preparations has shown that there is an orderly functional association between one melanocyte and a group of keratinocytes, the *epidermal-melanin unit*. Electron microscopy of this unit reveals that the melanocyte has a well-developed rough endoplasmic reticulum and many Golgi complexes. The cell lacks tonofilaments, desmosomes, and hemidesmosomes. The abutting keratinocytes also lack desmosomes and hemidesmosomes, which may lead to shrinkage during tissue processing. In such a unit, only one melanocyte serves as the source of pigment for a given number of epidermal cells. The number of melanocytes per unit area shows no sex or race differences; racial differences in skin color are due to differences in the number and size of melanosomes in keratinocytes. Cutaneous pigmentation probably depends on a number of influences, including hereditary, hormonal, and environmental factors. Genetic factors influence the size of

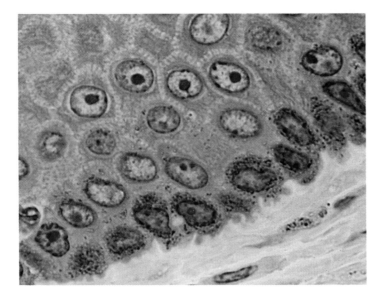

*Figure 10–11.* Epidermis showing the presence of melanin (brown) granules in the cytoplasm of many of the keratinocytes. H and E. Medium power.

the epidermal-melanin unit and of the melanosome and the production of melanin. Melanocyte-stimulating hormone (MSH) stimulates the migration of melanosomes into dendritic processes and the transfer to keratinocytes. Corticotropin moderately stimulates melanogenesis. Estrogen strongly stimulates the melanocytes in the pigmented skin surrounding the nipple (*areola*) and genital organs. Environmental factors, such as exposure to ultraviolet light, increase the enzymic activity of melanocytes and thus lead to increased melanin production and deposition in keratinocytes and to tanning.

The greater production of melanin in Mongoloids and Negroids is due to a greater number of melanosomes (not to number or distribution of melanocytes) than is present in Caucasoids. The former individuals have a lower incidence of skin cancer.

### Langerhans's Cells

The third cellular population within the epidermis is composed of Langerhans's cells (Fig. 10–12). These star-shaped cells, with numerous dendritic processes, are found principally within the stratum spinosum. Although they appear as "clear" cells by light microscopy, they are sharply delineated after impregnation with gold chloride. On electron microscopy, the cells exhibit an indented nucleus, a well-developed Golgi complex and rough endoplasmic reticulum, and a relatively clear cytoplasm without tonofilaments, desmosomes, or melanosomes. The cytoplasm does contain rod-like or racket-shaped inclusions, the *Birbeck granules*. These cells also have been described in other stratified epithelia, including that of the oral mucosa, esophagus, and vagina, and in hair follicles, sebaceous and apocrine glands, thymus, and lymph nodes. The wide distribution of these cells suggests that they may be a circulating population, and evidence is accumulating to indicate that they are of immunological importance. Recently, they have been shown to bear surface antigens common to most B and some T lymphocytes and monocytes. It is believed that they belong to a system of cells that fix and process exogenous antigens. Since they arise from bone marrow precursors, most authors include them in the mononuclear phagocyte system. They function in connection with the occurrence of *contact dermatitis* (the development of contact sensitivity in the skin).

### Merkel's Cells

Merkel's cells constitute the fourth cellular population within the epidermis (Fig. 10–13). These cells have a wide epidermal distribution and commonly are found in or near the stratum germinativum, often in association with intraepithelial nerve endings. They have irregularly shaped nuclei, and their cytoplasm is less electron-dense than that of adjacent keratinocytes. The cytoplasm contains loose bundles of tonofilaments and numerous small, dense granules. The granules are similar to those of catecholamine-containing cells and are concentrated in the basal region of the cell. Unlike Langerhans's cells, Merkel's cells are attached to neighboring keratinocytes by numerous desmosomes.

Although the function of Merkel's cells remains unclear, they are believed to function as mechanoreceptors. Because of the character of their granules, the cells also have been implicated as having APUD (amine precursor uptake and decarboxylation) cell–like activity. These granules are concentrated at the dermal border where axons arise in the dermis.

### The Dermis

It is difficult to define the exact limits of the dermis, since it merges into the underlying subcutaneous layer (hypodermis). However, the average thickness varies from 0.5 mm to 3 mm or more. The dermis determines the developmental pattern of the overlying epidermis. Transplanted dermis from the sole induces the formation of thick skin. The dermis repairs itself through fibroblastic activity and deposition of collagen. Defective formation of the latter fibril may lead to an abnormal increase in the extensibility of the skin, *cutis laxa*. The dermis is composed of dense irregularly arranged connective tissue and is subdivided into two strata: (1) the *papillary layer*, superficially, and (2) the *reticular layer*, beneath.

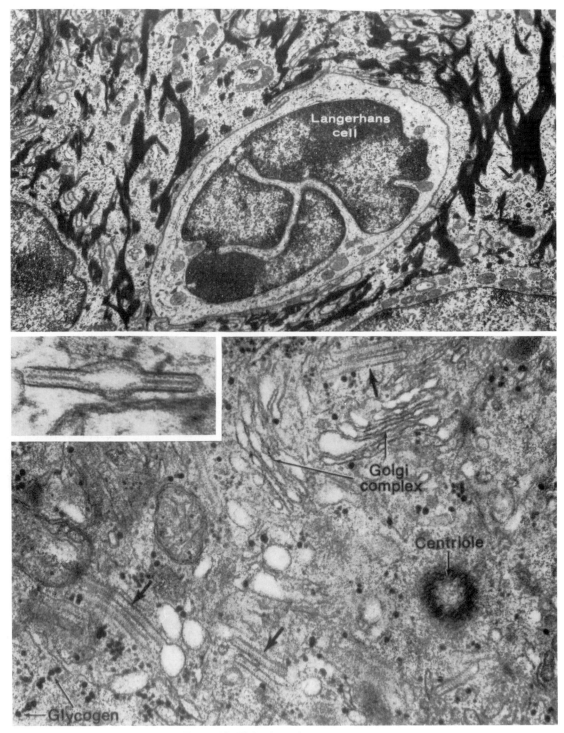

*Figure 10–12* See legend on opposite page

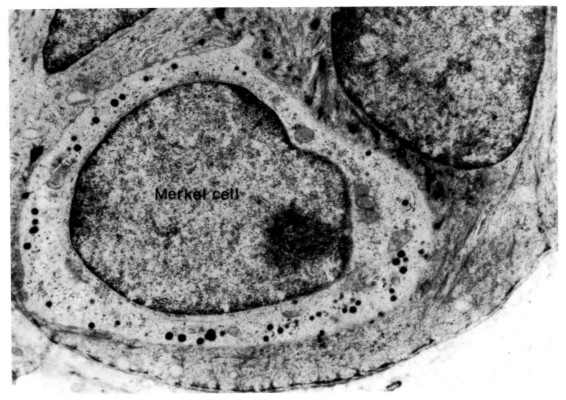

**Figure 10–13.** Electron micrograph of the base of the human epidermis, showing a Merkel's cell surrounded by keratinocytes. Notice its pale cytoplasm and characteristic dense granules. (Courtesy of G. Szabo and D. W. Fawcett, from Fawcett, D. W.: Bloom and Fawcett: A Textbook of Histology, 11th ed. Philadelphia, W. B. Saunders Co., 1986.)

**Papillary Layer.** The papillary layer includes the ridges and papillae that protrude into the epidermis. Papillae tend to occur in double rows and often are branched. Some papillae contain special nerve terminations (nervous papillae); others possess loops of capillary blood vessels (vascular papillae). The papillary layer is composed of thin collagenous, reticular, and elastic fibers arranged in an extensive network. Just beneath the epidermis, reticular fibers of the dermis form a close feltwork of fibrils that insert into the basal lamina beneath the epidermis and extend perpendicularly into the dermis as anchoring fibrils.

**Reticular Layer.** The reticular layer is the main fibrous bed of the dermis (Fig. 10–14). It consists of coarse, dense, interlacing collagenous fibers, in which are intermingled a few reticular fibers and numerous elastic fibers. The large amount of collagen endows the dermis with considerable mechanical strength and is the basis for the commercial tanning of the skin into leather. The predominant direction of all fibers is parallel to

**Figure 10–12.** Electron micrograph of the Langerhans's cell. Top: A Langerhans's cell surrounded by keratinocytes containing dense bundles of filaments. The polymorphous appearance of the nucleus is typical. The stellate form of the cell is not evident here because none of the processes is included in the plane of section. Bottom: A small area of cytoplasm of a Langerhans's cell, including one of the pair of centrioles, the Golgi complex, and several vermiform granules (at heavy arrows). One of these is shown at higher magnification in the inset. The dense granules in the cytoplasmic matrix are glycogen. (Courtesy of G. Szabo and D. W. Fawcett, from Fawcett, D. W.: Bloom and Fawcett: A Textbook of Histology, 11th ed. Philadelphia, W. B. Saunders Co., 1986.)

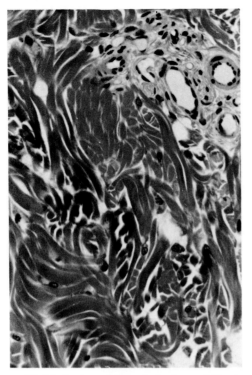

*Figure 10–14.* Section of the reticular layer of the dermis. Note the coarse interlacing collagenous fibers. Small blood vessels, components of the rete subpapillare, are present at the junction between the papillary and reticular layers of the dermis (top right). Plastic section. Medium power.

the surface. Owing to the direction of the fibers, lines of skin tension, *Langer's lines*, are formed. The direction of these lines is of surgical importance, since incisions made parallel with the lines gape less and heal with less scar tissue than incisions made at right angles to or obliquely across the lines.

The ground substance of the dermis is an amorphous matrix that embeds the collagenous and elastic fibers and, additionally, the skin appendages. The three principal glycosaminoglycans of skin are hyaluronic acid, dermatan sulfates, and chondroitin sulfates, and their proportions vary in different regions. They are markedly hydrophilic and form a gel. The decrease in the flexibility of the skin with time is due to a decrease in the amounts of water and glycosaminoglycans, not to a decrease in elastin.

**Cellular Elements.** The predominant cellular elements of the dermis are *fibroblasts* and *macrophages*. In addition, *fat cells* may be present, either singly or in groups. Apart from the usual types of connective tissue cells, pigmented, branched, connective tissue cells, *chromatophores*, may be present. They are numerous only in areas where the overlying epidermis is heavily pigmented, for example, in the areola of the nipple and the circumanal region. They do not elaborate their pigment, but obtain it apparently from melanocytes. True *dermal* melanocytes are rare. These, like the melanocytes of the epidermis, are dopa-positive. They may accumulate in the sacral region, where they form the "mongolian spot," or in certain tumors of the dermis (blue nevi). Generally, the papillary layer contains more cells and smaller and finer connective tissue fibers than does the reticular layer.

**Muscle Fibers.** Smooth muscle fibers may be found in the dermis. They are arranged in small bundles in connection with hair follicles (*arrector pili* muscles) and are scattered throughout the dermis in considerable numbers in the skin of the nipple, penis, scrotum, and parts of the perineum. The arrector pili muscles are innervated by the sympathetic division of the autonomic nervous system. Contraction of the fibers gives the skin of these regions a wrinkled appearance. In the face and neck, fibers of some skeletal muscles terminate in delicate elastic fiber networks of the dermis.

**Hypodermis.** The subcutaneous layer (superficial fascia) is not part of the skin but appears as a deep extension of the dermis. The line of demarcation between the dermis and the underlying subcutaneous layer is rarely clear-cut. The latter forms a link between the skin and the underlying deep fascia, or periosteum, and has important functions as a fat store and insulating layer. The density and arrangement of the subcutaneous layer determine the mobility of the skin. Depending upon the region of the body and the general state of nutrition of the organism, varying numbers of fat cells occur in the hypodermis. The fat is laid down in the reticular tissue formed in fetal life. The thickness of the fat layer is also predetermined at that time. The hypodermis contributes to the thermal insulation of the body. When continuous lobules of fat are present, the hypodermis forms a fat pad, the *panniculus adiposus*. On the abdomen, this layer may reach a thickness of 3 cm or more. In the eyelids, penis, and scrotum the subcutaneous layer is devoid of fat. The superficial zone of the hypodermis contains parts of the hair follicles and sweat glands.

## THE NAILS

The nails are horny plates that form a protective covering on the dorsal surface of the terminal phalanges of the fingers and toes.

## Structure

The structure and relationship of the nails to the epidermis and the dermis are understood best if consideration is given to their early development (Figs. 10–15 and 10–16). Toward the end of the third month of intrauterine life, the epidermis over the dorsal surface of the terminal phalanx of each finger and toe invades the underlying dermis. Unlike the early development of a gland, which is a tubular ingrowth of epithelial cells into the underlying connective tissue, in the case of the nail, the invasion occurs along a transverse curved line and slants proximally with relation to the surface. The invading plate of epidermis later splits to form a *nail groove*, and the epidermal cells of the deep (distal) wall of the groove proliferate to form the matrix of the nail. With continuing proliferation and differentiation of cells in the lower part of the matrix, the forming *nail plate* is pushed out of the groove and slowly advances over the dorsal surface of the digit toward the distal end. The epidermis immediately beneath the nail plate constitutes the *nail bed*. The nail plate itself is contained within the nail groove, which becomes U-shaped as seen from the dorsum, flanked by a skin fold, the *nail wall*. The nail bed, which underlies both the exposed and concealed portions of the nail, consists of only the deeper layers of the epidermis and the underlying dermis, which is ridged longitudinally. It

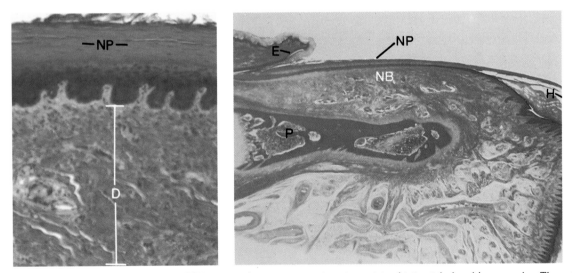

*Figure 10–15.* Nail. Left: *The nail plate (NP) appears homogeneous, since it consists of intimately fused horny scales. The nail bed, which underlies the nail plate, consists of the deeper layers of the epidermis (dark red) and the dermis (D), which lacks sweat glands and hair follicles. The dermis is grooved longitudinally, and thus in transverse sections, the junction between dermis and epidermis appears markedly irregular. Transverse section. H and E. High power.* Right: *Shown in this section is the distal phalanx of a finger (P) and the nail bed (NB), with the nail plate (NP) above. A portion of the proximal nail wall extends onto the free surface of the nail plate as the eponychium (E), and a portion of distal nail wall is thickened below the free margin of the nail to form the hyponychium (H). Longitudinal section. H and E. Low power.*

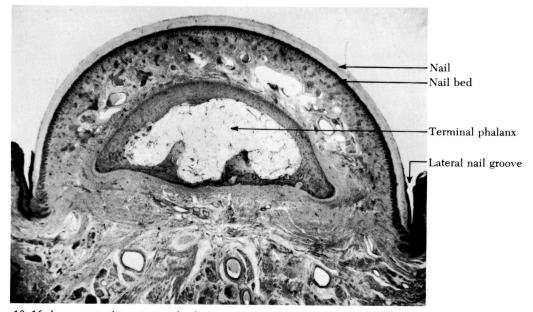

**Figure 10–16.** *Low-power photomicrograph of a cross section through a child's finger, showing the nail and nail bed. Low power.*

lacks sweat glands and hair follicles. The epidermis of the nail bed, the matrix, is thickest proximally, and it is here that nail growth chiefly occurs and the rate of cell division is rapid. Component cells contain numerous cytoplasmic fibrils that are lost at a later stage as the cells become homogeneous, cornify, and join the nail plate. At no time can keratohyalin granules be recognized in cells of the matrix, and the keratin of the nail is termed hard. In its deeper layers, the matrix contains melanocytes, and the nail plate may be pigmented, especially in darker races.

Epidermis of the nail bed is continuous distally with epidermis of the fingertip under the free edge of the nail. At the junction, the stratum corneum of the epidermis is thickened. This thickened epidermis is known as the *hyponychium*. The nail plate itself consists of intimately fused epidermal scales that do not desquamate. The body of the plate is translucent and transmits the pink color of blood vessels in the nail bed. The root is more opaque than the body, since cornification and drying are incomplete. The root becomes continuous with the body of the nail over a crescentic margin, a portion of which junction is visible distal to the nail groove. This is the *lunule*. The nail groove is lined by modified epidermis of the nail wall. Cells of the stratum corneum extend from the nail wall onto the free surface of the nail plate as the *eponychium*, or cuticle.

### Growth

The addition of newly keratinized cells to the nail root results in a slow movement of the nail plate over the nail bed. The nail bed continuously grows without the addition of a resting phase. The nail bed does not contribute to the structure or to the growth of the nail plate. On the average, nails grow at the rate of about 0.5 mm a week; growth is quicker in the fingernails than in the toenails. If a nail is removed forcibly, a new nail will grow if the matrix is not destroyed. Loss of the nail impairs touch perception.

### THE HAIR

Hairs are elastic keratinized threads that develop from the epidermis. They are distributed over the entire skin except for the palms, soles, dorsal surfaces of the distal phalanges, and the region of the anal and urogenital apertures. Each hair has a free *shaft* and a *root* embedded in the skin. Enclosing the hair root is a tubular *hair follicle*, which consists of epidermal (epithelial) and dermal (connective tissue) portions. At its lower end, the follicle expands into a *hair bulb*, which is indented at the basal end by a connective tissue *papilla*. Associated with the hair follicle are one or more sebaceous glands and a bundle of smooth muscle fibers. Together, these structures form a *pilosebaceous unit* (Fig. 10–17). The muscle, the *arrector pili*, is attached, at one end, to the connective tissue sheath of the follicle and, at the other, to the papillary layer of the dermis. By its contraction, it causes erection of the hair, since the hair is not set perpendicularly to the skin surface but slopes at an obtuse angle. Contraction of these muscle fibers also assists in the release of sebum from the sebaceous gland and depression of the skin where the muscles attach to the dermis. This muscle is absent in the eyebrows and eyelashes.

### Structure of the Hair

The hair consists of epidermal cells arranged in three concentric layers (Fig. 10–18):
1. The medulla.
2. The cortex.
3. The cuticle.

**Medulla.** The medulla forms the loose central axis and consists of two or three layers of shrunken, cornified, cuboidal cells that are separated partially by air spaces. The medulla is absent in fine short hairs of the downy type and is missing also from some of the hairs of the scalp and from "blonde" hair. The cells often contain pigment. The keratin of medullary cells is of the "soft" type, which has a low sulfur content and is characterized by the shedding of small visible particles. This shedding of particulate matter is typical of soft-keratinization, which goes through a granular morphogenesis.

**Cortex.** The cortex makes up the main bulk of the hair and is composed of several layers of long, flattened, spindle-shaped cornified cells in which the keratin is of the "hard" type. The keratin fibrils are oriented parallel to the long axis of the hair, and pigment granules are found in and between cells. Black hair contains pigment

that is oxidized. Air also accumulates in the intercellular spaces of cortical cells and modifies the hair color.

**Cuticle.** Superficially, there is a single layer of thin clear cells, the cuticle. These are cornified cells that, except for those in the base of the root, have lost their nuclei. The cells overlap, like shingles of a roof, with their free edges directed upward (Fig. 10–19). The appearance of hair in cross section varies according to race (that of Chinese, Eskimos, and American Indians appears round in cross sections; the wavy hair of many people, including Caucasians, appears oval; and the wooly hair of blacks appears elliptical, or reniform).

### Structure of the Hair Follicle

The hair follicle is a compound sheath consisting of an external connective tissue sheath (the *dermal root sheath*), derived from the dermis, and an internal *epithelial root sheath*, from the epidermis (Figs. 10–20 and 10–21). The epithelial root sheath is subdivided into inner and outer components. Toward its deep end, the follicle is expanded into a hair bulb where the hair root and its sheath blend in a mass of primitive cells, the matrix. The base of the bulb is invaginated by a connective tissue papilla, and it is in relation to the papilla that the hair root and its sheaths merge. The hair papilla, although much larger, is similar in structure to other dermal papillae and contains delicate connective tissue fibers, cellular elements, and a rich plexus of blood vessels and nerves. Not all layers of the follicle are found at all levels, but they are represented best in the portion of the follicle between the bulb and the entry of a sebaceous gland.

**Dermal Root Sheath.** The dermal root sheath is composed of three layers, corresponding to similar strata of the dermis. The outer layer is poorly defined and consists of coarse bundles of collagen fibers running in a longitudinal direction. It corresponds to the reticular layer of the dermis. The middle layer is thicker and corresponds to the papillary layer of the dermis. It is cellular and contains fine connective tissue fibers, circularly arranged. The inner layer is a homogeneous narrow band, the *glassy membrane*, corresponding to the basal lamina beneath the epidermis. It

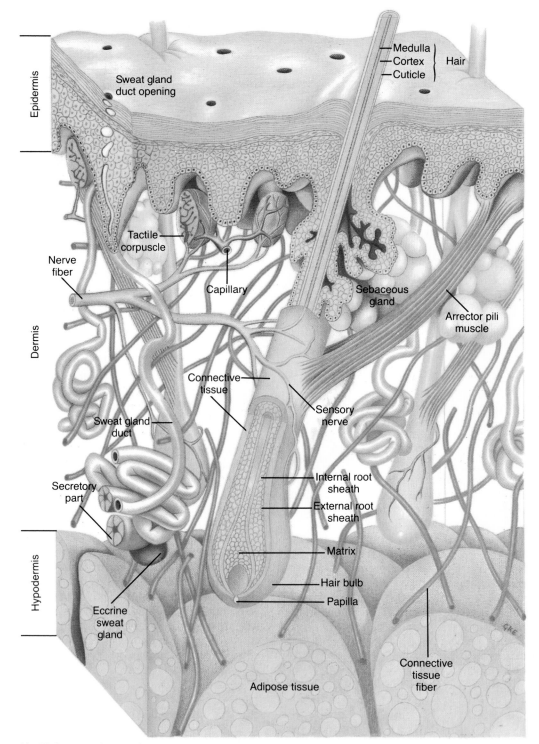

**Figure 10–17.** Diagram showing the general relationships of eccrine sweat glands and a pilosebaceous unit. The latter consists of a hair follicle, its associated sebaceous glands, and the arrector pili muscle.

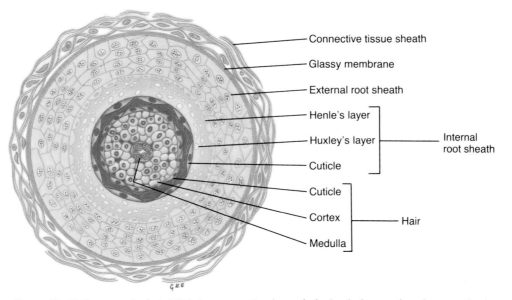

**Figure 10–18.** *Diagram of a hair follicle in cross section beneath the level of entry of a sebaceous gland.*

consists of reticular fibers and amorphous ground substance.

**Epidermal (Epithelial) Root Sheath.** The epidermal root sheath has an outer component, continuous with the deeper layers of the epidermis, and an inner component, which corresponds to the more specialized, superficial layers.

**Outer Sheath.** The outer epithelial root sheath possesses a single row of tall cells directly in relation to the glassy membrane and an inner stratum of polygonal cells (with cell contacts) that resemble cells of the stratum spinosum of the epidermis. The cells in the lower portion of the outer sheath contain an abundant supply of glycogen and appear clear in a hemotoxylin and eosin preparation. The cells in the upper portion have very little glycogen and resemble epidermal cells. The total thickness of the outer sheath increases from base to apical portion of the hair follicle.

**Inner Sheath.** The inner epithelial root sheath is a keratinized sheath enveloping the growing hair root, and like the hair, it is pushed up by addition of cells from the bulb. It elaborates "soft" keratin with a keratohyalin stage that is similar to that found in epidermis. The inner sheath does not extend above the point of entry of the duct

of the sebaceous gland into the follicle. It has three distinct strata:

1. *Henle's layer*, directly in relation to the outer epithelial root sheath, is a single layer of flattened, clear cells that contain hyaline fibrils.

2. Immediately internal to this is *Huxley's layer*, which consists of several rows of elongated cells whose cytoplasm contains *trichohyalin* granules, much like keratohyalin, and bundles of tonofibrils. In the deeper portion of the hair follicle, the cells contain nuclei, but superficially nuclei are pyknotic or absent.

3. The *cuticle of the root sheath* lies against the cuticle of the hair and is similar to the latter in structure. It is a single layer of transparent, horny scales, the free edges of which project downward and interdigitate with the upward projecting scales of the hair cuticle. This interlocking explains why the inner root sheath is also removed when a hair is extracted. The cuticle of the root sheath interdigitates with the cuticle of the hair shaft to anchor the hair shaft in the dermis.

### Growth

Growth of the hair occurs following mitosis in cells of the undifferentiated matrix of epidermal

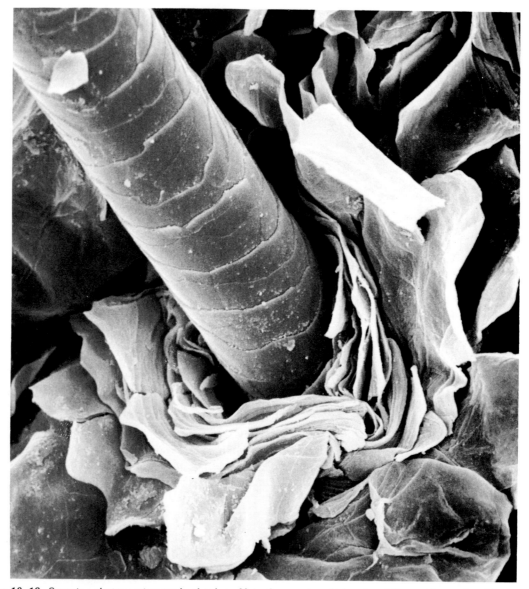

**Figure 10–19.** *Scanning electron micrograph of a hair. Note the way in which cells of the cuticle overlap. Monkey scalp.* × 1400. *(Courtesy of Dr. P. M. Andrews.)*

cells above and around the dermal papilla of the follicle. Cells immediately above the apex of the papilla form the medulla; those above the slope and sides form the cortex and cuticle of the hair, respectively. Cells immediately lateral to the papilla transform into the inner root sheath, which, like the hair root, grows upward. Cells at the

bottom of the follicle continue into the outer root sheath. The cells of the hair matrix are analogous to the malpighian layer of the epidermis in that the life cycle of each terminates with the formation of cornified cells. In the case of the epidermis, the product is soft keratinous material and the process is continuous. The product of matrix cells is a

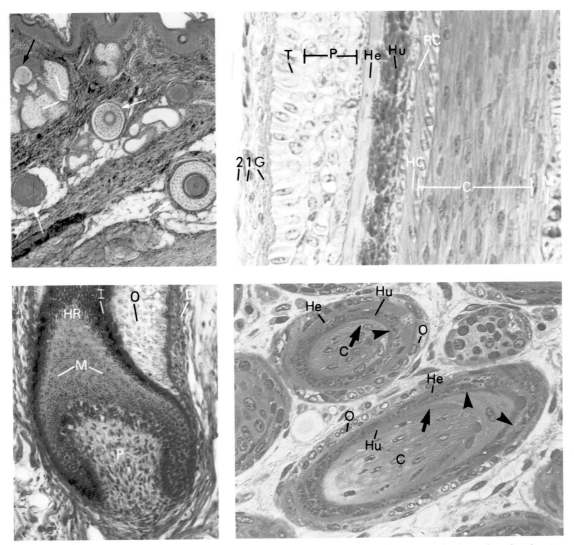

***Figure 10–20.*** *Hair follicle. Top left: Numerous hair follicles (arrows), sectioned transversely, lie within the dermis and hypodermis. One follicle near the surface of the dermis is associated with alveoli of sebaceous glands (S). Masson. Low power. Top right: This section shows portions of the hair root (right half of field) and the hair follicle. The hair exhibits the medulla (M), the cortex (C), and the cuticle (HC), a single row of cornified cells with their free edges directed upward. The inner component of the epidermal root sheath consists of the cuticle of the root sheath (RC), similar in structure to the hair cuticle but with the free edges projecting downward; Huxley's layer (Hu), the cells of which contain trichohyalin granules (deep red); and Henle's layer (He), a single row of clear cells (pale pink). The outer component of the epidermal root sheath contains several rows of polyhedral cells internally (P) and a single row of tall cells externally (T). The dermal root sheath shows an inner glassy membrane (G) and two strata of connective tissue (1 and 2) that correspond to the papillary and reticular layers of the dermis. Longitudinal section. H and E. High power. Bottom left: The hair follicle is expanded into a hair bulb, where the root of the hair (HR) and its sheath blend into a mass of primitive cells, the matrix (M). The base of the bulb is indented by a connective tissue papilla (P). The hair root is surrounded by the hair follicle, composed of the inner (I) and outer (O) epidermal root sheaths and the dermal root sheath (D). Longitudinal section. Iron hematoxylin, aniline blue. Medium power. Bottom right: Numerous hair follicles, sectioned transversely or obliquely, lie within the dermis. The hair root exhibits only cortex (C) and cuticle (arrows). The inner epidermal root sheath, here sectioned on a deep level, consists of the cuticle of the root sheath (arrowheads), Huxley's layer (Hu), and Henle's layer (He). The outer epidermal root sheath (O) at this level is poorly developed and is composed of a single row of cells. No dermal root sheath is apparent. Transverse section. H and E. Medium power.*

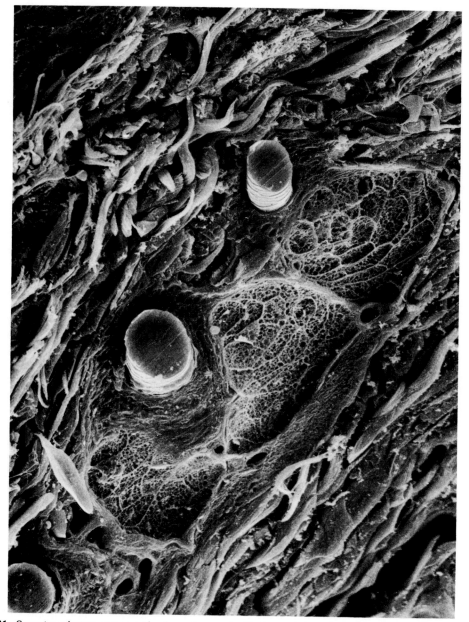

**Figure 10–21.** *Scanning electron micrograph of monkey scalp. Portions of three hair shafts and of the sebaceous glands associated with them are shown. They lie embedded in the coarse connective tissue of the dermis.* × *300. (Courtesy of Dr. P. M. Andrews.)*

hard keratinous material, and the process is intermittent and dependent upon an inductive influence by the dermal papilla. Pigment is acquired from melanocytes present within the matrix, in a manner similar to that occurring in the epidermis.

Hair has a definite period of growth that varies from region to region. It exhibits three phases of growth: *anagen* (the growth phase); *catagen* (the termination phase); and *telogen* (the resting phase). After telogen, the hair is lost and replaced periodically by a new one. The process is discontinuous, so that a particular area may contain growing hair follicles adjacent to resting hair follicles. The anagen phase for the head takes about two to four years and for eyelashes, only three to four months. Upon cessation of growth, multiplication of the undifferentiated cells at the base of the follicle ceases. The root of the hair then becomes detached from the matrix, and the hair either falls out or is pulled out. After a resting phase, the remaining cord of epithelial cells of the follicle undergoes a period of growth and contacts either the old papilla or a new one. A new germinal matrix develops, and a new hair begins to grow up the re-forming follicle. The mitotic activity of the follicle is stimulated by androgens and inhibited by estrogens. The estrogenic inhibition of hair growth occurs during pregnancy and lactation.

## GLANDS OF THE SKIN

Glands of the skin include *sebaceous, sweat,* and *mammary* glands. Mammary glands, which are specialized sweat glands, are described with the female genital system (Chapter 15).

### Sebaceous Glands

The sebaceous glands are, with a few exceptions, connected with hair follicles (Fig. 10–22). Usually, several drain into a single hair follicle; but where they are independent of hairs, their ducts open directly upon the free surface of the skin—for example, in the glans penis, labia minora, and tarsal (meibomian) glands of the eyelids. They are lacking entirely in the palms and the soles. Sebaceous glands are located in the dermis, where each gland is encapsulated by a thin layer of connective tissue. They are alveolar (saccular) glands that synthesize lipid. In most glands, several alveoli open into a short wide duct, which itself empties into the neck of a hair follicle. The most prominent sebaceous glands (located at the wings of the nose, neck, upper chest, and upper back) are associated with an enlarged follicle containing a reduced hair shaft. This results in the formation of a special pilosebaceous unit known as a *sebaceous follicle.* Its wide openings are termed "pores" and are subject to bacterial infections. The alveoli themselves are filled completely with a stratified epithelium. The epithelium of the lobular secretory portion lies upon a delicate basal lamina, on the internal surface of which is a single row of small cuboidal cells, continuous with the basal cells of the epidermis at the neck of the hair follicle. Like the basal cells of the epidermis, these cells are joined together by desmosomes. Basal cells acquire increased amounts of agranular endoplasmic reticulum before they become active in lipogenesis. Toward the center of the alveolus, cells become progressively larger, and the cytoplasm is distended with fat droplets. The droplets contain cholesterol, phospholipids, and triglycerides. Nuclei gradually shrink and then disappear, and the cells break down into a fatty mass and cellular debris. This is the oily secretion (*sebum*) of the gland, which is of the holocrine type, since it results from total destruction of epithelial cells. Sebum consists of lipids (60 per cent by weight) such as wax esters, squalene, and a great deal of free fatty acids and triglycerides. Unlike the epidermal cell, it does not contain great quantities of cholesterol and phospholipids.

Cells lost in the secretory process are replaced by proliferation from the basal cells and from cells close to the wall of the excretory duct. They are strongly basophil and comprise the regenerative cells of the gland. The short, wide duct of sebaceous glands is lined by stratified squamous epithelium continuous with the external root sheath of the hair and with the malpighian layer of the epidermis. Toward the alveolus, the layering decreases progressively until finally it merges with the row of low basal cells of the alveolus. Dis-

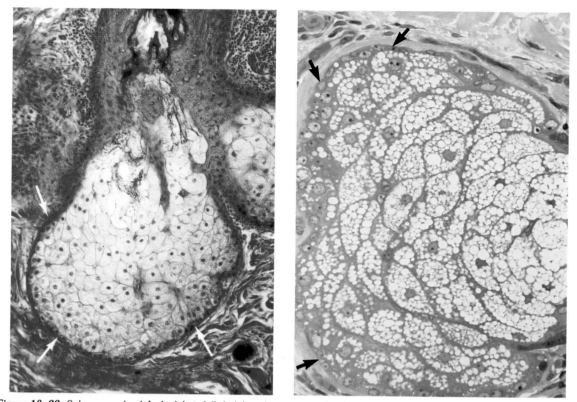

**Figure 10–22.** *Sebaceous gland. Left: A hair follicle (above) is associated with two sebaceous gland alveoli, embedded in dense connective tissue of the dermis (blue). A single row of low cuboidal cells (arrows), continuous with the basal cells of the epidermis at the neck of the hair follicle, surrounds the central alveolus. The alveolus is filled with a stratified epithelium, and toward the center, cells become progressively larger. The cytoplasm appears vacuolated (owing to the loss of fat droplets during preparation). Iron hematoxylin, aniline blue. Low power. Right: A single row of low cuboidal cells (arrows), surrounding the alveolus, is separated from the embedding dermal connective tissue by a wide, eosinophil basal lamina. Toward the center of the alveolus, cells become progressively larger, and the cytoplasm is distended with fat droplets. Nuclei appear shrunken and pyknotic. Plastic section. H and E. Medium power.*

charge of secretion is aided by contraction of the arrector pili muscle and by general pressure owing to an increase in the size of cells centrally within the alveolus.

Development and growth of sebaceous glands, particularly during puberty, are stimulated by androgens and inhibited by estrogens. Secretion of sebum occurs continuously. The significance of the secretion, with regard to maintenance of the health of skin, is unknown, and it has been suggested that sebum acts as a pheromone, since the scent glands of many primates are sebaceous in nature.

### Sweat Glands

The ordinary sweat glands (*eccrine* type) are unbranched, coiled, tubular glands distributed throughout the skin, except upon the nail bed, margins of the lips, glans penis, and eardrum (Fig. 10–23). They are most numerous on the palms and the soles. The secretory portion is situated deeply in the dermis, or in the hypodermis, and is coiled into a discrete mass. The excretory portion, or duct, rises to the epidermis by a slightly tortuous course, joins the epidermis, and spirals through it to reach the free surface, where it

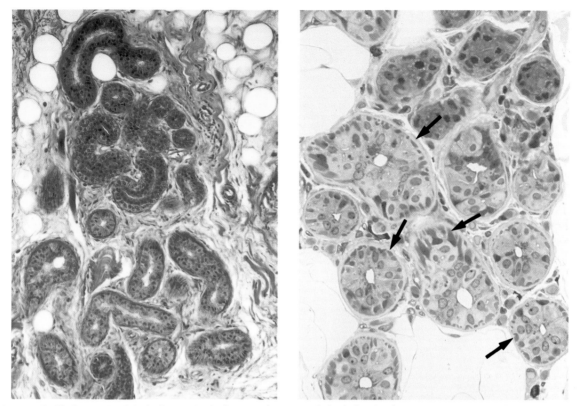

**Figure 10–23.** *Sweat gland. Left: Sweat glands, because they are coiled tubular glands, are cut in numerous planes in sections. Here, the secretory portion is seen below and the excretory portion above. The former is lined by a simple epithelium; the clear and dark cells are not differentiated by this stain. The excretory portion is lined by two layers of darkly staining cuboidal cells. The gland is surrounded by collagenous connective tissue of the hypodermis (blue) and by fat cells. Iron hematoxylin, aniline blue. Medium power. Right: Below are profiles of the secretory portion of this eccrine gland. The lining cells are pyramidal or columnar and possess a pale cytoplasm. Between the bases of the cells and the bounding basal lamina, cytoplasmic processes of myoepithelial cells, deeply acidophil, are visible (arrows). The excretory duct (above), represented by four profiles, is lined by a double layer of darkly staining cuboidal cells. Plastic section. H and E. High power.*

opens by a minute pit, the *sweat pore* (Figs. 10–24 and 10–25).

The coiled secretory portion of the gland is lined by a simple columnar or cuboidal epithelium supported by a distinct basal lamina. Two distinct cell types are present within the epithelium. The principal (clear) cells are *serous* and vary in height, depending on the activity of the gland. The nucleus is spherical and occupies a midposition in the cell. The cytoplasm is vacuolated and contains fat droplets and, occasionally, pigment granules. Secretory capillaries (intercellular canaliculi) occur between cells. The cells secrete a watery product containing solutes. Scattered between serous cells are *mucigenous* (dark) cells, which contain an extensive granular endoplasmic reticulum and small basophilic secretory granules. They produce a mucoid glycoprotein. Between the bases of the secretory cells and the bounding basal lamina, there is a layer of myoepithelial cells (Fig. 10–26). The nucleus of such cells is elongated, and the cytoplasm deeply acidophil. Contraction of these cells is believed to aid in emptying the gland of secretion. Additionally, these cells are thought to function as supportive structures, resisting changes in osmotic pressure that might

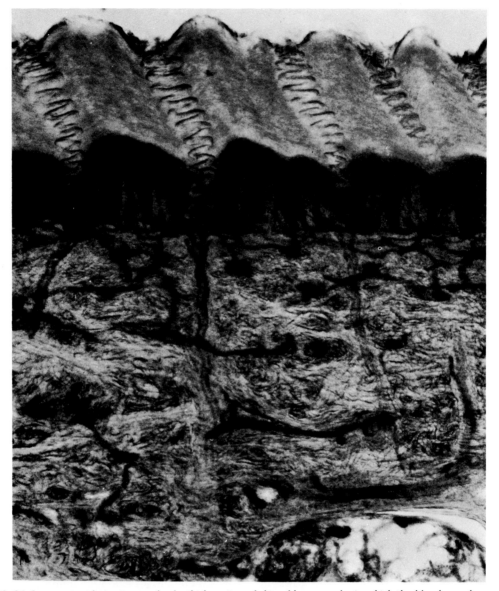

**Figure 10–24.** Low-power photomicrograph of a thick section of skin of human palm in which the blood vessels were injected with red gelatin. In this thick section, one also has a good demonstration of the spiral course taken through the epidermis by ducts of sweat glands. Low power.

endanger the structural integrity of the intercellular canaliculi.

The secretory tubule narrows into a slender excretory duct that is lined with a double layer of darkly staining cuboidal cells. The cells that form the inner layer of the duct wall bear a specialized fibrous border along their free surface, where the cytoplasm appears homogeneous and stains intensely because of the concentration of tonofilaments. The duct is surrounded by a basal lamina, but no myoepithelial elements are interposed between it and the lining epithelium. Where the

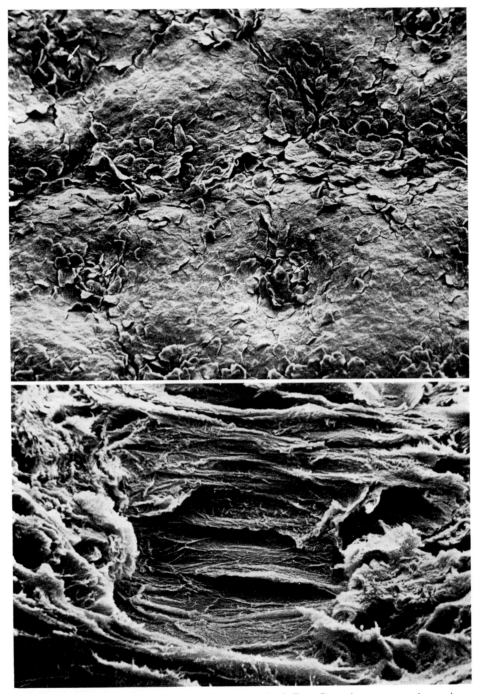

**Figure 10–25.** Scanning electron microscopic view of the sweat gland. Top: Several sweat pores (arrows) are seen on the surface of the sole. Each sweat pore is characterized by a rose-like concentration of scaly cells. × 200. Bottom: The spiral nature of a portion of a sweat gland duct is exposed. Note the wrinkled appearance of its wall. × 1900. (Reproduced with permission from Fujita, T., et al.: SEM Atlas of Cells and Tissues. New York, Igaku-Shoin, 1981.)

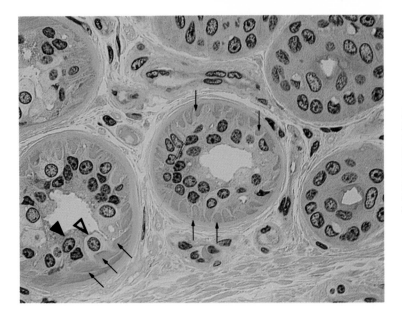

*Figure 10–26.* Photomicrograph of a sweat gland showing myoepithelial cells (small arrows) and two gland cell types, dark cell (dark arrowhead) and clear cell (light arrowhead). The apical portion of the dark cell is broad and circumscribes the lumen. The base of clear cell rests on the myoepithelial cell or directly on the basal lamina. Plastic section. H and E. Oil immersion.

duct joins the epidermis, it loses its own wall, becoming a specialized channel through the epithelium. Functionally, these glands play an important role in thermoregulation by providing a film of moisture on the skin surface for evaporative cooling. They also are responsive to nervous stress, particularly those glands in the palmar and plantar regions.

The ordinary sweat glands (eccrine type) are merocrine in their secretion, but certain large sweat glands found in the axilla, areola of the nipple, labia majora, and circumanal region produce a thicker secretion than the sweat formed by the smaller glands. The ducts, similar in structure to those of eccrine glands, frequently open into the upper portions of hair follicles. In the secretory portions, the apices of the gland cells frequently are broken off in the process of preparation. However, this is an artifact, and secretion is merocrine in type, although the glands traditionally still are called *apocrine* glands. No clear cells are present; the mucigenous (dark) cells are similar to those of eccrine sweat glands and contain secretory granules and numerous secondary lysosomes. These large sweat glands show less coiling than do ordinary sweat glands, and the lumen of the secretory portion is much wider. Myoepithelial cells are larger and form a more complete layer between the epithelial cells and the basal lamina. These glands begin to function only at puberty. The wax-secreting *ceruminous* glands of the external auditory canal and the

*glands of Moll* in the margin of the eyelid also belong to this group of larger sweat glands.

The larger sweat glands produce a viscous secretion in contrast with the more fluid discharge of the smaller sweat glands. The main fluid constituents of the smaller glands are water, sodium chloride, urea, ammonia, and uric acid. The secretion will last as long as the stimulus (cholinergic innervation) persists. The amount could reach up to 2 liters (L) of sweat per hour. An abnormal increase in the amount of sodium chloride in the sweat is diagnostic of the disease *cystic fibrosis*.

The number of sweat glands, in general, is very large at birth. Sweat glands may become functionally inactivated in persons who live in temperate regions. However, the number will remain high provided that the individuals are raised and remain in a tropical region up to adulthood. The latter phenomenon is referred to as *long-term acclimatization*.

### BLOOD VESSELS, LYMPHATICS, AND NERVES OF THE SKIN

The blood supply to the skin is from large arteries in the subcutaneous layer. These vessels send branches superficially to form a horizontally oriented network (*rete cutaneum*) at the junctional zone between dermis and hypodermis. From this network, branches pass on one side to supply the subcutaneous tissue (including sweat glands) and the deeper portions of hair follicles and on the other side to the dermis, where they form a further network between the papillary and reticular layers (the *rete subpapillare*). From the latter plexus, small arteries are given off to the papillae, where they break up into capillary networks to supply the papillae, sebaceous glands, and the intermediate portions of the hair follicles.

Veins collecting blood from the area supplied by the rete subpapillare form a network immediately beneath the papillae. This network communicates with a second plexus just deeper than the first and, via this, with a third plexus at the junction of the dermis and the hypodermis. Into the third plexus pass most of the veins from the fat lobules and sweat glands. From the third plexus, veins pass to a deeper network of large veins in the subcutaneous tissue which is drained by large veins accompanying the arteries. Arteriovenous anastomoses are common within the deeper layers of the dermis, where they play a role in temperature regulation (Fig. 10–27). Such anastomoses are especially numerous in the fingertips and toes.

The lymphatics begin in the papillae as endothelium-lined clefts, which pass to a horizontal network of lymph capillaries in the papillary layer. This network communicates with a network of larger lymph capillaries in the subcutaneous tissue, which also receives lymph from delicate plexuses surrounding sebaceous and sweat glands and hair follicles.

The skin, together with its accessory organs, receives stimuli from the external environment and, thus, is abundantly supplied with sensory nerves. These nerves arise from branches of the trigeminal and spinal nerves and differ as to size and degree of myelination. Therefore, sensory stimuli are conducted at various speeds. In the subcutaneous tissue, there are bundles of large nerves that send branches to several plexuses in the reticular, papillary, and subepithelial zones. In all layers of the skin and hypodermis, there are numerous nerve endings of various kinds (see Chapter 17). Apart from free endings of unmyelinated sensory fibers in or close to the epidermis, there are numerous fibers supplying hair follicles. In addition to sensory nerves, there are efferent sympathetic fibers supplying the blood vessels, the arrectores pilorum, and the secretory cells of the sweat glands.

## FUNCTIONAL SUMMARY

The skin is composed of two layers: the epidermis, a superficial layer devoid of blood vessels and lymphatics and composed of a stratified

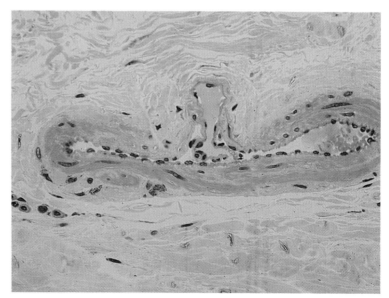

*Figure 10–27. Arteriovenous anastomoses seen within the deeper layers of the dermis. Plastic section. H and E. Oil immersion.*

squamous keratinized epithelium, and beneath this, the dermis, composed of a vascular loose (papillary layer) and an irregular dense (reticular layer) connective tissue, which corresponds to the lamina propria of a mucous membrane. Skin is commonly classified as thick or thin according to the depth of the epidermis (which consists of five robust strata) and not to the thickness of the skin as a whole. Compared with thin skin, thick skin is characterized by having a superficial layer of keratin (to increase the grip); fingerprints (to enhance the frictional force) that correspond to the high dermal papillae; no hair follicles with associated sebaceous glands (pilosebaceous units); and eccrine glands that are generally more abundant, with apocrine glands being less restricted in distribution.

The epidermis regenerates by regrowing from the residual portions of hair follicles and sweat glands. It is composed of four cell types: keratinocytes, melanocytes, Langerhans's cells, and Merkel's cells. The keratinocytes are arranged in five strata (germinativum, spinosum, granulosum, lucidum, and corneum) and are epithelial cells that eventually differentiate to produce nonmembranous, basophil (histidine-rich and cystine-containing protein) keratohyalin granules that have many phosphate groups. One of the functions of these granules seems to be to bind the tonofilaments and thus bring about a compartmentalization of these filaments within the cytoplasm. The keratin, the final end product, completely fills the scalelike cells of the stratum corneum and endows the skin with the following characteristics: impermeability to water and protection from mechanical damage, bacterial invasion, and dehydration. The tonofilaments insert into the desmosomes (cytoplasmic densities) and maintain cohesion while reducing the effects of abrasion among keratinocytes. The keratinocytes proliferate and acquire melanin granules from the melanocytes (the transfer process is injective and is called cytocrine secretion). The melanin is manufactured inside Golgi-derived tyrosinase-containing melanosomes. The tyrosinase, an enzyme that converts tyrosine to dopa and then into dopaquinone and eventually on to melanin, is made in the ribosomes and transferred to the Golgi-derived melanosomes. The manufacture of melanin is enhanced by ultraviolet (UV) light. The melanin protects the regenerative cells of the epidermis against chromosomal damage by capturing harmful free radicals produced by UV light. The presence of various amounts of melanin in the melanosomes is responsible for the shades of brown color of the skin. UV light exposure also stimulates the synthesis of vitamin D.

The epidermis also contains macrophages, called Langerhans's cells (derived from bone marrow precursors), that bear surface antigens common to most B and T lymphocytes and especially function in connection with the occurrence of *contact dermatitis* (development of contact sensitivity of the skin). Merkel's cells constitute the fourth cellular population within the epidermis and are believed to function as sensory mechanoreceptors. Neurites from the dermis form a terminal disc at the base of these cells where numerous dense-core osmiophil granules are concentrated. These cells attach themselves to keratinocytes via numerous desmosomes and have been implicated as having APUD (amine precursor uptake and decarboxylase) cell–like activity.

The dermis determines the developmental pattern of the overlying epidermis (transplanted dermis from the sole induces the formation of thick skin). The dermis repairs itself through fibroblastic activity and deposition of collagen. The collagen fibers of the loose connective tissue layer anchor the dermis to the epidermis. The defective formation of these fibrils may lead to abnormal increase in the extensibility of the skin, *cutis laxa*. The thicker reticular layer of the dermis contains many more type 1 coarse collagenous fibers and a thicker network of elastic fibers that together provide considerable mechanical strength. The predominant directional tendency of the collagenous fibers differ in different areas of the body (called cleavage lines of Langer). Surgical incisions that are made parallel to Langer's lines heal faster and produce less scar tissue. The dermal papillae, whose height varies directly with the thickness of the epidermis, increase the surface contact with the epidermis and thereby the diffusive nourishment to this avascular superficial layer. Encapsulated sensory organs (Meissner's and Vater-Pacini corpuscles) constitute an important part of the sensory apparatus found in the dermis. The eccrine sweat glands play a decisive role in the regulation of body temperatures, since unlike apocrine sweat glands, their secretion persists as long as the cholinergic stimulation lasts.

In addition, eccrine glands open onto the surface not into hair follicles, and their watery secretion contains sodium chloride. The concentration of sodium chloride may serve as a diagnostic tool for identifying cystic fibrosis. It is believed that the secretions of the apocrine sweat glands may act as pheromones (sexual attractants). Sebaceous glands usually are associated with a hair follicle and empty their holocrine secretory product (sebum) into the upper part of the hair follicle. The significance of the secretion, with regard to the maintenance of the health of the skin (as a lubricant, antidrying agent; water-sealant of the skin) is unknown, and it has been suggested that sebum acts mainly like a pheromone.

Hair, a hard and compact keratinized structure, has a definite period of growth. The erection of the hair by the arrector pili muscles gives the skin a wrinkled appearance. In humans, hair is mainly concerned with the sensory function of the skin. The hypodermis contributes to thermal insulation. Injuries to the dermal papillae result in the loss of hair. The mitotic activity in hair follicles is under the control of androgens. Dietary protein deficiency rapidly leads to atrophy and degeneration of the hair roots. The hair is anchored to the follicle via the interdigitation of the upward-directed keratinized scales of the hair cuticle and the downward-directed ones of the cuticle of the inner root sheath. The color of the hair is produced principally by the epidermal melanocytes located at the tip of the papilla.

The nails are plates of hard keratin whose cells originate from the nail matrix cells in a noncyclic manner. Damage to the nail matrix will end nail production. Growth is quicker in the fingernails than in the toenails. Nails have a protective function and a tactile role.

# The Digestive System

## GENERAL ORGANIZATION

The digestive system is made up of a long tube (the digestive tract), extending from the mouth to the anus, and associated glands such as salivary glands, the liver, and the pancreas, located outside the tube but passing their secretions into it by duct systems. Digestion involves, first, the breakdown of food material to a small particulate size, accomplished by the cutting and grinding action of the teeth and by the action of hydrochloric acid and digestive enzymes. The enzymes aid in the splitting, or hydrolyzing, of proteins, carbohydrates, and fat into basic components such as amino acids, monosaccharides, and glycerides. Second, these components (and fluid) are absorbed into the circulation. It should be appreciated that any material in the lumen of the digestive tract virtually is outside the body and thus has to pass through the lining of this tube to enter the

**11**

circulation. *Thus, digestion is the process whereby food material is converted into substances that can be absorbed into the circulation.* Useless materials, and some that are even toxic, are eliminated by fecal excretion.

The digestive system will be described in three major sections:

1. The oral cavity (including the salivary glands and oropharynx).
2. The tubular digestive tract (esophagus, stomach, small intestine, large intestine, rectum, and anal canal).
3. The major digestive glands (pancreas, liver, and biliary passages).

# The Oral Cavity

### THE LIP AND CHEEK

The oral cavity is closed anteriorly by apposition of the upper and lower lips. In lips and cheek, the substance, or core, is composed of striated muscle embedded in elastic fibroconnective tissue. Externally is a covering of skin with hair follicles, sebaceous glands, and sweat glands. Internally is a mucous membrane (mucosa) composed of stratified squamous nonkeratinizing epithelium lying upon a connective tissue lamina propria with high papillae (Figs. 11–1 and 11–2). Numerous sensory nerve endings lie in the lamina propria and in the dermis of the red lip margin, together with a blood capillary plexus, particularly rich beneath the latter. The submucosa contains elastic fibers that are continuous with both those around striated muscle of the core and those of the lamina propria. They serve to bind the mucous membrane quite firmly to the muscle, thus preventing folds of mucous membrane being formed and bitten between the teeth when the

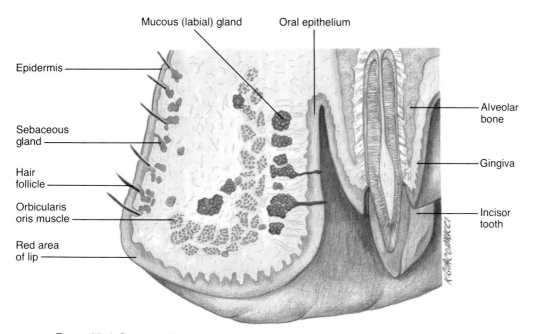

**Figure 11–1.** *Diagram of a vertical section through the upper lip and central incisor tooth.* × 6.

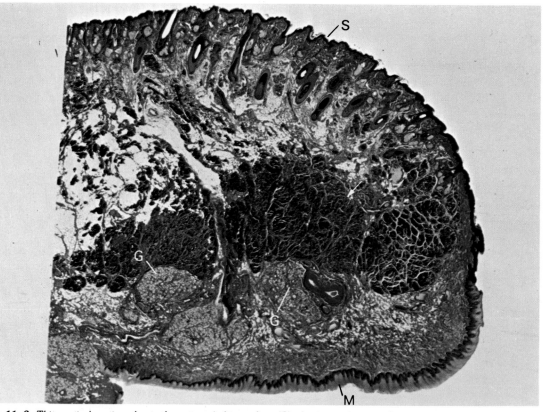

**Figure 11–2.** This vertical section shows the external skin surface (S), the internal mucosal surface (M), and the free margin (right) of the lip. The external surface is covered by thin skin with obvious hair follicles, sebaceous glands, and sweat glands; the epithelium is stratified, squamous, and keratinizing in type. As the free margin is approached, hairs and glands disappear and dermal papillae become tall. At the free margin, there are no glands, and the surface is kept moist by licking. The epithelium of the mucous membrane on the internal surface is nonkeratinizing and is supported by a lamina propria (blue) with high papillae. Within the connective tissue here are several small mucous (labial) glands (G, pink). In the core of the lip are masses of striated muscle arranged in bundles (arrows) and here cut transversely. This is muscle of the orbicularis oris. Iron hematoxylin, aniline blue. Low power.

jaws are closed. The submucosa contains many small mucous and mucoserous salivary (labial) glands, the secretion of which passes to the surface via short ducts.

At the lip margin, the epidermis is modified by a high content of keratohyalin and a thick stratum lucidum that make it more translucent. With an underlying dermis showing high papillae and with a rich vascular plexus, the free margin appears red. There are no hairs, sweat glands, or sebaceous glands in this region, and the surface epithelium is kept moist by licking with the tongue.

## TONGUE

The tongue consists of a freely movable portion (the body) located in the oral cavity and a base, or root, attached to the floor and forming part of the anterior wall of the pharynx. On the upper, or dorsal, surface of the tongue is a V-shaped groove, the *sulcus terminalis*, with the apex of the V directed posteriorly. This sulcus divides the tongue into anterior and posterior regions. The tongue is covered by a mucous membrane, and its bulk consists of striated muscle fibers and glands. The muscle fibers are both intrinsic and extrinsic; that is, some are confined to the tongue, whereas others originate outside, principally on the mandible and hyoid bone, and pass into the tongue. Between muscle fibers are glands. These glands are mainly *mucous* in the base of the tongue, their ducts opening behind the sulcus terminalis; *serous* in the body of the tongue, their ducts opening anterior to the sulcus (near circumvallate papillae); and *mixed acini* near the tip, their ducts opening on the inferior surface of the tongue.

The posterior third of the tongue has a nodular, irregular surface owing to the presence of lymphatic nodules (the lingual tonsil). Between the protrusions are cleft-like depressions of the surface epithelium termed *crypts*. Here, the epithelium is infiltrated with numerous lymphocytes.

The mucous membrane on the undersurface of the tongue is smooth and underlain by a submucosa. On the upper surface, the mucosa shows numerous small protuberances called *papillae*, which give the tongue a "furred" or roughened, appearance (Fig. 11–3). Four types of papillae are present:

1. *Filiform papillae*, located over the entire tongue surface mainly in rows parallel to the V-shaped sulcus, are of a slender, conical shape and 2 to 3 mm in height, each with a primary core of connective tissue of the lamina propria, with secondary papillae that end in tapered points (Fig. 11–4). The covering epithelium is often partially keratinized and quite hard. The keratinized epithelium gives the tongue its grayish color. The filiform papillae are hard enough to produce a rasp-like structure on the dorsal surface of the tongue of some animals.

2. *Fungiform papillae* are disposed singly among the rows of filiform papillae and are more numerous toward the tip of the tongue (Fig. 11–5). The shape is like a mushroom (fungus) with a short stalk and a broader cap. The connective tissue core shows secondary papillae, and the covering epithelium is quite thin, so that the rich vascular plexus within the lamina propria imparts a pink or reddish tinge to the papillae. Taste buds are found in the epithelium.

3. *Circumvallate papillae* (L. *vallum*, a wall) number only 10 to 14 in humans and are located along the V-shaped sulcus. Each protrudes slightly from the surface and is surrounded by a moat-like, circular furrow with numerous taste buds in the epithelium of the lateral wall (in the side of the circular furrow). Opening into the depths of the furrow are the ducts of serous (Ebner's) glands, which are located more deeply in the tongue. The thin serous secretion of these glands washes away food material from the furrow, permitting reception of new gustatory stimuli by the taste buds present along the sides of this papilla.

4. *Foliate papillae* appear as leaf-like folds on the posterolateral margins of the tongue, with taste buds in the grooves between the folds. As in circumvallate papillae, serous glands drain into the bottom of the trenches. These papillae are rudimentary in humans but well developed in rabbits.

All papillae contain numerous sensory nerve endings for touch; taste buds are associated with all except the filiform type.

## TASTE BUDS

Containing gustatory (taste) receptor cells, taste buds lie in the oral (stratified squamous) epithelium, mainly in relation to papillae but also elsewhere in the oral cavity, palate, and epiglottis. They are recognized easily on light microscopy as pale, barrel-shaped bodies lying in the epithelium, extending from its basal lamina through to the surface, but at the surface they are slightly depressed at the *taste pore*, a small aperture providing communication with the exterior.

Three cell types are present. *Supporting*, or *sustentacular, cells*, the first type, lie mainly at the periphery of the taste buds, arranged like staves of a barrel. Between them, and more centrally, lie lighter-staining *neuroepithelial taste cells*, the second cell type, usually only 10 to 14 in each taste bud. Both types have long apical microvilli, or taste hairs, projecting into the taste pore; the microvilli lie in amorphous polysaccharide material that is probably secreted by the sustentacular cells. It is possible that the amorphous polysaccharide provides a polyelectrolyte surface film for the binding of ions, which causes a change in the charge distribution that can be detected by the

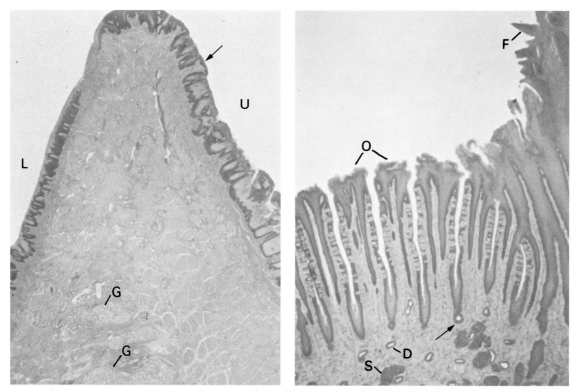

**Figure 11–3.** Tongue. Left: This is a section through the tip of the tongue with upper (U) and lower (L) surfaces covered by stratified squamous epithelium with very irregular connective tissue papillae. This irregularity is greater on the upper surface owing to the presence of fungiform papillae. Papillae are small protuberances responsible for the "furred," or roughened, appearance of the tongue. Fungiform papillae are shaped like a mushroom (fungus) with a short stalk and a broader cap (arrow). The connective tissue core usually shows secondary papillae, over which the epithelium is quite thin. A rich vascular plexus in the core imparts a reddish tinge to the structure. Within the tongue are striated muscle fibers, running vertically, transversely, and longitudinally, and some mixed salivary glands (G). H and E. Low power. Right: This is a section of the upper surface and shows filiform (F) and foliate (O) papillae. The filiform papillae have conical, pointed cores of connective tissue with a covering epithelium that, while not fully keratinized, is hard. (In some animals it is keratinized.) Foliate papillae, similar to circumvallate papillae of the human, are large, with a core of connective tissue and a surrounding depression, or trench. Taste buds are located in the sides of the papillae, that is, in the walls of the trench, and appear as pale-staining, barrel-shaped structures. Serous glands (S) lie in the connective tissue with their ducts (D) opening into the floors of the trenches (arrow). Plastic section. Methylene blue. Low power.

apical microvilli, or receptor hairs, within the cavity of the taste pore. The neuroepithelial cells function as transducers to initiate impulses in the dendrites of the afferent nerve fibers clasping them. They are chemoreceptors that are stimulated by substances dissolved in the saliva. The third type, *basal cells*, lying peripherally near the basal lamina, is believed to be the stem cell for the other cell types. There is a relatively rapid turnover of cells, with a life span in the order of ten days, and it may be that the sustentacular cell

is an intermediate stage in the differentiation of the sensory cells. Chemical stimuli are received by the sensory cells and transmitted by neurotransmitters to club-shaped nerve endings lying between the cells. As described previously, serous glands in relation to taste buds of vallate and foliate papillae wash away food material and permit new taste stimuli, and similar serous glands act in a like manner in relation to taste buds located elsewhere.

Only four fundamental taste sensations can be

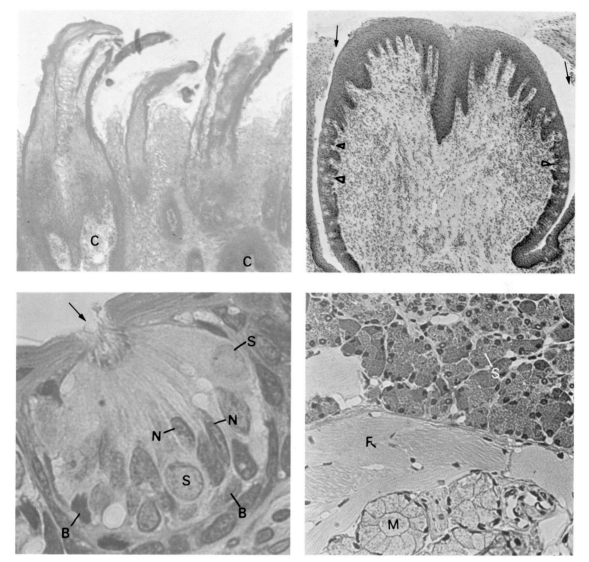

***Figure 11–4.*** *Tongue, taste buds, and glands.* Top left: *Filiform papillae. The conical form of the connective tissue core (C) of the filiform papillae with covering epithelium is seen. Note that papillae protrude for 2 to 3 mm from the surface. H and E. Medium power.* Top right: *Circumvallate papilla. These number only 10 to 14 in humans and are located along the V-shaped sulcus between the anterior and posterior parts of the tongue on its upper surface. Each protrudes slightly from the surface and is surrounded by a moat-like, circular furrow (arrows; a vallum is a wall). Secondary papillae are seen with taste buds on the lateral wall (arrowheads). H and E. Medium power.* Bottom left: *Taste bud. This is the lining epithelium from the side of a circumvallate papilla and is clearly stratified squamous in type. Located in the epithelium is a taste bud. This is barrel-shaped and composed of cells that are curved, fusiform, and arranged like the staves of a barrel. Apically, a taste pore is present (arrow), filled with hair-like processes, the taste hairs. Within the taste bud are sustentacular, or supporting, cells and neuroepithelial taste cells. The former are pale-staining, with ovoid, pale-staining nuclei (S). The latter are more slender and darker-staining, and they have darker, ovoid nuclei (N). A third cell type, the basal cell (B), is present and may be a stem cell for the other two types. Plastic section. H and E. Oil immersion.* Bottom right: *Tongue, glands. The bulk of the tongue is composed of striated muscle fibers (F), serous glands (S), and mucous glands (M). Plastic section. H and E. High power.*

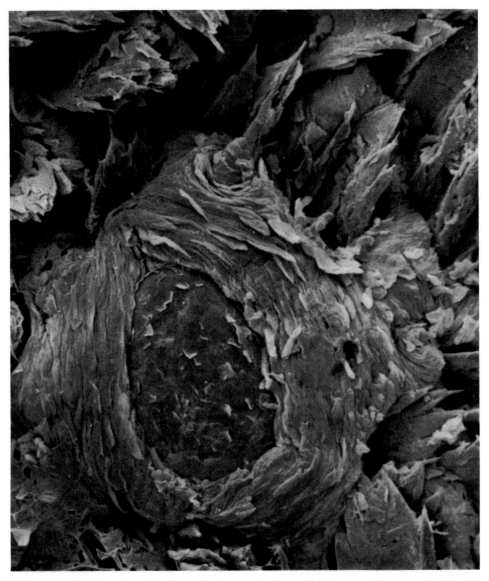

**Figure 11–5.** *Scanning electron micrograph of monkey tongue to show a fungiform papilla surrounded by filiform papillae.* × 80. *(Courtesy of P. M. Andrews.)*

detected, and there is a regional sensitivity on the tongue. Sensations of *sweet* and *salt* are appreciated at the tip, *sour* (acid) at the sides, and *bitter* in the region of the circumvallate papillae. The many different kinds of tastes must result from a synthesis of combinations of these four primary taste modalities. Recently, it has been demonstrated, however, that a single taste bud (and a single papilla) can respond to all four basic taste qualities; certainly, no structural differences have been found to explain differences in sensitivity. Nevertheless, there exists a different strength in various taste buds for a particular primary taste modality that forms the basis for the ability to discriminate between sweet, sour, salty and bitter. Nerves from taste buds in the anterior two thirds of the tongue pass in the chorda tympani branch of the facial nerve; those from the taste buds in the posterior third pass in the glossopharyngeal nerve, and those carrying taste sensation from the epiglottis and lower pharynx pass in the vagus nerve. All nerves lose their myelin before reaching taste buds. The musculature of the tongue is innervated by motor fibers in the hypoglossal nerve.

## TEETH

Basically, a tooth is derived from ectoderm and mesoderm, the latter forming most of the tooth. Teeth are actually elaborate papillae of the lamina propria, being constructed in part by a flint-like material—the hardest substance in the body. Teeth are embedded in bone of the upper and the lower jaws and are arranged in two arcs, the upper being larger than the lower, so that the lower teeth are overlapped slightly by the upper. In humans, two sets of teeth are distinguished. The *primary* (milk, or deciduous) teeth of childhood number five in each half jaw (total 20), erupting over a time period of about 6 months to 2 years of age. They are shed between 6 years of age and 12 to 13 years, being gradually replaced by the *permanent* set of adulthood. This set numbers eight in each half jaw (total 32); the anterior five replace milk teeth, and the posterior three are not represented in the primary dentition.

All teeth show a similar structure, although individual teeth are modified in shape for specific functions (e.g., incisors for biting, molars for grinding) (Fig. 11–6). A visible *crown* projects above the gum, or *gingiva*, with a *root* (or roots) buried in the alveolus of maxilla or mandible; the crown and root meet at the *neck* (Fig. 11–7). Each tooth has a *pulp cavity*, filled with connective tissue. The pulp cavity communicates via one or more small pores, or *apical foramina*, with the surrounding connective tissue, or *periodontal membrane*, that holds the tooth in its socket, or alveolus. This arrangement of a calcified tooth held in a bony socket by fibroconnective tissue is classified as a peg-and-socket type of fibrous joint, or *gomphosis*, and permits slight movement. The hard tissues of the tooth are *dentin*, surrounding the pulp cavity and forming the bulk of the tooth; *enamel*, covering the dentin of the crown; and *cementum*, covering the dentin of the root. The lower edge of enamel contacts cementum at the neck. Soft tissues are *pulp*, occupying the pulp cavity; *periodontal membrane*; and *gingiva* (or gum).

### Components of the Teeth

The hard components of the tooth comprise the dentin, enamel, and cementum. The soft components of the tooth are the pulp, the periodontal membrane, and the gingiva (Fig. 11–8).

*Dentin.* This forms the bulk of the tooth and is a calcified tissue similar to bone but harder because of a greater content of calcium salts (80 per cent) in the form of hydroxyapatite crystals. Dentin has no cells embedded in it—only the long processes of the odontoblasts. The organic intercellular material (20 per cent) is composed mainly of collagen fibers and glycosaminoglycans, synthesized by cells called *odontoblasts* (Fig. 11–9). Odontoblasts lie as a single row of cells at the periphery of the pulp on the inner aspect of dentin. Of mesenchymal origin, odontoblasts are tall, columnar-like cells with basal nuclei, basophilic cytoplasm with much granular endoplasmic reticulum, and a large supranuclear Golgi apparatus. The outer surface of the Golgi apparatus is close to the granular endoplasmic reticulum and forms the immature face (*cis* face) of the apparatus. The mature face (*trans* face) faces the center and contains enlarged vacuoles and prosecretion granules. Mature secretion granules are also seen in the long, tapered odontoblast process. Apically, toward the dentin, the cells show a cell web with junctional complexes and long, slender, cytoplasmic processes, called *Tomes's dentinal fibers*. These fibers penetrate through the full thickness of the dentin, lying in small canals in the dentin called the *dentinal tubules*. Peripherally, at the junction of dentin and enamel (crown) or dentin and cementum (root), the fibers branch, but centrally there are no branches; the fibers are 3 to 4 microns, or micrometers ($\mu$m) in diameter. The presence of dentinal tubules gives the dentin a radial striation, the tubules following a somewhat wavy course in the form of an open S. The dentin immediately around each tubule is more refringent and is called the *sheath of Neumann*.

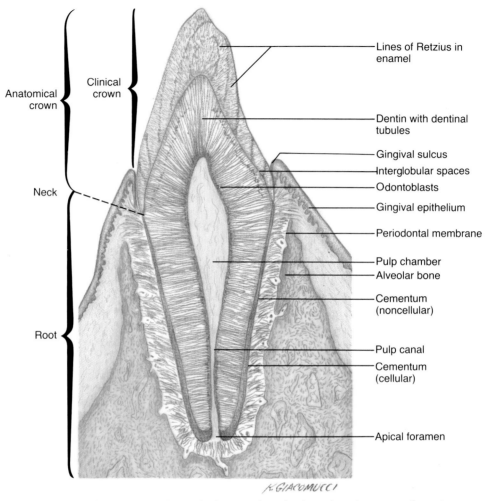

Lines of Retzius in enamel

Dentin with dentinal tubules

Gingival sulcus

Interglobular spaces

Odontoblasts

Gingival epithelium

Periodontal membrane

Pulp chamber

Alveolar bone

Cementum (noncellular)

Pulp canal

Cementum (cellular)

Apical foramen

Anatomical crown

Clinical crown

Neck

Root

K. GIACOMUCCI

*Figure 11–6. Diagram of a longitudinal section through a lower lateral incisor tooth. × 6.*

Young, immature dentin forms a layer in relation to the bases of the odontoblast processes and is called *predentin*. This layer essentially is nonmineralized and stains differently than does dentin. The thickness of this predentin layer is uniform in any tooth at a given moment of development. It contains ground substance and collagen fibrils formed by the odontoblasts. Collagenous fibrils tend to course parallel to one another and appear as closely packed wavy lines in the ground sections of the dentin. At the junction of predentin and dentin (the mineralization front), mineralization occurs, and the collagen fibrils become

masked by aggregations of *crystallites* of hydroxyapatite. These heavily encrusted calcified collagenous fibrils of mature dentin remain randomly woven, with no apparent pattern except in their longitudinal orientation to the odontoblast process. Variations in the degree of calcification of dentin are seen in small local regions, especially in the crown. Small areas, called interglobular spaces, that are noncalcified or partially calcified may remain in the dentin. Dentin formation is cyclic and not regular, and in the fully developed tooth, there are growth (incremental) lines (of Owen) that appear as growth rings in transverse

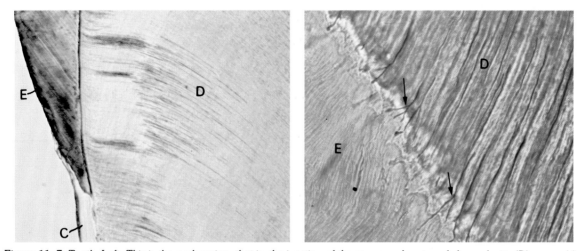

**Figure 11-7.** Tooth. Left: This is the neck region, that is, the junction of the crown and root, and shows dentin (D) covered by enamel (E) over the crown and acellular cementum (C) over the root. A regular, radial striation in the dentin is due to the presence of fine dentinal tubules. The striation in the enamel represents enamel prisms—each unit of hexagonal outline extending through the entire thickness of enamel and formed by a single ameloblast. Between prisms is interprismatic, calcified matrix. Both prisms and interprismatic substance are composed of apatite crystals with a little organic matrix. Cementum is similar to bone and is noncellular near the neck of the tooth. Ground section. Medium power. Right: This also is a ground section. Within the enamel (E) are curved, slightly sinuous enamel prisms. Only peripheral dentin (D) is seen. The thin dark lines within it are dentinal tubules, in life occupied by dentinal fibers or processes of odontoblasts. Between the tubules is a meshwork of collagenous fibers (not seen here) embedded in a calcified matrix. Note that some dentinal tubules branch (arrows) at their extremities. Ground section. High power.

section. These rhythmical growth patterns account for the incremental lines, often seen coursing at right angles to the dentinal canaliculi.

Dentin is sensitive to heat, cold, hydrogen ion concentration, and touch. It is believed that these stimuli are received by the dentinal fibers and transmitted to nerve fibers in the pulp. Odontoblasts persist throughout life, and if they are stimulated by excessive wear or periodontal disease, for example, they can lay down new, "reparative" dentin. This reparative dentin contains dentinal canaliculi filled with calcified matrix. This forms a more homogeneous and less sensitive dentin. If the odontoblasts are destroyed, dentin—unlike bone—persists for a long time. It is thus possible to maintain teeth whose pulp and odontoblasts have been destroyed by infection.

**Enamel.** This covers only the crown of the tooth, is of epithelial (ectodermal) origin, and is the hardest material of the body. Enamel is 99 per cent inorganic material, mainly calcium phosphate in the form of apatite crystals, and 1 per cent organic matrix material. The organic matrix contains not collagen but a protein called *enamelin*, which contains aspartic acid, serine, glycine, proline, and glutamic acid. This mature enamel protein contains smaller peptides that may have been formed from the breakdown of the larger proteins. Also, free sugars, glycoproteins, and phosphoproteins may be present.

The structural unit of enamel is the *enamel prism*, or *rod*, with *interprismatic substance* between prisms, both composed of apatite crystals in an organic matrix (Fig. 11-10). Each prism lies perpendicular to the surface of the dentin, extending from the dentinoenamel junction to the tooth surface, but is somewhat spiral centrally. Each prism is formed by a single *ameloblast*, is about 6 μm in diameter, and in cross section appears scale-like and basically hexagonal (Fig. 11-11). Ameloblasts are tall columnar cells, their apices (toward the dentin) elongated as Tomes's processes. These processes form the rods where the elongated apatite crystals are large and lie mainly parallel to the rod; in interprismatic substance, the crystals lie mainly perpendicular to the

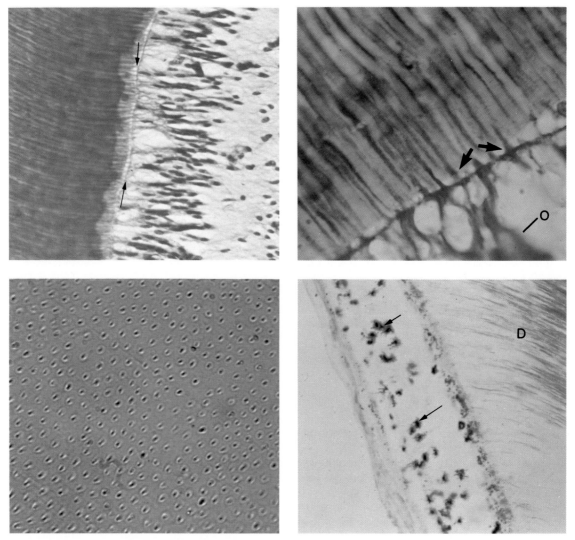

**Figure 11–8.** Tooth: pulp, dentinal fibers, dentin, and cementum. Top left: In this section of decalcified tooth, dentin lies to the left, pulp to the right. The pulp is composed of connective tissue with small, stellate cells, a few fine collagen fibrils, and relatively large amounts of mucoid intercellular substance. It resembles embryonic mesenchyme but lacks the potentiality of mesenchyme. It also contains blood vessels and nerves, which enter and leave the tooth through the apical canal. The periphery of the pulp shows a single row of tall columnar epithelium-like cells. These are odontoblasts, which have slender apical processes (Tomes's dentinal fibers) entering dentinal tubules (arrows). The paler staining of dentin (pink) adjacent to odontoblasts represents predentin. Romanes's stain. Medium power. Top right: Dentin stains dark blue with paler-staining dentinal tubules passing through it. Odontoblasts (O) are partially destroyed but show apical, pink, slender dentinal fibers or processes extending into dentinal tubules (arrows). Mallory. High power. Bottom left: The small, dark spherical dots are dentinal tubules, in life occupied by dentinal fibers. Immediately surrounding them is a lightly stained area called the sheath of Neumann (peritubular sheath). This area of the matrix contains less collagen and is more highly calcified than the remainder of the dentin matrix. The visible striation in the matrix indicates bundles of collagenous fibers, oriented in the long axis of the tooth at right angles to the dentinal tubules. Ground transverse section. High power. Bottom right: Cementum of the root is thicker toward the apex, and cellular. The cells, or cementocytes (arrows), occupy lacunae within the matrix, with delicate processes extending from them and lying in slender canaliculi in the matrix. This arrangement is similar to that of bone, and Haversian canals with blood vessels may occasionally be found in regions or conditions where cementum is very thick. Dentin (D) with dentinal tubules also is seen. Ground section. High power.

*Figure 11–9.* Drawing of an odontoblast. The odontoblasts are of mesodermal origin and cover the dental papilla, which later becomes the pulp cavity and underlies the dentin. They are believed to be responsible for the formation of the organic matrix of dentin called the predentin. Predentin consists of collagen fibers in a ground substance containing a mucopolysaccharide. The predentin then becomes calcified to form dentin. The cells are highly columnar, with a basally situated nucleus. The rough-surfaced endoplasmic reticulum is extensive and occupies much of the cytoplasm. Many of the cisternae are elongated, while others are shorter and more dilated. The central region of the cell is occupied by an extensive Golgi apparatus (G). The Golgi complex is composed of several stacks of membranous cisternae and small vesicles; dense granules (Gr) are situated near it. There are granules and mitochondria throughout the cell. Cytoplasmic filaments are common and, at the apex of the cell, form a terminal web. An odontoblastic process (top of plate) extends from the terminal web area into the dentin. These processes, or Tomes's fibers, fill the dentinal tubules, which are minute canals radiating from the pulp cavity to the periphery of the dentin. The cytoplasmic process is devoid of most organelles but contains a few dense granules, filaments, and microtubules. Vesicles are abundant, and many are fused with the plasma membrane. (From Lentz, T. L.: Cell Fine Structure. Philadelphia, W. B. Saunders Co., 1971.)

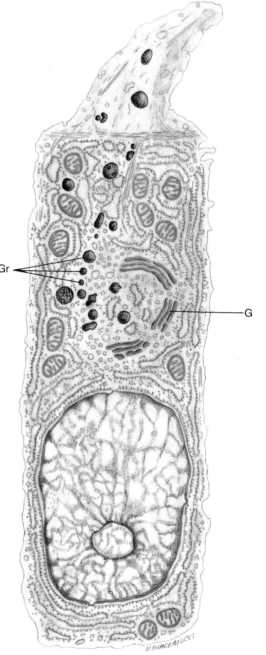

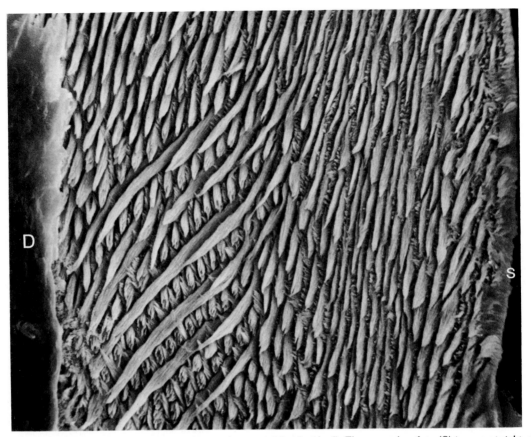

*Figure 11–10.* Scanning electron micrograph of rat molar enamel (acid-etched). The enamel surface (S) is seen at right, dentin (D) to the left. In the enamel, enamel prisms decussate in the inner enamel (left) and are parallel in the outer enamel (right). × 1250. (Courtesy of S. Risnes.)

enamel surface. As rods run obliquely through inter-rod enamel, the crystals of the two are nearly perpendicular to each other; otherwise, however, the enamel of prism and interprismatic substance is identical.

Like dentin, enamel is laid down rhythmically, and cross sections of the tooth crown show concentric, parallel, incremental lines (of Retzius). After the enamel is fully formed and mineralized, the ameloblasts persist for a short while as small, cuboidal cells, forming the *enamel cuticle* covering the enamel surface, but this cuticle is worn off with tooth eruption. With the loss of ameloblasts, further enamel formation obviously is not possible.

**Cementum.** This covers dentin of the root of the tooth, from the neck to the apex, and serves to attach the tooth to the periodontal membrane. Histologically, it is similar to bone, with coarse bundles of collagen fibrils in a calcified matrix. However, Haversian systems are usually absent, and nourishment is provided by blood vessels in the surrounding periodontal membrane. In general, it is thin and acelullar in the upper third, but bone cells (*cementocytes*) are present in the lower part, the cells lying in lacunae interconnected by canaliculi. The coarse bundles of collagen are continuous with fibers from the periodontal membrane that penetrate the cementum as *Sharpey's fibers*. These do not calcify, and thus they appear as clear canals in ground section.

Cementum, like bone, is a labile tissue that reacts to stresses and, under certain circumstances, can undergo resorption or hyperplasia. In-

**Figure 11–11.** *Drawing of an ameloblast. Secreting ameloblasts (ganoblasts) of the enamel organ are tall, extremely narrow cells of ectodermal origin, first situated in a layer next to the odontoblasts but then separated from them by the enamel and dentin. An oval nucleus with a nucleolus occupies the lower third of the cell. Some short, basal microvilli (Mv) extend into the stratum intermedium at the base of the cell. A cytoplasmic web of fine filaments (Fl) runs immediately below the plasma membrane. A cluster of mitochondria and masses of glycogen granules (Gly) are situated in the basal cytoplasm between the cytoplasmic web and nucleus. A large Golgi apparatus (G) is located in the supranuclear portion of the cell. The complex is oval and is composed of peripheral stacks of membranous cisternae surrounding a central core of cytoplasm. The Golgi cisternae are flattened in the inner regions of the stacks but are more dilated and sacculated on the outer sides. The cytoplasm enclosed by the Golgi membranes contains small, membrane-bounded secretory granules, vesicles, and both smooth- and rough-surfaced cisternae of endoplasmic reticulum. Dense granules like those in the Golgi region are common in the distal portion of the cell. The content of the granules is similar to the deposits of dense material in the extracellular spaces adjacent to the distal end of the cell. Enamel crystallites first appear in contact with the dense extracellular material. It is thought, therefore, that the ameloblasts elaborate the enamel matrix, which subsequently calcifies. Fully developed enamel consists mostly of apatite crystals and little organic material, and it is the hardest substance occurring in the body. Small vesicles are common in the apex of the cell, and some are in continuity with the plasma membrane. Larger secretory granules and multivesicular bodies, some with a dense matrix, are found in the vicinity of the Golgi complex. The cytoplasm lateral to the Golgi apparatus is largely filled with elongated cisternae of rough-surfaced endoplasmic reticulum that branch and anastomose. Free ribosomes occurring in clusters are common. Microtubules (Mt) and bundles of fine filaments (Fl) run parallel to the long axis of the cell. These filaments extend into the basal web of filaments and into a similar web at the distal pole of the cell. An ameloblastic process called Tomes's process (top of plate) extends from the tip of the cell beyond the terminal web region into the enamel. The process has no major organelles but contains microtubules, secretory granules (SG), and vesicles. When the enamel is formed, the ameloblasts atrophy and disappear. (From Lentz, T. L.: Cell Fine Structure. Philadelphia, W. B. Saunders Co., 1971.)*

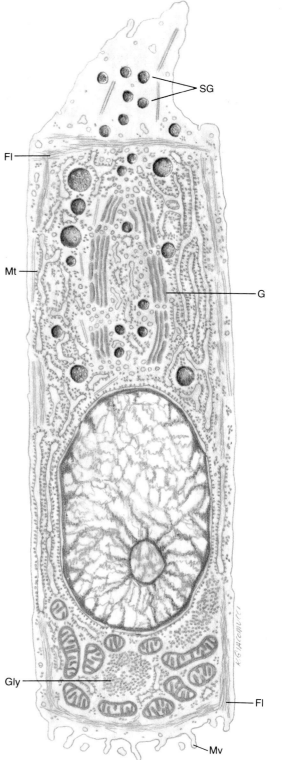

crease in thickness, which may develop near the apex in old age, occurs by appositional growth, that is, by addition of new layers to its surface. Occasionally, the thickness is such that Haversian systems with blood vessels will form. Destruction of cementum occurs rarely (e.g., in periodontal membrane disease). Cementum seems more resistant to resorption than bone. Osteoclastic activity is only seen in root resorption during replacement of the deciduous dentition.

**Pulp.** The *pulp* of the tooth is mesenchymal in origin and fills the main pulp chamber and the root canal(s). It consists of cells and intercellular material composed of fine collagen fibrils and ground substance containing glycosaminoglycans. The main cell type is stellate and resembles mesenchyme but does not have the same potentiality. Processes of these pulp cells appear to contact each other to form a reticulum, and they form the extracellular material. Other cells, such as lymphocytes, macrophages, and plasma cells, are present in limited numbers, and, as described previously, at the periphery of the pulp is a layer of dentin-producing odontoblasts.

Usually, a single thin-walled arteriole and two venules enter the pulp cavity through the root canal(s), branch, form a capillary plexus underlying and even extending between odontoblasts. Lymph vessels are difficult to identify. All pulpal blood vessels are thin-walled and thus pressure-sensitive, lying as they do in an unexpandable chamber. Thus, relatively mild inflammation and edema can cause occlusion of the blood vessels and consequent death of the pulp. Nerves also pass to .the pulp, supplying blood vessels and odontoblasts. Small unmyelinated fibers pass between odontoblasts and even along their processes into predentin and dentin, mediating the sensation of pain. In this manner, odontoblasts may be thought of as neuroepithelial receptors that function as transducers for the dendrites that envelop them.

**Periodontal Ligament.** The *periodontal membrane*, or *ligament*, is a special type of dense fibrous connective tissue that lies between alveolar bone and the tooth and also supports the gingiva at the neck of the tooth (Fig. 11–12). It functions not only as periosteum of the alveolar bone but also as the suspensory ligament of the tooth in its socket. Strong, thick bundles of collagenous fibers pass between alveolar bone and cementum, ex-

tending into bone and cementum as Sharpey's fibers. The fiber bundles are not taut and run a slightly wavy course, being attached somewhat deeper to the root of the tooth than to bone. Thus, the tooth is "slung" in its socket, and occlusal forces are transmitted to bone via the ligament fiber bundles. Therefore, it acts as the suspensory ligament of the tooth and permits slight movements in each direction. Groups of epithelioid cells are sometimes seen in the periodontal membrane. These seem to be remnants of the epithelial root sheath of the developing tooth. Occasionally, they give rise to cysts. The ground substance around the collagen contains glycosaminoglycans. Fibroblasts, and a few osteoblasts, lie between the fibers, forming and maintaining them, and the turnover rate of collagen is high, permitting remodeling (and orthodontic procedures). Spaces between the fiber bundles are occupied by blood vessels, nerves, and lymphatics, these supplying the tissue (and the teeth). Their location between the fiber bundles protects them from forces applied to the bundles. Small nerves distribute myelinated fibers, some coming from proprioceptive pressure end-organs, which serve to regulate the force of the bite, or from tactile receptors. Unmyelinated fibers function in a vasomotor capacity. The periodontal membrane is a very cellular, vascular, and metabolically active tissue that provides for a vital tooth suspensory apparatus in that it can rapidly renew its components when faced with a pathogenic invader.

**The Gingiva.** The *gingiva,* or *gum,* surrounds each tooth like a collar and is the oral mucous membrane extending between and connected to the periosteum of alveolar bone at its crest and the tooth above its neck. Near the tooth, the gingiva extends around the tooth as the gingival crest, between the summit of which and the tooth is a narrow gingival crevice. More deeply at the bottom of the gingival crevice, the gingiva is attached around the circumference of the tooth crown. This attachment is to enamel cuticle, and it extends deeply to the upper part of the cementum. The attachment to the enamel is not firm, and with age, the gingival sulcus deepens until the gingiva is attached only to cementum, thus exposing the entire crown.

The connective tissue papillae underlying the stratified squamous epithelium of the gingiva are

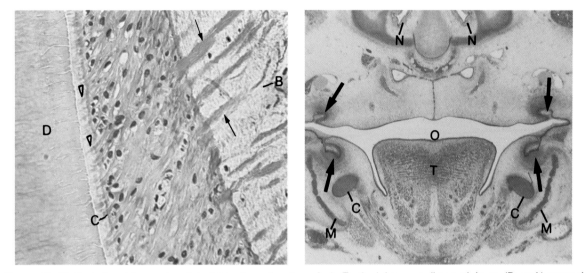

**Figure 11–12.** *Periodontal ligament and dental laminae of embryo. Left: To the left is a small part of dentin (D, pink) covered by acellular cementum (C), here quite thin. To the right is alveolar bone (B), with osteocytes in lacunae. Between cementum and bone is the periodontal membrane, consisting of collagen fibers and fibroblasts and with numerous small blood capillaries. Note that bundles of collagen fibers run obliquely between bone and cementum, thus "slinging" the tooth in its socket and that these fibers extend into matrix of both bone (arrows) and cementum (arrowheads) as Sharpey's fibers. Plastic section. H and E. High power. Right: This coronal section through the head of an embryo shows nasal cavities (N), oral cavity (O), tongue (T), and developing mandible (M) with Meckel's (first arch) cartilage (C). In each half jaw, at the angles of the mouth, an early enamel organ and dental lamina are seen (arrows). The dental lamina appears as a thickening of the oral ectoderm with a bud-like enamel organ, embedded in condensing mesenchyme (connective tissue) termed the dental sac. H and E. Low power.*

high. The connective tissue itself consists of interlacing bundles of collagenous fibers with relatively few fibroblasts and numerous blood capillaries that form a rich vascular network immediately below the epithelium. It is the blood in this network that is responsible for the pink color of the gums.

### Development of the Teeth

Each tooth has a mesodermal and an ectodermal component, the latter forming only the enamel. At five to six weeks, the oral ectoderm develops horseshoe-shaped linear thickenings in the upper and lower jaws. These *labiodental laminae* are at first solid and bifid, extending deeply into underlying mesoderm. The outer labial limb soon splits to form the groove between the lip and the alveolar process of the jaw (the future vestibule) while the inner limb, the dental

lamina, develops a series of bud-like thickenings, or *tooth germs*, numbering five in each half jaw, one for each deciduous tooth. Later, starting at 10 to 12 weeks, a second series of tooth germs develops on the lingual side, these numbering eight in each half jaw (five to replace deciduous teeth plus three to form the molars, which are not preceded by deciduous teeth). Each tooth germ of the two dentitions develops further in identical fashion (Fig. 11–13).

Each epithelial tooth germ, still attached above to the dental lamina by a cord of the cells, is at first "cap"-shaped but becomes invaginated from below by a mesenchymal papilla to become the "bell stage," or enamel organ, the whole embedded in connective tissue (the dental sac) (Fig. 11–14). Soon, this completely invests the developing tooth when the connection to the dental lamina breaks down and disappears. The peripheral part of the enamel organ is formed by a single layer of epithelial cells that are low cuboidal on the convexity of the bell (the outer enamel, or dental,

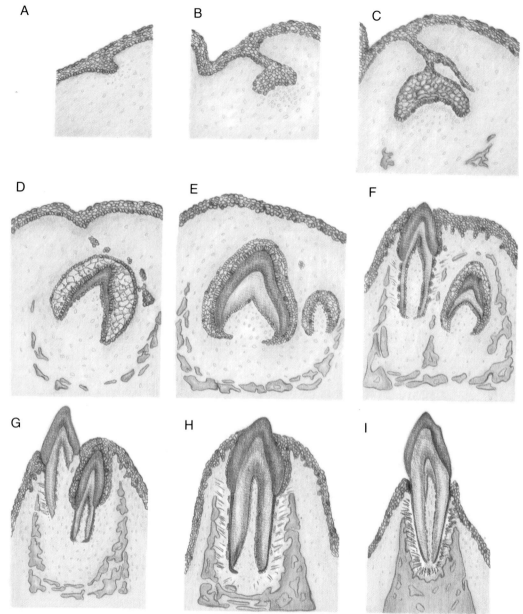

**Figure 11–13.** *Diagram illustrating stages in the development of the lower central incisor. The approximate age is indicated in parentheses. A, Dental lamina formation from oral epithelium (six weeks intrauterine). B, Early formation ("cap" stage) of the enamel organ of the deciduous tooth, with condensation of underlying mesenchyme (seven to eight weeks intrauterine). C, Early "bell" stage of the enamel organ with extension (to the right) of the dental lamina, indicating formation of the permanent tooth. Alveolar bone is forming (ten weeks intrauterine). D, Advanced "bell" stage with a cap of dentin now formed at the tip of the dental papilla. Connection between the tooth bud and the oral epithelium now is discontinuous (16 weeks intrauterine). E, The crown of the deciduous tooth is complete with enamel formation, and the permanent tooth is in the bell stage (birth). F, Early eruption of the deciduous tooth, the root of which now is formed, with the crown of the permanent tooth nearly completed, showing enamel and dentin (six months postnatal). G, The deciduous tooth shows resorption of the root and the process of shedding is commencing. In the permanent tooth, root formation is complete (six to seven years). H, The permanent tooth now is erupting (seven to eight years). I, In the permanent tooth, early attrition is shown with some recession in the neck and formation of secondary dentin (after 20 years). Stages A to E drawn at higher magnification than were stages F to I. (Based on diagrams supplied by J. G. Dale and K. J. Paynter.)*

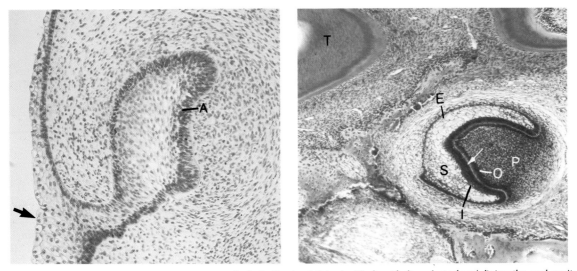

**Figure 11–14.** *Dental lamina and developing tooth. Left: To the left is stratified epithelium (ectoderm) lining the oral cavity, thickened to form the dental lamina (arrow). This extends deeply (to the right) into mesenchyme to form a bell- or cap-like expansion, the tooth germ. The central, pale area of the germ will become the stellate reticulum; the deepest cells (right) are the inner enamel epithelium. Cells here differentiate into ameloblasts (A) and later will form enamel. Note too the "condensation" of mesenchyme around the tooth germ. Those mesenchymal cells in relation to ameloblasts will differentiate into odontoblasts and later will form dentin. H and E. Medium power. Right: This section shows part of an erupted tooth of the "milk," or deciduous, dentition (T) and, enclosed in alveolar bone, a developing tooth in the late "bell" stage. Identifiable are outer enamel epithelium (E); stellate reticulum (S); inner enamel epithelium (I), or ameloblasts; odontoblasts (O); and mesenchyme of the developing pulp (P). Predentin is seen as a thin, pink-staining layer (arrow) between odontoblasts and ameloblasts. H and E. Low power.*

epithelium) and more columnar in the concavity (the inner enamel, or dental, epithelium). The two meet at the rim of the bell, the cervical area or neck, this marking the future cementoenamel junction. Internally in the bell, the cells are stellate and are separated by intercellular spaces (the stellate reticulum) but form a more regular layer called the *stratum intermedium* adjacent to the inner enamel epithelium. It is the cells of the inner enamel epithelium that become the enamel-forming ameloblasts.

By the time the ameloblasts are differentiated, the peripheral mesodermal cells of the dental papilla adjacent to them became arranged in a regular manner, one cell thick, as the odontoblasts, the two separated only by basal lamina material that later breaks down. By about 20 weeks of gestation, the hard tissues of the tooth begin to form. Uncalcified predentin is formed first and increases in thickness by apposition on the internal surface. The predentin extends down toward the neck, and as it increases in thickness, cytoplasmic processes of the odontoblasts are

formed as the dentinal fibers. The odontoblasts form collagen and matrix, mainly glycosaminoglycans, and calcification then follows in the first-formed matrix, transforming predentin to dentin. Because mineralization occurs after the formation of fibers and ground substance, there always is a thin layer of predentin adjacent to the odontoblasts. Once dentin formation has been initiated, ameloblasts commence to form enamel on the dentin surface. The first enamel formed is 70 per cent minerals and 30 per cent organic matrix, whereas mature enamel is 99 per cent mineral. Thus, the matrix is necessary for crystallite deposition and/or orientation, and later it is lost almost completely. With an increase in thickness of the enamel, the ameloblasts recede from the dentin (Figs. 11–15 and 11–16).

The development of the tooth as previously described accounts for only the formation of the crown. At the periphery of the enamel organ in the future neck region (i.e., at the edge of the bell), where inner and outer enamel epithelia come together, a fold of epithelial cells develops

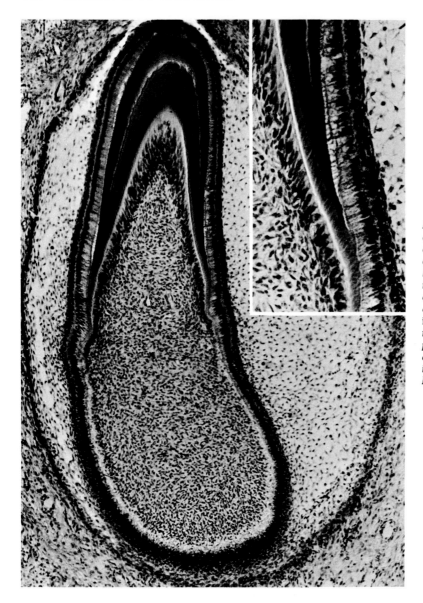

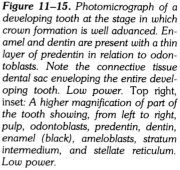

**Figure 11–15.** *Photomicrograph of a developing tooth at the stage in which crown formation is well advanced. Enamel and dentin are present with a thin layer of predentin in relation to odontoblasts. Note the connective tissue dental sac enveloping the entire developing tooth. Low power. Top right, inset: A higher magnification of part of the tooth showing, from left to right, pulp, odontoblasts, predentin, dentin, enamel (black), ameloblasts, stratum intermedium, and stellate reticulum. Low power.*

and grows downward toward the root. This is the *epithelial root sheath* (of Hertwig). Root development occurs shortly before tooth eruption and gradually progresses as the crown emerges through the gingiva. Odontoblasts develop in relation to the epithelial sheath of Hertwig and form dentin. Cementum develops from mesen-chyme of the periodontal membrane. The epithelial sheath of Hertwig disappears only when the root is formed completely.

During eruption of a permanent tooth, the deciduous tooth superficial to it gradually is resorbed by growth pressure, osteoclasts being prominent during the process. The deciduous

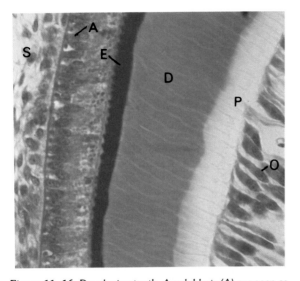

*Figure 11–16. Developing tooth. Ameloblasts (A) are seen as a row of tall columnar cells with basal nuclei and extensive, granular apical cytoplasm, lying on a (pink) basal lamina that separates them from a layer of small cuboidal cells (the stratum intermedium) and the stellate reticulum (S). A thin layer of dark, purple-stained enamel (E) lies adjacent to pink-staining dentin (D) in which dentinal tubules are seen. Predentin (P) stains pale and is opposed to a row of odontoblasts (O). H and E. High power.*

tooth when finally shed consists of only the upper portion of the crown, the remainder having been resorbed.

## THE MAJOR SALIVARY GLANDS

To moisten the mucous membrane of the oral cavity, vestibule, and lips, saliva is secreted continuously from numerous small glands associated with the oral cavity. In addition, the parotid, submandibular (submaxillary), and sublingual glands secrete copiously after mechanical, thermal, chemical, psychic, or olfactory stimuli from the presence, or anticipated presence, of food. These large, extrinsic, paired glands pass their secretions into the mouth via ducts. Each is a compound tubuloalveolar gland secreting in a merocrine fashion. These compound tubuloalveolar glands secrete proteins, glycoproteins, proteoglycans, electrolytes, and water into the oral

cavity. (For a general description of exocrine glands, refer to Chapter 2). A brief description of the major salivary glands follows (Figs. 11–17 through 11–19).

### Parotid Gland

This gland is located below and anterior to the ear, between the ramus of the mandible and the mastoid process, with an extension onto the face below the zygomatic arch from which the main (Stensen's) duct passes forward to penetrate the cheek and open into the vestibule opposite the second upper molar tooth (Fig. 11–20). The parotid gland is the largest of the salivary glands and is affected especially in mumps, *epidemic parotitis*. The gland is enclosed in a fascial sheet and contains serous acini composed of pyramidal-shaped cells and intercalated and striated ducts. From a fibrous capsule septa pass into the gland to divide it into lobes and lobules, these septa often containing fat cells. Slips of fine connective tissue surround and support acini and ducts, with numerous blood capillaries contained in this tissue.

The parotid is described as a compound, tubuloalveolar, serous gland. Acini (alveoli) are enclosed in a basal lamina with myoepithelial cells, and the pyramidal-shaped acinar cells show spherical, basally located nuclei with infranuclear cytoplasmic basophilia and apical secretory droplets. The acinar cells have a moderate number of ribosomes in their basal regions as compared with the pancreatic exocrine cell. The myoepithelial cells are basket-like contractile elements that are located between the acinar cells and basal lamina and function to expel the primary secretion. The secretory product has a high amylase activity and is rich in proteins and polysaccharides (sialomucin and sulfomucin). The initial section of the duct system, the intercalated duct, is long and therefore prominent in sections and is lined by squamous or low cuboidal epithelium, often with myoepithelial cells. The intercalated ducts drain to the larger striated ducts, both being intralobular in position. The striated ducts, lined by simple columnar epithelium, are so called because of a basal striation visible on light microscopy. On electron microscopy, they show vertically oriented

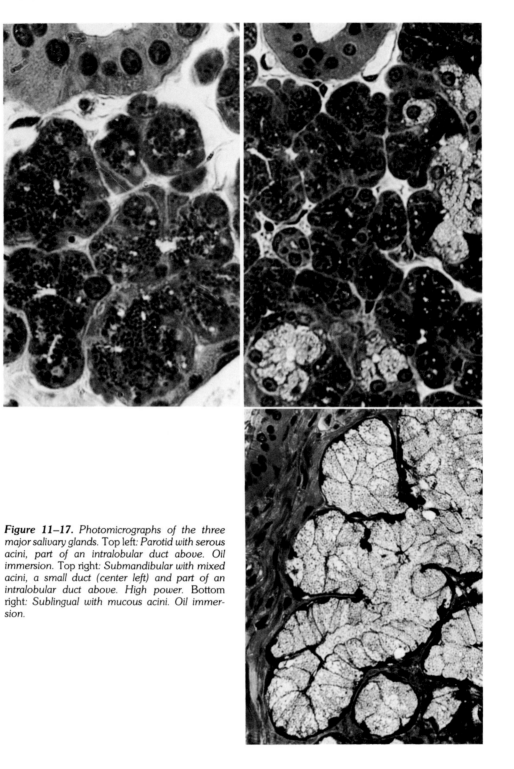

**Figure 11–17.** Photomicrographs of the three major salivary glands. Top left: Parotid with serous acini, part of an intralobular duct above. Oil immersion. Top right: Submandibular with mixed acini, a small duct (center left) and part of an intralobular duct above. High power. Bottom right: Sublingual with mucous acini. Oil immersion.

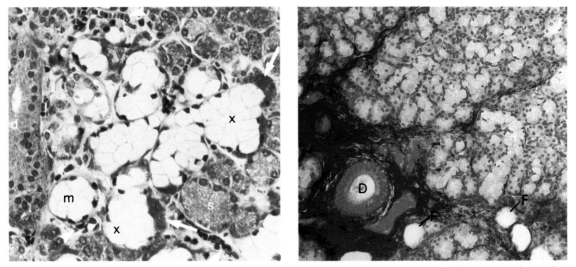

**Figure 11–18.** *Salivary glands with mixed acini. Left: Submandibular gland. This major salivary gland is compound, mixed, and acinar in type with serous (s), mucous (m), and mixed (x) acini, the last showing a serous crescent, or demilune (arrows). Also seen are an intralobular duct (d) and blood vessels containing erythrocytes (arrowheads) in the interacinar connective tissue. Plastic section. Azan trichrome. Medium power. Right: Sublingual gland. The sublingual salivary gland is really a collection of several small glands, each with a separate duct opening into the floor of the oral cavity. It is a compound, acinar, mucous gland, although a few mixed acini and, rarely, a few serous acini may be present. This section shows portions of several lobules separated by interlobular connective tissue (blue). Secretory units are mucous, with an interlobular duct (D) lying in relatively dense connective tissue and accompanied by small blood vessels. Fat cells (F) also are present. Mallory. Low power.*

mitochondria lying in basal compartments formed by infoldings of the basal plasma membrane and interdigitation of processes from adjacent cells. This type of specialization, seen also in distal convoluted tubules of the nephron, is characteristic of epithelia involved in rapid ion and water transport. Larger, interlobular ducts drain these intralobular (intercalated and striated) ducts and lie in connective tissue septa. They are lined first by a columnar, then pseudostratified, epithelium with occasional goblet cells. In the main duct, near its orifice, a stratified columnar or stratified squamous epithelial lining is found.

### Submandibular (Submaxillary) Gland

This gland lies in the floor of the mouth beneath the body of the mandible, extending below its lower border into the side of the neck, with a duct (Wharton's) that opens beneath the tip of the tongue. Like the parotid, this is a compound tubuloalveolar gland, but whereas most acini are serous, it also contains mucous and mixed acini

(i.e., mucous acini with serous crescents, or demilunes). Serous cells contain secretory granules that are PAS-positive and rich in sialoglycoproteins. The mucous cells contain either sialomucin or sulfomucin, or both. It has a capsule, septa, and a prominent duct system, similar to that of the parotid but with shorter and less prominent intercalated ducts and more conspicuous striated ducts. In the larger ducts, the pseudostratified epithelium modifies the composition of the saliva by secretion of mucus from scattered goblet cells and serous fluid from the principal columnar cells. Basically, saliva from this gland has a weak amylase activity, with lysozyme secreted by the serous demilune cells; this enzyme breaks down the walls of bacteria.

### Sublingual Gland

This really is not a single gland but a collection of glands lying in close relation to the duct of the submandibular gland beneath the mucous membrane of the floor of the mouth. Each part has a

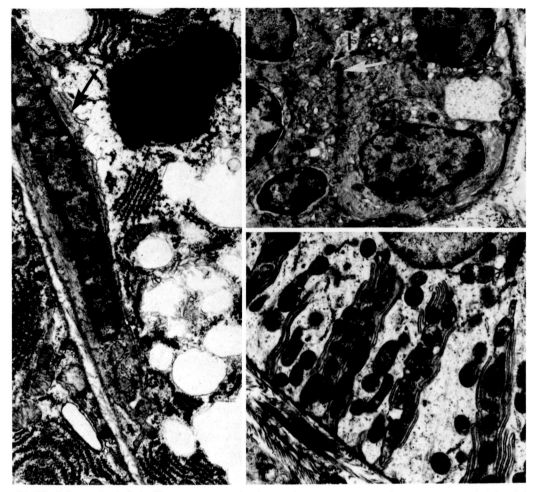

**Figure 11–19.** Salivary gland. Left: Electron micrograph of part of a mucous acinus showing a myoepithelial cell (arrow). × 9000. Top right: A small intralobular duct showing small lumen and junctional complexes (arrow) with desmosomes. × 7200. Bottom right: Part of a cell of a striated duct showing basal infoldings of the plasmalemma. × 7200.

separate duct opening beneath the tongue. It is a compound mixed tubuloalveolar gland; the majority of the acini are mucous, some with serous demilunes. The major constituent of the abundant mucous secretions are sulfated polysaccharides. Pure serous units are rare and, when present, contain sulfated glycoproteins. Myoepithelial cells are associated with acini. Both intercalated and striated ducts are short and thus less prominent than in the other glands, and the capsule is less thick, with fewer septa.

## SALIVA

Saliva is the mixed secretions of *all* the salivary glands and may amount to 1000 ml in 24 hours. It is a dilute aqueous fluid that serves several functions, and it is not an ultrafiltrate of the blood, as it differs in the concentration of hydrogen ions, glucose, proteins, and other components as well. It constantly moistens the oral cavity and aids in cleaning the mouth of food debris that otherwise would provide a culture medium for bacterial

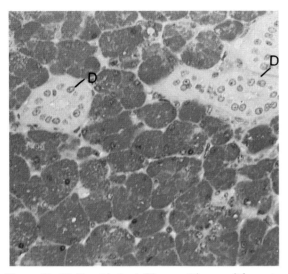

*Figure 11–20. Parotid gland. The parotid, one of the major salivary glands, is a compound, tubuloalveolar serous gland. Most of the field is occupied by serous acini, the cytoplasm of the cells filled with pink secretory droplets or granules. Also present are small intralobular ducts (D) lined by simple high cuboidal epithelium. Plastic section. H and E. Medium power.*

tion occurring when the body is dehydrated, giving rise to a sensation of thirst. This secretory activity is controlled almost entirely by the autonomic nervous system. Sympathetic stimulation produces a more viscous protein-rich saliva than does parasympathetic stimulation. The latter produces a more voluminous watery saliva. Sympathetic stimulation creates a dry sensation in the oral cavity. Much of the fluid in saliva, of course, is returned to the circulation by absorption in the digestive tract. Finally, saliva contains so-called salivary corpuscles, these being desquamated squamous epithelial cells from the oral epithelium together with a few lymphocytes and granulocytes.

## PALATE

The roof of the mouth, or palate, is also the floor of the nasal cavity. The anterior part, termed the *hard palate*, contains bone (palatine processes of maxillae and palatine bones) and thus is rigid. The posterior portion, called the *soft palate*, has a core of strong fibroconnective tissue and thus is movable. The hard palate provides a rigid surface against which the tongue, a powerful muscular organ, can bring force to mix food material and expedite the swallowing mechanism. The oral surface of the hard palate correspondingly is covered by stratified squamous keratinizing epithelium, the lamina propria of which blends with the periosteum. Within the lamina propria are numerous small glands and some fatty tissue. In the midline, the lamina propria is thin and is attached to a median ridge of bone. This linear region is called the *raphe*.

The soft palate functions to close off the nasopharynx from the oropharynx during swallowing, thus preventing aliment from entering the nasal cavity. It is covered inferiorly by stratified squamous nonkeratinizing epithelium, the lamina propria of which contains numerous glands. A layer of striated muscle (the musculus uvulae) lies between the lamina propria and the palatine aponeurosis, a sheet of fibroconnective tissue. On the nasal side, the soft palate is covered by the pseudostratified ciliated columnar epithelium of the nasal cavity, although posteriorly the oral type

growth. Obviously, it moistens food, and this permits both ease of swallowing and the appreciation of taste, for the chemical substances responsible for taste must be in solution to cause stimulation of the taste buds. Saliva also contains amylase and maltase, which commence digestion of some carbohydrates, and, as part of the oral antibacterial system, lysozyme and some RNase and DNase. Also present are gamma globulins, particularly immunoglobulin A (IgA) (which may also be part of the defense mechanism against oral bacteria that always are present in the mouth). This immunoglobulin is resistant to enzymatic digestion and is secreted by the plasma cells. It complexes with a unique protein produced by the serous acinar, intercalated duct, and striated duct cells. This unique protein is called a secretory piece, and the IgA complex is called *secretory IgA*. The latter is resistant to proteolysis. Peroxidase has also been identified in saliva. It, along with IgA, constitutes part of the immunologic defense system.

The secretion of saliva is also important in the maintenance of fluid balance, a decreased secre-

of epithelium extends around the posterior border of the soft palate and onto its superior, nasal surface. The lamina propria of this epithelium also contains a few glands.

## TONSILS

The oral cavity is continuous with the oropharynx through a region termed the *fauces*. There are two mucosal folds, each containing a muscle, on each side between the palate and the side of the tongue and pharynx, respectively. These are called the *palatoglossal* and *palatopharyngeal folds*, and between them is a depression in which is located a mass of lymphoid tissue. This is the *palatine tonsil*. Lymphoid tissue also is present in the nasopharynx (adenoids), around the openings of the pharyngotympanic (eustachian) tubes ("tubal tonsil"), and in the posterior part of the tongue ("lingual tonsil"). The parts of the pharynx are discussed in Chapter 12.

# The Tubular Digestive Tract

## LAYERS OF THE DIGESTIVE TRACT

Although the digestive tract is composed basically of four major parts, or organs (esophagus, stomach, small intestine, and large intestine), separated one from another by muscular valves or sphincters, all parts show four layers, or *tunicae* (Fig. 11–21):

1. The mucosa.
2. The submucosa.
3. The muscularis.
4. The serosa (adventitia).

## Mucosa

The *mucous membrane (tunica mucosa)* is composed of

1. A wet, surface epithelial membrane, lubricated by mucus and resting upon a basal lamina.
2. An underlying supporting layer of loose areolar connective tissue, the lamina propria. This layer carries both blood and lymphatic capillaries close to the epithelial surface, so that the products of digestion do not have to travel great distances to either type of capillary.
3. A thin, outer layer of smooth muscle, the muscularis mucosae, usually arranged in two layers oriented as inner circular and outer longitudinal. Its contractility produces folding of the mucous membrane, and, in the small intestine, contraction alters the extension of the villi and thus aids digestion and absorption. It may also function to relieve the pressure on submucosal veins brought about by partial contraction (tonus) of the muscularis externa.

In most regions, the mucosa is irregular and shows finger-like projections into the lumen, the *villi*, that greatly increase surface area, and deep epithelium-lined invaginations into the lamina propria, the *intestinal glands*, or *crypts*. These glands, which make the lamina propria difficult to identify as a separate entity, increase secretory capacity. Contained within the lamina propria are numerous blood and lymph capillaries into which absorbed food materials pass. The mucosa produces antibodies, especially IgA, in response to antigens and microorganisms in the gut lumen. This is accomplished by lymphatic tissue located mainly in the lamina propria as diffuse lymphatic tissue, solitary nodules, or aggregate nodules. Large lymphatic masses may spread into the submucosa. Diffuse lymphatic tissue in the lamina propria is found in the stomach and intestines with lymphocytes, plasma cells, macrophages, and, commonly, eosinophils and mast cells. The secretory IgA and other antibodies produced in these cells are bound to a secretory protein formed by epithelial cells of the mucosal surface and pass into the lumen to combine with antigens, enterotoxins, and bacteria to protect against viral and bacterial invasion.

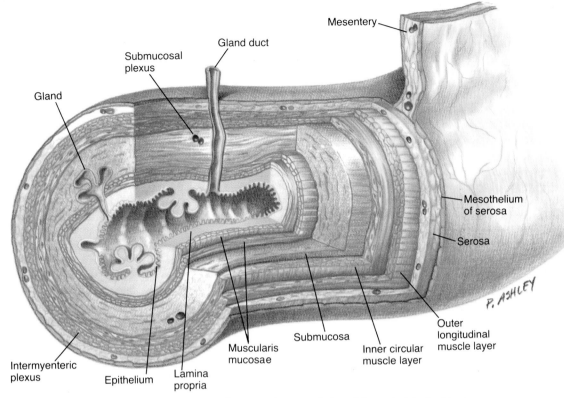

**Figure 11–21.** *Diagram illustrating the general plan of the gastrointestinal tract.*

## Submucosa

The *submucosa (tunica submucosa)* extends between the mucosa and the muscularis; consists of coarse areolar connective tissue with quite prominent elastic fibers but with fewer cells than the lamina propria; and often contains accumulations of lymphatic tissue. It permits mobility of the mucosa and contains plexuses of larger blood vessels and nerves with some ganglion cells, all of which are parasympathetic. The nerves mostly are postganglionic sympathetic, nonmyelinated fibers with some preganglionic parasympathetic fibers from the vagus nerve. The postganglionic fibers innervate the muscularis mucosae and the mucosal glands. This is termed the *submucosal plexus (of Meissner)*. This plexus is not easy to find in routine sections, since it contains relatively few ganglion cells. In some regions (e.g., the

duodenum), there are submucosal glands and, quite frequently, accumulations of lymphatic tissue.

## Muscularis Externa

The *muscularis externa (tunica muscularis)*, or, simply, the muscularis, consists of at least two layers of smooth muscle fibers, although there is striated muscle in the upper esophagus and the anal sphincter. The muscle is arranged as an inner circular layer and an outer longitudinal layer, the former constricting the lumen, the latter shortening the gut (and widening the lumen). In fact, the layers are actually arranged in a spiral fashion, the inner following a tight helix and the outer a very open helix. Between the layers is a vascular plexus and a nerve plexus associated with numerous small ganglia. This is *Auerbach's myenteric plexus*, and it mostly is parasympathetic with some postganglionic sympathetic fibers. The muscularis propels food material in the lumen of the digestive tube onward, a process termed *peristalsis,* and aids in mixing the food with digestive enzymes by churning movements. The peristaltic waves are coordinated by efferent impulses from the myenteric plexus and are of two kinds: slow and rapid ones called *peristaltic rushes.* Disturbances of the digestive tract motility could result from injury to the digestive tract plexuses in certain diseases (esophageal achalasia), producing emotional problems, and enlargement of the esophagus with collected food that often becomes infected with bacteria, causing ulcers to develop in the esophageal wall. Muscularis externa varies in thickness with the region; for example, a third layer is identified in the stomach wall.

### Serosa (Adventitia)

The *serosa* or *adventitia* (*tunica serosa* or *adventitia*) is the outermost layer formed by relatively dense and elastic areolar connective tissue. Often, it blends with the connective tissue of surrounding structures and is termed an *adventitia*; in many regions, however, it is covered by peritoneum (i.e., by a single layer of squamous mesothelial cells) and here is called a *serosa.* Blood and lymphatic vessels are present and pass through it to the other levels. Gut *mesenteries* are covered on both sides by peritoneal mesothelium and have a core of a thin layer of loose connective tissue.

Developmentally, the epithelial lining of the digestive tube is derived from endoderm, with the exception of the external parts of the oral cavity and the anal canal. These are ectodermal in origin. The connective and muscular tissues are derived from splanchnic or visceral mesoderm.

### THE ESOPHAGUS

The esophagus, about 25 cm long, is a relatively straight tube, continuous above with the pharynx at the lower border of the cricoid cartilage

and passing through the lower neck and thoracic mediastinum to perforate the diaphragm and terminate by opening into the stomach. Its wall shows the four layers as described previously (Fig. 11–22).

The *mucosal epithelium* is stratified squamous nonkeratinizing in type, continuous with that lining the pharynx, and is thick (about 300 μm), with mitotic figures in its basal layer, indicating a constant shedding and renewal of cells. Cells of the superficial layer contain keratohyalin granules, although they are not truly cornified. Complete keratinization may occur in humans subjected to excessive trauma. However, in animals that swallow rough material (herbivores), the keratinized type is normally present. Characteristically, this epithelium is indented by peg-like protrusions of the underlying lamina propria. At the lower end, it shows an abrupt transition to the simple columnar epithelial lining of the stomach. The supporting lamina propria is relatively acellular with scattered lymphocytes and a few lymphatic nodules. The muscularis mucosae is very thick, with most of its fibers longitudinal, and continuous with the elastic layer of the pharynx at the level of the cricoid cartilage.

The *submucosa* shows relatively coarse collagenous and elastic fibers that permit distension during swallowing. In the empty esophagus, it shows several longitudinal folds, giving the lumen a characteristic irregular outline. As the esophagus dilates to allow passage of a food bolus, these longitudinal folds are "ironed out." The muscle fibers of the *muscularis* are entirely skeletal, striated muscle in the upper third of the esophagus, often variable in orientation. In the middle third, smooth muscle bundles are mixed with striated fibers, and the proportion increases gradually until only smooth muscle is present in the lower third, where the usual arrangement into inner circular and outer longitudinal layers is more apparent. At upper and lower ends of the esophagus, a superior (pharyngoesophageal) and an inferior (esophagogastric) sphincter are formed. The latter functions to prevent reflux of gastric contents into the esophagus. Both sphincters seem to be primarily physiological in nature, since no significant increase in the number of circular muscle fibers can be anatomically demonstrated. It is a matter, in part, of increased muscle tone

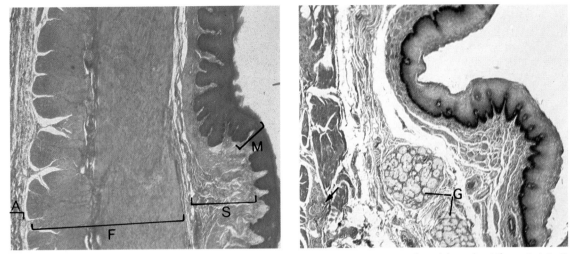

**Figure 11–22.** Esophagus. Left: This is a vertical section and shows the four tunics, or coats, found throughout the gastrointestinal tract. The mucosa (M) is formed by a stratified squamous epithelium and its lamina propria with a thin muscularis mucosae. Note the irregular but deep papillae of the lamina propria. The submucosa (S) is formed by quite dense areolar connective tissue and does contain glands, not seen here. The muscularis (F) shows a thick inner circular layer and outer longitudinal layer of muscle. Here the muscle is smooth, but striated muscle forms the muscularis in the upper esophagus. Externally, there is an adventitia (A) of loose connective tissue. H and E. Low power. Right: Similar to the companion photomicrograph, this transverse section shows mucous glands (G) in the submucosa and nerve fibers of the myenteric (Auerbach's) plexus, between the layers of muscle in the muscularis (arrow). H and E. Medium power.

that assists in closing off the esophagus, along with the intra-abdominal pressure on the lower portion of the esophagus below the diaphragm as well as cholinergic, adrenergic and peptidergic nerve stimulation. Failure to do so (*esophageal achalasia*) has been related to low levels of a vasoactive intestinal peptide (VIP). External to the muscularis, an *adventitia* blends with surrounding structures, while the short segment of the esophagus below the diaphragm is covered by a serosa.

Before rapidly traversing the esophagus, food material has been mixed with saliva, so that little additional lubrication is required. However, the esophagus does contain, throughout its length, scattered small, submucosal tubuloalveolar mucous glands and, at upper and lower ends, the so-called *cardiac glands* (Fig. 11–23). These mucus-secreting glands are confined to the lamina propria and resemble the cardic glands of the stomach. In the upper end, they facilitate the swallowing process, and in the lower end, they protect the mucosa from the backflow of the acid gastric juices.

## THE STOMACH

When empty, the stomach is of a caliber only slightly larger than that of the large gut, but it is capable of considerable distention to accommodate 2 to 3 liters of material when full. As indicated, there is an *esophagogastric,* or *cardiac, sphincter* at its entrance, and a more powerful *pyloric sphincter* at its junction with the small intestine. The stomach is flattened anteroposteriorly and is J-shaped with upper (right) concave and lower (left) convex borders called the *lesser* and *greater curvatures.* Above and to the left of the cardia (esophageal opening) is a bulge called the *fundus,* with the main *body* of the stomach below it and passing into a region called the *pyloric antrum.* This, in turn, is continuous with the *pyloric canal,* which narrows to the *pylorus,* the opening into the duodenum. In the empty, contracted stomach, the mucosa and submucosa are thrown into longitudinal folds, or *rugae,* that disappear with distention.

Food enters the stomach as boli (*bolus,* a ball)

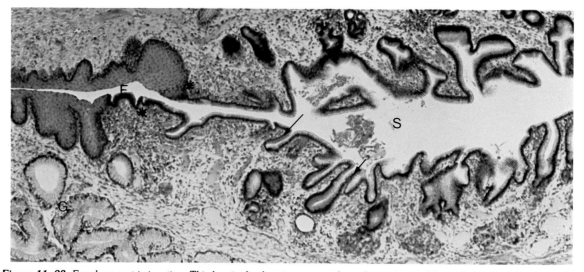

**Figure 11–23.** *Esophagogastric junction. This longitudinal section passes through esophagus (E), cardiac orifice of the stomach, and the cardiac portion of the stomach (S). Only the mucosa and submucosa are seen. The esophageal epithelium is stratified squamous, and this changes abruptly (stars) at the esophagogastric junction to a simple, columnar, mucus-secreting cell type with simple tubular or branched tubular glands (arrows). In the submucosa of both terminal esophagus and upper cardia are collections of mucus-secreting glands (G). These are called cardiac glands of the esophagus because they resemble the cardiac glands of the stomach. Similar glands are found in the lamina propria of the upper esophagus and in the submucosa of the esophagus throughout its length. H and E. Low power.*

of semisolid, masticated material, partially moistened by saliva, but leaves it intermittently after a period of three to four hours as a semifluid, pulp-like mass termed *chyme.* The thick muscularis of the stomach functions to churn the contained material, mixing it thoroughly with the digestive juices secreted by the stomach. The *gastric juice* contains hydrochloric acid, enzymes, and mucus. One of the enzymes, *pepsin*, in an acid medium commences the digestion of proteins; *renin* functions to curdle milk; and *lipase* starts fat digestion. In addition, the gastric mucosa secretes a factor necessary for the absorption of vitamin $B_{12}$ (essential for hemopoiesis). This factor is a glycoprotein called *intrinsic factor* and is produced by the parietal cells. It binds to vitamin $B_{12}$, thereby protecting and permitting the absorption of vitamin $B_{12}$ to take place in the ileal part of the small intestine. In the case of peptic ulcer, removal of the major portion of the stomach will result in a defective erythropoiesis (pernicious anemia). The stomach also forms several hormones, including gastrin. Gastrin is released from the gastrin-producing (G) cells via stimulation by the vagal

gastrin-releasing neuropeptide (*bombesin*), by distention of the stomach, or by alcohol or caffeine. Gastrin stimulates the secretion of acid by the parietal cells, the secretion of three types of pepsinogens (precursors of type I, II, and III pepsins) by chief cells, and the growth of the gastric mucosa. Some absorption occurs, although this is limited to salts, water, glucose, alcohol, and some drugs.

The stomach wall is composed of four layers.

### Mucosa

The mucosa of the living stomach is of a pale, grayish-pink color and is lined by simple columnar epithelium (Fig. 11–24). It is thick (0.5 to 1.5 mm) because of the presence of a mass of *gastric glands*, opening on the surface by *gastric pits*, or foveolae, several glands opening into each pit. While the pits mainly are tubular, they may appear also as linear crevices. The gastric glands are simple tubular or branched tubular, extending deeply to the muscularis mucosae, and between them is the lamina propria, difficult to recognize as a separate entity because it is split up to occupy the spaces between pits and glands.

On the basis of differences in the glands and the pits, three zones are recognized:

1. *Cardiac* glands form a narrow, ring-shaped area around the cardia. These glands appear to be more coiled and dilated than pyloric glands. The gastric pits are not as deep as those found in the pyloric region.

2. *Gastric* (main, or fundic) glands lie in the fundus and main body of the stomach and possess different cell types that readily distinguish them from the other two types of stomach glands.

3. *Pyloric* glands are found in the pyloric antrum and canal, which extend more proximally on the lesser than on the greater curvature.

There are some 15 to 20 million glands in the stomach.

**Cardiac Glands.** Cardiac glands extend for only about 2 to 4 cm from the cardiac orifice (Fig. 11–25). The pits in this region extend from the surface for one quarter to one third of the thickness of the mucosa, with the simple or branched tubular glands accounting for the remainder. The glands have a relatively wide lumen, and they are often coiled, particularly in the deeper zone. The cells forming the glands are predominantly mucus-secreting and resemble the cardiac glands of the esophagus, but a few acid-secreting parietal cells and some enteroendocrine cells also are present (to be described later). The function of these glands is unknown, but they may produce lysozyme.

**Gastric Glands.** Gastric glands occupy the largest area of the stomach and produce most of the enzymes and acid secreted by the mucosa of the stomach (Figs. 11–26 through 11–28). Pits here are relatively short, occupying about one quarter of the mucosal thickness, while the simple branched tubular glands are long and straight. The epithelium of the glands is formed by different cell types secreting acid, enzymes, mucus, and hormones (parietal, chief, mucous neck, enteroendocrine; these will be described later). It is usual to describe three regions to the glands:

1. The *isthmus* superficially at the base of the gastric pit.
2. The *neck*.
3. The *base*.

**Pyloric Glands.** Pyloric glands of the distal part of the stomach show deep pits extending to half the thickness of the mucosa (Fig. 11–29). Thus, the glands are short, usually of relatively wide diameter, and coiled, so that rarely are they sectioned along their lengths. A few parietal and hormone-secreting enteroendocrine cells are present; however, most are mucus-secreting, similar to the mucous neck cell of the gastric glands, with pale cytoplasm, indistinct granulation, and a flattened basal nucleus.

**Lamina Propria.** In all three mucosal regions of the stomach, the *lamina propria* is scanty, consisting of a delicate meshwork of collagenous and reticular fibers with a few fibroblasts or reticular cells. Scattered in the meshwork are lymphocytes, sometimes present in small local nodules, these being more obvious at cardiac and pyloric regions, with plasma cells, mast cells, and white blood cells. As mentioned previously, the lamina propria is not extensive owing to the masses of glands, being limited to slender spaces around and between the glands. It is more obvious toward the mucosal surface where spaces between pits are more extensive. Occasional smooth muscle cells are found in the lamina, these passing from the muscularis mucosae.

The *muscularis mucosae* itself is not thick. It is arranged into inner circular and outer longitudinal laminae, in some regions with a third external, oblique coat. Slips of muscle may extend from the muscularis mucosae into the lamina propria between glands.

## Epithelial Cells of the Stomach

**Surface Epithelial (Mucous) Cells.** The simple columnar epithelium that lines the entire stomach also extends into the pits, or foveolae (Fig. 11–30). It commences abruptly at the cardia, adjoining the esophageal stratified squamous epithelium, and at the pylorus is continuous with the intestinal epithelium. Nuclei of these cells are situated toward the bases of the cells and are ovoid, with some basal cytoplasmic basophilia present as a result of granular endoplasmic reticulum. The Golgi apparatus lies in a supranuclear position with apical cytoplasm occupied by dense, ovoid or spherical, discrete mucin granules,

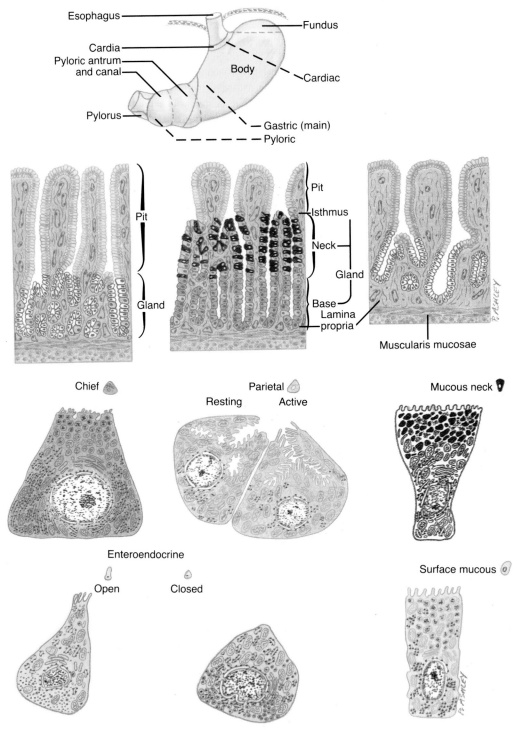

*Figure 11–24* See legend on opposite page

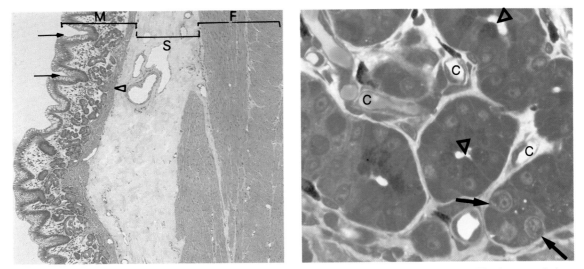

**Figure 11–25.** *Stomach, cardia. Left: The mucosa (M), submucosa (S), and muscularis (F) are seen. The lining epithelium is simple columnar and mucus-secreting and shows invaginations, or pits (arrows). Simple tubular and branched tubular glands open into the pits and extend the full depth of the mucosa, that is, deeply to the muscularis mucosae (arrowhead). The lamina propria is a cellular, loose (areolar) connective tissue. In the submucosa are some blood vessels. The muscularis is thick and in basically three layers—outer longitudinal, middle circular, and inner oblique. The cardiac glands are mucus-secreting, but a few parietal (acid-secreting) cells are present, interspersed among the mucus-secreting, columnar cells. Plastic section. H and E. Low power. Right: The bases of cardiac glands are coiled and thus cut in oblique-transverse section, rather than through their lengths. The major cell type is mucus-secreting, with apical secretory, mucin granules (arrowheads). A few parietal cells (arrows) also are seen. The lamina propria contains numerous capillary blood vessels (C). Plastic section. Methylene blue, azure A, basic fuchsin. High power.*

formed within the Golgi complex. These granules are stained poorly, by light microscopy, and the apical cytoplasm thus appears foamy in some preparations. The granules are positive for periodic acid–Schiff (PAS) stain and contain a viscid, alkaline mucin, which adheres to the gastric mucosal surface, forming a 1-mm thick protective layer that binds bicarbonate ions. Substances, such as aspirin, can cause disruption of this protective layer and cause an ulceration. At the cell periphery, tight junctions are prominent apically with numerous spot desmosomes; on the luminal border, stubby microvilli are present.

The neutral glycoprotein mucus secreted by the surface epithelial cells forms a film to protect the mucosa from acid; in its absence, the mucosa becomes ulcerated. The mortality rate of the surface epithelial cells is high, and they are replaced by mitosis of less differentiated cells lying in the depths of the foveolae. These more deeply situated cells contain fewer mucin granules than do the surface cells.

**Chief (Zymogenic) Cells.** This cell type lies in the bases of gastric glands and has the typical appearance of a protein (zymogen)-secreting cell (see Figs. 11–26 through 11–28). Cells extend from the basal lamina of a gastric gland to the lumen and, in cross section of a gland, are pyramidal in shape. A spherical nucleus lies toward the base, and the basal cytoplasm is baso-

**Figure 11–24.** *Diagram summarizing the main features of the gastric mucosa. Top: The three histological (shaded) areas of the stomach. Center: The light microscopical appearance of the three areas. Note the relation between depth of pit and gland, relative tortuosity of the glands (more in pyloric region), and cell composition. Bottom: The electron microscopical appearance of the cell types. The main mucous cell of the pyloric region is similar to the mucous neck cell; that of the cardiac region is also mucus-secreting but differs from other types (these two cells are not illustrated). See text for full description.*

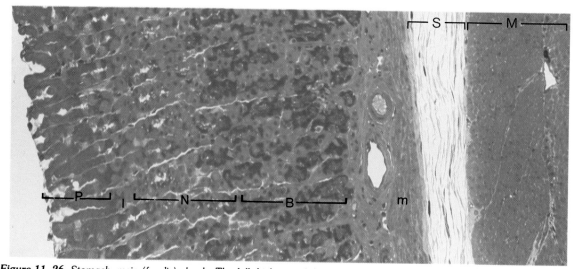

**Figure 11–26.** Stomach, main (fundic) glands. The full thickness of the stomach is seen with muscularis (M) covered by serosa (right), submucosa (S), and mucosa (left). In the mucosa, note the thick muscularis mucosae (m) at its base, the remainder occupied by glands between which are slips of lamina propria. The surface epithelium is simple columnar and shows shallow pits (P). Opening into the pits are long, simple tubular glands divided into base (B), neck (N), and isthmus (I). Dark-staining chief, or zymogenic, cells are confined to the bases of glands, and scattered among them are pink-staining parietal cells. Other cell types are not clearly identifiable at this magnification. Plastic section. H and E. Low power.

philic, containing granular reticulum and mitochondria. A Golgi apparatus lies above the nucleus, with the apical cytoplasm filled with acidophilic zymogen granules that often are not well preserved. The granules form in the Golgi apparatus and are released into the gland lumen by exocytosis. Chief cells secrete pepsinogen, which, in the acid medium of the stomach, is transformed to the active enzyme pepsin, the function of which is the hydrolysis of proteins to smaller peptides. Unlike other proteolytic digestive enzymes, it can extensively degrade collagen and functions at a pH optimum of about 2. Three types of pepsinogens have been isolated from the human gastric mucosa, giving rise to three types of pepsins with only slightly different chemical properties.

**Parietal (Oxyntic) Cells.** Parietal, or oxyntic (i.e., acid-forming), cells are scattered singly and in small groups between other cell types from the isthmus to the base of gastric glands, but they are more numerous in the neck and isthmus regions (Fig. 11–31). A few are found in pyloric glands and, although very few in number, are also present in cardiac glands. Characteristically, they are large, spherical or pyramidal cells with acidophilic or pale cytoplasm, and they appear to bulge into the surrounding lamina propria. The nucleus is spherical and centrally located, usually with the Golgi apparatus below or to the side of it. The cytoplasm contains numerous mitochondria with prominent cristae. An unusual feature is the presence of intracellular canaliculi, these being deep invaginations of the luminal surface with associated microvilli—a modification that obviously greatly increases surface area. In ordinary preparations, the canalicular system appears as an irregular, unstained area; by the use of chemical indicators, it has been shown to have an extremely acid pH, while the cytoplasm, as a whole, has a neutral pH. The hydrochloric acid is secreted into the intracellular canaliculi as chloride and hydrogen ions by an active process. The chloride ion originates from the chlorides present in the blood, and the hydrogen ion results from the action of the enzyme *carbonic anhydrase*. The latter enzyme forms carbonic acid, which dissociates into hydrogen ions and bicarbonate ions. The bicarbonate ion is returned to the blood as indicated by an increase in blood pH during

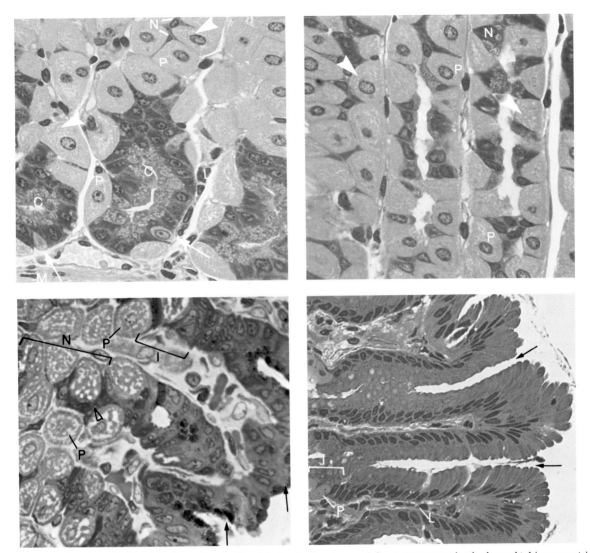

**Figure 11–27.** *Stomach.* Top left: *Base of main (fundic) glands. The bases of the main gastric glands show chief (zymogenic) cells (C) with basophil cytoplasm, apical (unstained) secretory droplets, and prominent nucleoli—features of protein (enzyme-) secreting cells. Interspersed among them are pale-staining parietal cells (P), some showing clear, intracellular canaliculi (arrowheads). Enteroendocrine cells also are present (arrows) and, in the neck region of the glands (above), mucous neck cells (N). Between glands are slips of lamina propria (L) with the muscularis mucosae (M) below. Plastic section. Alcian blue, nuclear red. High power. Top right: Necks of main glands. The glands are cut longitudinally (indicating that they are straight and not coiled) and show parietal cells (P), some showing clear intracellular canaliculi (arrowheads), and mucous neck cells (N)—cells of irregular outline, "squashed" between the adjacent cells, and with clear, unstained, apical secretory droplets. Plastic section. Alcian blue, nuclear red. High power. Bottom left: Pits and apex of main glands. This shows mucus as dark-purple secretory droplets present in surface epithelial cells (arrows) at the surface and in pits, and in mucous neck cells (arrowhead) in the necks of gastric glands. Parietal cells (P) are seen in both isthmus (I) and neck (N). The meshwork of clear, intracellular canaliculi within the cytoplasm of parietal cells is seen clearly. Plastic section. Toluidine blue and safranin. High power. Bottom right: Pits and apex of main glands. This is a higher magnification of Figure 11–26. The simple, tall columnar surface epithelium is mucus-secreting and extends to line pits (arrows). Opening into the bases of the pits are gastric glands at the isthmus (I), where parietal cells (P) are interspersed with surface epithelial cells. Slips of connective tissue of the lamina propria (L) are seen. Plastic section. H and E. Medium power.*

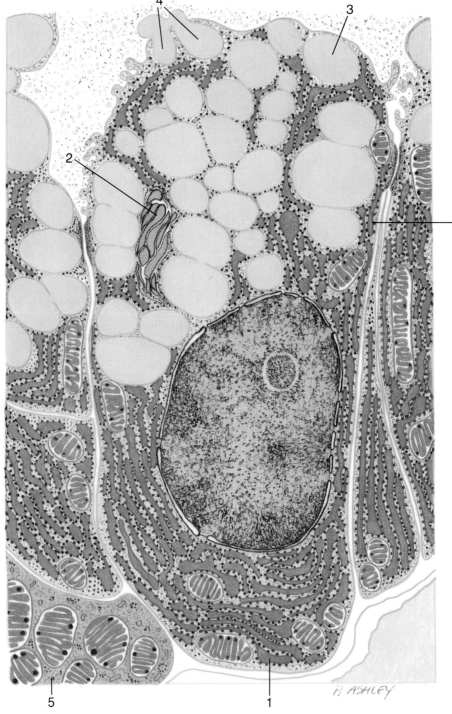

*Figure 11–28* See legend on opposite page

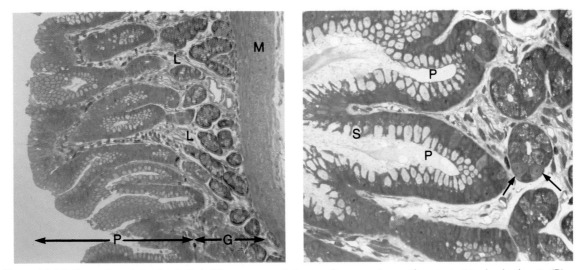

**Figure 11–29.** Stomach, pyloric glands. Left: The mucosa only is seen. In comparison with main gastric glands, the pits (P) are deep and the glands (G) are short and coiled. The main cell type in the glands is mucus-secreting, similar to the mucous neck cell. Between glands and pits is the lamina propria (L), with a thick muscularis mucosae (M) at right. Plastic section. Methylene blue, azure A, basic fuchsin. Low power. Right: A higher magnification of the accompanying micrograph, this shows the surface epithelial cells (S) with clear, apical secretory material. This cell extends to line the gastric pits (P). The pyloric glands are formed by mucus-secreting cells with apical mucin droplets, but a few parietal cells (arrows) and enteroendocrine cells (not seen here) also are present. Plastic section. Methylene blue, azure A, basic fuchsin. High power.

digestion. Prominent in the cytoplasm is the presence of closely packed tubulovesicles, particularly adjacent to canaliculi. The smooth membrane of the tubulovesicle system resembles the surface plasma membrane and probably represents a membrane reserve. In a resting parietal cell, the tubulovesicles are numerous, and canaliculi are dilated with relatively few microvilli. During acid secretion, microvilli become more numerous and tubulovesicles decrease, suggesting membrane interchange between tubulovesicles in the cytoplasm and microvilli at the surface. Actin filaments that surround the tubulovesicles play a prominent role in the interaction between these vesicles and

the cell membrane. Hydrochloric acid secretion occurs at this large membrane surface and is stimulated through cholinergic nerve endings, histamine, and gastrin. The hydrochloric acid that is secreted has a pH that may be as low as 0.8 and kills almost all bacteria that are ingested with the food, thus producing a generally sterile chyme. Parietal cells also secrete intrinsic factor, a glycoprotein that binds with vitamin $B_{12}$ and aids its absorption in the small intestine. Vitamin $B_{12}$ is necessary for red blood cell formation. A deficiency of $B_{12}$ results in pernicious anemia—a disease that appears to be autoimmune in character, since the blood of patients having this

**Figure 11–28.** Chief cell in the gastric gland of the rat. A further example of protein-synthesizing cells with elaborate rough ER (endoplasmic reticulum) is given by the chief cells of gastric glands proper. These cells, which secrete pepsinogen, contain a large number of predominantly parallel lamellae (l) of rough ER, called ergastoplasm. Between the lamellae are numerous free ribosomes. Above the nucleus, with its distinct nucleolus, note the distended Golgi apparatus (2) and the presence of secretory granules (3), some of which are being discharged from the cell (4). The cell is flanked by two similar cells, while a portion of a parietal cell (5) is present at the lower left. × 1500. (Reproduced with permission from Krstic, R. V.: Ultrastructure of the Mammalian Cell. New York, Springer-Verlag, 1979.)

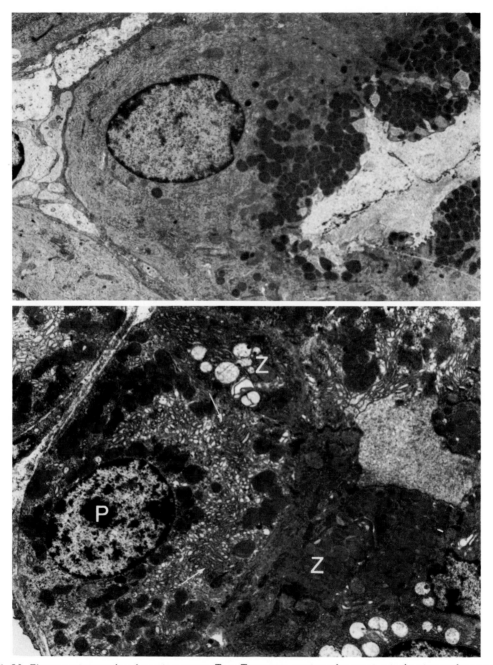

**Figure 11–30.** *Electron micrographs of gastric mucosa. Top: Transverse section of a gastric pit showing surface mucous cells with apical secretory droplets.* × *6500. Bottom: Transverse section through the base of a gastric gland showing a parietal cell (P) with canaliculi (arrows) and parts of chief (zymogenic) cells (Z).* × *6500.*

anemia is rich in antibodies against parietal cell proteins.

**Mucous Neck Cells.** These cells are located in the necks of gastric glands in small groups and as single cells. They tend to be of irregular shape, as though deformed by the cells (mainly parietal) around them, usually with a slender base and expanded apex, although others are more pyramidal in shape. The nucleus is basally located; basal cytoplasm is basophilic, with quite prominent granular reticulum; and a well-developed Golgi apparatus lies in a supranuclear position. Apical granules stain well with both PAS and mucicarmine; on electron microscopy, these granules are dense and vary in shape and size. The cells have stubby, apical microvilli with a characteristic "fuzz" of fine filamentous material. These cells produce an acid mucus, unlike the neutral mucus formed by surface mucous cells. Their secretion granules are larger and less dense than those of the surface mucous cells. Undifferentiated cells are also found in the neck region. These low columnar cells, which contain many free ribosomes, a prominent Golgi apparatus, and a prominent nucleolus, exhibit mitoses and can differentiate into gastric pit and mucous surface cells in about a week's time. By a slower downward migration, they may also form mucous neck cells, parietal cells, chief cells, and enteroendocrine cells.

**Enteroendocrine Cells.** Several different types of enteroendocrine cells are found in stomach glands (Fig. 11–32). They are particularly numerous in the pyloric antrum and are more usually found in the bases of the glands. All resemble the peptide-secreting cells of endocrine glands. They are found in not only the stomach mucosa but also the epithelia of small and large intestine, the lower esophagus (cardiac) glands, and, to a limited extent, the main ducts of the liver and pancreas. Generally, they are small pyramidal cells with clear, unstained cytoplasm. Granules in basal cytoplasm have been demonstrated by light microscopy. In some (the argentaffin cells), ammoniacal silver nitrate solution results in silver precipitation; in others (the argyrophilic cells), silver is precipitated only in the presence of a reducing agent. Many of the cells can be stained by potassium dichromate and have been called *enterochromaffin cells*.

By electron microscopy, all cells of the group are similar, but two main types have been recognized: (1) the "open" type has a broad base with a slender apical extension that reaches the gland lumen and usually shows a few microvilli, and (2) the "closed" type contacts the basal lamina but does not extend to the lumen. In both types, cytoplasmic organelles are sparse with basally located, small secretory granules. The granules are released into the lamina propria and thus to the vascular system. The size, shape, and density of the granules show variations probably associated with the type of peptide secreted.

Most of the cells have the characteristics of the so-called APUD cells (amine *p*recursor *u*ptake and *d*ecarboxylation), which are widespread in the body and are concerned in the production and release of polypeptides and proteins with hormonal activity. These active principles, the *regulatory peptides*, can be produced and released by both endocrine and neural tissues and may act as circulating hormones, local regulators, neurotransmitters, or all of these. ("Regulatory peptides" describes active peptides capable of producing their effects in one or more of these three ways.) Enteroendocrine cells produce some true peptide hormones (e.g., secretin, gastrin, and cholecystokinin), all of which pass via the blood stream to their target organs of pancreas, stomach, and gallbladder. The secretin-producing (S) cells are scattered on the villi of the duodenal and jejunal mucosa and in the intestinal glands. The gastrin-producing (G) cells occur in the glands of the gastric antrum, and the cholecystokinin-producing (CCK) cells are in duodenal and jejunal intestinal glands. Cholecystokinin stimulates secretion of pancreatic enzymes and enhances their action. Secretin stimulates secretion of pancreatic juice with high amounts of bicarbonate and water but a low amount of enzymes. The latter effect is on the pancreatic duct cell system via augmentation of its cyclic AMP mechanism. The presence of acid chyme in the duodenum and protein breakdown products stimulates secretin secretion. Cholecystokinin also increases the secretion of enterokinase and enhances gallbladder contraction. An example of a local regulator is *somatostatin*, which has its effect on nearby tissues. The somatostatin-producing (D) cells are found in the glands of the gastric antrum; somatostatin inhibits gastrin secretion in a paracrine manner. Somatostatin was first demonstrated in the hypothalamus as an inhibitor of the growth process. It has been demonstrated in the nerve fibers and neurons belonging to the myenteric and submucosal plexi and may function as a modulator or even as a neurotransmitter. The distribution, throughout the gastrointestinal tract, of these cells that produce different peptides is precise. In the stom-

ach, gastrin-producing (*G*) cells are found mainly in the pylorus, glucagon-producing (*A*) cells in proximal and distal parts but not the midportion, whereas serotonin production occurs throughout the mucosa in the *EC* cells, which represent the majority of cells that histologists describe as argentaffin cells. The latter function by increasing gut motility and inhibiting the secretion of gastric acid. Other types of argentaffin cells include the

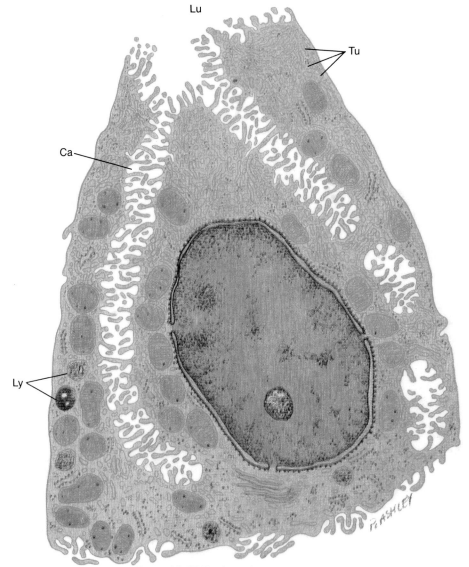

*Figure 11–31* See legend on opposite page

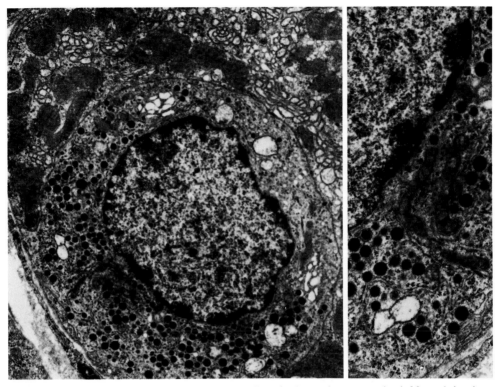

**Figure 11–32.** Electron micrographs of an enteroendocrine cell in the base of a gastric gland. Most of the dense secretory granules lie in basal cytoplasm (to the left), that is, infranuclear (right, below). In the left micrograph, part of a parietal cell is seen above. Left, × 900; right, × 18,000.

**Figure 11–31.** Drawing of a parietal cell. Parietal, or oxyntic, cells are pyramidal or triangular and occur singly in gastric glands. One of the striking morphological specializations of this cell is secretory canaliculi (Ca) that extend from the apex of the cell and pass lateral to the nucleus almost to the base of the cell. The canaliculus takes the form of a sinuous tubular channel, or it may form a deep indentation that is completely concentric with the nucleus. Numerous microvilli extend into the lumen of the canaliculus. In some places, strands of cytoplasm extend across the lumen. The canaliculi open into a common outlet that is continuous with the lumen (Lu) of the gland. Thus, the extensive surface area of the canaliculi is exposed to the glandular lumen. Microvilli also occur on the surface of the common opening and apical region of the cell. The lateral surfaces are relatively smooth in contour, but the basal surface is thrown into villi or plications. Another unusual structural feature of this cell is a system of cytoplasmic tubules (Tu). These tubules are sometimes so extensive that they crowd the other organelles into basal or lateral positions. The tubules are limited by smooth membranes, and the enclosed space is electron-lucent. In places, these tubules may be continuous with the surface plasma membrane of the canaliculus, in which case they should be regarded as complex invaginations of plasma membrane instead of smooth-surfaced endoplasmic reticulum. Mitochondria are relatively large, and spherical or oval. Cristae are closely packed and traverse over half the width of the organelle. Lysosomes (Ly) are present, as well as a few short cisternae of rough-surfaced endoplasmic reticulum. Free ribosomes occur in the cytoplasm, and a small Golgi apparatus is located near the base of the cell, sometimes in an infranuclear position. Parietal cells secrete the hydrochloric acid of gastric juice, but the relationship of the structural specializations to acid secretion is not well understood. One possible mechanism is that sodium chloride is secreted into the canaliculi, whereupon the sodium is exchanged for hydrogen ions across the membrane. (From Lentz, T. L.: Cell Fine Structure. Philadelphia, W. B. Saunders Co., 1971.)

*Mo cells* of the jejunum and ileum, which are responsible for the secretion of *motilin*. The latter stimulates the secretion of gastric acid and gastric motility. *K cells* are present in the crypts of duodenum and jejunum and produce a gastric inhibitory polypeptide (*GIP*) that inhibits gastric secretion and gastric motility and stimulates insulin secretion. *GIP* is stimulated by fat and glucose in the duodenum. A subtype of the D cell (with similar distribution) called the $D_1$ *cell* produces (within its smaller medium-dense granules) a vasoactive intestinal peptide (*VIP*), which stimulates ion and water secretion by the intestinal mucosa. *P cells* are present in the duodenal intestinal crypts and possibly may produce *bombesin* (a gastrin-releasing peptide).

Knowledge of these enteroendocrine cells still is incomplete, and their interrelation with the nervous system requires further clarification. However, it must be appreciated that, although the nervous system controls secretory activity and muscle action in the digestive tract, there is a complex interaction with many of the hormones produced by enteroendocrine cells. Scattered throughout the tract, these cells do not appear very impressive histologically, but together they constitute a relatively large endocrine organ.

### Others Layers of the Stomach

**Submucosa.** The submucosa extends into the rugae, or longitudinal folds, present in the contracted stomach and consists of loose connective tissue with collagenous and elastic fibers. In addition to fibroblasts, accumulations of lymphocytes and plasma cells occur, particularly near the cardia and the pylorus, with mast cells and usually some fat cells. Clusters of fat cells commonly occur with age. The layer contains blood and lymph vessels and peripheral nerves of the submucous plexus.

**Muscularis.** The muscularis is formed by three layers of smooth muscle: (1) an *outer longitudinal* and (2) a *middle circular layer* are continuous with the two layers of muscle of the esophagus but are supplemented by (3) an *inner oblique layer* in the form of loops of muscle passing from the cardia around the fundus and corpus. The oblique layer is best developed at the cardiac end

and the body of the stomach. At the pylorus, the middle circular layer is thickened as the pyloric sphincter. The longitudinal layer is best developed along the curvatures. Ganglion cells and nerve fibers (Auerbach's plexus) occur between the longitudinal and circular layers that coordinate contractions of the muscularis externa, thus churning and homogenizing ingested food.

**Serosa.** The serosa at the greater and lesser curvatures is continuous with the greater and lesser mesenteries (omenta). The greater omentum hangs down from the stomach like an apron and usually becomes increasingly adipose with age. Major vessels to and from the stomach course in the omenta.

### THE SMALL INTESTINE

The small intestine extends from the pyloric orifice, where it is continuous with the stomach, to the ileocecal junction, where it continues into the large intestine. It is about 720 cm in length, is much coiled within the abdominal cavity, and is divided into three parts (Figs. 11–33 and 11–34). (1) The *duodenum* is only 20 cm long. It is relatively fixed to the posterior abdominal wall, since it has no mesentery throughout the greater part of its length and thus is retroperitoneal. The remainder of the small intestine is divided into (2) the *jejunum*, the next two fifths of the length, and (3) the *ileum*, the remaining three fifths. The jejunum and ileum are suspended from the posterior abdominal wall by the *mesentery* (intraperitoneal), although the terminal ileum again is fixed to the posterior abdominal wall. The functions of the small intestine are to transport food material (chyme) from the stomach to the large intestine, to complete digestion by the secretion of enzymes from its wall and from accessory glands, to absorb the final products of digestion into blood and lymph vessels in its wall, and to secrete certain hormones.

To subserve these functions, particularly of absorption and digestive secretion, the small intestine shows certain specializations that increase the surface area of its mucosa (Figs. 11–35 through 11–38).

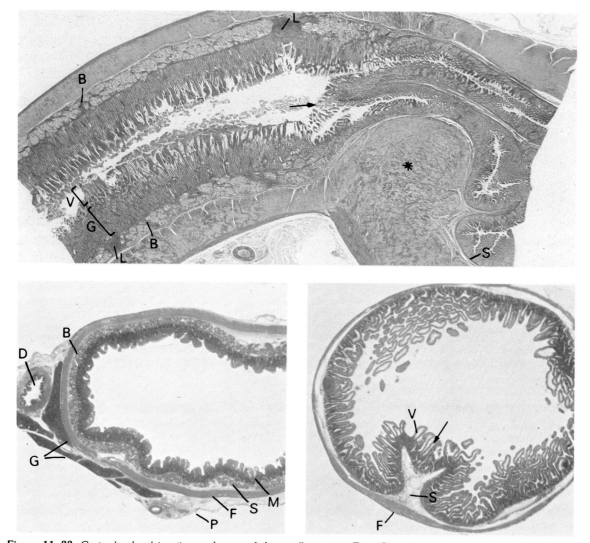

**Figure 11–33.** *Gastroduodenal junction and most of the small intestine. Top: Gastroduodenal junction. To the right is the terminal part of the stomach (pyloric canal), with the duodenum on the left. At the pyloric antrum, the middle (circular) layer of smooth muscle of the muscularis is thickened to form the pyloric sphincter (asterisk). The submucosa of the stomach (S) is thick, and the mucosa shows complex folds, or rugae, one of which is sectioned in such a manner that it appears to protrude through the pyloric orifice (arrow). The duodenal mucosa is thick and shows numerous villi (V), finger-like processes with a core of lamina propria, and intestinal glands (G), or crypts of Lieberkühn. The submucosa of the duodenum is thick and contains pale-staining glands (of Brunner, B). Two small lymphoid follicles (L) are seen. H and E. Low power. Bottom left: Duodenum. This transverse section also shows part of the pancreas (G) and the common bile duct (D). In the duodenum, the serosa (P), muscularis (F), submucosa (S), and mucosa (M) are seen. In the submucosa are glands of Brunner (B), and the mucosa shows villi protruding from the surface and intestinal glands (darkly staining). H and E. Low power. Bottom right: Jejunum. Cut in transverse section. This shows all layers. Villi (V) are long, and glands stain dark in the mucosa. A plica circularis (arrow,) bifid at its apex, is seen and has a core of submucosa (S). The muscularis (F) is quite thin. H and E. Low power.*

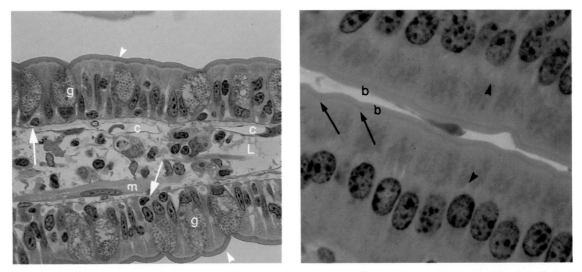

**Figure 11–34.** *Small intestine. Left: Ileum, villus. The connective tissue core of lamina propria (L) contains blood capillaries (c) and a variety of connective tissue cells. Also present is a small bundle of smooth muscle (m). On the surface, the simple columnar (absorptive) cells show a brush border (arrowheads). Scattered among them are goblet, or mucous (g), cells of characteristic shape, filled with secretory droplets. Enteroendocrine cells also are present in this epithelium. Arrows indicate cells that may be of this type. Plastic section. Methylene blue, azure A, basic fuchsin. Medium power. Right: Intestinal epithelium. The simple columnar (absorptive) epithelium here is seen covering villi of the duodenum. Note that no goblet cells are visible (although they are present); this indicates that the section was from the duodenum. Goblet cells increase in number from duodenum to terminal ileum. The columnar cells or enterocytes show elongated nuclei, the cytoplasm is basophilic, and in a supranuclear position, the Golgi apparatus is seen as a negative image (arrowheads). Apically, there is a brush border (b), and on some lateral cell interfaces near the lumen, a dense pink dot indicates a junctional complex or terminal bar (arrows). The basally located cell with dark irregular nucleus at bottom may be an enteroendocrine cell. Plastic section. H and E. Oil immersion.*

## Mucosal Surface Specializations

These specializations increase the surface area and include plicae circulares, or circular folds; villi that cover the surface of the plicae circulares; crypts, or intestinal glands, that originate by an invaginatory process from the surface epithelium; and microvilli, which are finger-like projections of the apical surface of the intestinal cells (Fig. 11–39).

**Plicae Circulares (Valves of Kerckring).** These are permanent circular or spiral folds of the entire thickness of the mucosa, with a core of submucosa. Any one fold may extend two thirds or more around the circumference of the intestine, but rarely do the folds completely encircle the lumen. Branching of some plicae occurs. The plicae commence in the duodenum within 2.5 to 5 cm of the pylorus, reach their maximum development in terminal duodenum and proximal jejunum, and thereafter diminish, disappearing in

the distal half of the ileum. These permanent circular folds increase the surface area of the mucosa by about three times and, when viewed under the electron microscope, consist of some 800 incomplete ridges within the submucosa.

**Villi and Crypts.** *Villi* are small finger- or leaf-like projections of the mucous membrane, 0.5 to 1.5 mm long, found only in the small intestine (Fig. 11–40). Each is covered by epithelium and has a core of cellular lamina propria, many cells being of the immune system. In the core are an arteriole and venule with a capillary network and a central lymphatic or lacteal. The capillary network is denser than that around the crypts, which are more deeply placed within the mucosa, and the capillaries in villi are fenestrated and are permeable to macromolecules. Villi vary in form and height in different regions. Those of the duodenum are broad, spatulate structures, but they become finger-like in the ileum. By contraction of smooth muscle cells that lie in the core,

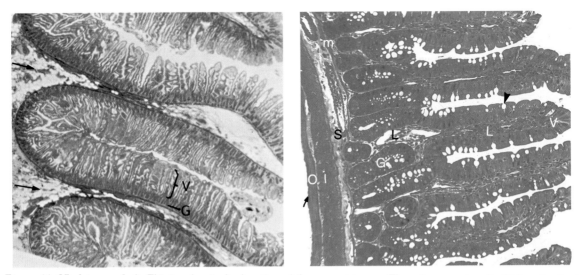

**Figure 11–35.** *Jejunum. Left: This is a longitudinal section of the upper jejunum. The submucosa is quite thick and extends into the cores of two plicae circulares (arrows). In the mucosa, villi (V) and glands (G) are seen clearly. It is obvious that the surface of the gut lining is increased greatly by plicae, villi, and glands. Mallory. Low power. Right: All four layers are seen—the serosa, at the arrow; outer (O) and inner (I) layers of the muscularis; the submucosa (S); and as parts of the mucosa, the muscularis mucosae (m) and lamina propria (L) lying between intestinal glands (G) and in the cores of villi (V). In the epithelium of glands and villi, clear-staining goblet cells are present (arrowhead). Plastic section. H and E. Low power.*

villi can contract and shorten, thus aiding in lymphatic drainage. Generally, villi shorten with distention and the state of contraction of the smooth muscle fibers of the intestine. These evaginatory processes increase the surface area of the mucosa by some five to ten times in humans and represent a total population of some 4 million, with about 10 to 40 per square mm. Their number directly varies with the extent of the absorptive work—up to 40 per square mm in the duodenum. Between the villi are small openings of simple tubular glands called crypts.

*Crypts*, or intestinal glands (of Lieberkühn), are tube-like structures opening between the bases of villi, are 0.3 to 0.5 mm in depth, and extend deeply to the muscularis mucosae. The epithelium that lines the crypts is continuous with that which covers the villi. Crypts are not packed as closely as the gastric glands, the spaces between them being filled with connective tissue of the lamina propria. Crypts also are present in the large intestine, although villi are not, and thus it is important for identification of sections that the student be able to recognize differences between villi and crypts when cut in cross section. Villi

appear as circular or oval profiles with a core of connective tissue (lamina propria) covered by epithelium. A crypt in cross section appears as a central lumen lined by epithelium, the whole embedded in connective tissue of the lamina propria, and represents a further increase of the mucosal surface. The generative and secretory functions of the crypt are reflected by the nature of its cell types, which include some absorptive cells, undifferentiated cells, Paneth's cells, mucous cells, and enteroendocrine cells, as will be described later.

**Microvilli.** To further increase surface area, the columnar absorptive cells covering villi and lining crypts have a brush or striated border composed of numerous microvillous processes (Fig. 11–41). The absorptive cell has about 3000 microvilli (1 mm square of mucosa has about 200 million), with each measuring 1.0 to 1.5 μm high and 0.1 μm wide (Fig. 11–42). These apical protrusions are seen under the light microscope as a 1-μm wide refractile zone that effectively amplifies the surface area some 20 to 30 times. Each microvillus is covered by an extension of the plasma membrane, the outer lamina of which is associ-

*Text continued on page 443*

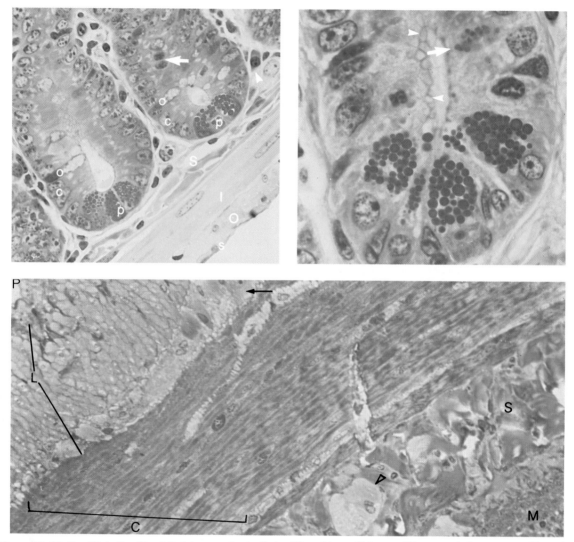

**Figure 11–36.** *Small intestine. Top left: Jejunum, glands. Outer (O) and inner (I) layers of the muscularis are covered by a thin serosa (s), with submucosa (S) internally. In the bases of intestinal glands, or crypts, there are immature columnar (stem) cells (c) that show negative Golgi apparatuses in a supranuclear position, some in mitosis (a telophase is indicated by arrow); immature goblet (oligomucous) cells (o); and Paneth's cells (p), clearly distinguished by apical, eosinophilic, secretory droplets. Note the plasma cell (arrowhead) in the lamina propria. Plastic section. H and E. High power. Top right: Paneth's cells. The base of one jejunal gland, or crypt, contains Paneth's cells, serozymogenic in type and with spherical, apical, secretory droplets, varying in size. These cells produce lysozyme. The cell indicated by the arrow, lying higher in the crypt with a few, small secretory droplets, probably is an immature Paneth's cell formed in the "stem cell zone." Columnar epithelial cells, where cut obliquely through their apices, show prominent terminal bars (arrowheads). Plastic section. H and E. Oil immersion. Bottom: Intestinal nerve plexuses. This is a section through the outer portion of the ileum to show the myenteric (Auerbach's) and submucosal (Meissner's) plexuses. At top left is serosa (P) covering the outer longitudinal (L) and inner circular (C) layers of smooth muscle of the muscularis. To the right is submucosa (S) extending up to the muscularis mucosae (M). Between the two layers of the muscularis is a collection of ganglion cells and nerve fibers of Auerbach's plexus (arrow), with a similar collection of Meissner's plexus (arrowhead) in the submucosa. Plastic section. Toluidine blue, aldehyde fuchsin. Medium power.*

*Figure 11–37.* Intestinal glands, mitosis. This is a transverse section through the bases of two intestinal glands in the terminal ileum. The tubular glands are lined by simple columnar epithelium. Several "mitotic figures" (cells undergoing mitosis) are seen. For cell division, which is active in the intestinal lining, cells round up, pass toward the lumen, and undergo mitosis to form two daughter cells. The visible stages are a late telophase (T), metaphase plates (M), an anaphase (A), and an early telophase ($T_1$). H and E. High power.

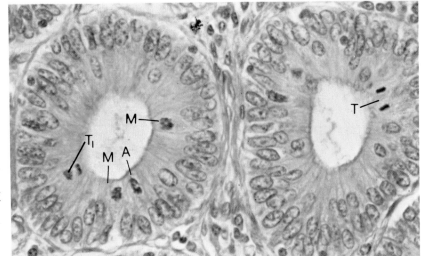

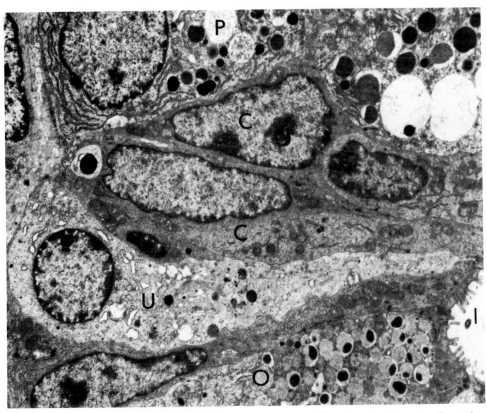

*Figure 11–38.* Electron micrograph of the base of a jejunal gland, with lumen (l) to the right. At top is a Paneth's cell (P) with prominent granular reticulum and apical secretory granules. In addition to columnar cells (C), or enterocytes, one cell probably is a young columnar or undifferentiated cell (U), and at bottom is an oligomucous, or early goblet, cell (O) × 3500.

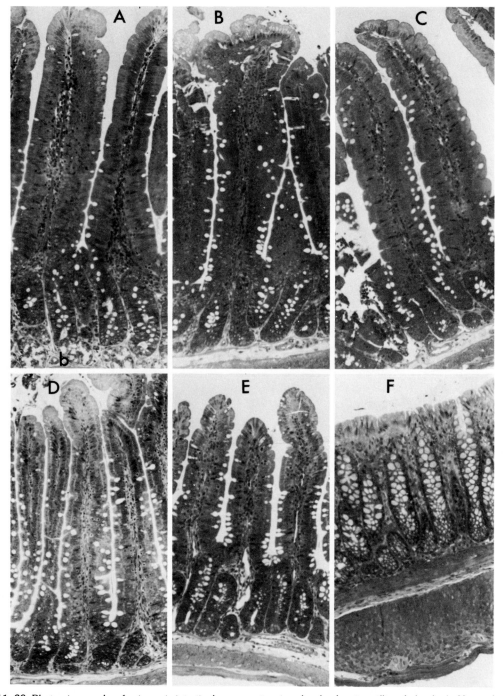

*Figure 11–39.* Photomicrographs of guinea pig intestinal mucosa at various levels, showing villi and glands. A: Upper duodenum, with Brunner's glands (b) below. B: Lower duodenum. C: Upper jejunum. D: Lower jejunum. E: Ileum. F: Colon. Note that villi decrease in length, goblet cells (pale-staining) increase in number from above down, and the colon shows only glands. All low power.

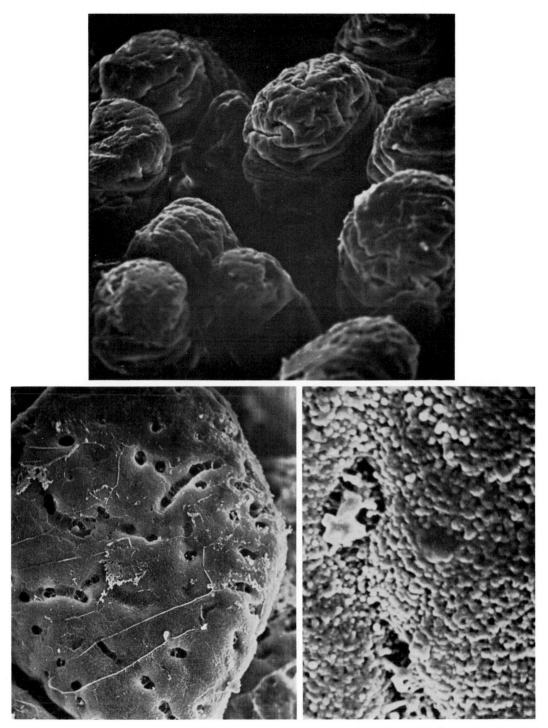

**Figure 11–40.** Scanning electron micrographs. Top: *Low power, showing finger-like villi.* × *536.* Bottom left: *A single finger-like villus showing goblet cell orifices with interconnecting troughs and strands of mucus (white) on the surface.* × *1070.* Bottom right: *Cell surface showing microvilli and two goblet cells with mucus.* × *10,300. (Courtesy of N. M. Marsh, J. A. Swift, and E. D. Williams.)*

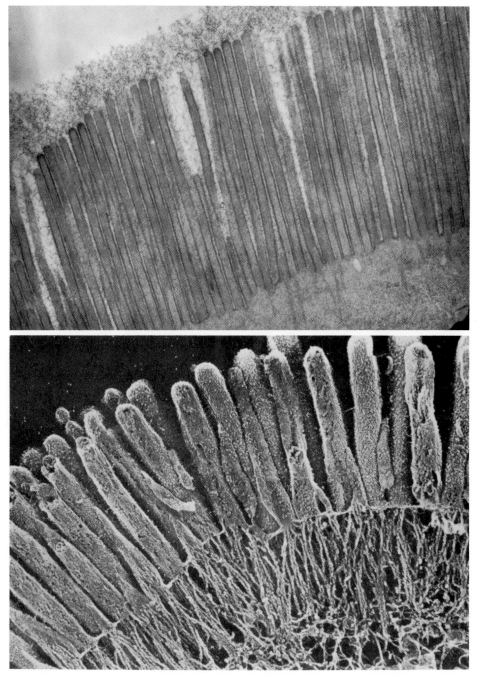

*Figure 11–41.* Intestinal microvilli. Top: Electron micrograph of the intestinal microvilli of the hamster shows a thick, mat-like coat called the glycocalyx. It is associated with the apical border of the microvillus membranes. The uniform microvilli contain bundles of actin microfilaments that project into the terminal web of the cytoplasm. × 23,500. (Courtesy of Dr. H. N. Tung.) Bottom: Brush border of an intestinal absorptive cell prepared by quick-freezing, deep-etching, and rotary shadowing. Bundles of actin filaments can be seen extending from the cores of the microvilli downward into the meshwork of filaments making up the terminal web. (Courtesy of N. Hirokawa and J. Heuser.)

ated with a feltwork of fine filaments giving a fuzzy appearance. This filamentous coat, which occupies the spaces between microvilli and at their tips, forms a continuous surface layer, contains a glycoprotein, and is resistant to proteolytic and mucolytic agents. In the cores of microvilli are thin, longitudinally oriented filaments that at the bases are continuous with the filaments of the terminal web (these will be described later).

To the food material in the lumen of the small intestine are added the secretions of many glands. These are of three main types:

1. *Intestinal glands.* As just explained, these are found in both the small and the large intestines.

2. *Submucosal glands.* These are located in the duodenum, are compound tubular in type, and are termed the *duodenal glands* (*of Brunner*). Usually, they are more extensive in the first part of the duodenum near the pylorus.

3. *Glands situated outside the digestive tract but passing their secretions into its lumen by a duct system.* These glands are the *liver* and *pancreas*, and both deliver their exocrine secretions into the duodenum.

### Epithelium

The epithelium of the intestinal mucosa is simple columnar in type but differs from the surface epithelium of the stomach in that more than one

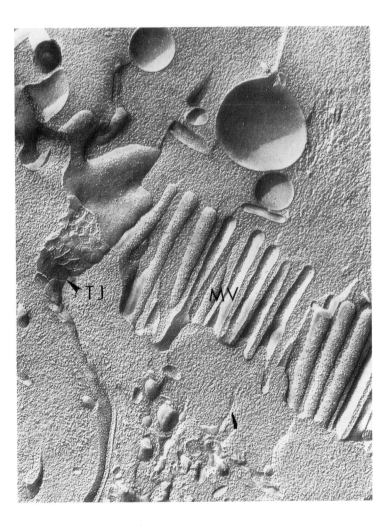

**Figure 11–42.** Electron micrograph of replica of freeze-fractured intestinal absorptive cells. Note microvilli (MV) and tight junction (TJ). × 35,800. (Courtesy of Dr. H. N. Tung.)

cell type is present. There are columnar cells with a striated border, Paneth's cells, goblet cells, enteroendocrine cells, and others.

**Columnar (Absorptive) Cells.** These tall columnar cells rest upon a basal lamina (Fig. 11–43). Nuclei are ovoid and are located toward the base. Mitochondria are elongated and numerous and are oriented longitudinally, particularly in the base of the cell. Some free ribosomes are scattered throughout, while the endoplasmic reticulum forms a continuous network of canaliculi and fenestrated saccules throughout the cell, with mainly canaliculi lying below the nucleus and saccules above the nucleus. The reticulum is predominantly granular, but the reticulum in the apex is agranular, the two types being in conti-

nuity. The Golgi apparatus is well developed and supranuclear in position; lysosomes also are present, particularly in older cells near a villus tip. Each cell has a striated, or brush, border formed by closely packed, parallel microvilli, about 1.5 μm tall on cells near the villus tip, but shorter on cells at the villus base. The interdigitation of the branching filamentous material at the tips of the microvilli results in the formation of a continuous *surface coat* on the striated border. This border is PAS-positive as a result of the glycocalyx associated with the microvilli and varies from 0.1 to 0.5 μm in width, depending on the species and being well developed in humans. The glycocalyx is resistant to proteolytic and mucolytic agents and has the effect of increasing the surface area

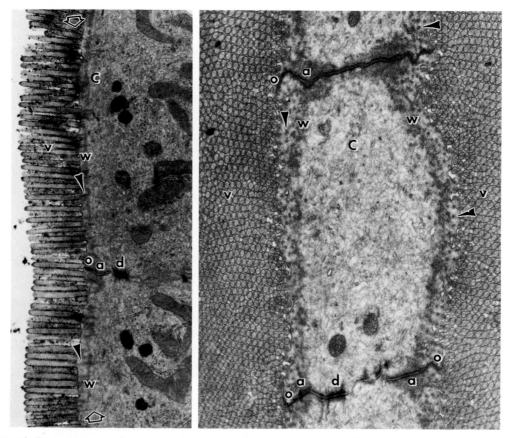

**Figure 11–43.** Electron micrographs of duodenal columnar cells cut longitudinally (left) and transversely at the apex (right, the plane of section indicated by open arrowheads on the left picture). In both, note microvilli (v) of the brush border, with core filament bundles (arrowheads) extending into the terminal web (w) of apical cytoplasm (C). At cell interfaces, junctional complexes show zonulae occludentes (o) and adherentes (a), with spot desmosomes (d). Both, × 18,000.

about 30-fold. The glycoprotein coat is formed by the columnar cells and contains digestive enzymes such as disaccharidases and dipeptidases that break down sugars and peptides. Other enzymes such as alkaline phosphatase and enterokinase also are found in the surface coat, having been formed by columnar cells, and pancreatic enzymes are absorbed into it from the lumen. In addition to its intraluminal digestive role, the glycocalyx may have specific binding sites for substances that are selectively absorbed in a particular portion of the small intestine. The microvilli contain fine filaments, mainly actin, in their cores, and these blend into the terminal web, which contains myosin. As explained in Chapter 2, it is believed that a myosin-actin interaction results in contraction/shortening of the microvilli. At the cell periphery and near the apex, junctional complexes bind adjacent cells together, and lateral cell interfaces show interdigitation of adjacent plasmalemmae (Fig. 11–44).

These columnar cells absorb sugars and amino acids from the gut lumen; these substances pass through the cells to the blood capillaries in the subjacent lamina propria. Their passage between cells is blocked by the zonula occludens. Both the sugars and the amino acids are absorbed into the cell by an active process and leave the basal area of the cell via a passive diffusion into the extracellular space. Lipid absorption also is a function of the columnar cells (Figs. 11–45 and 11–46). In the latter process, lipids are first taken up by intraluminal micelles of bile salts, which stabilize them in an emulsion and transport them to the brush border, where the hydrolyzed products diffuse through the cell membrane as fatty acids and monoglycerides. Fatty acids that contain more than 12 carbons are re-esterified into triglycerides by enzymes located in the smooth endoplasmic reticulum located near the apex of the cell. Then they are bound to a glycoprotein component (apoprotein) in the Golgi apparatus. The lipoprotein droplets, or chylomicrons, so formed are passed laterally into the intercellular spaces and travel down and pass through the basal lamina, to enter lymphatic vessels (lacteals) in the lamina propria. Lipid absorption is most efficiently carried out by villous absorptive cells of the jejunum.

Columnar cells are "mature" only when they reach a villus tip, being formed in crypts and migrating up crypts and along villi to the tips, where eventually they are shed. Immature cells show shorter, less regular microvilli and have less enzyme activity and a lower absorptive capacity.

**Undifferentiated (Stem) Cells.** Stem cells lie in the bases of intestinal glands (crypts) and are the source of other cells both in crypts and on villi. They are columnar but somewhat irregular, showing features of immature cells (such as few mitochondria, poorly developed endoplasmic reticulum, and a small Golgi apparatus but numerous free ribosomes and polysomes). Apical microvilli are shorter, less regular, and less numerous than those of the columnar absorptive cells. These cells are capable of, and undergo, frequent mitosis not only to maintain their population but also to form cells that differentiate into columnar, goblet, Paneth's, and enteroendocrine cells. In the differentiation of columnar cells, radioautography has shown that a differentiating cell passes from crypt to villus tip in about four to five days and then is shed; thus, there is a constant renewal of the intestinal epithelium, with a constant migration upward of cells from crypt bases to villi. The sloughing of cells at the apex of the villus occurs in an area called the extrusion zone, marked by an infolding of the epithelium that contains compressed degenerating cells. This upward migration applies to columnar, goblet, and enteroendocrine cells, each differentiating to maturity in its travel, but migration of maturing Paneth's cells appears to be downward from a so-called stem-cell zone situated a little above the actual base of the crypt.

**Paneth's Cells.** Found only in the bases of crypts in the small intestine, Paneth's cells are pyramidal in shape, with a broad base and a narrow apex. They show all the features of protein-secreting cells with basal endoplasmic reticulum, a large supranuclear Golgi complex, and apical secretory droplets that are acidophilic and are released at a slow rate. However, secretion is accelerated after feeding. They produce lysozyme, an enzyme that digests some bacterial cell walls, and have been reported as capable of phagocytosing some bacteria. Although their function is uncertain, it may be in regulating the microbial flora of the intestine. Although only a few Paneth's cells are found in the base of each crypt, collectively throughout the small intestine they constitute a considerable mass of cells. As indicated, the mature Paneth's cell with a full content of

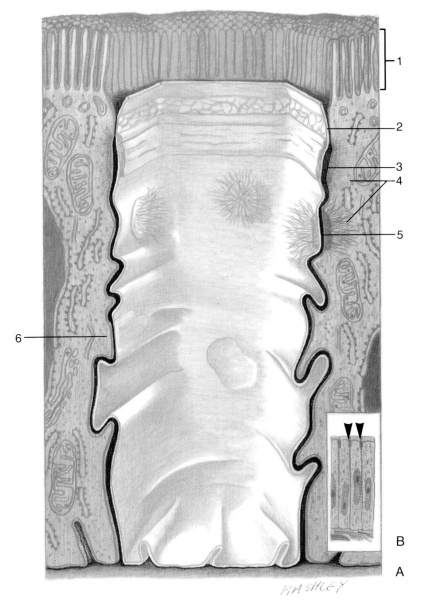

KM ASHLEY

**Figure 11–44.** *Junctional complex of a jejunal epithelial cell. Three-dimensional representation. A: The union of cells into structural units is ensured by various specialized devices of the cell surface, such as extensive junctional complexes. In order to illustrate these, a jejunal epithelial cell is shown emptied of cytoplasm. Just beneath the microvilli (1) appear zones where the cell membranes have fused, forming the zonula occludens or tight junctions (2). Below it lies the zonula adherens (3), where neighboring cells are separated by an intercellular cleft 150–200 Å wide. On its cytoplasmic side, the zonula adherens is dense and reinforced by short tonofilaments (4). Both zonulae, occludens and adherens, girdle the apical cell portion without interruption. Desmosome halves or maculae adherentes (5), from which tonofilaments (4) radiate into the cytoplasm like the hairs on a brush, are scattered over the plasmalemma. Every desmosome half of one cell corresponds to a similar one of the contiguous cell. Unlike zonulae occludentes and adherentes, desmosomes are circumscribed, button-like sites of attachment. Since their function requires the utilization of energy, several mitochondria are located nearby. × 6000. B: By light microscopy, the three structures described above are visible together as terminal bars (B, arrowheads). × 1000. (Reproduced with permission from Krstic, R. V.: Ultrastructure of the Mammalian Cell. New York, Springer-Verlag, 1979.)*

**Figure 11–45.** A drawing of an intestinal epithelial cell showing fat absorption. Following fat administration to an animal, no morphological changes can be detected in the microvilli of the intestinal epithelial cells. Similarly, apical pits and apical vesicles are unchanged in number or structure, except for the rare occurrence of a fat droplet in an apical pit. Striking alterations, on the other hand, occur in the endoplasmic reticulum. The smooth endoplasmic reticulum (SER) becomes much more prominent and occupies a greater proportion of the apical cytoplasm, while cisternae of rough-surfaced endoplasmic reticulum become shorter and reduced in number. Fenestrations occur along the margins of the rough cisternae. Lipid droplets are found in tubules, bulbous expansions, and isolated vesicles of the smooth endoplasmic reticulum. Continuities persist between the smooth and rough cisternae, and sometimes a lipid droplet is seen in a rough cisterna. The Golgi apparatus (G) is also conspicuously enlarged during fat absorption. Initially, Golgi vacuoles contain several fat droplets the size of those within the smooth endoplasmic reticulum. The small droplets apparently fuse to produce larger droplets. Eventually, each Golgi vacuole contains one large droplet of liquid. Vesicles containing single lipid droplets are abundant along the lateral margins of the cell. The intercellular spaces are enlarged and contain lipid droplets, or chylomicrons (Chy). A few coated pits border the intercellular spaces and may represent vesicles that have fused with the plasma membrane and discharged their contents. (From Lentz, T. L.: Cell Fine Structure. Philadelphia, W. B. Saunders Co., 1971.)

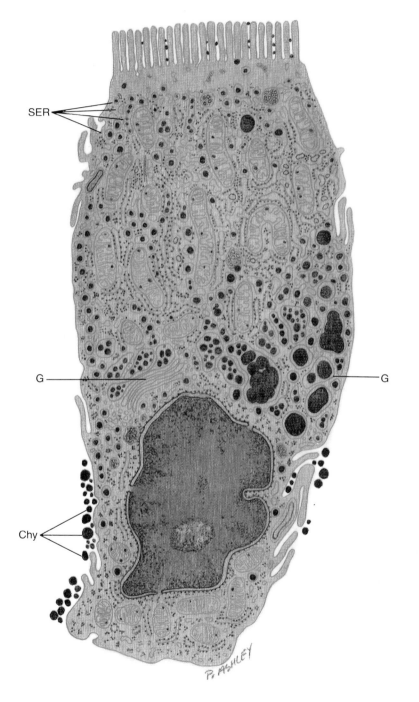

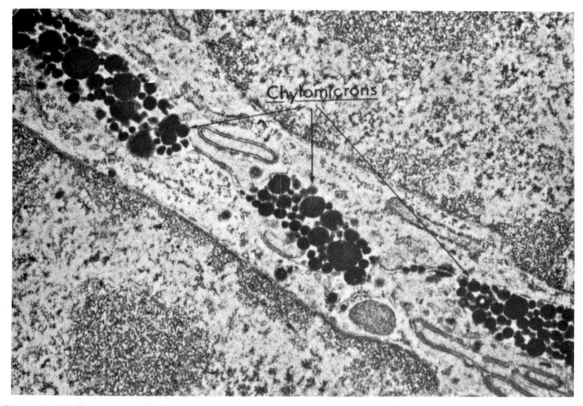

**Figure 11–46.** *Electron micrograph of the boundary between two rat intestinal epithelial cells during lipid absorption. The absorbed lipid has been discharged through the lateral cell surfaces and is seen to have accumulated here as aggregations of chylomicrons in the intercellular spaces. × 30,000. (Courtesy of S. L. Palay and J. P. Revel.)*

granules lies in the very base of the crypt, with less mature cells lying slightly higher in the crypt. Paneth's cells show a slower renewal rate (of 30 to 40 days) than those of columnar and goblet cells. In inflammatory diseases, these cells may appear in other regions of the gastrointestinal tract.

**Mucous (Goblet) Cells.** Goblet, or mucus-secreting, cells are scattered between the columnar cells, their numbers increasing from the duodenum to the terminal ileum (Figs. 11–47 through 11–50). Generally, the cells have a slender base that is darkly staining and contains the nucleus, and an apex that is expanded to the typical shape by the accumulation of mucous secretory granules. The excreted mucus is an acidic glycoprotein and forms a protective film lying on the glycocalyx of the microvilli of the columnar cells. These cells are formed by stem cells through an intermediate stage called the *oligomucous cell*. This cell is found in the crypt and contains a prominent Golgi apparatus with few secretory granules. At this stage, the cell probably is capable of mitosis; however, with the accumulation of more mucous granules, the capacity for division is lost. Like columnar cells, the goblet cells migrate from the crypt to the villus; they accumulate more secretory granules, become more goblet-shaped, and are shed at the villus tip. Their replacement rate is similar to that of columnar cells.

**Enteroendocrine Cells.** These cells (already described in relation to the stomach) are found in crypts and on villi, and they secrete active, regulatory peptides concerned in gastric secretion, intestinal motility, pancreatic secretion, and gallbladder contraction.

**Other Epithelial Cell Types.** *Caveolated* cells are not common but are found in both crypts and

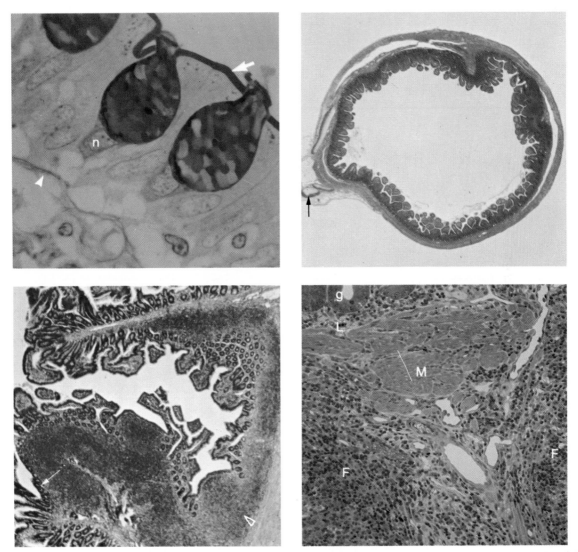

**Figure 11–47.** *Ileum.* Top left: *The epithelium of an ileal villus shows goblet cells, with the "stem" containing the nucleus (n), and the apex expanded to the goblet shape with mucous secretory granules. The mucus is an acidic glycoprotein. Also staining positively (magenta) with the periodic acid–Schiff (PAS) technique is the brush border of the columnar cells (arrow), as a result of the glycocalyx and, faintly, the basal lamina (arrowhead). Plastic section. PAS. Oil immersion. Top right: All layers are seen with the mesentery (arrow). Villi here are short and closely packed, and the lumen is smaller than that of the duodenum or jejunum. H and E. Low power. Bottom left: Peyer's patches. Here, masses of lymphoid tissue occupy the lamina propria and infiltrate the submucosa (arrowhead). Such masses may be visible to the naked eye. They are located on the antimesenteric border. Where follicles are large, there are no villi, and there may be no glands, the follicles being separated from the lumen only by a simple columnar epithelium (arrow). H and E. Medium power. Bottom right: Lymphatic tissue in the Peyer's patch infiltrates the lamina propria (L) and muscularis mucosae (M) and forms follicles (F) in the submucosa. Above, the bases of intestinal glands (g) are visible, but villi and glands may not be present over a Peyer's patch. Plastic section. Methylene blue, azure A, basic fuchsin. High power.*

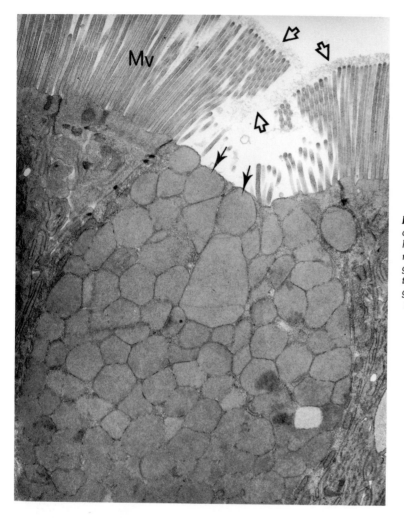

**Figure 11–48.** An electron micrograph of a goblet cell from the jejunal epithelium at higher magnification. This cell contains numerous osmiophilic-mucopolysaccharide granules (dark arrows), which upon secretion form a protective film lying on the glycocalyx (clear arrows). (Mv, microvilli.) × 19,500. (Courtesy of Dr. H. N. Tung.)

villi of the small intestine, the large intestine, and the stomach, and in other endoderm-derived tissues, such as bronchi. They are piriform in shape, with a base wider than the apex, and are characterized by long, apical microvilli containing prominent bundles of filaments extending deeply into apical cytoplasm. Between these bundles are irregular invaginations of the apical plasmalemma (caveolae). Their function is unknown, although it has been suggested that they are chemoreceptors.

Also found in intestinal epithelum are *migrating cells*, mainly lymphocytes, and less commonly, other leukocytes. Finally, found in the epithelium overlying Peyer's patches is the *M cell*. This specialized epithelial cell has an apical surface with microfolds or pleats, and its basal surface is closely related to lymphocytes lying within the epithelium. This cell transports macromolecules from the lumen to these lymphocytes, where responses to foreign antigens can be undertaken.

### Lamina Propria

The lamina propria extends between intestinal glands and into the cores of villi. Its character is quite distinctive, with a network of reticular fibers and many features of loose lymphatic tissue. It is best described, perhaps, as a loose, areolar connective tissue with lymphoid tendencies. Present in the meshwork of reticular fibers are primitive

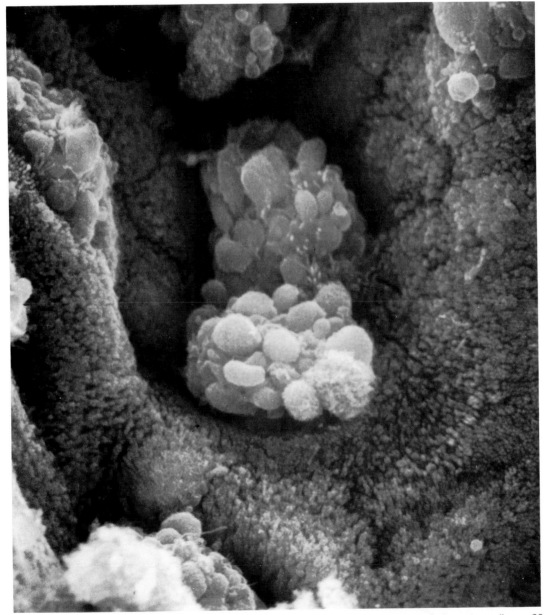

*Figure 11–49.* Scanning electron micrograph showing the apical portions of goblet cells and absorptive cells. × 20,500. (Courtesy of R. Blumershine and the Electron Microscopy Facility of Southern Illinois University School of Medicine.)

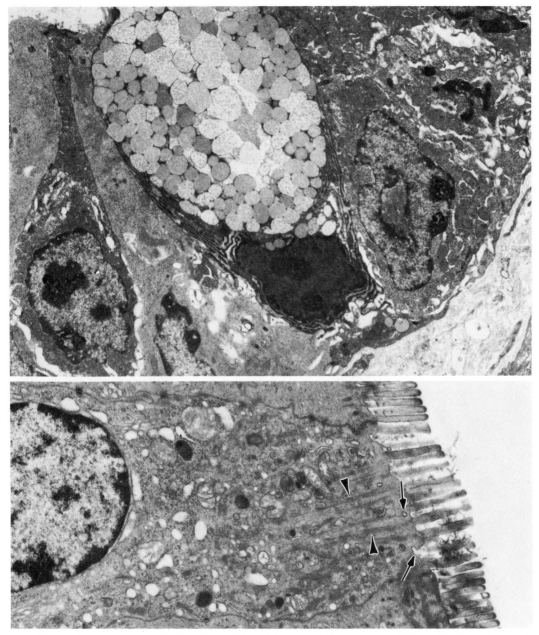

**Figure 11–50.** Top: *Electron micrograph of a goblet cell from jejunal epithelium.* × *4500.* Bottom: *Electron micrograph of the apical portion of a caveolated cell showing apical, long microvilli containing filament bundles extending deeply into apical cytoplasm (arrowheads), with caveolae between them (arrows).* × *9000.*

reticular cells with large, oval, pale-staining nuclei, lymphocytes, macrophages, and plasma cells. Eosinophil leukocytes, in particular, are evident, these having migrated from blood vessels. Single smooth muscle cells oriented lengthwise in the cores of villi usually are related closely to lymphatic capillaries. These start blindly in villi, contain absorbed fat after a meal, and thus appear white in fresh or living tissue. They are called *lacteals*.

In addition to scattered lymphocytes, there are present in the lamina propria large numbers of *solitary follicles* or isolated lymphatic nodules, more numerous distally in the intestine. If large, they may occupy the entire thickness of the mucosa and bulge the surface. There are no villi and may be no crypts on the surface of large follicles, which are then separated from the lumen only by a simple columnar epithelium. In many regions, but mainly in the ileum, follicles may be so numerous and close together as to aggregate into large masses of lymphoid tissue visible to the naked eye. They vary in size from 12 to 20 mm long and 8 to 12 mm wide, the longer axis lying along the length of the intestine. Always they are situated on the antimesenteric border (i.e., on the side away from the attachment of the mesentery). These are the *Peyer's patches*, or aggregated nodules.

From the immunological point of view, the lamina propria is important, with lymphoid cells and macrophages providing a barrier between the body and antigens, microorganisms, and other foreign materials that always are present in the intestinal lumen. This gut-associated lymphoid tissue (GALT) contains both T and B lymphocytes, although T cells are more numerous. Many of these cells are not permanent residents of the mucosa but circulate. B cells mature and proliferate in lymphatic nodules and Peyer's patches, and many become plasma cells producing antibodies (mainly IgA). IgA is also found in the parotid, submandibular, mammary, tracheobronchial, and gastrointestinal glands. As mentioned earlier, it is produced by plasma cells that exist as free cells in the lamina propria in all of the previously mentioned glands. The differentiation of B cells into mature plasma cells that produce IgA antibody is believed to be initiated by M cells that are associated with lymphoid nodules, such as those of Peyer's patches, and are specialized for the endocytosis and transcellular movement of intestinal luminal antigens. The frequent association of macrophagic pseudopods juxtapositioned near plasma cells within the lamina propria is believed to actively promote a strong antigenic response. The intestinal epithelium produces a glycoprotein secretory component that protects and carries the dimeric form of IgA and allows this so-called *secretory IgA* to coexist with the intestinal proteolytic enzymes. This immunoglobulin complex is transported across the epithelial cell in vesicles and is released to take up residence in the glycocalyx. Here, it is strategically positioned to combine with antigens, microorganisms, and toxins to prevent their attachment to the cell membrane and subsequent penetration into the epithelium. This effect thus produced is called *immune exclusion*. Certain bacteria (e.g., *Neisseria gonorrhoeae*) have evolved an IgA protease that can split the immunoglobulin complex and thus lead to its ultimate destruction and to the loss of the epithelial cell's function as a barrier and local immune modulator. In addition to dimeric secretory immunoglobulin, plasma cells produce monomeric immunoglobulin A (*serum IgA*), which is present in the blood and lymphatic circulation, and other similar forms—*IgE* and *IgG*. IgE can bind to the cell membrane of mast cells in the lamina propria, which renders the latter more sensitive to particular intestinal antigens. IgG is the antibody that mediates general humoral immunity. Both *IgE* and *IgG* primarily enter the lymphatic circulation.

The muscularis mucosae, submucosa, muscularis, and serosa do not merit a separate description, although it should be noted that the submucosa usually is infiltrated with lymphocytes in the region of Peyer's patches.

### Duodenal Glands (of Brunner)

These submucosal glands of the duodenum are composed of tall cuboidal cells with dark, flattened, basal nuclei and a clear, vacuolated cytoplasm (Figs. 11–51 and 11–52). The glandular portions continue into ducts lined by low cuboidal cells, and these penetrate the muscularis mucosae to open into intestinal glands. Often, the muscularis mucosae does not form a complete layer over the glands, and slips of smooth muscle

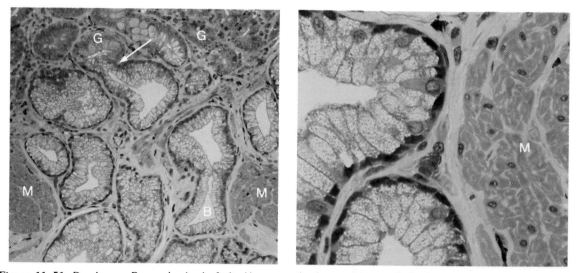

**Figure 11–51.** *Duodenum, Brunner's glands. Left: Above are the bases of intestinal glands, or crypts (G), below are the submucosal glands of Brunner (B). This gland secretes a neutral or alkaline mucus with a high bicarbonate content. The ducts of the gland pass through the muscularis mucosae (M) to drain into the bases of the crypts, as seen at arrow. Plastic section. Methylene blue, azure A, basic fuchsin. Medium power. Right: A higher magnification of Figure 11–33, this section shows smooth muscle (M) of the muscularis mucosae in transverse section with parts of two secretory acini of Brunner's glands. The cells are tall and columnar, nuclei are basally located, and the extensive apical cytoplasm is pale-staining and filled with mucous droplets. Plastic section. Methylene blue, azure A, basic fuchsin. Oil immersion.*

extend in the connective tissue between the glandular units. Occasionally, Brunner's glands extend into the upper part of the jejunum and, more commonly, may be found in the pyloric region of the stomach. These glands secrete an alkaline (pH 8.2 to 9.3) mucus. The acidic gastric secretion could cause erosion of the duodenal mucosa, and the secretion of the submucosal glands protects against this by its mucus, by its alkalinity, and presumably by the buffering capacity of its bicar-

**Figure 11–52.** *Drawing of a Brunner's gland cell. These cells comprise the Brunner's glands found in the submucosa of the duodenum. The cells are cuboidal to low-columnar; the basal nucleus contains a nucleolus and evenly dispersed chromatin material. Microvilli extend from the free surface of the cell. Laterally and apically between adjacent cells, small intercellular channels or secretory canals (Ca) may occur. Toward the base, complex interdigitations are found. The gland cells contain a well-developed endoplasmic reticulum that is most extensive in the basal portion of the cell. The rough-surfaced cisternae range from short tubular profiles to elongated cisterns that extend in parallel. Free ribosomes occur singly and in clusters, in the cytoplasm. These cells have an extensive Golgi system (G) that is dispersed over a wide area above the nucleus. Flattened, smooth membranous lamellae occur in parallel aggregations. The outermost cisternae are flat and empty, while the innermost are distended by material similar to that comprising early secretory granules. Vesicles are dispersed around the margins of the lamellar stacks, especially laterally and distally. Vesicles are also abundant near rough-surfaced cisternae of endoplasmic reticulum that face the Golgi region, and some appear to bud off from the cisternae. Vacuoles (Vac) containing secretory material are numerous along the inner face of the Golgi. Small spherical secretory granules (SG) with a dense content are found in the Golgi zone. The granules are larger in the distal areas of the cell and accumulate in the apex. Mitochondria are large, and round or oval. Some are partially surrounded by cisternae of endoplasmic reticulum. Multivesicular bodies are sometimes found in the Golgi zone. Brunner's glands secrete a clear, viscous, alkaline fluid that may protect the duodenal mucosa from the action of acid gastric fluid. It has been suggested that the protein component of the secretory product is synthesized in the rough-surfaced endoplasmic reticulum, while synthesis of a carbohydrate component and its combination with the protein moiety may occur in the Golgi complex. (From Lentz, T. L.: Cell Fine Structure. Philadelphia, W. B. Saunders Co., 1971.)*

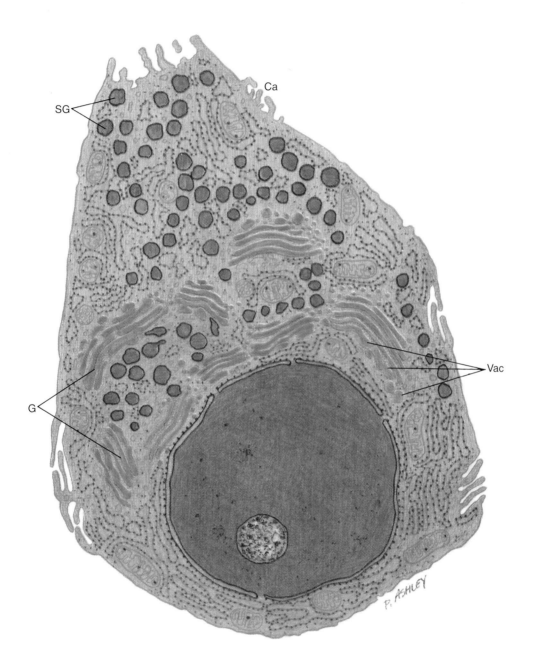

bonate content, which reacts with the hydrochloric acid to form sodium chloride and carbonic acid. The net result is the formation of a neutral salt in the intestine. In a similar manner, pancreatic secretions neutralize the acidity of the chyme coming from the stomach. It has been shown by immunofluorescence that the cells of Brunner's glands contain urogastrone, a peptide that inhibits the secretion of hydrochloric acid in the stomach and also stimulates epithelial proliferation. The latter may function to stimulate the rapid renewal of the epithelial cells within the intestinal crypts.

## THE LARGE INTESTINE

The large intestine is about 180 cm in length and consists of the *cecum*, continuous with the ileum at the ileocecal valve; the *appendix*, a small diverticulum from the cecum; the *colon*, continuous with the cecum and divided into the ascending, transverse, and descending parts; and then the *rectum* and the *anal canal*, terminating at the *anus* at the body surface. Food material enters the cecum in a semifluid state; it becomes semisolid, the consistency of *feces*, in the colon. Thus, one function of the large intestine is absorption of fluid. Other functions are secretion of mucus (lubrication becomes more important as fluid is absorbed and the fecal mass becomes harder and thus more likely to damage the mucosa) and digestion, accomplished by enzymes present in the food material and by putrefaction by bacteria always present in the large intestine. No digestive enzymes are secreted by the large intestine.

The large intestine lacks plicae and villi, and thus the surface epithelium is more obvious than it is in the small intestine. Intestinal glands, or crypts, are present, and are longer than those of the small intestine and more closely packed. As in the small intestine, stem cells give rise to columnar, goblet, and enteroendocrine cells. The columnar and goblet cells are removed from the luminal mucosa at extrusion zones situated midway between intestinal gland openings. At the luminal surface, enteroendocrine cells are not in contact with the lumen but remain closely applied to the basal lamina. When situated in the crypts, the latter cells are held together by tight junctions,

and since their average life span is approximately three times that of the other two cell types (21 days as compared with 6 days), they must migrate independently within the crypts. Epithelial cell types are identical to those of the small intestine, but the goblet (mucus-secreting) cells are more numerous.

### Ileocecal Junction

At the ileocecal junction, there is an abrupt change in the character of the mucosa, which is thrown into anterior and posterior folds to form two *valves*. These folds consist of mucosa and submucosa, supported by a mass of circular smooth muscle, a thickening of the inner layer of the muscularis; because of their position, the ileocecal orifice has the form of a vertical slit.

The ileocecal junction is located at the lower right side of the abdomen and is fixed to the posterior abdominal wall (i.e., the terminal ileum has no mesentery). The cecum is a small blind pouch hanging down from the ileocecal junction and has a structure identical to that of the colon.

### Appendix

The appendix is a small, slender, blind diverticulum of the cecum arising about 2.5 cm below the ileocecal valve (Fig. 11–53). It is in a good position to sample microbial flora leaving both the small and the large intestines, particularly in the case of the large intestine, where the content of bacteria is far greater than in other portions of the digestive tract. In cross section, the lumen is small and usually of irregular outline, often contains cellular debris, and may be completely occluded. Villi are absent, and intestinal glands are few and of irregular length. The surface epithelium is mainly composed of columnar, striated border cells, with only a few goblet cells. In the crypts, there are a few Paneth's cells, and enteroendocrine cells are numerous and mainly of the EC type (particularly, those that secrete serotonin). Carcinoid tumors in the appendix produce large amounts of this indolamine. The lamina propria is occupied by a mass of lymphoid nodules that are similar to those of the palatine tonsil and are more or less confluent. The muscularis mucosae

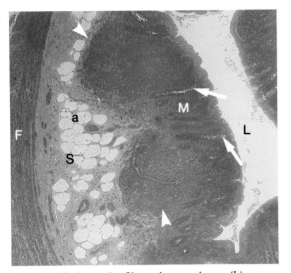

*Figure 11–53. Appendix. Shown here are lumen (L), mucosa (M), submucosa (S), and part of the muscularis (F). In the mucosa, there are no villi and the glands (arrows) are few and lined by a simple columnar epithelium in which goblet cells (clear-staining) are numerous. The lamina propria is very cellular because of lymphoid infiltration with lymph nodules (arrowheads) extending into the submucosa through an incomplete muscularis mucosae. Note fat cells (a) in the submucosa. Plastic section. Methylene blue, azure A, basic fuchsin. Low power.*

usually is incomplete. The submucosa is thick and contains blood vessels and nerves, and the muscularis is thin but shows the usual two layers without the presence of taeniae coli. The serous coat is identical to that covering the remainder of the intestine.

The appendix so commonly is the site of acute and chronic inflammation that it is difficult to obtain a completely normal appendix. Usually, some eosinophils and neutrophils are present in lamina propria and submucosa. If present in large numbers, they are evidence of chronic and acute infection, respectively.

### Cecum, Colon, and Rectum

The depth of intestinal glands is greater in the large intestine than in the small intestine. Also, these glands are packed more closely in the large intestine compared with the small. They increase in depth to 0.75 mm in the rectum, being 0.5 mm in the colon (Figs. 11–54 and 11–55). Goblet

cells are numerous. Enteroendocrine cells are occasional in the depths, but Paneth's cells usually are not present. Most of the cells in the depths of the glands are undifferentiated epithelial cells that undergo rapid mitosis. These cells contain some secretory granules, which are discharged before the cells reach the surface of the mucosa (Figs. 11–56 and 11–57). The secreted material forms part of the glycocalyx. The lamina propria between glands is similar in appearance to that of the small intestine and contains scattered lymphatic nodules that extend deeply into the submucosa. The muscularis mucosae is well developed but may be irregular or deficient at the sites of the lymphatic nodules. In the cecum and colon, the outer longitudinal coat of the muscularis is not a complete layer and is present as three longitudinal bands, the *taeniae coli*. In the rectum, it again becomes a complete layer. The serous coat shows, on the surface not attached to the posterior abdominal wall, small, taglike protuberances composed of adipose tissue, the *appendices epiploicae*. In the transverse colon, there is a true mesentery.

### Rectoanal Junction

In the lower end of the rectum, the intestinal glands become short and disappear in the anal canal. Here, the mucous membrane is thrown into a series of longitudinal folds termed the *rectal columns of Morgagni*. Below, adjacent rectal columns are united by a series of crescentic mucosal folds termed *anal valves*. These valves together with their enclosed blind concavities (termed *anal sinuses*, or *crypts*) form the *pectinate line*. This line delineates the endoderm-derived component of the anal canal (*anatomical anal canal*) from the ectoderm-derived component (*clinical or true anal canal*). Above the anal valves, the columnar epithelium abruptly reverts to a moist stratified squamous epithelium whose junctional ring is termed the *line of Hilton*. Below the rectal columns, the muscularis mucosae becomes broken up into a series of bundles and finally disappears, so that there is no distinction between lamina propria and submucosa. In this region, there are numerous longitudinal, thin-walled veins that, if dilated and convoluted, cause protrusion of the mucous membrane over them. Such a condition consti-

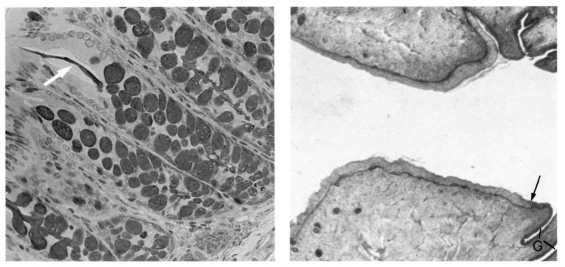

**Figure 11–54.** *Large intestine. Left: Colon. The simple tubular glands of the mucosa contain numerous goblet cells. The secretory mucin granules are stained magenta. The mucus is discharged to lie in the lumen near the surface (arrow). The surface epithelium is simple columnar with interspersed (and dying) goblet cells. There are no villi in the large intestine. Plastic section. PAS. High power. Right: Rectoanal junction. In the terminal rectum, there are a few simple tubular glands (G) with a simple columnar epithelial lining. The columnar epithelium then changes abruptly (arrow), in this longitudinal section, to a stratified squamous epithelium lining the anal canal. This is short, and at the anal orifice the epithelium changes again to epidermis. At the anus, the epithelium is keratinized, and deep to it are the branched, tubular, circumanal glands (darkly staining). H and E. Low power.*

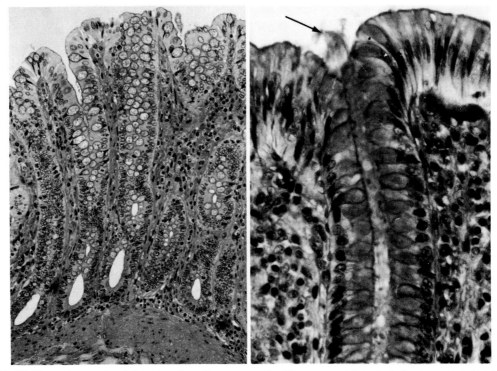

**Figure 11–55.** *Photomicrographs of the colon show the mucosa. No villi are present, intestinal glands are straight tubules, and goblet cells are abundant. The arrow indicates mucus discharged from one gland. Plastic section. Left, low power; right, medium power.*

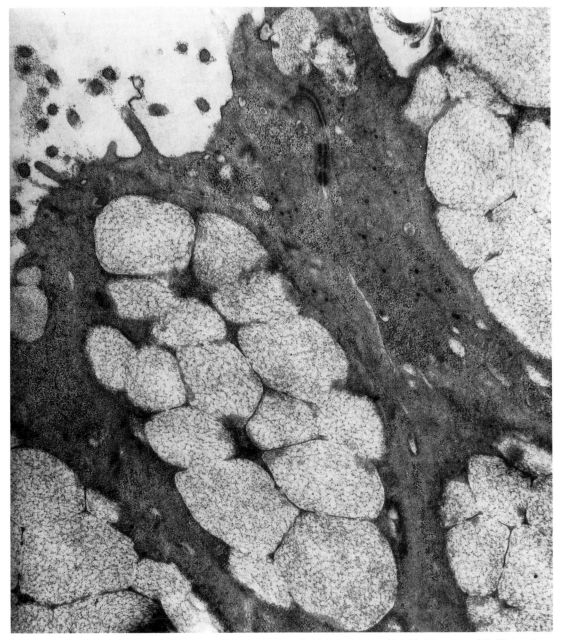

**Figure 11–56.** An electron micrograph showing mucus-secreting cells of the colon. × 19,000. (Courtesy of R. Blumershine and the Electron Microscopy Facility of Southern Illinois University School of Medicine.)

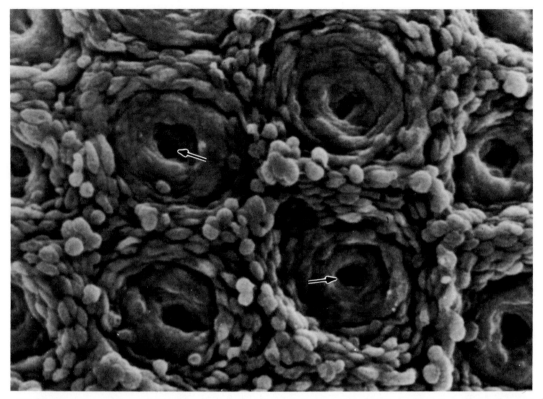

**Figure 11–57.** *Scanning electron micrograph of monkey colon showing openings (arrows) of crypts to the surface.* × 890. *(Courtesy of R. D. Specian and M. R. Neutra.)*

tutes *internal hemorrhoids,* or *piles.* About 2.5 cm above the anal orifice, the columnar epithelium abruptly changes to a stratified squamous epithelium that extends downward for a short extent only as a transitional zone between intestinal epithelium and skin. At the anus, the epithelium is keratinized, and beneath it are branched tubular glands termed the *circumanal glands.*

The muscularis at the rectoanal junction shows certain modifications. In the lower rectum, the longitudinal layer appears to be shorter than the length of the rectum and thus causes the mucosa to bulge into the lumen as transverse shelves termed the *plicae transversales;* there are two such shelves on the right and one on the left. These may aid in the support of feces but also are thought to help the separation of feces from flatus. In the lower rectum and anal canal, the internal layer of the muscularis is thickened as the *internal sphincter* of the anus. Surrounding the anal canal are bundles of striated muscle, the *external sphincter* of the anus.

**Figure 11–58.** *Diagrams of distribution of blood vessels (A and B) and of lymphatics (C and D) in the small intestine of the dog. B and D are drawn on a larger scale to show details. CM, circular muscle; Cr, crypt; F, follicle; LM, longitudinal muscle; Mm, lamina muscularis mucosae; PF, perifollicular plexus; Smp, submucous plexus; Sub, tunica submucosa; V, villus. (Courtesy of Dr. D. W. Fawcett.)*

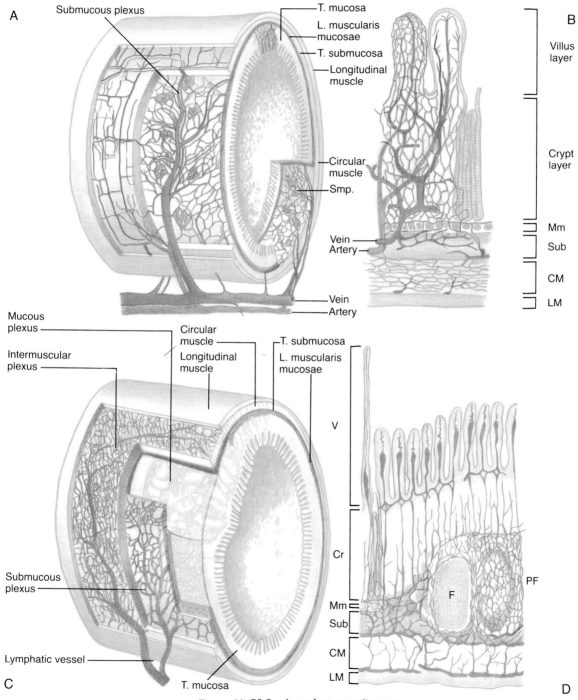

A

Submucous plexus

T. mucosa
L. muscularis mucosae
T. submucosa
Longitudinal muscle

Circular muscle
Smp.

Vein
Artery

Vein
Artery

B

Villus layer

Crypt layer

Mm
Sub
CM
LM

Mucous plexus

Intermuscular plexus

Circular muscle
Longitudinal muscle

T. submucosa
L. muscularis mucosae

Submucous plexus

Lymphatic vessel

T. mucosa

C

V

Cr

Mm
Sub
CM
LM

F

PF

D

*Figure 11–58* See legend on opposite page

## INTESTINAL ABSORPTION

The digestion of food material within the intestinal lumen involves the reduction of foodstuffs to molecular size. This is accomplished by the secretions of the major digestive glands (pancreas and liver) and by secretions of intestinal juice, produced mainly by the intestinal glands (of Lieberkühn). Bile from the liver reduces lipid to triglycerides, while pancreatic juice contains lipolytic, proteolytic, and carbohydrate-splitting enzymes. Intestinal juice contains lipase, maltase, and peptidase. In the adult, amino acids resulting from the intraluminal digestion of proteins are absorbed by the intestinal epithelium. The majority of lipid is absorbed as micelles of fatty acids and monoglycerides that are re-esterified to triglyceride in the agranular reticulum of apical cytoplasm. The triglyceride then is combined with protein to form *chylomicrons*, which later enter the lacteals. This protein is hydrophilic, which prevents the chylomicrons from sticking to each other and to the walls of the lacteals.

## BLOOD VESSELS

Generally, throughout the digestive tract, the arrangements of blood and lymph vessels are similar (Fig. 11–58). Basically, arteries entering the tract pass through the muscularis to form an extensive submucous plexus. From this plexus, branches pass toward the lumen and supply capillaries to the muscularis mucosae and capillary networks throughout the mucosa and around the glands. Venous return commences superficially, from the mucosal capillary plexus, as large-caliber vessels that form an extensive venous plexus just internal to the muscularis mucosae. From here, veins pass outward into the submucosa, where there is a second extensive plexus that is drained by large veins passing through the muscularis to the serosa. These large veins run with the entering arteries.

In the small intestine, the arterial pattern is more extensive than that just described (Fig. 11–59). In addition to capillary networks around the intestinal glands, other arterioles originate in the submucous plexus and are destined specifically to supply villi, each villus receiving one or more such arterioles. Having entered the base of a villus, these arterioles break up into a dense capillary network situated adjacent to the basal lamina of the epithelium. Small veins arise from this superficial capillary network at the tip of a villus and pass outward to join the venous plexus internal to the muscularis mucosae.

Lymphatic capillaries form an extensive system surrounding glands in the superficial layers of the mucosa, and in the small intestine this plexus is joined by lacteals. Lacteals start blindly in the apices of villi and run axially in the cores of villi.

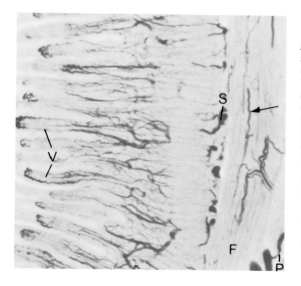

*Figure 11–59.* Small intestine, blood vessels injected. This is a transverse section of the jejunum. The arterial system was injected with red gelatin to demonstrate the blood supply. Terminal branches (vasa recta) of arterial arcades from the superior mesenteric artery lie in the connective tissue of the serosa (P). They give a few branches to serosa and muscularis and then pass through the muscularis (F) to form an extensive submucosal plexus (S). In the muscularis, blood vessels run parallel to muscle fibers; that is, they are circular in the inner layer (arrow). From the submucous plexus, vessels run radially and extend into villi (V) to form extensive capillary networks. Indeed, capillary plexuses here are so extensive as to clearly outline villi. Venous return, not demonstrated here, starts in mucosal plexuses and then passes to an extensive submucosal plexus. Large veins drain this plexus and pass through muscularis and serosa to run with arteries and join the portal vein to pass to the liver. Low power.

From the mucosal plexus, branches pierce the muscularis mucosae and form a plexus of lymphatics in the submucosa, from which larger lymphatics pass outward through the muscularis and follow blood vessels to the retroperitoneal tissues. In the muscularis, lymphatics receive many tributaries from another lymphatic plexus located in the muscularis.

# The Major Digestive Glands

There are two large abdominal organs that connect to the digestive tract by duct systems. These are the *pancreas* and the *liver*.

## THE PANCREAS

The pancreas (Gr. *pan*, all; *kreas*, flesh) is a large, elongated organ lying in the concavity of the duodenum and extending behind the peritoneum of the posterior abdominal wall toward the left to reach the hilum of the spleen. It is both an exocrine and an endocrine organ, the two func-

tions being performed by different cell types (Figs. 11–60 and 11–61).

In the fresh condition, it is pale-pink or white and has no definite fibrous capsule but is covered by thin areolar tissue from which thin septa extend into the gland to divide it into obvious lobules. This thin connective tissue capsule places the pancreas in a vulnerable position with regard to invasive diseases. More support is gained internally via the associated dense connective tissue layers of its large excretory ducts, which course through the head and body of the pancreas. Fine, delicate connective tissue surrounds individual acini.

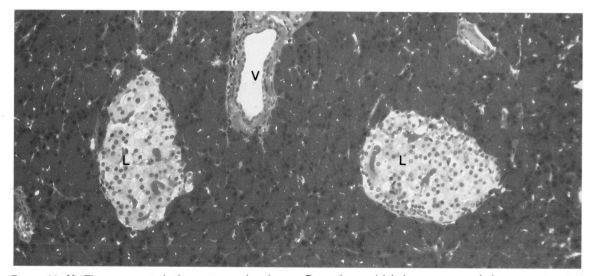

**Figure 11–60.** *The pancreas is both exocrine and endocrine. Parts of several lobules are seen, with fine connective tissue between lobules. The secretory units, or acini, are not clearly distinguished at this magnification but are formed by cells with basophil cytoplasm and pink-staining secretory droplets. In the more extensive connective tissue are some large blood vessels (V). Located in lobules among the acini are two pale-staining, spheroidal clumps of cells (L). These are the endocrine islets of Langerhans. The exocrine pancreas is classified as a compound acinar serous gland, secreting digestive enzymes. The islets secrete insulin, the antidiabetic hormone, and glucagon, which increases the level of blood sugar. Plastic section. Low power.*

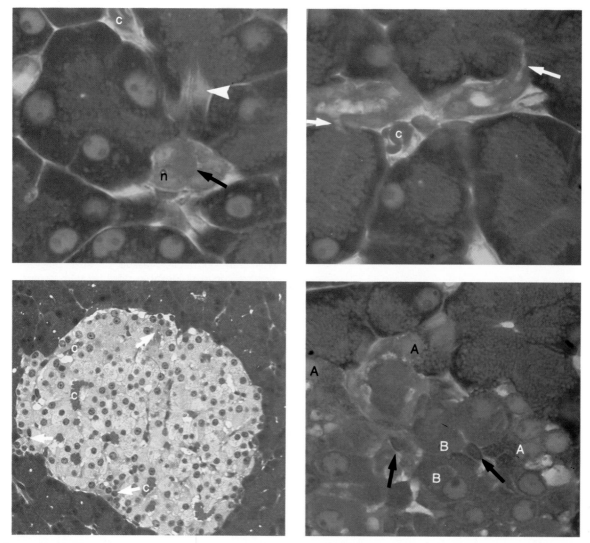

**Figure 11–61.** *The exocrine (top micrographs) and endocrine (bottom micrographs) portions of the pancreas. Top left: Pancreas, exocrine. Several acini are seen with sparse connective tissue between them in which there is a blood capillary (c). Acinar cells show the features of protein (enzyme) secretion with vesicular nuclei with prominent and often multiple nucleoli, intense cytoplasmic basophilia, and discrete, apical secretory droplets (pink). A centroacinar cell (arrowhead) is seen in one acinus, and beneath it is an intercalated duct lined by simple, low cuboidal epithelium, the cells with pale-staining nuclei (n), and the lumen containing pink-staining secretory material (arrow). Plastic section. Methylene blue, basic fuchsin. Oil immersion. Top right: Pancreas, exocrine, The exocrine cells show features similar to those in the companion micrograph; note, however, that the lumina of two acini show continuity with intercalated ducts at the arrows, the ducts lined by squamous or low cuboidal epithelium. A capillary (c) also is seen. Plastic section. Methylene blue, basic fuchsin. Oil immersion. Bottom left: Endocrine pancreas. The field mainly is occupied by an islet of Langerhans, surrounded by exocrine acini. In the islet, the endocrine cells are large, polygonal, and pale-staining with centrally located nuclei and are arranged in cords and clumps between blood capillaries (c) containing erythrocytes (red). Most of the cells are insulin-secreting B cells. Cells with pinker cytoplasm at the periphery of the islet are glucagon-secreting A cells (arrows). Plastic section. H and E. High power. Bottom right: Endocrine pancreas. A portion of an islet of Langerhans shows large polygonal cells with fine secretory granules, much smaller than the pink-staining granules in the adjacent exocrine cells (above). Most of the islet cells stain purple and are insulin-secreting B cells (B), but a few at the periphery show more red-colored granules and are glucagon-secreting A cells (A) and perhaps D (somatostatin-secreting) cells. All endocrine cells contact a capillary blood vessel, of which two are seen in the area. (The nuclei of lining endothelial cells are arrowed.) Plastic section. Methylene blue, basic fuchsin. Oil immersion.*

## Exocrine Portion

The pancreas can be classified as a large, lobulated, compound, tubuloacinar gland (Fig. 11–62; see Figs. 11–60 and 11–61).

### ACINI

Acini, or alveoli, are tubular or pear-shaped, are surrounded by a basal lamina that is continuous with that investing the ductules, and are composed of five to eight pyramidal cells arranged around a small central lumen (Fig. 11–63). Myoepithelial cells are not present. Between acini is delicate connective tissue containing blood ves-

sels, lymphatics, nerves, and excretory ducts. The acini are packed in an irregular fashion, and thus in any section, they will be cut in every possible plane. Obviously, the lumen of all will not be sectioned. In addition, the caliber of the lumen varies with the secretory phase, and the lumen may contain small cells. These, the *centroacinar cells*, belong to the duct system, which often commences not from the terminations but from the central parts of acini (Fig. 11–64).

In an acinar cell, the nucleus is spherical, lies toward the base, and contains abundant chromatin and one to three large nucleoli (Fig. 11–65). The basal cytoplasm is basophil and may show a longitudinal striation owing to the pres-

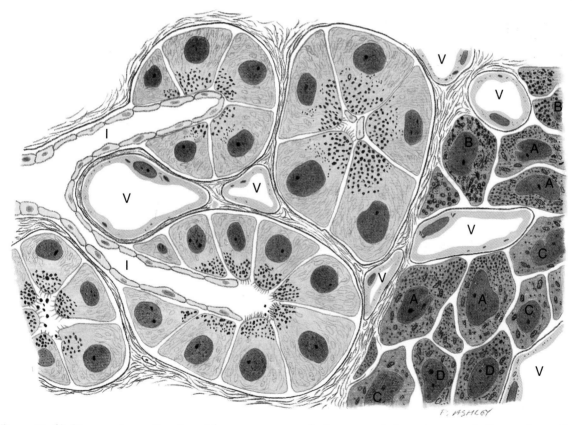

**Figure 11–62.** Diagram of a small portion of the pancreas as seen by low-power electron microscopy. In the exocrine portion (left), parts of four acini are illustrated. Two are drained by intercalated ducts (I) and one (top center) shows two centroacinar cells. In a typical exocrine cell, identify the following features: nucleus with nucleolus, basal ergastoplasm and mitochondria, supranuclear Golgi zone (clear space) and apical zymogen and prozymogen droplets. In the endocrine islet of Langerhans (right), A, B, C, and D cells are labeled. Note the variation in type of secretory granules and their relation to capillary blood vessels (V). Approximately × 1500.

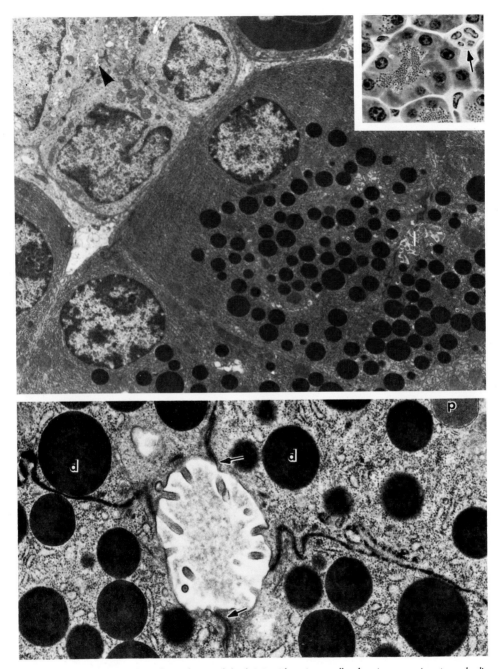

**Figure 11–63.** *Exocrine pancreas.* Top: Inset *(top right):* Acini with acinar cells showing prominent nucleoli, cytoplasmic basophilia, apical secretory droplets, and a small duct *(arrow).* × 250. *The electron micrograph shows a similar area: part of an acinus with lumen (l); masses of granular reticulum; and spherical, dense secretory droplets. The small intralobular duct (top left) shows lumen (arrowhead) lined by small cuboidal cells.* × 4500. *Bottom: The lumen of an acinus is seen with a few microvilli. Zymogen (d) droplets are very dense, part of a prozymogen droplet (p) is less dense. Cell interfaces (here black due to the use of lanthanum as a "tracer") show zonula occludens (arrows) near the lumen.* × 24,000.

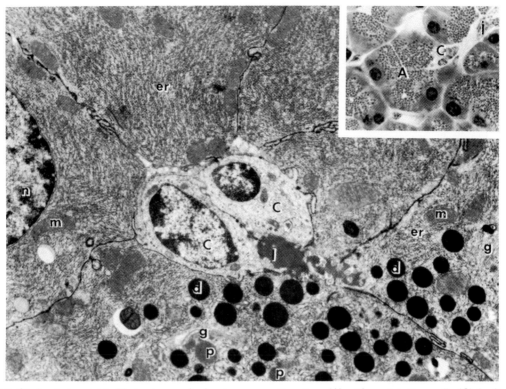

**Figure 11–64.** Inset, top right: *Photomicrograph showing pancreatic acinus (A) with centroacinar cells (C) leading to an intercalated duct (i).* × *250. Electron micrograph of a similar area shows an acinar lumen (l) filled with dense, secretory material and partially bordered by two centroacinar cells (C). In acinar cells, note nucleus (n), granular reticulum (er), Golgi apparatus (g), zymogen (d) and prozymogen (p) droplets, and mitochondria (m). Cell interfaces (black) have been filled with the tracer lanthanum.* × *6500.*

ence of numerous elongated mitochondria. The apical cytoplasm contains acidophil secretion (zymogenic) droplets or granules that are highly refractile. In a supranuclear position also is an extensive Golgi apparatus, sometimes visible as a clear area among the zymogen granules. By electron microscopy, acini are seen to be enclosed by a thin basal lamina supported by reticular fibers. The main features of these cells are the specializations for protein secretion (see Chapter 1). The cytoplasm is filled largely with flattened sacs of granular endoplasmic reticulum (ergastoplasm), particularly prominent in the basal region but extending also into the supranuclear zone. The membranes of the granular endoplasmic reticulum constitute approximately 60 per cent of the total surface formed by the acinar cell's mem-

branes. Mitochondria are quite numerous, usually elongated, and mainly oriented perpendicularly in the basal cytoplasm. A well-developed Golgi zone is located in a supranuclear position, and the vacuoles of this zone have a content of varying density representing formative stages of zymogen granules. Zymogen granules are large, spherical, and homogeneously dense, with a limiting membrane (Fig. 11–66). Some with a less dense matrix have been termed prozymogen granules. The secretion of enzymes as inactive proenzymes serves to protect the acinar cell from autodigestion. A *trypsin inhibitor*, also secreted by these cells, blocks the activation process (tryptic cleavage) and prevents premature activation of the proenzymes, thus allowing enterokinase, an enzyme of the intestinal brush border, the final

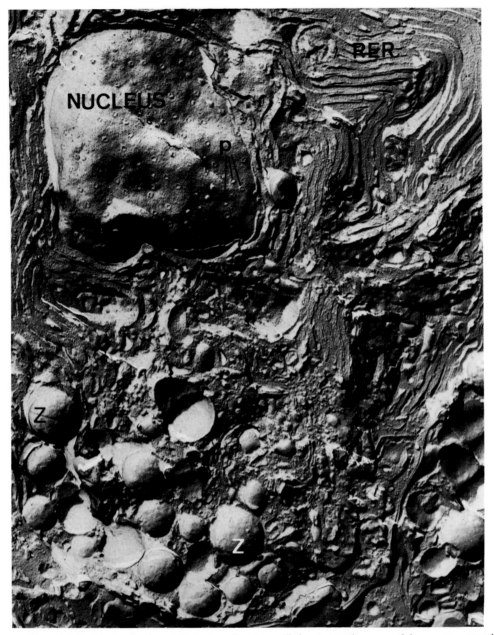

**Figure 11.–65.** *Freeze-etch micrograph of part of a pancreatic acinar cell showing nuclear pores (p), zymogen granules (Z) and rough endoplasmic reticulum (RER). The lumen lies below. × 15,000. (Courtesy of L. Orci.)*

conversion step in the chemical transformation of trypsinogen to trypsin. The premature activation of the proenzyme in the acinar cells leads to a disease called *acute pancreatitis*, which results in autolysis of pancreatic tissue. The presence of tight junctions contained within the junctional complex of the acinar cells prevents the egress of material into the intercellular spaces. Further

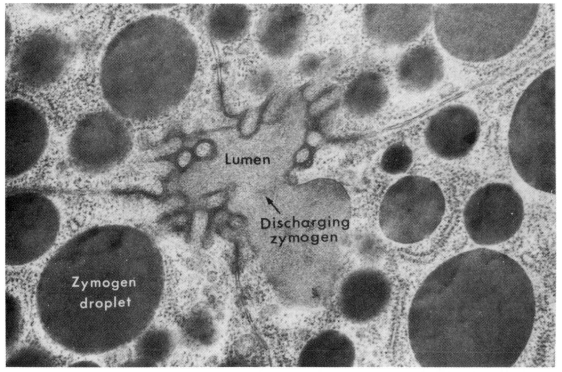

**Figure 11–66.** Electron micrograph of the lumen of an acinus and the apical portions of four acinar cells. Large, dense zymogen droplets or granules are found in the cell apex. The limiting membrane of one of these has fused with the cell membrane, and its zymogen is being discharged into the lumen. The free surface of the acinar cells bears short microvilli. (From Fawcett, D. W.: Bloom and Fawcett: A Textbook of Histology, 11th ed. Philadelphia, W. B. Saunders Co., 1986.)

down, the junctional complex also contains zonula adherens and desmosomes (for cell-to-cell adhesion) and gap junctions (for electrical and metabolic coupling of acinar cells). The remainder of the lateral border shows none of the extensive lateral interdigitations exhibited by salivary gland acinar cells. A few short microvilli are present at the apex.

The formation and secretion of zymogen granules have been studied by radioautography after injection of tritiated leucine, glycine, and methionine. Such studies confirm the theory of protein secretion as explained in Chapter 1. Radioautographic label appears rapidly in the endoplasmic reticulum (about five minutes after injection); shows up later in the Golgi zone (in about 10 to 12 minutes), where protein is built into prozymogen granules; and appears still later in zymogen granules (in 30 to 40 minutes). The life span of a zymogen granule in an acinar cell is estimated at only 50 minutes. These figures give some indication of the extreme activity of the pancreatic acinar cells. Thus, in summary, it is believed that the digestive enzymes of the pancreas are synthesized in the basal region of the cytoplasm and accumulate in the canals of the endoplasmic reticulum. From there, the enzymes pass in a vectorial manner to the Golgi region, where they are segregated in membrane-bound vesicles and are concentrated into typical zymogen droplets. These droplets later pass to the cell surface, where they are discharged by a process of exocytosis. In exocytosis, the membrane bounding the zymogen droplet fuses with the luminal plasmalemma, thus permitting extrusion of the contents of the droplet. Secretion and discharge of the excretory products from the acinar cells are discontinuous and quantal and subject to neural and particularly hormonal regulation (Fig. 11–67). Hence, the presence of a storage granule is

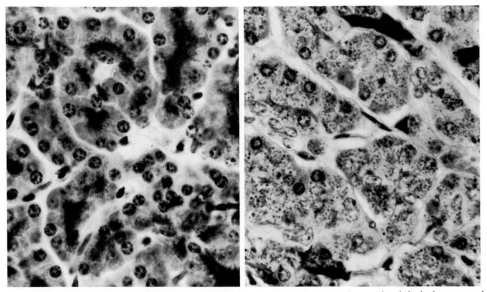

**Figure 11–67.** *Photomicrographs of the pancreas stained to show secretion (zymogen) granules, left, before a meal, and right, after a meal. Note that the majority of the granules has been secreted after feeding. Iron hematoxylin, osmic acid. × 350. (Courtesy of Dr. D. W. Fawcett.)*

required. The concentration of the pancreatic secretory protein, before release, is brought about by the electrostatic interaction of the positively charged secretory proteins and a negatively charged proteoglycan (a large protein-linked polysaccharide that is sulfated in the Golgi apparatus), which produces an osmotically inactive precipitate, causing the passive efflux of water. Secretory vesicles fuse with only the apical portions of the plasma membranes because of the information contained within the clathrin-coated recyclable transport vesicles.

The pancreatic juice contains proteolytic enzymes (e.g., trypsin and chymotrypsin), which split proteins; carboxypeptidase, which cleaves peptides; ribonuclease (RNase) and deoxyribonuclease (DNase), which break down ribonucleoprotein (RNP) and deoxyribonucleoprotein (DNP); amylase, which hydrolyzes starch and other carbohydrates; lipase, which hydrolyzes neutral fat to glycerol and fatty acids; and cholesterol esterase, which splits cholesterol esters into cholesterol and fatty acids. In addition to these digestive enzymes, pancreatic juice contains large amounts of sodium bicarbonate, which reacts with the hydrochloric acid present in the chyme and produces the neutral or alkaline pH necessary for the pancreatic digestive enzymes to function in an optimal way.

## DUCTS

Three regions of the duct system are described. The cells of all three show close similarities. These regions are, in order, (1) the centroacinar or centroductular cells, (2) the intercalated (intercalary) ductules, and (3) the intralobular to interlobular to main or accessory ducts. The centroacinar cells, which surround the centroacinar lumen, are responsible for the initiation of the alkalinization of the pancreatic juice (as evidenced by the abundant mitochondrial population) and for solubilizing the contents of the zymogen granules during exocytosis. These cells, in addition to most of the excretory duct cells, modify the electrolyte and the bicarbonate content (alkaline pH of 8.4 and in amounts five times that found in plasma) to neutralize the gastric products and correct pH for pancreatic enzyme activity. The transitions from one region of the duct system to the next are gradual, with the epithelium increasing in height from squamous through cuboidal to columnar. By light microscopy, in all regions cytoplasm is pale-staining, and nuclei show little chromatin. Organelles are not prominent. The main features, as shown by electron microscopy, are thin basal lamina, lateral plasma membrane interdigitations with desmosomes and junctional complexes, indented nuclei, and apical microvilli. The interlobular and larger ducts lie in fibroconnective tissue, only fine connective tissue with reticular fibers surrounding intercalated and intralobular ducts. The relation of centroacinar cells and intercalated ducts is illustrated in Figure 11–59.

Although some pancreatic secretion is induced by vagal stimulation, secretion appears to be controlled mainly by two hormones secreted by the duodenal mucosa and triggered by the passage of stomach contents into the duodenum. One, secretin, causes release of abundant, nonenzymatic, bicarbonate-rich fluid, presumably from ductal cells, while the other, cholecystokinin, acts on acinar cells with release of enzyme-rich pancreatic juice and causes the gallbladder to contract. The latter function releases the bile salts that enhance the hydrolytic activity of the pancreatic lipase, with its emulsification of lipids into smaller units. Cholecystokinin is liberated from the enteroendocrine cells of the intestinal crypt by the presence of fatty acids and L-amino acids in the chyme. It also has a trophic effect on the pancreas and increases the secretion of enterokinase. The acid pH of the chyme seems to act as the releasing factor for secretin. The latter also enhances the action of cholecystokinin and inhibits the release of the gastric hydrochloric acid, thus preventing excess acid build-up in the upper small intestine.

### Endocrine Portion

The endocrine portion of the pancreas, the *islets of Langerhans*, is scattered throughout the pancreas as irregular, spheroidal masses of pale-staining cells with a rich vascular supply (Fig. 11–68). They are delineated incompletely from surrounding exocrine tissue by fine reticular fibers, with few fibers within islet tissue. In the islet, cells are arranged in irregular cords, between which are capillaries. No granules are seen in ordinary hematoxylin and eosin (H and E) preparations, since the granules are soluble in alcohol and would be washed out. Special staining methods demonstrate three main cell types called A (*alpha*), B (*beta*) and D (*delta*) *cells*, with a few nongranulated C (*clear*) *cells* (Figs. 11–69 and 11–70). All are irregular, polygonal cells with central, spherical nuclei, small rod-like mitochondria, and a small Golgi apparatus; by electron microscopy, they show differences in respect of their cytoplasmic granules. Within islets, B cells usually are more numerous (comprising about 70 per cent of the islet cell population) and are centrally located, whereas A and D cells are fewer (20 per cent and 5 per cent, respectively) and lie peripherally. It should be pointed out that there is a considerable variation of cell type numbers from islet to islet. However, there is in the pancreas a regional variation in cell content of the islets, those in the head containing fewer B and D cells, and often very few A cells, but numerous cells that produce pancreatic polypeptide (PP). All hormones except insulin (secreted by B cells) are produced also by intestinal cells lying in the gastrointestinal mucosa (enteroendocrine cells). Some invertebrates also show B cells in their digestive tracts.

The *B cell* contains numerous 300-nm granules characterized by a crystalloid core of rhomboid or polygonal shape, the crystalloid probably being insulin, with species differences being recognized by the shape of these crystals. Mitochondria are numerous, small, and spherical. The *A cell* contains secretory vesicles of 250 nm, with an electron-dense core surrounded by less dense material, and the nucleus frequently is of irregular outline. *D cells*, usually located adjacent to A cells, are somewhat larger than A cells and contain secretory vesicles that show a variation in size from 300 to 350 nm, with a homogeneous, granular content of low to medium density. A variant, the $D_1$ *cell*, contains small, 150- to 200-nm homogenous, granular vesicles. Another cell type, more common in islets of the head of the pancreas, is the *PP cell*, identified by small homogeneous, granular vesicles only 140 to 200 nm in diameter. This cell type can be found outside the islets among acinar cells and within the epithelia of pancreatic ducts. *C cells* are pale-staining, generally lack granules, and lie centrally among B cells. Their function is unknown, but they may represent a reserve or resting cell. All endocrine cell types tend to show a polarity with

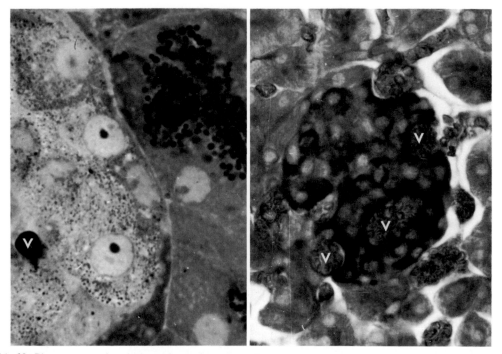

**Figure 11–68.** Photomicrographs of islet of Langerhans. Left: The islet cells contain discrete, dust-like granules (left), much smaller than zymogen granules of acinar cells (right). Right: An islet stained to demonstrate B cells. Note the extreme vascularity of islets (blood capillaries labeled v). Left: × 1000; right, aldehyde fuchsin stain; × 450.

respect to capillaries, the majority of their granules being adjacent to the capillaries. Diseases that affect the thickness of the basal lamina readily inactivate these cells.

Each cell type secretes a different hormone. The B cell produces insulin, which acts on cell membranes (particularly liver and muscle) to facilitate glucose transport into the cell, with a subsequent lowering of the blood sugar level. The B cell actually synthesizes preproinsulin, which is converted to proinsulin by splitting off a 23 amino acid residue from the C terminal backbone, thus allowing it to fold back on itself and connect via disulfide bonds. The proinsulin contains 35 amino acid moieties more than insulin. This 35 amino acid connecting peptide (C peptide) is cleaved off in the Golgi apparatus and immature vesicles, producing insulin and C peptide. The insulin consists of an A chain (21 amino acids) and a B chain (30 amino acids) coupled by two disulfide linkages in the form of a zinc complex. The concentration of insulin within the granule is

caused by reduction of its osmotic activity with the zinc complex, the protein precipitates, resulting in the passive efflux of water from the granule. When insulin is no longer formed in adequate amounts, the disease is called *diabetes mellitus.* This is accompanied by a reduction in the number of B cells. Tumors located in B cells (*insulinoma*) produce more B cells, with a subsequent increase in insulin levels. Insulin release is stimulated by a raised blood sugar level. This seems to be brought about, in part, by the gastroinhibitory polypeptide (*GIP*), which is produced by cells located in the middle zone of the glands of the duodenum and jejunum and by the A cell. Stimulation of insulin is accompanied by inhibition of gastric acid and pepsin secretion. The A cell forms glucagon, its release being stimulated by a low blood sugar level. Glucagon causes glucose release (mainly from the liver) by glycogenolysis, thus raising blood sugar levels. There is evidence that A cells also release other active peptides, including adrenocorticotropic hormone (ACTH) and endor-

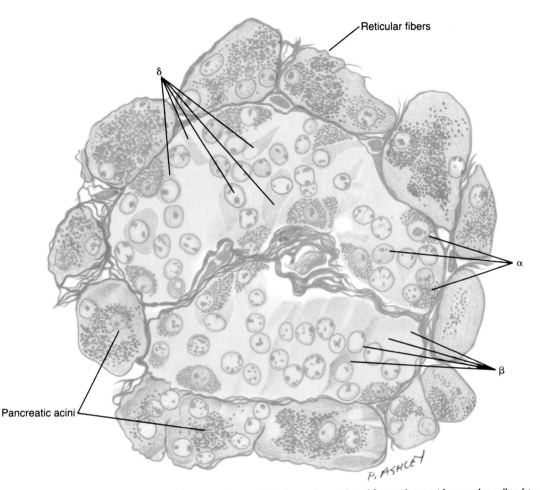

**Figure 11–69.** *Section of human pancreas. The central part of the figure is an islet of Langerhans with granular cells of types alpha, beta, and delta. Mallory-azan stain. × 960. (After Bloom, 1931.) (From Fawcett, D. W.: Bloom and Fawcett: A Textbook of Histology. Philadelphia, W. B. Saunders Co., 1975.)*

phin, or their common precursor. D cells release somatostatin, which may inhibit the secretion of both insulin and glucagon and the pancreatic polypeptide and probably produces its effect in a paracrine manner. The $D_1$ cell secretes vasoactive intestinal peptide (VIP), which, like glucagon, causes lysis of glycogen but which also affects motility and secretory activity of the gut by inhibiting the acid secretion in the stomach. It stimulates secretion of electrolytes and water by the mucosa of the intestine and causes dilation of blood vessels. The pancreatic polypeptide produced by the PP cell stimulates enzyme secretion by the stomach.

### Blood Vessels and Nerves

The pancreas receives a rich arterial supply by branches of the celiac and superior mesenteric arteries, with venous return to the portal system. Major vessels run in interlobular connective tissue, with fine vessels passing into the lobules. From these intralobular vessels, arterioles pass to the islets and break up into an extensive capillary network, this system first supplying the peripherally located A and D cells and then the more centrally placed B cells.

Blood from the islets passes then to supply exocrine tissue. By this arrangement, a large

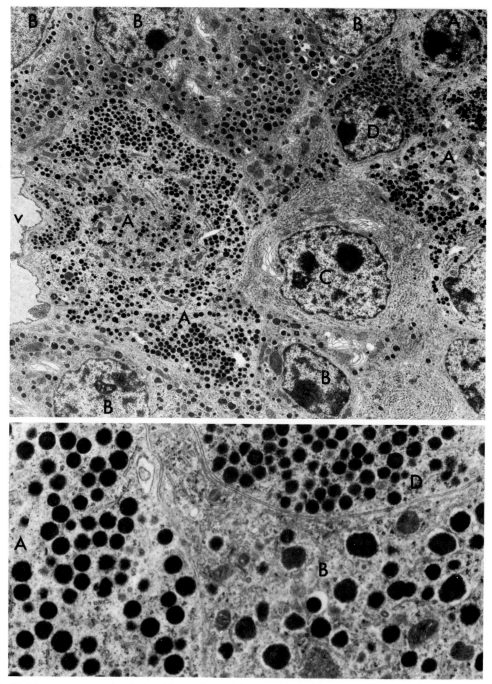

**Figure 11–70.** Electron micrographs of islet of Langerhans of the guinea pig, showing all cell types labeled A, B, C, and D, with their characteristic granules and a capillary blood vessel (v, left, in upper figure). Top, × 3000; bottom, × 28,000.

proportion of the pancreatic blood supply passes first to the islets and permits interaction between islet cells and between the islet cells and acinar tissue. Peptide hormones of the islets do influence acinar function (e.g., insulin increases the flow of pancreatic juice, glucagon stimulates enzyme secretion, and both somatostatin and pancreatic peptide inhibit enzyme secretion).

Autonomic nerve supply to the pancreas is from the celiac ganglion (sympathetic) and the vagus (parasympathetic), with a few ganglion cells present in interlobular connective tissue.

### Development

The pancreas arises from two diverticula, ventral and dorsal, from the junction of foregut and the midgut. The diverticula fuse, the epithelial lining branching to form acini connected to the primary outgrowths by a duct system. Some epithelial buds lose their connection to the duct system and differentiate into islet tissue. However, it has been suggested that some of the islet cell types may arise from cells of the neural crest that migrate into the pancreas early in development. While new islet tissue can regenerate from the proliferation of cells from the duct system, acinar tissue has a very limited regenerative capacity. During development, the duct systems of the two diverticula become interconnected, so that although the dorsal diverticulum forms the bulk of the pancreas, its secretion passes to the ventral outgrowth, the duct of which becomes the main pancreatic duct (of Wirsung). The proximal part of the duct of the dorsal diverticulum remains as the accessory pancreatic duct (of Santorini), which opens into the duodenum at a higher level than the main duct. The latter has a common opening into the duodenum with the common bile duct from the liver.

### THE LIVER

The liver is the heaviest gland in the body, weighing 3 or more pounds (1.5 kg), is of soft consistency, and is situated beneath the diaphragm in the upper abdomen (Fig. 11–71). It is dark red or reddish brown in the fresh condition, the color being caused mainly by a very rich blood supply. It not only receives an arterial supply from the celiac artery but also receives blood from the intestinal tract via the portal vein. Its venous drainage returns to the inferior vena cava, and thus it lies interposed along the venous drainage of the intestinal tract. It receives all the material absorbed from the intestinal tract with the exception of lipid, most of which is transported in the lymphatic system. In addition to the digested and absorbed material that is assimilated and stored in the liver, the portal blood also carries to the liver various toxic materials, which then are detoxicated in, or excreted by, the liver. Bile from the liver drains via a duct system into the duodenum and is partly a secretion, in that it contains bile salts that are important in digestion, and partly an excretion, in that it contains waste and even harmful materials for ultimate evacuation in the feces. The portal vein and hepatic artery enter, and the hepatic (bile) ducts leave, the liver at a region called the *porta hepatis*, a transverse fissure on the inferior surface. The remainder of the liver is covered by a fibroconnective tissue capsule (of Glisson) from which thin connective tissue septa enter the substance of the liver at the porta hepatis to divide it into lobes and lobules. In some animals (e.g., the pig), the content of connective tissue is much greater than it is in the human. Over a large area, the capsule is covered by peritoneum, although there is an area (the "bare area") in direct contact with the diaphragm and viscera of the posterior abdominal wall.

### General Histological Plan

In a section examined under low power, the liver is seen to be composed of masses of epithelial, parenchymal cells (hepatocytes) arranged in anastomosing and branching plates that form a three-dimensional lattice. Between plates are sinusoidal blood spaces. In this respect, the liver has the structure of an endocrine gland. Also present are areas termed the *portal areas*, or *portal canals*, each comprising branches of the portal vein, hepatic artery, and bile duct, often also with a lymphatic vessel, lying in a small amount of connective tissue. The portal areas are so arranged as to delineate lobules of liver tissue. Such a lobule, the *classic,* or *hepatic, lobule,* has several portal canals at its periphery, and in its center is a central vein, a tributary of the inferior vena cava, from which plates of parenchymal cells

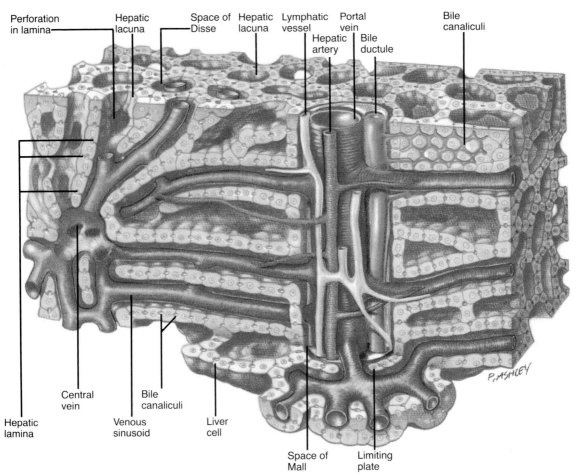

**Figure 11–71.** *Diagram of hepatic structure. (After Prof. H. Elias.) (Courtesy of Dr. D. W. Fawcett; reproduced from Gray's Anatomy. 35th ed. Edinburgh, Churchill Livingstone, 1973.)*

radiate like the spokes of a wheel from a central hub (Fig. 11–72). This unit of structure is repeated thousands of times. With the afferent vessels (portal vein and hepatic artery) at the periphery of the lobule and the efferent vessels (the central vein) at the center of the lobule, it is obvious that blood flow is from the periphery through the sinusoidal channels between plates of liver cells to the central vein (Fig. 11–73). Bile secretion, on the other hand, is from the liver cells to the small bile ducts at the periphery. Closer examination of a section at higher magnification reveals that each cord or plate of liver cells is composed of one to two rows of liver cells, between which are tiny channels, the bile canaliculi, that drain peripherally in a lobule to bile ducts (Fig. 11–74).

These bile canaliculi are simply spaces between adjacent liver cells and have no other lining epithelium. The sinusoidal spaces between liver plates are lined by reticuloendothelial cells, cells lying in a meshwork of fine reticular fibers. Thus, cells in a liver lobule are either parenchymal (hepatic) cells, cells associated with the walls of hepatic sinusoids, or blood cells in the lumina of sinusoids.

## Lobulation

The *classic,* or *hepatic, lobule* has just been outlined. It is a polygonal prism measuring about 1 to 2 mm and usually appears hexagonal in

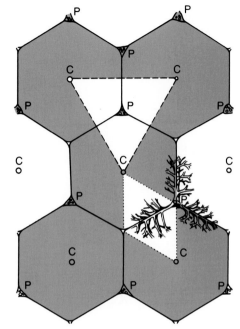

**Figure 11–72.** Diagram of hepatic lobules. The classic hepatic lobule is outlined with solid lines, the portal lobule with an interrupted line, and the liver acinus, or functional unit, with a dotted line. The branches of a portal vein and a hepatic artery (solid) from one portal area are shown at lower right. Portal areas are labeled "P," central veins "C." × 40.

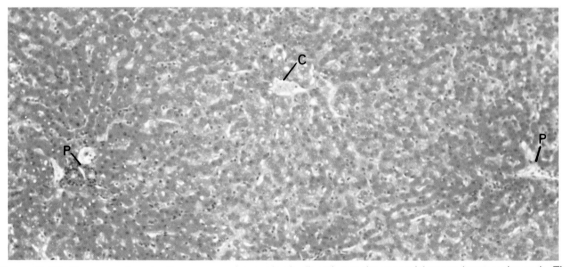

**Figure 11–73.** Liver parenchymal cells are arranged as cords of cells with vascular sinusoidal spaces between the cords. The cords radiate from central veins (C)—tributaries of the hepatic veins—and these are the centers of classic hepatic lobules. Lobules are polygonal prisms, and at their peripheries are portal canals (P), these composed of branches of the portal vein, hepatic artery, bile duct, and lymphatics. Lobules are not delineated by connective tissue. In a lobule, blood enters the periphery from portal vein and hepatic artery radicles and passes radially in the sinusoidal channels between cords of parenchymal cells to the central vein, and then to hepatic veins and the inferior vena cava. H and E. Low power.

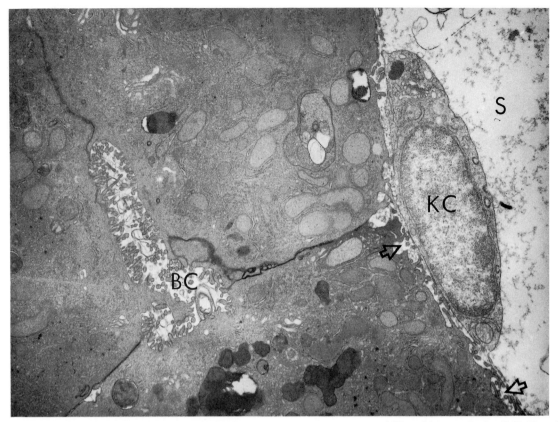

**Figure 11–74.** *Electron micrograph of several hepatocytes disposed between a sinusoid (S) and bile canaliculus (BC). Note the presence of a Kupffer's cell (KC) and perisinusoidal space of Disse (arrows). × 7900. (Courtesy of Dr. H. N. Tung.)*

cross section, with a central vein at its center and portal canals peripherally at the corners. It is not delineated by connective tissue in humans, although it is in some mammals (e.g., pigs). Rarely in humans are portal canals found at each of the six corners of the hexagon. It is obvious that such a lobule does not correspond to, for example, a lobule of an exocrine gland, in which a lobule is the collection of tissue that drains into a duct or is clearly demarcated by fibrous tissue. However, the classic liver lobule is of some functional significance in that it is a unit of structure from which the blood supply drains to a lobule (central) vein. Because its morphological determination is made by its vascular supply, it will be obvious to the student that the peripheral parts of a lobule (i.e., those nearest the portal vein and hepatic artery)

will be best supplied with food materials and oxygen. The central area will not be as well supplied. The hepatic lobule is one of three concepts of liver lobulation that emphasize the endocrine function of the liver and is a useful tool to better understand the structural changes that accompany a centrolobular necrosis occurring in, for example, carbon tetrachloride poisoning.

Other criteria have been used for demarcating functional units in the liver. A *portal lobule* has at its center a portal canal and consists of the tissue draining bile into the bile duct of that portal area. Such a unit is triangular in cross section, contains parts of three adjacent classic lobules, has a central vein peripherally at each corner, and brings the histological organization of the hepatic lobule more in line with most exocrine glands

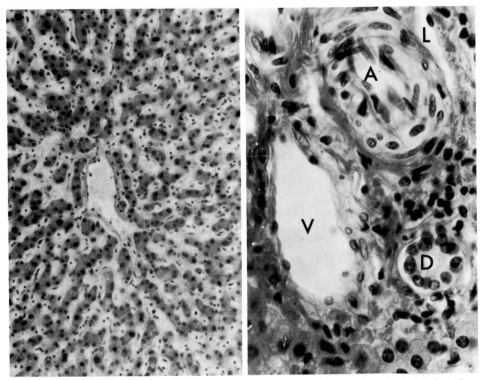

**Figure 11–75.** *Photomicrographs of the human liver showing (left) the central area of a classic lobule with a central vein (× 250) and (right) the portal area with a branch of the hepatic artery (A), a branch of the portal vein (V), a small bile duct (D), and a lymphatic vessel (L). × 750.*

(Fig. 11–75). Pathologically, however, liver damage usually is related to blood supply, and a smaller unit of liver structure now is recognized on this basis. This is the *liver acinus*, or the *functional unit*. As just explained, it is rare to find a portal canal at each corner of the classic lobule. Such deficient areas are supplied by branches from an adjacent area that leave parent vessels, at a right angle, and course along the border between adjacent classic lobules. The vessels supply and the bile ductule drains an area of diamond shape in cross section, with two central veins at two opposite corners and the portal canal branches coursing transversely between them. The liver acinus directly correlates blood supply with metabolic activity, sets up a zonation of gradient activity, and helps to explain a particular pattern in the regeneration process.

### Parenchyma (Hepatic Cells)

The parenchymal, or hepatic, cells (hepatocytes) are arranged in a series of branching and anastomosing perforated plates, or laminae, to form a spongework or labyrinth, between which are the sinusoidal spaces (Fig. 11–76). These plates extend from the periphery of the classic lobule to the central vein at its center in a radial fashion. Except at the sites of anastomosis and branching, the plates usually are only one cell thick, although obviously any single parenchymal cell is bordered by several others within a plate. Around portal areas, the liver cells are arranged as a sheet, one cell thick, lying against the periportal connective tissue and termed the *limiting plate*. The limiting plate is composed of cells somewhat smaller than hepatic cells in the center

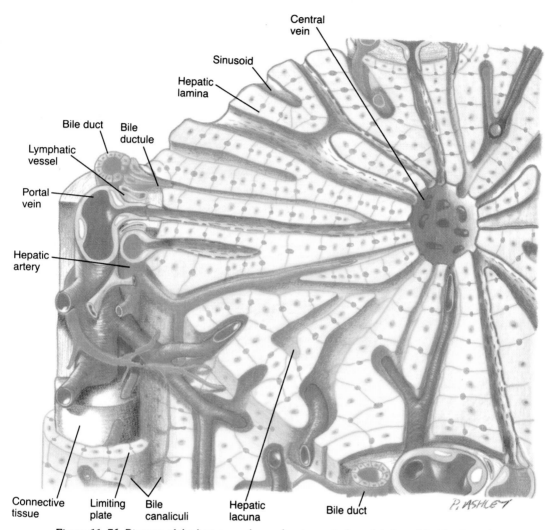

*Figure 11–76. Diagram of the liver parenchyma showing part of one lobule and its blood supply.*

of the lobule and is perforated by blood vessels (branches of the hepatic artery and the portal vein) and by branches of the bile ducts.

Hepatic cells are polygonal, with six or more surfaces, and are usually 20 to 35 μm in diameter, with a clearly defined cell membrane (Figs. 11–77 and 11–78). These cells make up about 80 per cent of the cell population in the liver. The surfaces are either external and related to a sinusoidal space, closely applied to the surface of an adjacent liver cell, or partially separated from

an adjacent cell to form a bile canaliculus (Fig. 11–79). Nuclei are spherical or ovoid, with a regular surface, and show considerable variation in size from cell to cell, a variation associated with the condition of polyploidy. Occasionally, binucleate cells are present (Fig. 11–80). Each nucleus is vesicular in type, with prominent, scattered chromatin granules and one or more nucleoli, and stains less intensely than nuclei of other cells in the liver. Mitosis is rare in adult liver cells (1 mitosis per 15,000 cells), but numerous mitotic

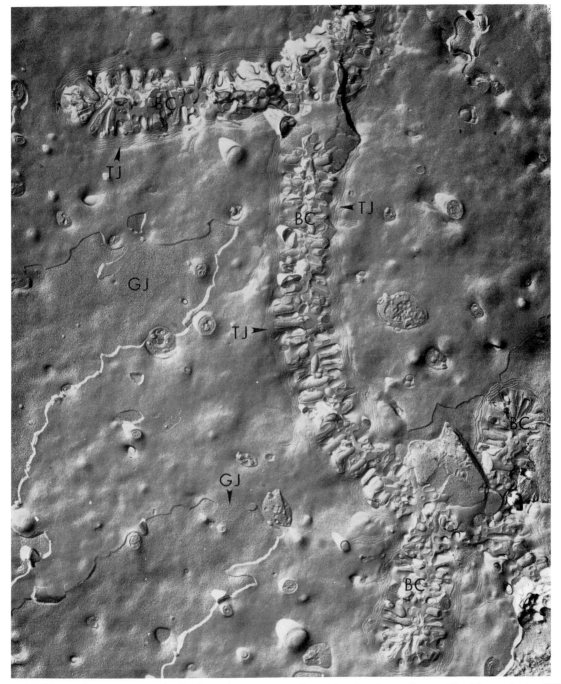

**Figure 11–77.** An electron micrograph of a freeze-fracture preparation of hepatocyte membranes. The bile canaliculus (BC), tight junction (TJ), and gap junction (GJ) are depicted. × 19,000. (Courtesy of H. N. Tung and R. Roberts.)

figures can be found during repair following injury.

The cytoplasm of hepatic cells shows considerable variation dependent upon functional activity, particularly in glycogen and fat storage. Both of these substances usually are removed during routine section preparation but are indicated by a lace-like appearance with spaces of irregular outline and by spherical vacuoles, respectively. Present in all cells are clumps of basophil material, usually of such an extent as to give the cytoplasm a slightly basophil reaction. However, after a prolonged fast, there is a decrease in the basophilic ribonucleoprotein and an increase in cytoplasmic eosinophilia. The latter is due to the presence of large numbers of mitochondria and,

to a lesser extent, to the smooth endoplasmic reticulum. Mitochondria are small but numerous throughout the cytoplasm, and the Golgi apparatus usually is demonstrable, situated either near the nucleus or peripheral and adjacent to a bile canaliculus.

Although all parenchymal cells show a similar structure, there are distinct variations in different regions and at different times in relation to feeding. This is dependent upon blood supply. The peripheral cells in a lobule have a good blood supply, but those near the central vein are farthest removed from their blood supply. After feeding, glycogen is deposited first in the peripheral zone. Only after a very heavy carbohydrate meal do the central cells show evidence of glycogen stor-

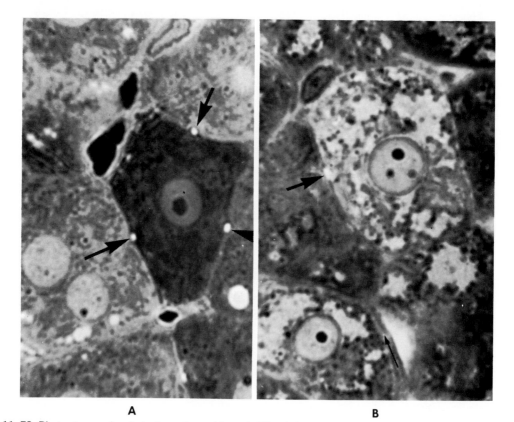

**A**　　　　　　　　　　　　　　　　　**B**

*Figure 11–78.* Photomicrographs of plastic sections of liver. A, The dark parenchymal cell at center right shows five surfaces, two short ones adjacent to sinusoids containing red blood corpuscles, and three longer sides adjacent to surrounding parenchymal cells. On each of these three interfaces is a bile canaliculus (arrows). Note also the binucleate cell (bottom left). × 1500. B, The central parenchymal cell here shows extensive unstained areas of glycogen and one bile canaliculus (broad arrow). At bottom center, the perisinusoidal space between a parenchymal cell and a sinusoid lining is visible (narrow arrow). × 1500.

Illustration continued on opposite page

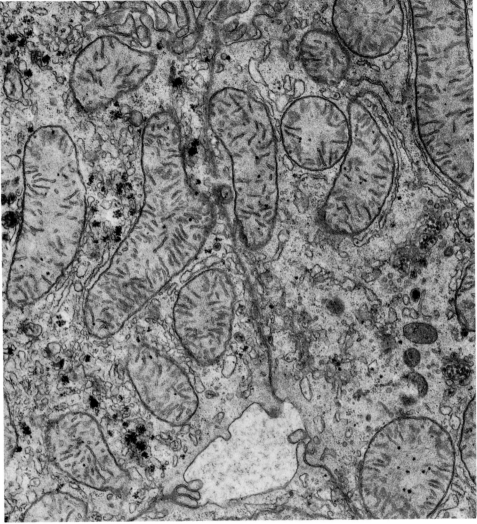

C

**Figure 11–78** Continued C, *Electron micrograph of a bile canaliculus (bottom) between three parenchymal hepatic cells. Microvilli at top center are in the space of Disse.* × *28,000. (Courtesy of J. Steiner and A.-M. Jezequel.)*

age (Fig. 11–81). Similarly, when glycogen is removed to increase a falling blood sugar level, glycogen first is removed from the central cells. Under certain conditions, fat too is deposited in parenchymal cells, and it always appears first in cells adjacent to central veins of lobules. The latter observation can be correlated to the significantly higher surface area of the smooth endoplasmic reticulum in the central cells as compared with the peripheral cells of the hepatic lobule. These variations between cells in a lobule are not restricted to inclusions, for mitochondria show distinct morphological changes associated with glycogen storage, being small and spherical in peripheral cells and more slender and elongated in central cells.

### Fine Structure

Hepatocytes show no special nuclear features, although, as already noted, there is marked vari-

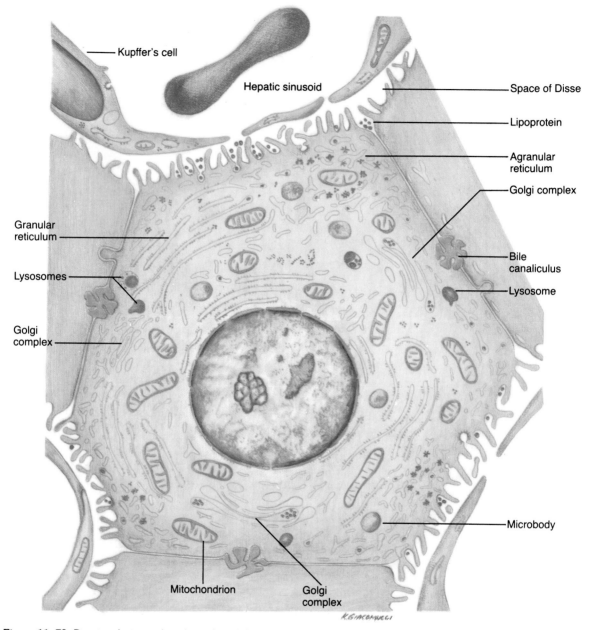

**Figure 11–79.** *Drawing depicting the relationship of the liver cells to each other and to the sinusoids and showing the principal components of the hepatic cell as seen in electron micrographs. (Drawing by Sylvia Colard Keene.) (From Fawcett, D. W.: Bloom and Fawcett: A Textbook of Histology, 11th ed. Philadelphia, W. B. Saunders Co., 1986.)*

ation in size, this being an expression of polyploidy, with up to 25 per cent of cells being binucleate. These binuclear cells arise from mononuclear cells through endomitosis when nuclear volume and DNA content have approximately doubled. With age, the cell size and incidence of polyploidy appear to increase. Gap junctions are frequently observed between hepatocytes. Both

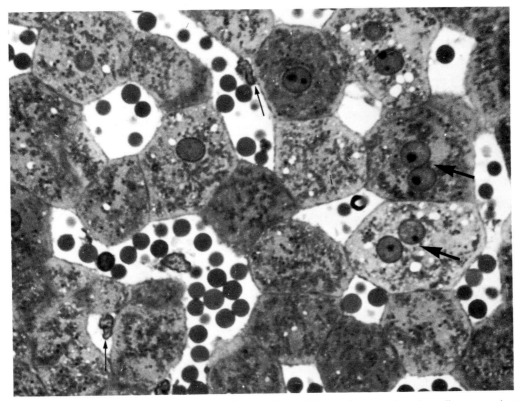

**Figure 11–80.** Photomicrograph of liver parenchyma showing plates of liver cells, some binucleate (large arrow), and with numerous mitochondria (dark dots) and some lipid vacuoles. Between them are sinusoids containing erythrocytes and lined by reticuloendothelium (small arrows). × 600.

granular and agranular endoplasmic reticula are prominent in the cytoplasm, with regions of continuity between the two types. Granular reticulum usually occurs as groups of 3 to 15 parallel cisternae, the ends of which tend to expand. In addition to ribosomes attached to these membranes, polysomes are present, both free and associated with the membranes. The smooth reticulum appears as a meshwork of branching and anastomosing tubules, often continuous with granular reticulum, and may contain globules, 30 to 40 nm in diameter, composed of low-density serum lipoprotein. The granular endoplasmic reticulum synthesizes the protein component of plasma lipoproteins, while the smooth endoplasmic reticulum produces the triglycerides and cholesterol. Plasma lipoproteins and plasma proteins (albumin, alpha and beta globulins, prothrombin) both pass to the prominent Golgi ap-

paratus, where they are packaged into secretory granules. The Golgi apparatus is usually multiple and located near the nucleus and adjacent to bile canaliculi, each formed by a few closely packed lamellae (Fig. 11–82). Near bile canaliculi and Golgi apparatus are membrane-limited, dense peribiliary bodies, about 0.2 to 0.5 µm in diameter, containing acid hydrolases. Peroxisomes, or microbodies, occur in the same area. These are spherical, 0.2 to 0.8 µm in diameter, and membrane-bound; in many species (but not humans), they contain a crystalline structure containing uricase and enzymes concerned with the oxidation of fatty acids. Lysosomes, which also are present, vary in appearance and may contain lipofuscin. These organelles may contain ferritin-like substances, which may be stored in large amounts in iron-storage diseases. Mitochondria are numerous and usually filamentous in form.

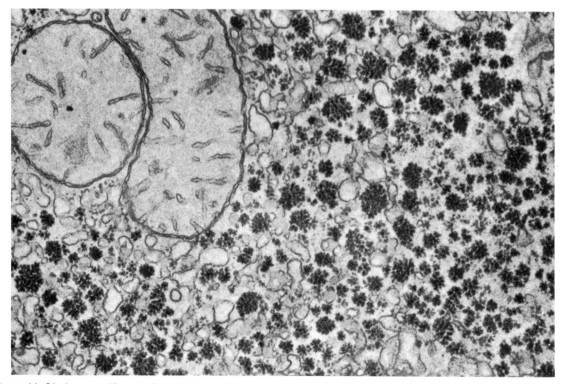

*Figure 11–81.* An area of hamster hepatocyte cytoplasm containing a high concentration of glycogen in aggregations of varying electron-dense sizes (alpha particles). The glycogen is closely associated with profiles of the agranular endoplasmic reticulum. (From Fawcett, D. W.: Bloom and Fawcett: A Textbook of Histology, 11th ed. Philadelphia, W. B. Saunders Co., 1986.)

Associated with smooth reticulum are glycogen particles, usually in aggregates or rosettes (alpha particles) up to 0.1 μm in diameter, composed of individual beta particles 20 to 30 nm in diameter. The enzyme glucose-6-phosphatase is located in the cisternal membranes of the smooth endoplasmic reticulum. This enzyme converts glucose-6-phosphate into free glucose. Lipid may be present as osmiophilic, spherical droplets of varying size. Fat metabolism and the turnover of sex hormones are other important functions associated with the smooth endoplasmic reticulum.

The plasma membrane of the hepatocyte, about 7.5 nm thick, shows specializations in certain regions. Adjacent to a sinusoidal blood space, the hepatocyte is separated from the wall of the vascular channel by a narrow *perisinusoidal space* (the space of *Disse*), and here the plasmalemma shows numerous long microvilli with vacuoles and vesicles in subjacent cytoplasm (Figs. 11–83 and 11–84). This provides a large surface area for absorption and secretion. In some regions, where connective tissue fibers are present in the perisinusoidal space, microvilli are lacking. Plasmalemmae of adjacent hepatocytes at an interface show some irregularity, with occasional spot desmosomes. At the so-called biliary pole, the two membranes of an interface separate to form an intercellular canal, the bile canaliculus, usually 1 to 2 μm across. Microvilli protrude from plasma membranes into the lumen of the canaliculus, and at each lateral border the interface usually is reinforced by a desmosome.

### Bile Canaliculi

Bile canaliculi can be seen occasionally in routine H and E preparations as tiny cavities between adjacent hepatic cells, but they can be better

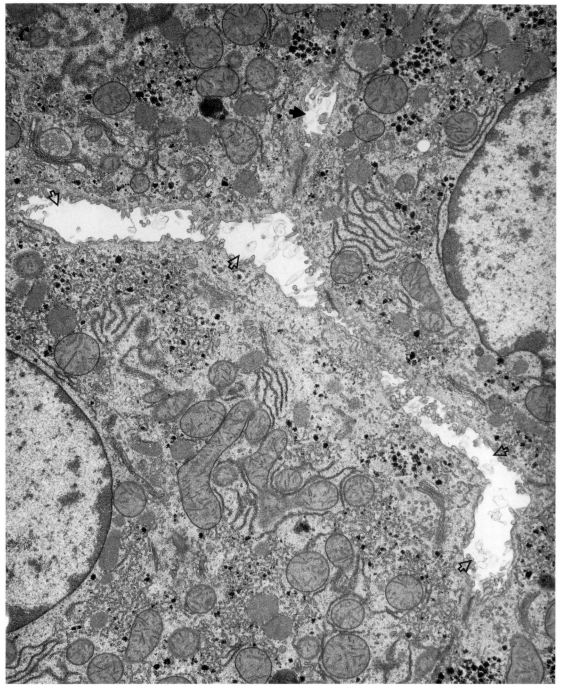

*Figure 11–82.* An electron micrograph of several hepatocytes showing multiple Golgi complexes adjacent to the bile canaliculi (arrows). × 14,400. (Courtesy of Dr. H. N. Tung.)

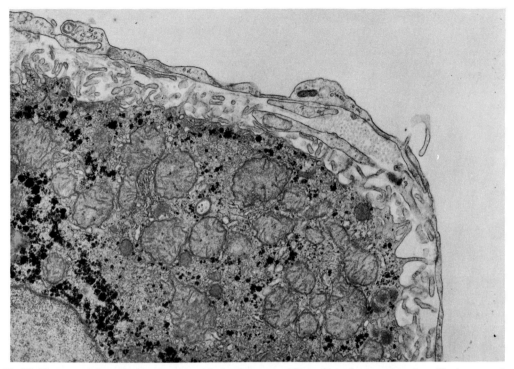

**Figure 11–83.** *Electron micrograph showing the perisinusoidal space of Disse. Note the irregular microvilli of a parenchymal cell protruding into the space that separates the parenchymal cell from reticuloendothelium lining sinusoids. There are a few collagen fibrils in the space. × 15,000. (Courtesy of J. Steiner and A.-M. Jezequel.)*

demonstrated by special staining methods (e.g., Gomori's reaction for alkaline phosphatase or silver impregnation). They form a three-dimensional network between liver cells, the walls of the canaliculi being adjacent parenchymal cells, as just described (Fig. 11–85). The junctions of bile canaliculi with bile ducts at the periphery of a lobule are not demonstrated easily. The junctions occur by means of an intermediate structure called the *ductule*, or *canal, of Hering*. At the periphery of a lobule, the parenchymal cells that form the wall of the bile canaliculus are replaced gradually by smaller, lighter-staining cells with dark nuclei and poorly developed organelles. These cells, the ductule cells, are underlain by a distinct basal lamina and represent the terminal interlobular ramifications of the bile duct system. These terminal bile ducts run along the lateral sides of the classic lobule along with the terminal branches of the hepatic artery and portal vein within an interlobular connective tissue cover. Blockage of the bile duct system may lead to an

intensive growth of these duct cells. The lumen of such a ductule eventually joins that of a bile duct in a portal area. The bile ducts are lined with a cuboidal or columnar epithelium and are surrounded with a well-developed connective tissue sheath. These ducts join at the porta hepatis to form right and left hepatic ducts that eventually leave the porta hepatis of the liver to form the common bile duct.

### Blood Channels within the Lobule

These blood channels consist of the sinusoidal spaces, central veins, and portal canals (Fig. 11–86).

**Sinusoidal Spaces.** As previously explained, the blood supply of the liver lobule is via the sinusoids, which form a very extensive spongework between the plates of hepatic cells. Blood enters the sinusoidal meshwork at the periphery of the lobule from interlobular branches of portal

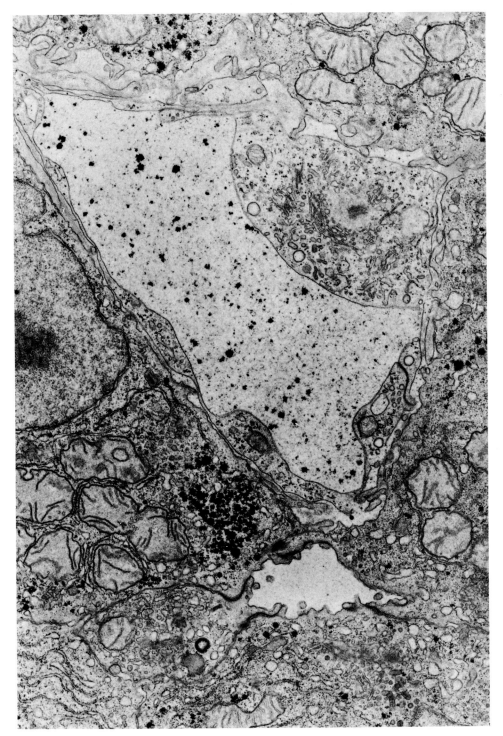

**Figure 11–84.** Electron micrograph of a hepatic sinusoid completely lined by parts of two sinus-lining cells. A narrow space (of Disse) separates it from surrounding parenchymal cells, between which a bile canaliculus is shown below the sinusoid. The small, very dense particles are glycogen, some of which are present also in the lumen of the sinusoid. × 17,000. (Courtesy of J. Steiner and A.-M. Jezequel.)

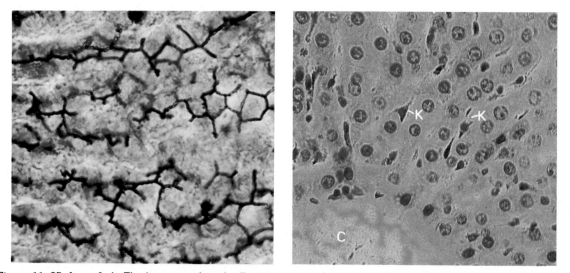

**Figure 11–85.** *Liver.* Left: *The liver parenchymal cells stain green and are arranged in cords with clear spaces of sinusoidal channels between. Bile canaliculi are seen as fine tubular channels arranged in a three-dimensional network, between the parenchymal cells. Their walls are formed by adjacent parenchymal cells, that is, they are simply spaces between cells and have no intrinsic cellular lining of their own. Drainage of bile in a classic lobule is from the center to the periphery. Injected specimen. Oil immersion.* Right: *Before death, an animal was injected with lithium carmine, a particulate, red dye. Here, part of a central vein (C) is seen with radiating cords of liver cells and sinusoidal spaces between them. Associated with liver sinusoids are endothelial-type cells and phagocytic (stellate) cells of Küpffer (K). The latter have picked up the dye material. Clearly, they are stellate in shape, with thin cytoplasmic arms, and lie in relation to sinusoidal spaces. Lithium carmine, toluidine blue. High power.*

vein and hepatic artery and passes in a radial fashion through sinusoidal spaces to drain from the lobule by the central vein.

Sinusoidal spaces differ from capillaries in that they are of greater diameter (9 to 12 μm) and their lining cells are not typically of endothelium. The basal lamina around sinusoids is incomplete. Two main types of cell, with intermediate forms, are present in the sinusoidal lining of the adult liver.

1. *"Endothelial" Type*—This cell has a small, elongated darkly staining nucleus and greatly attenuated cytoplasm. The cytoplasm may interdigitate with, or even overlie, cytoplasmic processes of adjacent cells of the same or other types. Organelles are few and small, although numerous micropinocytotic vesicles are present. The endothelial lining of the sinusoids appears to be incomplete, with gaps between adjacent cells producing intercellular clefts of up to 0.5 μm in diameter and fenestrations in the attenuated cytoplasm of up to 0.2 μm in diameter. These fenestrations occur in groups, producing areas that are sieve-

like. The fenestrae are larger than those found in type II endothelium of capillaries (about 100 nm in diameter) and are not closed by a diaphragm.

2. *Phagocytic (Stellate) Cell of Kupffer*—This cell has a larger, paler nucleus and more extensive cytoplasm with processes that may extend into or even across a sinusoidal space. The cells lie adjacent to the endothelial cells without the formation of junctional complexes and arise (like other macrophages) from bone marrow. The cells are actively phagocytic and frequently contain engulfed and degenerating erythrocytes, pigment granules, and iron-containing granules (Fig. 11–87). This property of phagocytosis can be demonstrated by intravital injections of dyes such as trypan blue and particulate matter (e.g., India ink).

Although not all sinusoid lining cells are phagocytic, in time of need the stellate cells of Kupffer are increased in number, perhaps by differentiation of the more primitive endothelial cells.

At the terminations of sinusoids into a central vein or a larger sublobular tributary of a hepatic

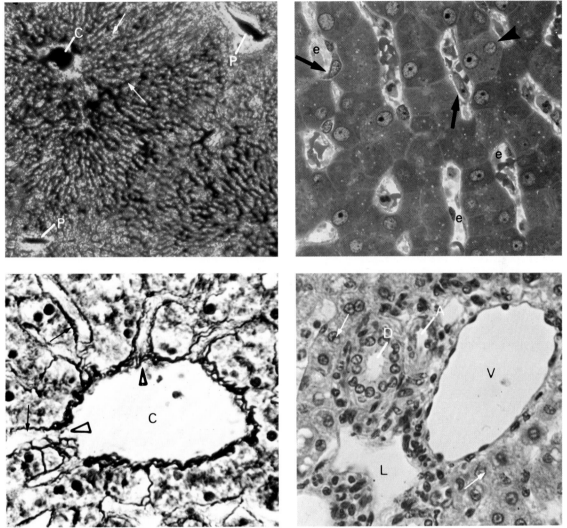

**Figure 11–86.** *Liver.* Top left: *This technique demonstrates blood vessels and sinusoidal spaces (black). Most of the field is occupied by part of one lobule. At its center is a central vein (C) with portal canals (P) at its periphery. Note the radial arrangement of the sinusoidal spaces (arrows) draining to the central vein. Parenchymal cells are arranged as cords or plates between the sinusoidal spaces. Kull's method. Low power.* Top right: *Liver parenchymal cells are arranged in anastomosing plates and cords. Their nuclei are vesicular, often with prominent nucleoli, and polyploidal or binucleate cells (arrowhead) are common. The cytoplasm is basophil and here shows several small, clear, spherical spaces that represent lipid as a cytoplasmic inclusion. Between the plates of parenchymal cells are blood sinusoids containing red and white blood corpuscles lined by cells of the endothelial (e) or phagocytic (Kupffer) types. The latter cannot be recognized with certainty in this preparation, but probable phagocytic cells are arrowed. Between each arrowed cell and the adjacent parenchymal cell is a slender space, the perisinusoidal space of Disse (also visible in other areas). Plastic section. Methylene blue, azure A, basic fuchsin. High power.* Bottom left: *This stain demonstrates reticular fibers (black). Parenchymal cells stain brown with black nuclei and are arranged in cords radiating from a central vein (C). Note that reticular fibers are found in the wall of the central vein and in the walls of liver sinusoids (arrows), the sinusoids draining into the central vein (arrowheads). Silver stain. High power.* Bottom right: *Portal areas, or canals, are surrounded by small amounts of connective tissue and contain the "portal triad" of hepatic artery (A), portal vein (V), and bile duct (D), usually with a lymphatic vessel (L). The bile duct is lined by simple cuboidal epithelium; the branch of the hepatic artery is an arteriole lined by endothelium and with a single layer of smooth muscle in its wall; and the branch of the portal vein is a large venule. Parenchymal cells lie as a plate around the portal area, this being called the limiting plate (arrows), and as radiating cords in adjacent liver lobules. H and E. High power.*

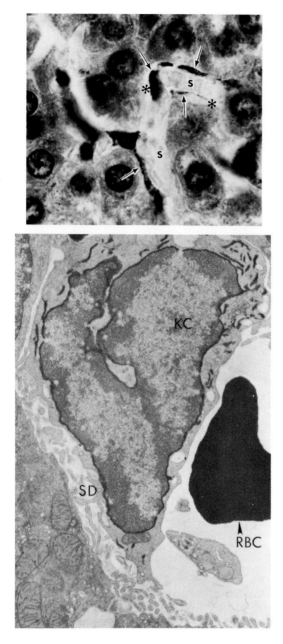

**Figure 11–87.** Top: *Photomicrograph of rat liver demonstrates phagocytosis by the cells of Kupffer after intravital injection of dye. Dye particles lie in the cytoplasm of Kupffer's cells (arrows) and partially outline a sinusoid (s). Note the space of Disse (asterisks). Medium power. Bottom: Electron micrograph of a Kupffer's cell (KC) showing a positive reaction for peroxidase in the nuclear envelope and cisternae of the endoplasmic reticulum. This reaction serves to distinguish Kupffer's cells from endothelial cells. The perisinusoidal space of Disse (SD) and an erythrocyte (RBC) also are indicated. (Courtesy of Dr. D. J. Fahimi, from The Journal of Cell Biology 47:247, 1970, and reproduced with the permission of The Rockefeller University Press.)*

vein, there is some evidence for a contractile, sphincteric mechanism that controls blood flow through the lobules.

One question concerning sinusoids is whether or not the lining is discontinuous. Discontinuities in the sinusoidal lining have been demonstrated by the electron microscope, using a variety of preparative techniques, and particulate material of small diameter (following injection into the portal vein) rapidly passes into the perisinusoidal space. As just noted, the basal lamina around sinusoids is incomplete, and thus there is no morphological barrier between sinusoids and the perisinusoidal space. There is direct access of plasma to the surface of the liver cell, a structural feature of great functional importance for active metabolic exchange between the liver and the blood. The perisinusoidal space itself is not a true lymph channel, for it is not lined by endothelium and is to be regarded as an interstitial space containing some formed reticular and collagenous fibers but in which fluid may circulate freely. It probably plays an important role in lymph production. Also contained in the perisinusoidal space are a few mesenchymal cells referred to as "pericytes," "fat-storing cells," lipocytes, or "extravascular reticular cells." In the adult liver, this cell is closely associated with reticular and collagenous fibers, probably being responsible for their formation, and possibly is involved in vitamin A turnover, since it can sequester exogenously administered retinyl esters in its lipid droplets. In fetal liver, this primitive mesenchymal cell probably is the stem cell for hemopoiesis. It differs from the two types of sinusoid lining cells not only in location but also in that it does not become phagocytic toward particulate material.

**Central Veins.** These are centrally located in lobules and are the smallest radicles of the hepatic veins. They drain into larger sublobular veins that, in turn, join to form collecting veins, which themselves are tributaries of hepatic veins. The last, drain directly into the inferior vena cava. Sinusoids normally drain into central veins, although a few probably open directly into sublobular veins.

**Portal Veins (Portal Areas).** These are surrounded by small amounts of fibroconnective tissue and contain the "portal triad" of hepatic artery, portal vein, and bile duct, usually with a lymphatic vessel. The largest structure usually is the branch of the portal vein and is thin-walled; the smallest is the artery or arteriole, a branch of the hepatic artery; and the bile duct is intermediate in size and is recognized by its lining of cubical epithelial cells. In that a portal area is a region of branching, multiples of the triad are commonly seen. Lymphatic vessels appear as slit-like spaces lined by endothelium. All components of a portal canal increase in size and are sur-

rounded by stronger fibroconnective tissue nearer the hilum. The larger bile ducts are lined by a columnar epithelium.

In small portal areas, the portal vein gives off smaller venules with lateral branches lying between lobules. From these arise the terminal twigs, which penetrate the limiting plate of hepatic cells and open directly into sinusoids. The terminal branchings of the hepatic artery are similar, although some are said to penetrate deeply into a lobule before opening into a sinusoid. Direct communications between terminal branches of hepatic artery and portal vein also are said to exist, but probably they are few in number and involve connecting interlobular vessels and connecting perilobular vessels (terminal portal venules and terminal hepatic arterioles).

The lymphatic drainage of the liver via the large vessels in the porta hepatis is profuse. The fine lymphatic channels in small portal areas appear to commence blindly in the connective tissue, and no direct communication with the perisinusoidal spaces has been established. However, the fluid of these spaces is discharged into interstitial spaces of the connective tissue to the periportal tissue *space of Mall*, which lies between the portal connective tissue and the limiting plate, and thus passes indirectly into the lymphatic capillaries. Presumably, flow in the perisinusoidal spaces is toward the periphery of the lobule, but this must be exceedingly sluggish and perhaps intermittent consequent upon variations in blood pressure in the sinusoidal spaces.

A few fine unmyelinated nerve fibers of the autonomic nervous system accompany the portal canals. Sympathetic (postganglionic fibers) come from the celiac ganglion, while parasympathetic (preganglionic fibers) emerge from the vagus nerve. Both innervate the arterial musculature within the portal triad. In addition, parasympathetic fibers enter the liver lobule to form plexuses near liver cells and sinusoids.

### Stroma

Connective tissue of the liver, a large organ, is sparse. Over the liver surface, covered in most areas by the mesothelium of the peritoneum, is the relatively dense fibroconnective tissue of Glisson's capsule, which at the porta hepatis is continuous with that around the portal canals. By this means, the entire organ is permeated by a fibroconnective tissue skeleton composed of collagenous fibers with relatively few cells, the majority of which are fibroblasts. Within the lobule, there is a fine meshwork of reticular and collagenous fibers around the sinusoids and within the perisinusoidal spaces, but only a few fibroblasts within the perisinusoidal space of Disse. The fibers here are elaborated and maintained by the sinus-lining cells and the pericytes of the perisinusoidal spaces. In particular, the fat cell within the perisinusoidal space, as in other tissues, may be transformed into fibroblasts and therefore may be the stem cell for the perisinusoidal fibroblast. The reticular network not only supports the liver parenchyma but also may aid in keeping the sinusoids open. Their retention following an injury ensures that the healing process proceeds in a rapid, orderly manner. This fine meshwork is continuous at the periphery of the lobule with the connective tissues surrounding the terminal branches of the components of the portal canals, whose size depends on their position in the connective tissue stroma. An excess in the amount of this supporting network is a good histological predictor of chronic liver diseases such as *hepatic fibrosis*. If this condition is allowed to continue, the excess connective tissue replaces the functional hepatocytes.

### Regeneration

After injury the liver shows quite a remarkable degree of regeneration. The organization of the repair process depends upon the nature of the injury, but remaining hepatic cells are capable of both hypertrophy and hyperplasia. Bile ducts also actively proliferate, and it is possible that new hepatic cells may arise from this source also. The cells in the liver probably synthesize a chemical messenger (termed a *chalone*) that regulates the mitotic activity by a negative-feedback mechanism, so that loss of tissue is balanced by regeneration of tissue. When liver tissue is removed or injured, the amount of chalone goes down, so that a marked increase in mitotic activity occurs. The completion of the regeneration process brings about an increase in chalones and a return to a normally low turnover rate.

### Functions

The liver is essential to life, and because of its unique position interposed in the venous drainage of the digestive tract, it is susceptible to damage from absorbed toxic materials. It subserves several functions. It is important in the maintenance of blood glucose concentration. Parenchymal cells take up blood glucose and store it as glycogen. Glycogen also is formed from other compounds such as lactic and pyruvic acids. Stored particles of glycogen are frequently seen near the smooth endoplasmic reticulum, which is distributed diffusely throughout the liver cell cytoplasm. This organelle houses the enzyme glucose-6-phosphatase, which converts glucose-6-phosphate to free glucose that can readily diffuse out of the liver cell and into the sinusoids. The liver also is important in lipid metabolism in that lipid is transported in the blood as lipoprotein, this substance being formed in the liver. The protein is made in the granular endoplasmic reticulum, and the lipid component is synthesized by the well-developed smooth endoplasmic reticulum. This lipoprotein, along with the plasma proteins (see later), are transported in secretory vesicles packaged by the Golgi apparatus for discharge into the sinusoids. It stores also vitamins A and B and heparin (originating in mast cells) and secretes bile salts into the biliary system and fibrinogen (an antianemic factor) and plasma albumins into the blood. Also, the liver synthesizes cholesterol, excretes bile pigments from the breakdown of hemoglobin of damaged erythrocytes, and produces urea (a by-product of protein metabolism). Detoxification of various toxic materials circulating in the blood, phagocytosis of particulate material by the cells of Kupffer, and hemopoiesis in the fetus and newborn are additional functions. In the case of detoxification, the enzymes that can oxidize, methylate, or conjugate with various drugs (barbiturates, antihistamines, and anticonvulsants) are present in the smooth endoplasmic reticulum. For example, the enzyme glucuronyl transferase (an enzyme that can conjugate bilirubin to glucuronic acid after its dissociation from its albumin carrier) will also inactivate barbiturates via conjugation. All of the drugs previously mentioned can induce enzyme production in this organelle. This forms the structural and biochemical basis for what is termed *drug* tolerance.

Finally, the bilirubin that is excreted in the bile salts originated from the degradation of hemoglobin by phagocytic cells of the reticuloendothelial system. The albumin carrier is removed, and glucuronic acid is conjugated to it (so-called bilirubin glucuronide) by a smooth endoplasmic reticulum enzyme—glucuronyl transferase. This new conjugated complex is water soluble and passes into the intestine where it is reduced to *urobilinogens* by bacteria. The latter contributes to the color of the feces. The abnormal increase in bilirubin (caused by obstruction of the bile duct, destruction of red blood cells, and viral impairment of smooth endoplasmic reticulum) produces a condition called *jaundice*. A type of impairment in infants (*neonatal hyperbilirubinemia*) can be rectified with a treatment by phenobarbital (a barbiturate), which stimulates immature smooth reticulum to produce glucuronyl transferase.

## Development

The liver develops as a ventral diverticulum (endoderm) of the foregut and midgut junction and extends anteriorly into the mesenchyme of the septum transversum. Proliferation of the endodermal cells gives rise to the cords and plates of hepatic cells, which at first are tubular in arrangement with cells arranged around a central lumen. The sinusoids develop from vascular tissue associated with the vitelline veins, which themselves form the portal vein. Mesenchyme associated with the portal vein and that of the septum transversum develops into the connective tissue and the capsule of the organ

The original diverticulum of the gut and its main branches remain tubular as the bile and hepatic ducts. The gallbladder and cystic duct develop as a diverticulum from the main duct.

The liver, as stated before, is one of the main blood-forming organs in the fetus and retains this potentiality in the adult (Fig. 11–88).

### Extrahepatic Biliary Passages

The arrangement of the major biliary passages is illustrated in Figure 11–89.

**Extrahepatic Ducts.** These all are lined by a tall columnar epithelium that secretes mucus. There is a layer of subepithelial connective tissue with a preponderance of elastic fibers and a marked lymphoid tendency. Many lymphocytes and occasional granulocytes are found migrating through the epithelium into the lumen. In the subepithelial layer, there may be accumulations of tubuloacinar glands, mostly mucous in type, and blood vessels and nerves are prominent. In the common bile duct, there is also a layer of smooth muscle, at first composed of isolated

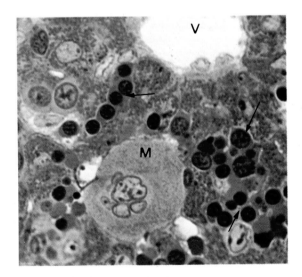

*Figure 11–88. Embryonic liver: hemopoiesis. Blood cells are formed in different sites at different stages during development, and in the fetus, they appear successively in the yolk sac, mesenchyme, liver, spleen, and lymph nodes. Blood formation commences in the liver at about six weeks and gradually diminishes during the middle of fetal life. This section demonstrates active hemopoiesis within the liver. Hepatic cells are large and contain large vesicular nuclei. The cells are arranged in plates that radiate from the central vein (V). Between the plates of liver cells are numerous hemopoietic elements (arrows), principally of the red cell series. A large megakaryocyte (M), with a complex lobed nucleus and finely granular cytoplasm, also is present. With the development of bone marrow (during the third fetal month), hemopoiesis wanes in the liver. Plastic section. Paragon. High power.*

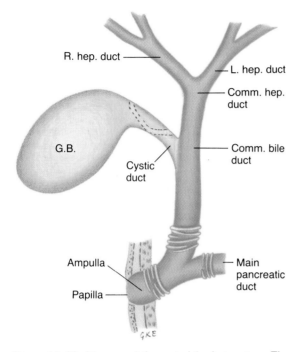

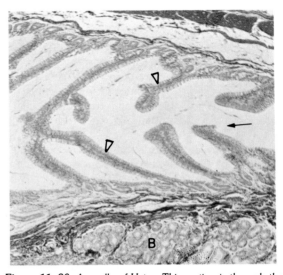

**Figure 11–90.** *Ampulla of Vater. This section is through the combined opening of the common bile duct and main pancreatic duct as it passes through the wall of the duodenum. The mucosa, with a simple columnar epithelium, is thrown into valve-like folds (arrowheads). Also seen are glands of Brunner (B) in the submucosa of the duodenum. Fluid flows in the combined duct in the direction of the arrow. Masson. Low power.*

**Figure 11–89.** *Diagram of the main bile duct system. The sphincter muscles and the spiral valve of the cystic duct are indicated.*

bundles of smooth muscle fibers but, near the duodenum, forming a complete investment of oblique and transverse fibers. This layer, particularly the circular fibers, is thickened at the termination of the common bile duct (the sphincter of Boyden) and around the ampulla of the conjoined bile and pancreatic ducts just proximal to the ampullary opening into the duodenum (the sphincter of Oddi). At the opening into the duodenum (the ampulla of Vater), the mucosa shows valve-like folds protruding into the lumen (Fig. 11–90). Because the common bile duct traverses the lesser omentum, it is covered also by peritoneum.

### THE GALLBLADDER

The gallbladder is a blind, pear-shaped diverticulum of the common hepatic duct, to which it is connected by the *cystic duct*. Occasionally,

embryonic bile ducts, *Luschka's ducts*, are seen in the connective tissue that opens into the bile duct of the liver. These embryonic remnants never communicate with the lumen of this organ. The gallbladder is approximately 3 inches (8 cm) in length and 1.5 inches (4 cm) in diameter but is capable of considerable distention. Its wall is composed of three layers:

1. The mucous membrane.
2. The muscularis.
3. The adventitia (serosa).

### Mucous Membrane

When empty, the mucosa is thrown into many folds, or rugae, and thus is irregular in section, often with the appearance of simple glands (Figs. 11–91 and 11–92). All epithelial cells are similar, tall, columnar cells, with basally located nuclei. Electron microscopy demonstrates a fine, microvillous apical border, with lateral borders nearest the lumen exhibiting zonula occludens, and basal borders showing folds. The cells are supported

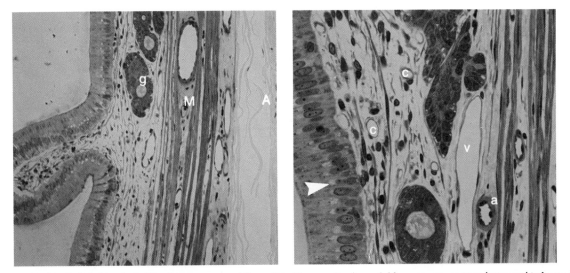

**Figure 11–91.** Gallbladder. Left: The lining mucosa of the gallbladder usually shows folds, or rugae, as seen here, and is formed by a simple columnar epithelium with supporting lamina propria. In the lamina, small mucous glands (g) may be present, particularly at the neck region. There is no true submucosa. External to the lamina is the muscularis (M), composed of slips of smooth muscle with an external adventitia (A). Plastic section. Methylene blue, basic fuchsin. Medium power. Right: This is a higher magnification of the left photomicrograph. Note the simple, tall columnar epithelium. In these cells, a "negative" Golgi apparatus is seen clearly in a supranuclear position (arrowhead). The lamina propria is loose (areolar) connective tissue, containing an arteriole (a), a venule (v), and capillaries (c), with mucous glands. The smooth muscle slips of the muscularis are cut longitudinally (right). Plastic section. Methylene blue, azure A, basic fuchsin. High power.

by a fine basal lamina and a lamina propria of delicate, reticular connective tissue with numerous small blood vessels provided by the cystic artery and cystic veins, with some of the venous blood being returned to the sinusoids of the liver. Occasional small lymph nodules are present, with a few mucous glands at the neck of the gallbladder. These glands occur more frequently in individuals with chronic inflammation of this organ along with abnormal folds of the epithelium, *Rokitansky-Aschoff sinuses*. The latter are not glands and may extend as far as the perimuscular connective tissue layer.

### Muscularis

There is no submucosa in the gallbladder, and external to the mucosa is a layer of smooth muscle, irregular in thickness and orientation of its component bundles. In any section, smooth muscle will be cut in all possible planes, for the muscularis is a meshwork of interlacing bundles of smooth muscle fibers between which are collagenous, reticular, and some elastic fibers.

### Adventitia, or Serosa

The gallbladder lies on the inferior surface of the liver, and its outer coat of dense fibroconnective tissue blends in some regions with that of Glisson's capsule. Elsewhere, the adventitia is covered by peritoneum.

The neck of the gallbladder continues into the cystic duct, and here the mucous membrane is thrown into a spiral fold with a core containing smooth muscle. This is termed the *spiral valve of Heister* and is believed to prevent sudden changes in capacity of the gallbladder following changes of pressure. The gallbladder itself functions as a reservoir for bile, secreted continuously by the liver but discharged intermittently into the intestine following contraction that is stimulated by cholecystokinin. Cholecystokinin is released in response to the presence in the duodenum of peptides and fatty acids consisting of more than

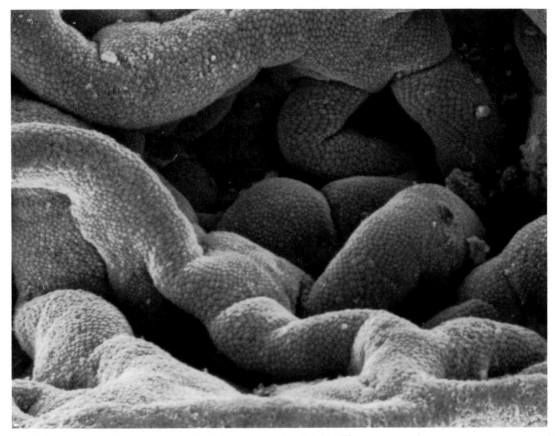

**Figure 11–92.** *Scanning electron micrograph of the contracted gallbladder.The mucosa is thrown up into many convoluted folds.* × *5000.*

ten carbons. This hormone initiates the reflex, and, along with contraction of the muscle layer of the gallblader, it relaxes the sphincters of Boyden and Oddi. In the gallbladder, bile is concentrated by absorption of fluid by the epithelium. The concentration, which is about five to ten times, is brought about by the absorption of water and electrolytes, using a mechanism similar to that employed by small intestinal epithelium.

## SUMMARY

The lip and cheek consist of a core material composed of skeletal muscle embedded in an elastic fibroconnective tissue. Internally, a mucous membrane consisting of a stratified squamous nonkeratinizing epithelium (except at the lip margin, or red lip) rests on a lamina propria with high papillae. The submucosa contains labial (mucoserous) glands and elastic fibers that bind the mucous epithelium firmly to the musculature. The lips control access to the oral cavity.

A tooth consists of a crown, neck, and root. Each tooth has a pulp cavity of connective tissue with a surrounding connective tissue called the periodontal membrane. The latter holds the tooth in the alveolus via a fibrous joint, or gomphosis. The hard tissues surrounding the pulp cavity are dentin; enamel, covering the dentin of the crown; and cementum, covering the dentin of the root. The dentin is made by the odontoblasts whose processes (Tomes's dentinal fibers) lie in small canals in the dentin called dentinal tubules. Enamel is made by the ameloblasts and is the hardest component of the human body. Cementum is made by the cementoblasts, and it contains fibers of the periodontal ligament. The latter binds the cementum of the tooth to the bony walls of its socket, the alveolus.

The tongue is covered by a mucous membrane, and its bulk consists of intrinsic and extrinsic striated muscle fibers and mucous, serous, and mixed glands. The tongue is important for both chewing and swallowing, and it is aided by the rigid dais of the hard palate. The skeletal musculature of the soft palate aids in sealing off the oropharynx. The sulcus terminalis divides the tongue into anterior and posterior regions. The tongue consists of the body (a freely movable portion) and a base that is attached to the floor of the pharynx. Four types of papillae are seen:

1. Filiform papillae are cone-shaped projections that are found in parallel rows along the entire tongue. They are covered with a hard partially keratinized epithelium with no taste buds.

2. Fungiform papillae are mushroom-shaped projections ("red dots") with a thin epithelium containing taste buds along their dorsal aspect.

3. Circumvallate papillae are located along the V-shaped sulcus and are surrounded by a circular furrow with taste buds along the lateral wall. The furrows are washed by the serous (Ebner's) gland that permits new gustatory stimuli to reach the taste buds.

4. Foliate papillae are leaf-shaped folds with taste buds in the grooves between the folds. They are present along the sides of the tongue.

The taste buds are pale, barrel-shaped bodies within the epithelium that communicate with the exterior via the taste pores. Three cell types are present in the taste bud—supporting, or sustentacular, cells; neuroepithelial taste cells; and basal cells. There are four fundamental taste sensations—sweet and salt at the tip, sour at the sides, and bitter in the region of the circumvallate papillae.

The major salivary glands include the parotid, submandibular (submaxillary), and sublingual glands that secrete saliva. The parotid gland is a compound, tubuloalveolar, serous gland. The submandibular gland is a compound tubuloalveolar gland that contains mostly serous acini, with mucous acini and mixed acini with serous demilunes. The sublingual gland has a similar anatomic structure, with mostly mucous acini with some serous demilunes. The sublingual gland has a thin capsule and short intercalated and striated ducts. The submandibular gland has shorter and less prominent intercalated ducts, but with more conspicuous striated ducts than the parotid gland. These glands secrete saliva, which aids in cleaning the mouth and renewing the sense of taste and contains enzymes (amylase and maltase) that begin carbohydrate digestion and lysozymes, peroxidases, and IgA for antibacterial action.

The tubular digestive tract consists of four organs (esophagus, stomach, small intestine, and large intestine). All of these parts show four tunicae: the mucosa, submucosa, muscularis externa, and serosa (or adventitia). The mucosa consists of an epithelial membrane with a basal lamina resting on a loose areolar layer, the lamina propria. Its outer border terminates as an inner circular and outer longitudinal smooth muscle layer (the muscularis mucosae). In some regions, the mucosa forms evaginated projections (villi) or invaginated epithelium-lined intestinal glands, or crypts. The mucosa produces antibodies, especially IgA, in response to antigens and microorganisms in the gut. The submucosa permits mobility of the mucosa and contains large blood vessels and a nerve plexus called the submucosal plexus of Meissner. The muscularis externa is arranged as an inner circular (or tight helical) and an outer longitudinal (or open helical) smooth muscle layer. The former constricts the lumen, and the latter shortens the gut. Auerbach's myenteric plexus is located between these two muscle layers and regulates the propulsion of food by a process termed peristalsis. A third inner oblique muscular layer is present in the stomach wall. The outermost layer ends in an elastic areolar connective tissue (termed an adventitia) or is covered by a layer of mesothelial cells (called a serosa).

The esophagus transports food that has been mixed with saliva, and has a mucosal epithelium that is nonkeratinizing stratified squamous type. It is indented by peg-like protrusions of the lamina propria and changes abruptly to a simple columnar epithelium upon entering the stomach. The muscularis mucosae is thick and is continuous above with the elastic layer of the pharynx. The submucosa contains coarse collagenous and elastic fibers and tubuloalveolar mucous glands. The muscularis externa can be entirely skeletal (upper third); skeletal and smooth (middle third); or only smooth (lower third) in nature. Contraction of the skeletal muscle rapidly transports the bolus of food into the esophagus. The circular muscle is thickened in the upper (pharyngoesophageal) and lower (esophagogastric) portions to form sphincters. The luminal pressures are higher in the region of the sphincters, thus preventing a backflow of the semisolid mass of food. Outside of the muscularis externa, an adventitia turns into a serosa below the diaphragm.

The stomach is lined by a columnar epithelium whose apical cytoplasm is occupied by PAS-positive, discrete mucin (neutral glycoprotein) granules from the Golgi complex. At the luminal border, tight junctions, spot desmosomes, and short microvilli are present. Linear crevices (foveolae) appear in the mucosa into which gastric glands communicate with the surface. Three zones are recognized on the basis of glands and foveolae: cardiac glands; gastric, or fundic, glands; and pyloric glands. Cardiac glands have a wide lumen and are branched tubular mucus-secreting glands that occupy about two thirds of the mucosa, with very few parietal cell and some enteroendocrine cells. Fundic glands occupy about three quarters of the mucosa and produce most of the gastric juice, which contains hydrochloric acid, pepsin (which commences protein digestion), renin (which functions to curdle milk), and lipase (which starts fat digestion). This gland consists of four cell types, which secrete acid (parietal cells), mucus (mucous neck cells), enzymes (chief cells), and hormones (enteroendocrine cells of the "open" and "closed" types). The pyloric glands open into gastric pits that extend to about one half of the mucosa. The cell types are mostly mucus-secreting, with a few parietal and enteroendocrine cell types present. The lamina propria is scanty, and the muscularis mucosae is thin. Several different types of enteroendocrine cells are found in stomach glands. Throughout the organ, argentaffin cells that secrete serotonin (produces smooth muscle contractions) and A-like cells that secrete glucagon (an antagonist to insulin) are found. In addition, the pyloric glands have argyrophilic cells that secrete histamine (which stimulates parietal cells); G cells of the pyloric antrum that produce gastrin (which also stimulates parietal cells); D cells in the midzone of the gastric glands that secrete somatostatin (which inhibits the release of the growth hor-

mone); and finally VIP cells of the fundus region (which secrete a vasoactive intestinal peptide that stimulates the pancreas to secrete alkaline juices and raise blood glucose levels). These enterochromaffin cells occur throughout the digestive tract and, to a lesser extent, in the main ducts of the liver and the pancreas.

The small intestine is divided into three parts: duodenum, jejunum, and ileum. It functions to transport food material (chyme) from the stomach to the large intestine; to complete digestion via its enzymes and those from accessory glands; to absorb the final products of digestion; and to secrete certain hormones. Certain specializations that increase the surface area of the mucosa are plicae circulares, villi, intestinal crypts, and submucosal glands (duodenal glands of Brunner) that secrete an alkaline fluid, rich in bicarbonate. The epithelium of the mucosa is simple columnar in type and consists of absorptive cells with a striated border (microvilli), Paneth's cells, goblet cells, and enteroendocrine cells. Stem cells are also present at the base of the crypts and are the source of the other cell types. The lamina propria extends between intestinal glands and into the cores of the villi, which contain blood vessels and a blindly ending lymphatic vessel (lacteal) that receives the chylomicrons. Lymphatic nodules surrounded by M cells (a cell that transports macromolecules from lumen to lymphocytes) are abundant in Peyer's patches in the ileum. Immunoglobulins are produced that protect against bacterial and viral invasions. The muscularis mucosae, submucosa, muscularis externa, and serosa do not merit a separate description. However, the following is a list of some of the regulatory peptides and proteins produced by enteroendocrine cells in this region: serotonin; endorphin (morphine-like action); histamine; gastroinhibitory polypeptide (GIP), which inhibits secretion of gastric acid and pepsin; somatostatin, which stimulates the exocrine pancreas to secrete bicarbonates and contracture of the pyloric sphincter; motilin, which stimulates contraction of stomach musculature; and cholecystokinin, which stimulates the flow of pancreatic secretion and bile flow.

The large intestine is composed of the cecum, continuous with the ileum at the ileocecal valve; the appendix, a diverticulum from the cecum; the colon, continuous with the cecum and divided into ascending, transverse, and descending parts;

the rectum; and the anal canal. The large intestine's functions are the absorption of water, the lubrication of the fecal mass, and digestion, which is accomplished by the enzymes present in the food material. Villi are absent, but the intestinal glands remain, with goblet cells becoming the most numerous cell type in the colon. The mucosa is thicker, with fewer Paneth's cells and enteroendocrine cells than that of the small intestine. The muscularis mucosae is well developed but may be deficient at the sites of lymphatic nodules. In the colon and the cecum, the outer longitudinal layer of the muscularis externa is not a complete layer and is present in three bands—taeniae coli. The serosa, on the surfaces not attached to the posterior abdominal wall, shows fat-filled pouches, the appendices epiploicae. The appendix has a lamina propria rich in lymph nodules with no taeniae coli. At the end of the rectum, the intestinal glands and muscularis mucosae disappear, and the epithelium changes to the stratified squamous type of the anal canal. Here are also present hair follicles, apocrine sweat glands (circumanal glands), and a large plexus of hemorrhoidal veins. The inner circular layer is thickened as the internal sphincter, and bundles of striated muscle that surround the anal canal form the external sphincter.

The pancreas is both an exocrine and an endocrine organ. The exocrine portion is arranged into lobulated, compound, tubuloacinar glands, with each acinus consisting of about eight pyramidal cells surrounding centroductular cells. Their apical cytoplasm contains acidophil zymogenic granules. The latter granules contain proteolytic enzymes (trypsin and chymotrypsin) and carboxypeptidase, ribonuclease, deoxyribonuclease, amylase, and lipases. The pancreatic juice is transported through centroductular, intercalated ductules and intralobular to interlobular to main and accessory ducts. Two hormones, secretin and cholecystokinin, stimulate acinar secretion that is bicarbonate-rich or enzyme-rich, respectively. The endocrine portion (islets of Langerhans) demonstrates the following cell types: alpha cells, which produce glucagon (which causes lysis of glycogen), adrenocorticotropin, and endorphin; beta cells, which produce insulin (which facilitates glucose transport into the cell); clear cells, which may represent a reserve or resting cell; and delta cells, which produce somatostatin (which inhibits

the secretion of insulin and glucagon). A variant of delta cells ($D_1$ cells) secretes VIP, which, like glucagon, causes lysis of glycogen and also effects motility and secretory activity of the gut. Pancreatic polypeptide cells (PP cells) represent another cell type, in the head of the pancreas, that stimulates enzyme secretion by the stomach.

The liver is covered by a thin fibroconnective capsule (of Glisson) that divides the parenchyma into lobes and lobules. The portal vein and the hepatic artery enter and the bile ducts and the lymphatic ductules leave the liver at the porta hepatis. Hepatocytes are arranged into branching plates, with sinusoidal blood spaces located between the plates. Portal canals (each comprising branches of the portal vein, hepatic artery, and bile duct) delineate a lobule of liver tissue called the classic, or hepatic, lobule, with a central vein in the center. A portal lobule incorporates a central vein peripherally at each corner and encompasses parts of three adjacent classic lobules. The liver acinus or the functional lobule, whose morphology is based on blood flow, is a diamond-shaped area that includes two neighboring central veins (along its long axis) and two neighboring portal areas (long its short axis).

The hepatic cells are hexagonal, with their surfaces related to a sinusoidal space or closely applied to adjacent liver cells or partially separated to form a bile canaliculus. The sinusoids are lined by endothelial and phagocytic cells (cells of Kupffer) along with a few fat cells and extravascular reticular cells. The endothelial lining is incomplete, with gaps between cells and nondiaphragmatic fenestrations in its attenuated cytoplasm. The junctions of bile canaliculi with the bile ducts occur via intermediate structures called the ductules or canals of Hering. The hepatocyte is separated from the wall of the sinusoid by a narrow perisinusoidal space of Disse. The liver functions in the fetus as a hemopoietic organ, and in the adult, in the maintenance of blood glucose, lipid metabolism, and the storage of vitamins A and B and heparin. It also secretes bile salts, fibrinogen, and plasma albumins into the blood, produces cholesterol, detoxifies toxic materials, and functions in the phagocytosis of particulate matter.

The gallbladder functions both to concentrate and to store bile. The discharge of bile occurs in response to cholecystokinin stimulation of the obliquely oriented muscularis layer. The mucosa is capable of considerable distention, and, at the neck of the gallbladder, it forms a spiral fold (or spiral valve of Heister) that protects against bile release due to sudden pressure fluctuations. The organ is covered partially by Glisson's capsule (adventitia), while the peritoneum (or serosa) covers the remaining surface. The cystic duct connects the gallbladder to the common bile duct. At the termination of the latter, the circular fibers are thickened to form the sphincter of Boyden. The conjoined bile and pancreatic ducts just proximal to the ampullary opening into the duodenum show the sphincter of Oddi.

# The Respiratory System

## INTRODUCTION

The main function of the respiratory system is to provide for the intake of oxygen (from inspired air) and the elimination of carbon dioxide (a toxic by-product of body metabolism) (Fig. 12–1). Oxygen, of course, is necessary for cell metabolism and is transported from the lungs to cells by the circulatory system, which, in turn, transports carbon dioxide from them back to the lungs. The respiratory system comprises the lungs and a series of respiratory passages that connect them to the exterior. The system has two parts. A *conducting portion* consists of the nose, the pharynx, the larynx, the trachea, and the bronchi and larger bronchioles; these passages are relatively rigid structures, being constantly patent. The *respiratory portion* consists of respiratory bronchioles, alveolar ducts, alveolar sacs, and alveoli; here gaseous exchange occurs between air and the blood. To perform this function, the barrier between air in respiratory tissue and blood in capillaries is extremely thin.

From the nasal cavity to alveoli in the lungs, the respiratory tract is a closed system, open to the exterior only at the

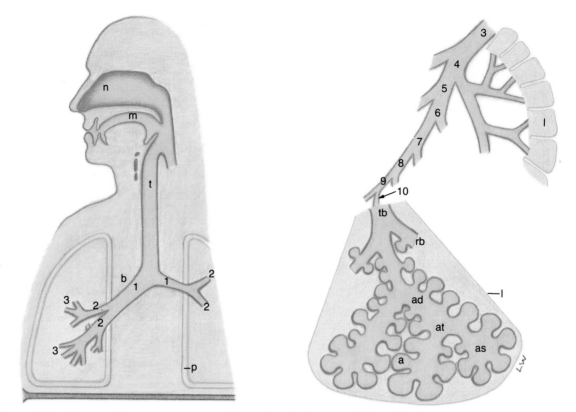

**Figure 12–1.** *Diagram of the respiratory system. The numbers indicate the divisions of the bronchial tree; n, nasal cavity; m, mouth; t, trachea; b, bronchus; p, pleural cavity; tb, terminal bronchiole; rb, respiratory bronchiole; ad, alveolar duct; at, atrium; as, alveolar sac; a, alveolus; l, lobule.*

nasal and oral orifices. The lungs are contained within the thoracic cavity, and thus, if the capacity of the thoracic cavity is increased, air will be drawn through the conducting system into the lungs. Such inspiratory movements are effective in drawing air into the lungs only if the passage to the exterior remains patent, which explains why the conducting portion of the system is rigid and constantly patent. In its passage through the conducting part of the respiratory system, air is conditioned or modified. It is warmed, moistened, and filtered, with the removal of particulate material. Important in this process of conditioning is the presence of *mucus*, which lines the luminal surface of most of the conducting portion of the tract. Secreted by glands in the walls of the conducting tubes and by goblet cells in the lining epithelium, mucus not only counters dehydration of the lining epithelium but also traps particulate matter in the inspired air and, together with the secretions of serous glands, moistens and warms

it. By the action of cilia in the lining epithelium, mucus is moved to the pharynx, where it is either expectorated or swallowed.

The respiratory system has additional functions to that of gaseous exchange. Water is lost in the expired air, and thus, the lungs also are excretory organs. In nasal cavities is located the olfactory mucosa, the receptor for smell, and the larynx functions in phonation, these two functions being dependent upon air movement in inspiration and expiration, respectively.

## CONDUCTING PORTION

### The Nose

The nose is divided by a midline septum into right and left nasal cavities, each communicating anteriorly with the exterior by an *anterior naris*, or nostril, and posteriorly with the nasopharynx. The wall of the anterior naris is of fibroconnective tissue and cartilage, and its dimensions can be changed by muscular action. The remainder of the nasal cavity has a rigid wall of bone and hyaline cartilage. Each nasal cavity is divided into a *vestibule*, the wider portion immediately internal to the anterior naris, the *respiratory* portion, and the *olfactory* portion.

**Vestibule.** Skin over the external surface of the nose is characterized by the presence of large sebaceous glands, and it extends into the anterior part of the vestibule, where it contains sweat and sebaceous glands and hair follicles with thick, stiff hairs. They project into the airway and filter out coarse particles of dust in the inspired air. Deeper in the vestibule, the lining epithelium becomes nonkeratinizing stratified squamous in type.

**Respiratory Portion.** The remainder of the nasal cavity is lined by a pseudostratified ciliated columnar epithelium with goblet cells that rests upon a basal lamina and is supported by a connective tissue in which mucous and serous glands are present (Fig. 12–2). Fluid from these glands and the goblet cells keeps the lining epithelium moist. In addition to ciliated and goblet cells, the respiratory epithelium also contains basal cells, believed to be stem cells capable of differentiation into other cell types, and a few "brush" cells, similar to those found in the olfactory mucosa (see later).

The connective tissue lamina propria of the respiratory epithelium contains small collections of lymphatic tissue, especially posteriorly near the nasopharynx. The deepest layer of the lamina blends into, and is continuous with, the periosteum or perichondrium of bone or cartilage in the wall of the nasal cavity, the mucosa being bound firmly to the periosteum or perichondrium as a *mucoperiosteum* or *mucoperichondrium*.

In frontal (coronal) section, the nasal cavity is pear-shaped and is divided by the median nasal septum. Protruding into the cavity from the lateral wall on each side are three slender, curved plates of bone covered by mucoperiosteum, the superior, middle, and inferior *turbinate bones*, or the *conchae* (L. *concha*, shell) (Fig. 12–3). The inferior turbinate is the largest and is covered by a thicker mucosa. In the lamina propria of the respiratory mucosa, in general, there is a rich

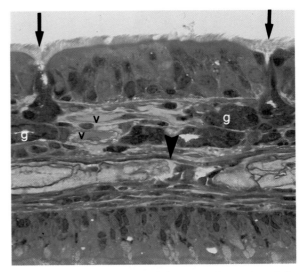

**Figure 12–2.** *The mucosa of the respiratory portion of the nasal cavity is formed by a pseudostratified ciliated columnar epithelium with basal, ciliated columnar, and goblet cells and by a lamina propria that forms a mucoperiosteum (periosteum of a nasal concha is indicated by an arrowhead). In the lamina propria are seromucous glands (g) from which ducts pass to the surface (arrows) and numerous venous channels (V) of the cavernous tissue. Methylene blue, azure A, basic fuchsin. High power.*

vascular plexus in which arteriovenous anastomoses are common, but over the conchae (and particularly the inferior one), there is an extensive, superficial venous plexus of large, thin-walled vessels termed *cavernous* or *erectile tissue*. While this resembles the true erectile tissue of the penis, it lacks muscle in septa between cavernous (blood) spaces. This tissue is capable of considerable engorgement, and at periodic intervals of 30 to 60 minutes, the tissue ("swell bodies") of one side of the nasal cavity automatically swells with blood, thus restricting air flow on that side and permitting the respiratory epithelium to recover from desiccation.

Not only do mucous and serous secretions keep the mucosal surface moist, but also they humidify inspired air, which is warmed by blood in the venous sinuses. Much of the blood, in fact, flows anteriorly, in a direction opposite to that of the inspired air, the whole forming a countercurrent system. Conchae cause turbulence in the air flow in addition to providing an increase in surface area, and this improves contact between the air and the mucous coat, trapping particulate material

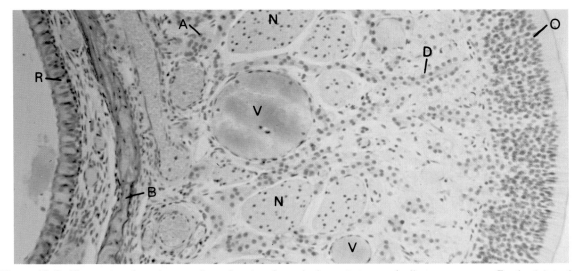

**Figure 12–3.** *This section through a nasal concha also shows both respiratory and olfactory mucosae. To the left is the respiratory mucosa with a pseudostratified, ciliated, columnar epithelium with goblet cells (R) and its lamina propria blended into periosteum of the concha (turbinate bone, B) as a mucoperiosteum. The olfactory epithelium (O) is very tall, pseudostratified columnar in type with a thick lamina propria containing acini (A) and ducts (D) of serous glands of Bowman, numerous small nerve bundles (N) of the fila olfactoria, and dilated venous channels (V) of the cavernous (erectile) tissue. H and E. Medium power.*

and absorbing pollutant gases such as ozone and sulfur dioxide. This mucous coat is moved posteriorly to the nasopharynx by ciliary action, where it is either expectorated or swallowed in the saliva.

*Paranasal air sinuses* are air-filled cavities within the bones of the skull. They are the maxillary, the frontal, the ethmoidal, and the sphenoidal, all communicating with the nasal cavity by openings and all lined by an epithelium continuous with, and identical to, that of the nose. The epithelium is pseudostratified ciliated columnar in type but is thinner than that in the nasal cavity, has fewer goblet cells, and shows a thinner lamina propria with fewer glands. Erectile tissue is not present. The deeper layers, like those of the nose, are continuous with periosteum. The paranasal air sinuses frequently are the site of infection, a condition called sinusitis, which may require surgical treatment.

**Olfactory Portion.** In the roof of each nasal cavity and extending down over the superior concha and the adjacent part of the septum is an area where the fresh mucosa is yellowish brown, in contrast with the pink color of the respiratory mucosa. This specialized area is the *olfactory mucosa* and contains the receptors for the sense of smell.

The *olfactory epithelium* is a tall, pseudostratified columnar epithelium about 60 μm in height, lacking goblet cells and with no distinct basal lamina (Figs. 12–4 and 12–5). Three main types of cell are present: supporting, basal, and olfactory. *Supporting*, or *sustentacular, cells* are tall, slender, cylindrical cells, broader at their apices and tapering basally. Their nuclei lie centrally and form a row lying more superficially than nuclei of olfactory cells. Apically, there is a prominent terminal web of filamentous material associated with terminal bars (junctional complexes) between the supporting and adjacent sensory cells, with numerous long slender microvilli that protrude into an overlying film of mucus. In apical (supranuclear) cytoplasm is a small Golgi apparatus and pigment granules that are similar to lipofuscin and are responsible for the yellowish-brown coloration of the mucosa.

*Basal cells* are small and conical in shape with dark, ovoid nuclei and branching cytoplasmic processes lying between the bases of supporting cells. They are believed to be stem cells capable of differentiating into sustentacular cells.

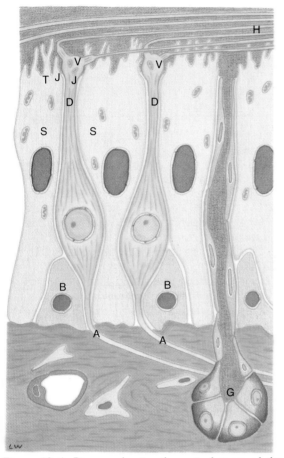

**Figure 12–4.** Diagram showing the main features of the olfactory epithelium. Olfactory hairs (H), or cilia, arise from the olfactory vesicles (V) and lie in a surface film of fluid (gray) produced mainly by Bowman's glands (G). From the olfactory vesicle, a functional dendrite (D) of the olfactory (sensory cell) extends to the cell body with nucleus lying basal to nuclei of sustentacular cells (S). From cell bodies of these olfactory (bipolar) cells, functional axons (A) pass deeply into the underlying lamina propria (green) where they are collected into bundles (fila olfactoria). Sustentacular and olfactory cells meet at junctional complexes (J), the former cells with well-developed terminal webs (T). Also present in the epithelium are basal (B) cells. The height of the epithelium has been reduced.

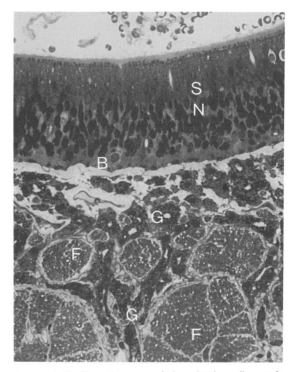

**Figure 12–5.** The olfactory epithelium (top) is tall, pseudostratified columnar epithelium. It is formed by sustentacular cells with their nuclei (paler-staining) forming a row lying apically (S) and by sensory (bipolar) cells (N) with darker-staining nuclei lying more basally. Also present are basal cells (B) and a few "brush cells," the latter not identifiable here. The axons of the sensory cells pass into the underlying lamina propria, where they collect into bundles, the fila olfactoria (F). Also present in the lamina propria are serous glands of Bowman (G). Methylene blue, azure A, basic fuchsin. Medium power.

*Olfactory,* or *sensory, cells* are distributed evenly between supporting cells and are modified bipolar cells with a cell body, a dendrite extending to the surface, and an axon that passes deeply into the underlying lamina propria. Their nuclei are spherical and lie more basally than those of sustentacular cells. The cytoplasm contains bun-

dles of neurofibrils, more prominent around the nucleus. Apically, there is a narrowing of the cell at the region of terminal bars. Above this, the dendrite expands into a small, bulb-like swelling termed the *olfactory vesicle,* from which radiate six to ten *olfactory cilia,* or *hairs,* with basal bodies in the cytoplasm of the vesicle. These are long and nonmotile and lie parallel to the surface, in a thick layer of mucus. These cilia appear to be the actual receptive elements for smell. Basally, the cell tapers to a slender, cylindrical process only 1 μm in diameter, which passes deeply into the underlying lamina propria as the axon. In the lamina propria, axons, or olfactory nerve fibers, are collected into small bundles, the *fila olfactoria,* which then pass superiorly through fine canals in the cribriform plate of the ethmoid bone to enter the olfactory bulb of the brain.

Also present in the olfactory epithelium are a few *brush cells* with thick, short, apical microvilli and apparently contacting nerve fibers originating in the trigeminal (fifth) cranial nerve. They probably receive ordinary sensation in the olfactory mucosa.

The lamina propria of the olfactory epithelium contains lymph and venous plexuses, the former communicating with the subarachnoid space via capillaries running with the fila olfactoria. Within the lamina also are branched tubuloalveolar serous glands (the *glands of Bowman*) that secrete a watery fluid, carried to the surface by slender ducts. This fluid acts as a solvent for odoriferous substances, and its continuous secretion serves to freshen the surface film of fluid and prevent repetitive stimulation of olfactory hairs by a single odor. Olfactory sensory cells frequently are damaged owing to repeated exposure to infection and other trauma, and there is a loss of some cells. Consequently, in the elderly, it is usual for the sense of smell to be diminished; in such people, the olfactory epithelium usually is atypical.

### The Nasopharynx

The pharynx is a chamber through which both food and air pass. It lies behind the nose, mouth, and larynx and is flattened anteroposteriorly. It is subdivided into the *nasopharynx*, lying below the base of the skull, behind the posterior nares of the nose, and above the soft palate; the *oropharynx*, behind the oral cavity and posterior surface of the tongue; and the *laryngopharynx*, behind the larynx.

The pharynx has muscular walls posteriorly and laterally and thus can dilate or, by muscular contraction, can be occluded, although the nasopharynx cannot be closed completely. However, its dimensions can change. By apposition of the soft palate with the posterior wall of the pharynx, the nasopharynx can be isolated completely from the oropharynx. This movement occurs in swallowing, and normally, no food material is permitted to enter the nasopharynx.

The epithelium lining the pharynx varies with location. Over much of the area there is a respiratory epithelium (i.e., a pseudostratified ciliated columnar epithelium with goblet cells), but in regions where the surface is subject to attrition when two surfaces come into contact during swallowing, the epithelium is stratified squamous in type. For example, this "wear and tear" epithelium is found over the posterior border of the soft palate and at the posterior wall of the pharynx. In the lamina propria, there is prominent elastic tissue with numerous small glands, mainly mucous in type, although serous and mixed glands also are found. Lymphatic tissue is prominent throughout the pharynx. True lymphatic follicles are present posteriorly in the nasopharynx (the adenoids, or pharyngeal tonsil), laterally around the openings of the pharyngotympanic (eustachian) tubes ("tubal tonsil"), laterally on each side at the junction of the oral cavity and the oropharynx (the palatine tonsil), and in the root of the tongue (the lingual tonsil) (see Chapter 9). In the lateral walls of the nasopharynx is a loose submucosa; elsewhere, the lamina propria extends to the muscular wall of the pharynx.

### The Larynx

The larynx is the segment of the respiratory tract that connects the pharynx and the trachea (Figs. 12–6 and 12–7). It is a cavity of irregular shape, with a "skeleton" of hyaline and elastic cartilages, some connective tissue, striated muscle, and mucous glands in its walls.

The major cartilages of the larynx—the *thyroid, cricoid,* and *arytenoids*—are hyaline; the smaller cartilages—the corniculates, cuneiforms, and tips of the arytenoids—are elastic, as is the cartilage of the epiglottis. Three large, flat membranes interconnect these cartilages and the hyoid bone, these composed of dense fibroconnective tissue in which many elastic fibers are present. These membranes are the thyrohyoid, the quadrates, and the cricovocals, the latter having the *vocal cords* (inferior thyroarytenoid ligaments) in their upper free edges, the cords containing prominent bundles of elastic fibers. The free lower borders of the quadrate membranes (superior thyroarytenoid ligaments, or false vocal cords) and the true vocal cords lie in an anteroposterior plane, and between them is the sinus and the saccule of the larynx, a small slit-like diverticulum of the

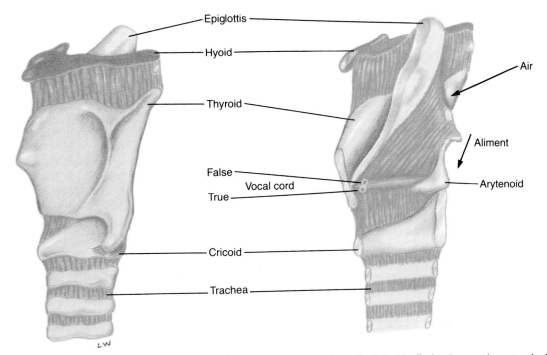

**Figure 12–6.** Diagrams of the larynx. Left: External appearance, as seen from the left side. Right: A sagittal section, looking toward the right half of the specimen. The rima glottidis, the narrowest part of the larynx, lies between the two true vocal cords.

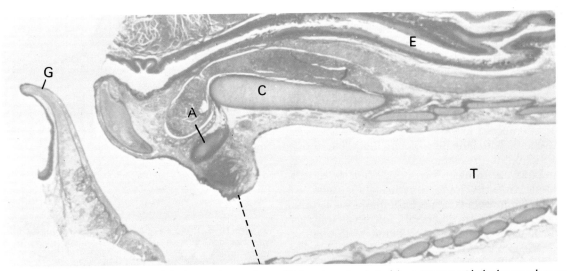

**Figure 12–7.** In this sagittal section of the larynx, the esophagus (E) lies above (posteriorly), continuous with the laryngopharynx, both lined by thick, stratified squamous epithelium, the two meeting at the lower border of the cricoid cartilage (C). The epiglottis (G) has a core of elastic cartilage with some mucous glands inferiorly (right) covered above (left) by stratified squamous epithelium and below (right) by thinner respiratory epithelium. The trachea (T) is lined by respiratory mucosa with tracheal rings of cartilage seen both anteriorly (below) and posteriorly (above) in its wall. The position of the vocal cord (inferior thyroarytenoid ligament) is indicated by a dotted line with part of the arytenoid cartilage (A) posteriorly. H and E. Low power.

general laryngeal cavity. The cricoid cartilage is in the shape of a signet ring, broader posteriorly, and the cavity within it is continuous below with the lumen of the trachea. Posterior to the cricoid and arytenoid cartilages, the posterior wall of the pharynx is formed by striated muscle of the pharyngeal constrictor muscles, which, at the lower border of the cricoid cartilage, are continuous with the intrinsic musculature of the esophagus. From the larynx, the air passage extends through the cavity of the cricoid to the trachea, while aliment passes over the posterior surface of the cricoid into the lumen of the esophagus. The laryngeal cavity is lined by a mucosa, the epithelium of which varies with location.

Much of the laryngeal cavity is lined by respiratory epithelium (i.e., pseudostratified ciliated columnar epithelium with goblet cells). A stratified squamous nonkeratinizing epithelium is located in areas subject to wear and tear, that is, over the anterior and upper half of the posterior surface of the epiglottis, the aryepiglottic folds (upper edges of the quadrate membranes), and the vocal cords. Patches of stratified squamous epithelium are not unusual in other locations in the larynx. Over the vocal folds, the lamina propria is bound firmly to underlying connective tissue of the vocal ligament. Elsewhere, it is thick and contains tubuloacinar glands, most of which are mucous, some with serous crescents. In the epiglottis, mixed salivary glands are found on both surfaces, mainly the posterior surface, lying in irregular depressions in the elastic cartilage. On the posterior, or laryngeal, surface, a few taste buds are found in the surface epithelium. Lymph nodes are scattered in the lamina propria. There is no true submucosa in the larynx.

Cilia of the laryngeal epithelium, like those throughout the respiratory passages, beat toward the pharynx, moving the surface film of mucus with its contained trapped particulate material.

Striated muscle is found throughout the larynx. Posterolaterally are fibers of constrictor muscles with fibers of intrinsic musculature of the larynx found in relation to quadrate and cricovocal membranes. These muscles are concerned with phonation, breathing, and swallowing.

The shape of the opening between the vocal cords (the glottis) varies greatly with breathing and in phonation. Air passing through the glottis causes vibrations of the vocal folds, and these can be altered by changing tension and the size of the glottal opening to produce sounds of varying pitch.

## The Trachea

The trachea is a tube about 10 to 12 cm long and 2 to 2.5 cm in diameter, continuous above with the cricoid ring and extending through the lower part of the neck to the superior mediastinum of the thorax, where it terminates by dividing into right and left main bronchi (Figs. 12–8 through 12–10). While it is semirigid, it is also flexible and is capable of elongation with respiratory and postural movements.

Patency in the trachea is maintained by a series of about 20 horseshoe-shaped *cartilages* (C-shaped rings) of irregular outline oriented one above the other, with the deficiencies posteriorly.

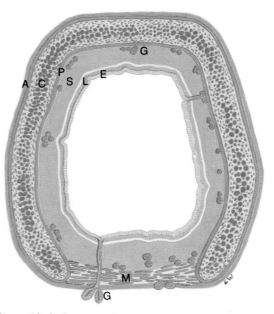

**Figure 12–8.** *Diagram of a transverse section of the trachea showing adventitia (A, dark green), a cartilage ring (C, light blue) with its perichondrium (P, midblue), the submucosa (S, light green) and the mucosa with its lamina propria (L, midgreen) and lining respiratory epithelium (E, pink). Posteriorly is smooth muscle (M, brown) of the trachealis muscle lying in elastic connective tissue (yellow), and present also are tracheal (submucous) glands (G, red), some extending through the muscle. A condensation of elastic tissue (yellow) lies at the junction of submucosa and lamina propria.*

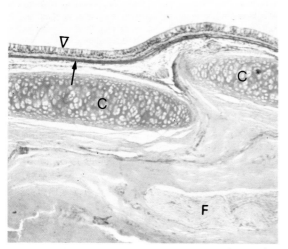

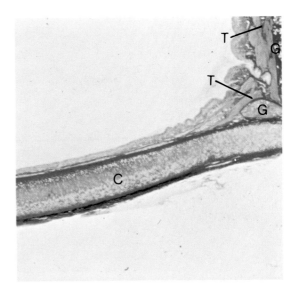

**Figure 12–9.** In this longitudinal section of the trachea, portions of two tracheal rings (C) are seen, and externally (below) is relatively dense connective tissue of the adventitia containing a nerve fiber bundle (F). Internal to cartilage is the submucosa of loose areolar connective tissue with a concentration of elastic fibers (arrow, brown) of the lamina propria where the two meet. The lining epithelium is pseudostratified ciliated columnar with goblet cells (arrowhead). Van Gieson, orcein. Low power.

**Figure 12–10.** This transverse section of the trachea shows part of one hyaline cartilage ring (C) with its perichondrium and other collagenous material stained blue. Submucosa and lamina propria are not distinguished clearly at this magnification, nor is the lining respiratory epithelium. Posteriorly (right) are slips of the trachealis (smooth) muscle (T) with some glands (G) and the duct of a gland opening to the surface. Mallory. Low power.

These cartilages are flat externally and slightly convex internally, and the gaps between them are bridged by fibroelastic connective tissue that blends with perichondrium of the rings. In the posterior gaps between the C-shaped cartilages, there are interlacing bundles of smooth muscle fibers (the *musculus trachealis*) oriented mainly transversely and attached to the free posterior ends of the cartilages and their associated elastic tissue. Contraction of this muscle diminishes the diameter of the trachea. External to the tube is loose fibroconnective tissue of the *adventitia* that contains small blood vessels and autonomic nerves that supply the trachea and its musculus.

A *submucosa* lies internal to the cartilages and is a layer of loose areolar fibroconnective tissue in which are numerous small mixed glands and some serous secretory units. The glands lie mainly between adjacent cartilage rings or posteriorly in their deficiencies, both within and external to the smooth muscle, their ducts piercing the lamina propria of the mucosa to open on the surface. Blood and lymph capillaries form rich plexuses in the submucosa.

Lining the trachea is a *mucous membrane* consisting of a pseudostratified ciliated columnar epithelium with goblet cells resting upon a basal lamina and supported by a connective tissue lamina propria (Fig. 12–11). Three common cell types, all identifiable by light microscopy, are present in the epithelium, and three less common cell types also are present but identifiable only by electron microscopy. Most common are the tall, columnar, *ciliated* cells with apically numerous cilia and microvilli. Interspersed among them are *goblet*, mucus-secreting cells, their expanded apices filled with mucigen granules (Fig. 12–12). *Basal* cells lie adjacent to the basal lamina, do not reach the lumen, and are small and pyramidal in shape. They are undifferentiated, reserve cells and are precursors (stem cells) of other cell types. Less common are the *brush* cells, which are tall, slender, columnar cells with large, blunt microvilli at their apices. Their function is not clear, and some appear to show synapses at their basal ends with intraepithelial nerve fibers. They are similar to the brush or caveolated cells found in intestinal epithelium (and in the olfactory mucosa) and may

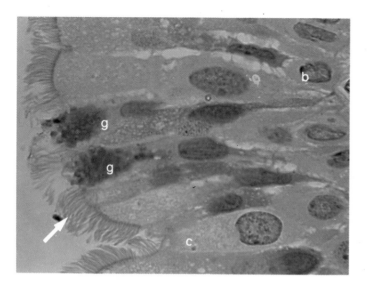

*Figure 12–11.* The tracheal lining respiratory epithelium is pseudostratified ciliated columnar with goblet cells. Seen here are the three main cell types as recognized by light microscopy—ciliated columnar (the arrow indicates apical cilia), goblet (g) with apical secretory (pink) granules, and basal (b). Also seen is a columnar nonciliated cell (c). Small granule and brush cells are not seen here. H and E. Oil immersion.

have a sensory function. Also present are a few *small granule* cells (argyrophilic cells), similar to the argentaffin (or APUD—*amine precursor up-take and decarboxylation*) cells of the gastrointestinal tract. Some reach the lumen, others do not, but all contain numerous, small, dense, secretory granules, 100 to 300 nm in diameter. Some appear to store catecholamines, others vasoactive peptide hormones. The last cell type is a tall *columnar* cell that may or may not have apical

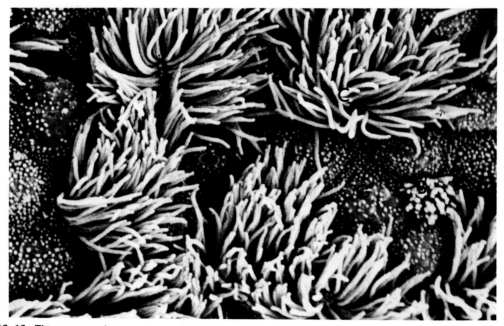

*Figure 12–12.* This scanning electron micrograph shows the surface of the tracheal epithelium with ciliated (C), goblet (G), and brush (B) cells. × 3600. (Courtesy of Dr. P. M. Andrews.)

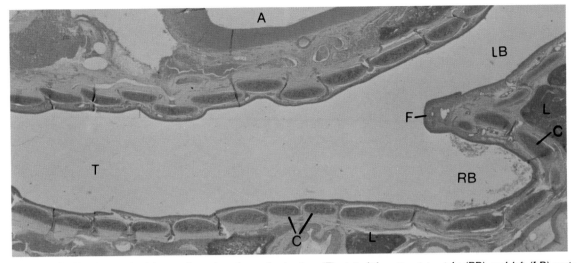

**Figure 12–13.** *This longitudinal (coronal) section shows the trachea (T) at its bifurcation into right (RB) and left (LB) main bronchi, with the carina (F). The main bronchi and the trachea are similar in structure, with cartilage rings (C) in their walls. Externally are several large blood vessels, including the aorta (A) and some lymph nodes (L), the largest at the bifurcation (right). H and E. Low power.*

microvilli, and may represent an intermediate or immature cell that later will differentiate into a ciliated or a goblet cell. Other similar cells may represent depleted goblet cells that have discharged their secretory granules and are resting. Additionally, migrating lymphocytes are seen frequently within the epithelium.

The lamina propria is relatively thin and contains many elastic fibers, condensed to form an indefinite layer at the junction with the submucosa. Most of the elastic fibers run longitudinally. Within the lamina propria, small accumulations of lymphocytes are common.

Characteristically, the lumen of the trachea is D-shaped in transverse section. As noted already, the trachea terminates by dividing into right and left main bronchi, which, shortly after their origin, enter the lungs, where the remainder of the conducting part and all of the respiratory portion of the system are located (Fig. 12–13).

### The Lungs

#### THE BRONCHIAL TREE

Centrally in the thoracic cavity is the *mediastinum*, which contains the heart and the major blood vessels, the esophagus, the lower trachea, and remnants of the thymus gland. On each side of the mediastinum lie the lungs, protected by the rib cage and separated from the abdominal cavity below by the muscular diaphragm. The thoracic cavity on each side is lined by a thin serous membrane, the *parietal pleura*, which at the *hilum*, or *root*, of the lung is reflected over the lung as the *visceral pleura*. The *pleural cavity* is the potential space between parietal and visceral pleura; it contains a small amount of watery, serous fluid. All structures that pass to and from the lung do so through the hilum. The thoracic cavity is virtually a closed space, then, containing the right and left lungs on each side of the central mediastinum, and connected to the exterior by the trachea, larynx, pharynx, and nasal and oral cavities. When the capacity of the thoracic cavity is expanded by spreading of the rib cage and descent of the diaphragm (by muscular action), air is inspired through the conducting passages into the lungs. Expiration occurs mainly by elastic recoil in a passive manner, although this can be aided actively by muscular action of the chest wall and contraction of abdominal musculature.

In the mediastinum, the trachea divides into right and left main or primary bronchi. Before entering the lung, the right *primary* bronchus divides into upper lobe and lower lobe (*secondary*) bronchi, with the right middle lobe bronchus arising from the latter within the lung. On the left side, the left primary bronchus usually divides into upper and lower lobe bronchi within lung tissue. In the lungs, there are three right and two left lobes, each supplied by a secondary bronchus. In each lobe, the secondary (lobe) bronchus divides further into *tertiary* bronchi, each of which supplies a *bronchopulmonary segment*; there are ten segments in each lung. Within each bronchopulmonary segment, further orders of dichotomous branching occur. It should be noted that the cross-sectional areas of the two daughter branches exceed that of the mother branch, and thus, air travels more slowly in the small branches. After about nine to twelve generations of branching, tube size is reduced to about 1 mm in diameter, and the tube now is termed a *bronchiole*, with a change in histological characteristics.

Each bronchiole supplies a *lung lobule*, the basic unit of structure of the lung. A lobule is pyramidal in shape, with the bronchiole entering at the apex that points toward the hilum and with a base of 1 to 2 cm, and a similar height. Lobules often are irregular in shape, with 30 to 60 in each bronchopulmonary segment. Within a lobule, the bronchiole branches further into, usually, four to seven *terminal bronchioles*, each of which divides into two *respiratory bronchioles*. A respiratory bronchiole may divide up to three times, and these branches continue as *alveolar ducts*. Two further divisions may occur before the ducts terminate as small dilations, or *atria*. In turn, atria open into *alveolar sacs* and *alveoli*. Gaseous exchange occurs from respiratory bronchiole to alveoli. It should be noted that pulmonary blood vessels also branch in a manner similar to that of bronchi and lie closely adjacent to them.

### Bronchi

*Extrapulmonary* bronchi closely resemble the trachea in structure, although they are of smaller diameter, and show cartilage rings that are incomplete, with the posterior deficiency occupied by smooth muscle (Fig. 12–14).

*Intrapulmonary* bronchi, however, differ. First, they are round and not D-shaped in outline owing

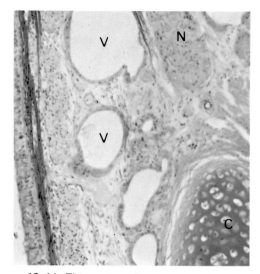

**Figure 12–14.** *This section of an extrapulmonary (main) bronchus shows a structure similar to that of the trachea with a lining respiratory epithelium, a concentration of elastic fibers (brown) in the lamina propria (at the junction with the submucosa), some venous channels (V) and a small nerve (N) in the submucosa, and part of a cartilage ring (C) and its perichondrium. Van Gieson, orcein. Medium power.*

to the presence of irregular plates of hyaline cartilage (and not C rings) distributed around the circumference (Figs. 12–15 and 12–16). Some of these plates completely encircle the lumen, but they are so irregular that on transverse section, the appearance is of several small pieces of cartilage, each being a protuberance from a large plate. The cartilage is surrounded by elastic fibroconnective tissue, and internal to it is a submucosa containing mixed mucoserous and mucous glands, the ducts of which pass centrally to reach the luminal surface. At the junction of submucosa and mucosa is a condensation of elastic fibers, as there is in the trachea and primary bronchi, but here reinforced by an outer sheet of smooth muscle fibers. These fibers are arranged in open spirals in interlacing bundles, and between them are elastic fibers. Their contraction results in narrowing of the lumen. Internally is a mucosa similar to that of the trachea, and characteristically in sections, it shows numerous longitudinal folds owing to contraction of the smooth muscle.

With successive branching of the bronchial tree, bronchi become smaller, but the basic structure

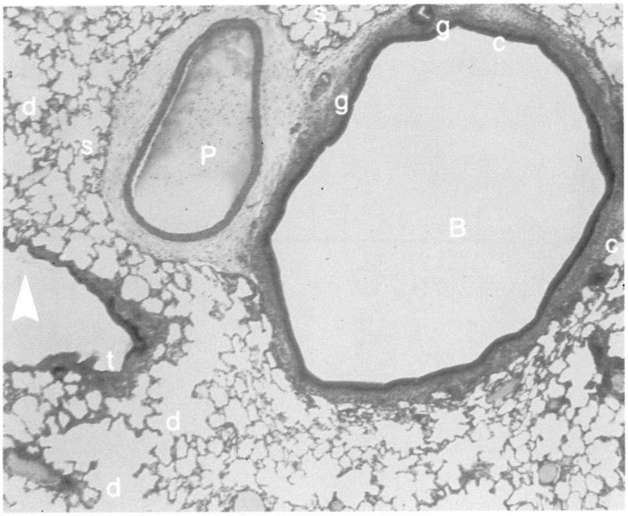

**Figure 12–15.** *This section of lung shows a large intrapulmonary bronchus (B) with cartilage (c) and glands (g) in its wall, with an accompanying branch of the pulmonary artery (P), the two lying in connective tissue. Present also is a terminal bronchiole (t) leading to a respiratory bronchiole (the arrowhead indicates the opening of an alveolus from the latter), alveolar ducts (d), alveolar sacs (s), and alveoli. H and E. Low power.*

remains unchanged (Fig. 12–17). The smallest bronchi contain less cartilage, and no longer are complete rings of it present. The lining epithelium becomes ciliated columnar with goblet cells and is of less height than the pseudostratified epithe-lium of the larger bronchi. All bronchi lie in connective tissue continuous with that of the hilum, with pulmonary blood vessels related closely to them and embedded in the same connective tissue.

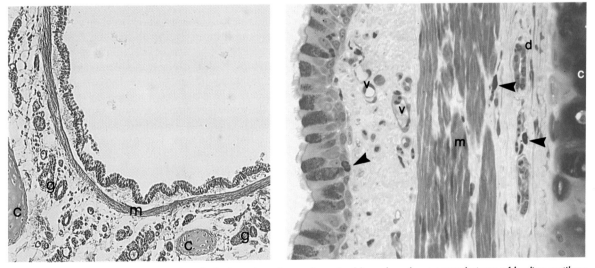

**Figure 12–16.** *Intrapulmonary bronchus. Left: A portion of a medium-sized bronchus shows several pieces of hyaline cartilage (c) in its wall, glands (g) in the submucosa, prominent bundles of smooth muscle (m) at the junction of submucosa and mucosa, a delicate lamina propria, a lining columnar, ciliated epithelium with goblet cells. H and E. Low power. Right: A similar bronchus shows similar features, cartilage (c) to the right, with a duct (d) of a submucosal gland. Numerous small blood vessels (v) are present in the lamina propria, and the lining epithelium is pseudostratified ciliated columnar in type (although not as tall as that of the trachea) with prominent goblet cells (dark-blue apical granules). The arrowheads point to mast cells in the connective tissue. Methylene blue, azure A, basic fuchsin. Medium power.*

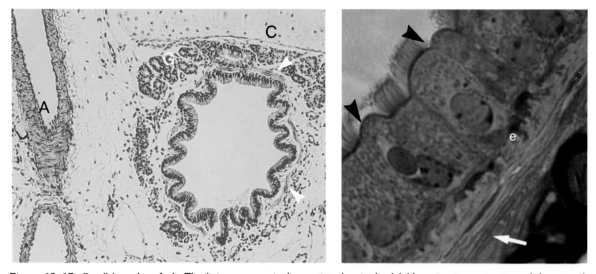

**Figure 12–17.** *Small bronchus.* Left: *The lining mucosa is thrown into longitudinal folds owing to contraction of the smooth muscle (arrowheads) located at the junction of lamina propria and submucosa. The epithelium is ciliated columnar with some goblet cells, and submucous glands (G) are present as is a piece of hyaline cartilage (C). The bronchus lies in delicate connective tissue, together with a branch of the pulmonary artery (A). Iron hematoxylin. Low power.* Right: *A bronchus of similar size is lined by ciliated columnar epithelium with some nonciliated cells (arrowheads). A few goblet cells, not seen here, also are present. At lower right is a small piece of cartilage with smooth muscle fibers (arrow) at the junction of submucosa and mucosa. Elastic fibers (e) lie just beneath the epithelium and stain dark purple. Methylene blue, basic fuchsin. Oil immersion.*

### Bronchioles

While no abrupt transition is seen between bronchi and bronchioles, a bronchiole is regarded as a conducting tube of 1 mm in diameter or less, embedded in little or no connective tissue, and surrounded by respiratory tissue (Figs. 12–18 and 12–19). Characteristically, cartilage, glands, and lymph nodes are absent, with only a thin adventitia of connective tissue. The lamina propria is occupied largely by prominent bundles of smooth muscle and elastic fibers. In larger bronchioles, the lining epithelium is ciliated columnar with a few goblet cells. With further divisions into smaller bronchioles (about 0.3 mm in diameter), the goblet cells disappear, and the ciliated cells are low columnar or cuboidal in type. Scattered between them are *Clara cells*, nonciliated and columnar with their dome-shaped apices protruding into the lumen. They show characteristics of secretory cells, with basal granular reticulum, supranuclear agranular reticulum, and apical granules. The granules are discharged by exocytosis to contribute to a bronchiolar fluid that contains protein, glycoprotein, and cholesterol. Their function is unknown, but probably they produce also a surfactant (surface-active agent) similar, but not identical, to that present in alveoli (see later). This functions to lower surface tension and thus to facilitate dilation of the air passages on inspiration. In terminal bronchioles, only small patches of ciliated cells are found in a basic nonciliated cuboidal epithelium. Throughout the bronchioles, a few brush and small granule neuroendocrine cells also are present in the epithelium.

Functionally, rigidity in the conducting tubes is essential to maintaining patency, this being achieved by the presence of cartilage from the trachea to the smallest bronchi. The tubes, however, can change in length and diameter, the latter controlled by smooth muscle supplied by the autonomic nervous system. The abundance of elastic tissue in the walls of the bronchi and throughout the lung permits expansion during inspiration and aids in contraction during expiration by elastic recoil. As in the nose, the mucous coat traps particulate material, which then is passed by ciliary action to the pharynx for elimi-

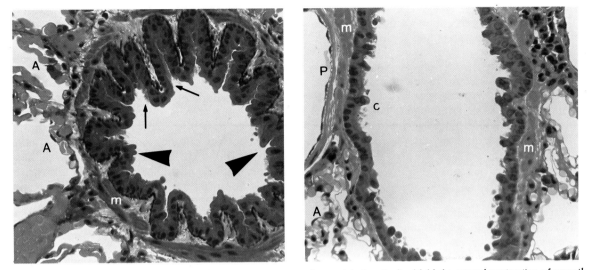

***Figure 12–18.*** *Bronchioles. Left: Characteristically, the mucosa is thrown into longitudinal folds by agonal contraction of smooth muscle in the lamina propria (and of elastic tissue). The epithelium of this large bronchiole is ciliated (arrows), low columnar with scattered Clara cells (arrowheads)—non-ciliated, with their domed apices protruding into the lumen. No goblet cells are present. Elastic fibers (black) and bundles of smooth muscle (m) are prominent in the lamina propria with a small amount of connective tissue. Alveoli (A) surround the bronchiole. Methylene blue, basic fuchsin, Weigert. Medium power. Right: A somewhat smaller bronchiole, sectioned longitudinally, is lined by ciliated cuboidal epithelium with numerous Clara (c) cells. Adjacent to it is a branch of the pulmonary artery (P) and alveoli (A). Methylene blue, basic fuchsin. Medium power.*

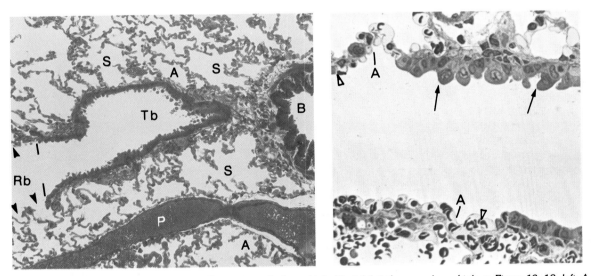

***Figure 12–19.*** *Terminal bronchiole. Left: The portion of a bronchiole (B, right) is the same bronchiole as Figure 12–18, left. A branch of this is a terminal bronchiole (Tb), cut longitudinally, with a simple cuboidal epithelium of which a few more proximal cells are ciliated, with numerous Clara cells protruding into the lumen. Externally are slips of muscle and elastic fibers. At the marked junction, this passes into a respiratory bronchiole (Rb, left) with outpocketing alveoli (arrowheads). Also seen are alveoli (A) and alveolar sacs (S) and a branch of the pulmonary artery (P). Methylene blue, basic fuchsin. Low power. Right: The transition from terminal bronchiole (right) with a simple cuboidal epithelium (with Clara cells, arrows) to the squamous epithelium of a respiratory bronchiole (left) is abrupt. Numerous capillary blood vessels (arrowheads) lie in the wall of the respiratory bronchiole and in interalveolar septa. Alveoli (A) open from the wall of the respiratory bronchiole. Toluidine blue. High power.*

nation. It should be noted that cilia extend further down the respiratory tree than do goblet cells and submucosal glands, preventing occlusion by mucus or waterlogging of respiratory tissue, the cilia constituting an internal drainage system. In the smallest bronchioles, and in the absence of cilia, macrophages by phagocytosis of material perform the function of internal drainage. Finally, mucous and serous secretions humidify the inspired air.

### RESPIRATORY PORTION

*Respiration* (i.e., gaseous exchange) can occur only where the barrier separating air and blood is very thin. Such an arrangement is found from the respiratory bronchioles to the alveoli.

### Respiratory Bronchioles

Terminal bronchioles end by branching into respiratory bronchioles (Figs. 12–20 through 12–23). These are short, about 1 to 4 mm long,

usually branch three times, and vary from 0.2 to 0.15 mm in diameter. The lining epithelium is at first cuboidal ciliated, with some Clara cells, becoming, with branching, simple low cuboidal and nonciliated. Externally, the epithelium is supported by interlacing bundles of smooth muscle and elastic fibroconnective tissue. However, respiratory bronchioles differ from terminal bronchioles in that their walls are interrupted by alveoli, saccular outpocketings lined by squamous epithelium (Fig. 12–24). At the openings of these alveoli, the cuboidal lining epithelium is continuous with the simple squamous alveolar lining. Gaseous exchange occurs in the alveoli, hence the term "respiratory bronchiole." The respiratory bronchioles continue into alveolar ducts.

### Alveolar Ducts

These are cone-shaped, thin-walled tubes with a squamous epithelial lining so thin that it is difficult to resolve with the light microscope. External to the epithelium is thin fibroelastic tissue. Around the circumference of the duct are the

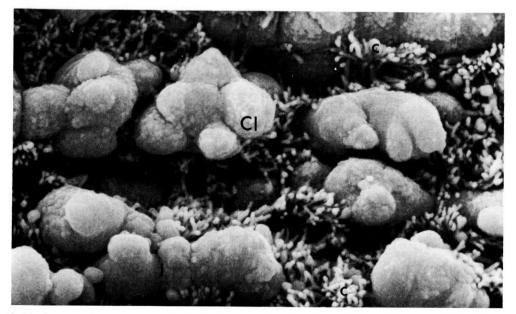

**Figure 12–20.** *Scanning electron micrograph of bronchiole showing ciliated (c) and Clara (Cl) cells. × 2000. (Courtesy of Dr. P. M. Andrews.)*

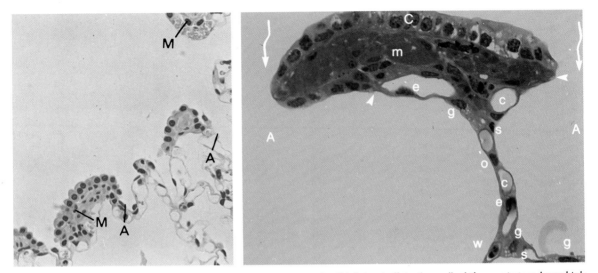

**Figure 12–21.** *Respiratory bronchiole. Left: In transverse section, the "deficiencies" in the wall of the respiratory bronchiole that open into alveoli (A) are more apparent. The epithelium is low cuboidal, supported by slips of smooth muscle (M) but changes abruptly to the squamous epithelium lining the alveoli. H and E. High power. Right: Above is the lumen of the respiratory bronchiole that is lined by simple cuboidal epithelium (C), interrupted by the openings (arrows) to two alveoli (A), and is continuous at the arrowheads with squamous epithelium lining the alveoli. Numerous capillaries (c) are present in the interalveolar septum and nuclei of several cell types: s, squamous, type I alveolar; e, endothelium; g, type II alveolar cell; w, white blood cell in capillary; O, unidentified, possibly type I. Methylene blue, azure A, basic fuchsin. High power.*

openings of numerous alveoli and alveolar sacs (clusters of alveoli), and, particularly at their orifices, smooth muscle fibers are prominent. The openings of alveoli from alveolar ducts are so numerous that it is difficult to delineate the wall of the duct, although this is more obvious in thick sections, where bundles of elastic, collagenous, and muscle fibers are visible, interweaving between and around the openings of alveoli along the wall of the alveolar duct.

Alveolar ducts branch two or three times to terminate in small chambers, or spaces, called *atria*. These are simply vestibules or irregular spaces from which *alveolar sacs* and *alveoli* diverge, usually with two or more alveolar sacs opening from each atrium. Alveolar sacs are multilocular, a collection or cluster of alveoli opening into a central, slightly larger chamber. Around the openings of atria and alveolar sacs (and also alveoli) is a supporting network of elastic and reticular fibers; the elastic fibers permit expansion of alveoli on inspiration and recoil-like contraction on expiration, while the reticular fibers prevent overdistention and damage to the delicate respiratory tissue.

## Alveoli

Alveoli are polyhedral or hexagonal spaces with one wall open to a respiratory bronchiole, alveolar duct, atrium, or alveolar sac to permit inflow of air (Fig. 12–25). If flattened out, all alveoli together represent an enormous surface for gaseous exchange, nearly 150 sq. m.

Alveoli are packed so tightly in the lung that each does not have a separate wall: Instead, adjacent alveoli are separated by an *interalveolar septum*, as are the "cells" in a honeycomb (Fig. 12–26). Each alveolus, however, is lined by a squamous epithelium that is greatly attenuated but complete, and two types of cell are present in this lining epithelium. An interalveolar septum must resist the pressure of air in the alveoli, a pressure that varies with the phase of respiration. The support of the septum is provided by a framework of reticular and elastic fibers, and located in the septa, and largely filling them, are capillary blood vessels arranged in an extremely rich plexus (Figs. 12–27 and 12–28). Thus, an interalveolar septum is covered on each surface by the attenuated epithelium lining alveoli, each

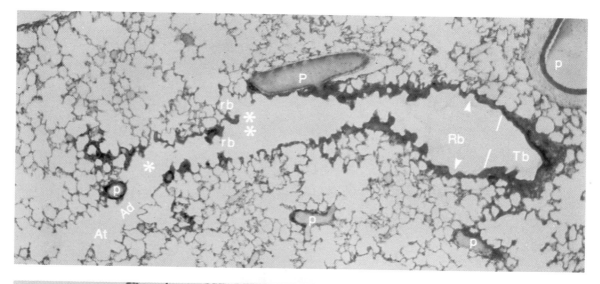

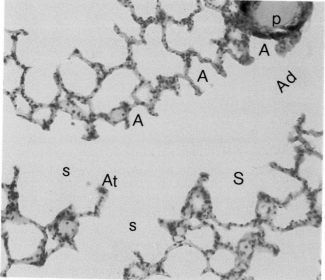

*Figure 12–22.* Lung. Top: *A terminal bronchiole (Tb, right) passes to a respiratory bronchiole (Rb) at the marked lines, with alveoli outpocketing from the latter (arrowheads). At the double asterisk, this respiratory bronchiole branches further into two smaller respiratory bronchioles (rb), one of which terminates at the single asterisk, where it passes into an alveolar duct (Ad). In turn, this duct terminates in an atrium (At). In passing from terminal bronchiole to alveolar duct, the lining epithelium changes from (ciliated) cuboidal to squamous, and the amount of supporting tissue (smooth muscle and elastic fibroconnective tissue) decreases. Also seen in the field are other alveolar ducts, alveolar sacs, and alveoli, and branches of the pulmonary artery (P, p). H and E. Low power.* Bottom: *This higher magnification of the lower left portion of the above shows the alveolar duct (Ad) with numerous openings from its wall of alveoli (A) and an alveolar sac (S). It terminates in a chamber, or atrium (At), from which open more alveolar sacs (s). Medium power.*

*Figure 12–23.* Top left: *Photomicrograph of lung showing terminal bronchiole (Tb) leading to respiratory bronchiole (Rb), which divides into two alveolar ducts (Ad). Also seen are alveolar sacs (S), alveoli (A), and branches of the pulmonary artery (e). The features of these structures are illustrated in the diagrams in both longitudinal and transverse section. The main diagram (top, right) shows a lung acinus (i.e., the parts supplied by a terminal bronchiole) and is an interpretation of the section with the left alveolar duct shown dividing further into two smaller ducts (asterisks) of which one terminates in an atrium (At) from which alveolar sacs and alveoli open. The section levels are indicated by numbers. Other labels are: b, type II cell; c, blood capillary; d, cell within an interalveolar septum; m, muscle; p, free alveolar phagocyte. The arrows indicate alveolar pores.*

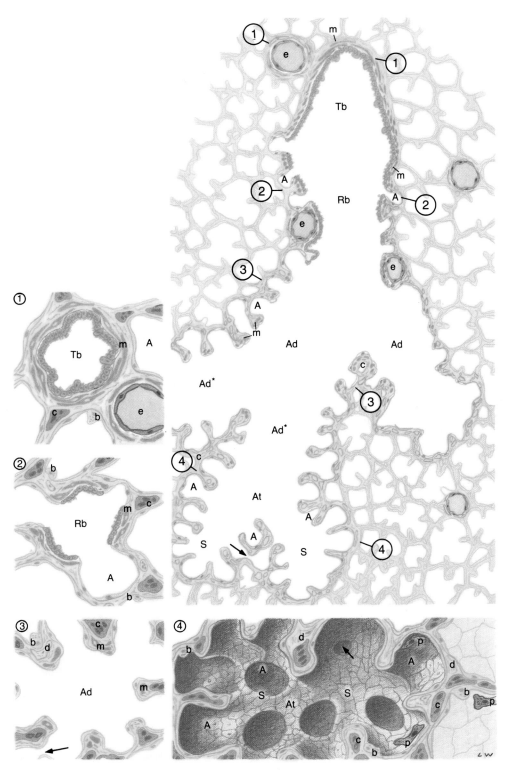

*Figure 12–23* See legend on opposite page

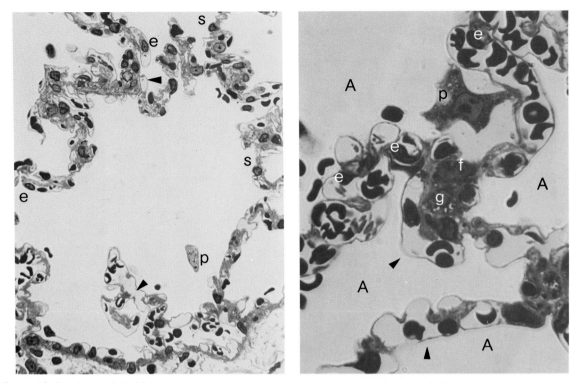

*Figure 12–24. Alveoli. Left: Most of one alveolus is seen, with portions of surrounding alveoli. The very rich capillary network lying in interalveolar septa is well seen, the capillaries containing erythrocytes (dark blue-black). At this magnification, nuclei of several cell types are seen, but not all are identifiable clearly. A few are endothelial cell nucleus (e), type I alveolar (squamous) cell (s), and free alveolar macrophage or phagocyte (p). In some places, the blood-air barrier is seen clearly and is extremely thin (arrowheads). Toluidine blue. Low power. Right: Portions of several alveoli (A) with interalveolar septa are seen. Capillaries in the septa contain erythrocytes (blue-black), and the blood-air barrier (arrowheads) is very thin. Cell types seen are endothelial (e), type II (great) alveolar (g), and alveolar macrophage (p). The cell labeled "f" probably is a septal (fibroblast) cell. Toluidine blue. High power.*

resting upon a basal lamina, and contains some connective tissue in which lies an extremely rich capillary network (Fig. 12–29).

Two main cell types are found in the alveolar epithelium.

1. The *type I alveolar cell*, or squamous surface epithelial cell, is the most common, lining over 90 per cent of the alveolar surface, but less than 0.2 μm thick. By light microscopy, their flattened nuclei can be resolved, but their cytoplasm is so attenuated that often it is beyond resolution. Electron microscopy demonstrates the presence of micropinocytotic vesicles at basal and apical surfaces and that the cells are held together by occluding (tight) junctions.

2. The *type II alveolar cell*, or great alveolar cell, occurs singly or in small groups between the squamous cells. They are cuboidal cells that may bulge into alveolar spaces but usually are situated in the corners or angles of alveolar walls. By light microscopy, they are recognized by their spherical, vesicular nuclei and vacuolated cytoplasm. On electron microscopy, they have the appearance of secretory cells with granular reticulum, a Golgi apparatus, mitochondria, a few apical surface microvilli, and secretory granules in apical cytoplasm. These granules are 0.2 to 1.0 μm in diameter and show a lamellar structure, with parallel membrane lamellae in their cores. They contain phospholipid and some protein. The granules are secreted by exocytosis and contain surfactant (described later), which upon release into the alveolar spaces forms myelin patterns (see Fig. 12–32) but later spreads out over the alveolar surface in a monomolecular film. Type II cells also appear to be capable of mitosis and are

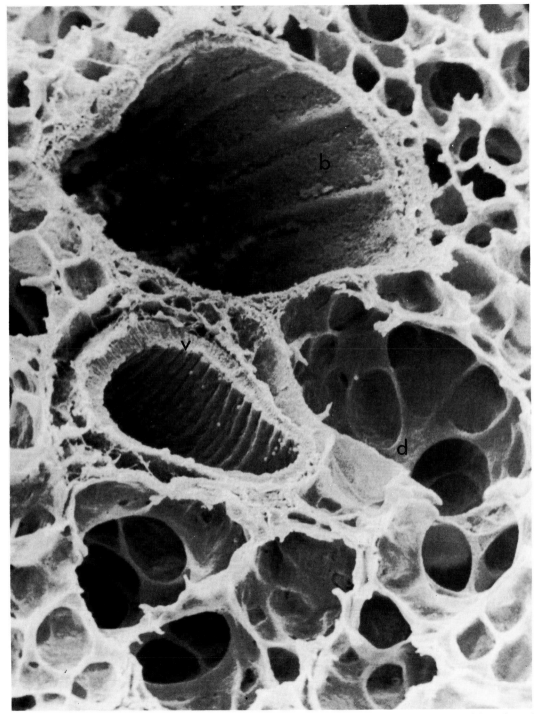

**Figure 12–25.** Scanning electron micrograph of rat lung showing a small bronchiole (b), a small artery (v), and an alveolar duct (d) with alveoli opening from its wall. Numerous alveoli with interalveolar septa occupy most of the field. × 200. (Courtesy of Dr. P. M. Andrews.)

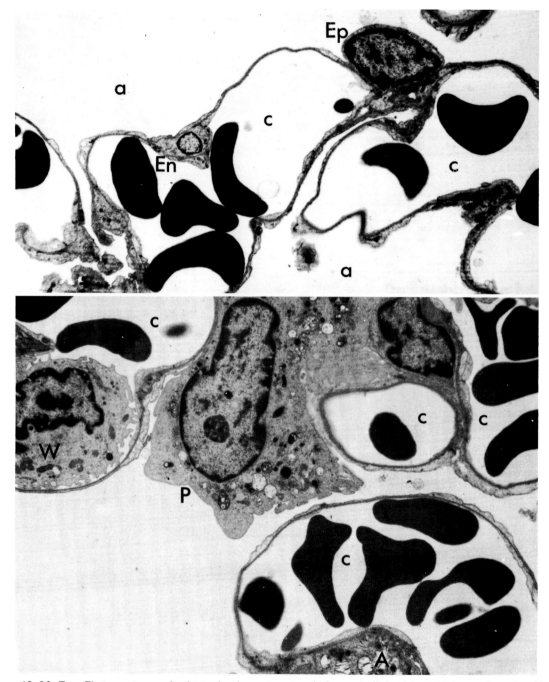

**Figure 12–26.** Top: *Electron micrograph of interalveolar septum, in which are capillaries (c) containing erythrocytes. Alveoli are indicated by "a." The two nuclei are of surface epithelial or type I (Ep) and endothelial (En) cells.* × 4200. Bottom: *This micrograph shows a white blood cell (W) in the lumen of one alveolar capillary, an alveolar phagocyte (P) with phagocytosed material, and part of an alveolar type II cell (A) containing lamellated bodies.* × 4500.

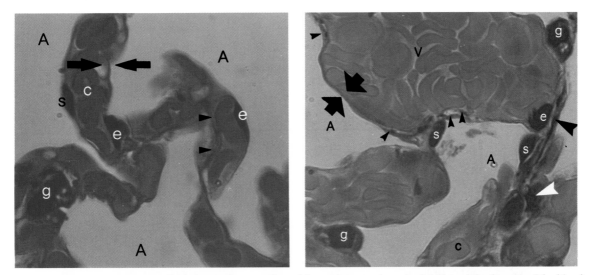

*Figure 12–27.* Interalveolar septa. Both figures show capillaries (c) containing erythrocytes (pink), and the thinness of the blood-air barrier (between arrows). Cell types identifiable are type I squamous alveolar cells (s) lining alveoli; type II alveolar cells (g) with vacuolated cytoplasm; and endothelial cells (e) lining capillaries. Small strands of elastic tissue (large arrowheads) are seen in interalveolar septa, and in the wall of the venule (V) (small arrowheads) in the right figure. "A" indicates alveoli. Methylene blue, basic fuchsin. Oil immersion.

involved in the repair of alveolar epithelium following injury.

Additionally, a few brush cells may be seen in alveolar epithelium, although they are not identified easily.

### INTERSTITIUM AND INTERALVEOLAR SEPTA

As already explained, between two layers of pulmonary epithelium lining adjacent alveoli is an interstitium, the whole forming an interalveolar septum. The interstitium is limited on each side by the basal laminae that underlie the alveolar epithelium, and this connective tissue space contains an amorphous ground substance in which cells and fibers are embedded. Cell types present include mast cells, monocytes, lymphocytes, and fibroblasts or *septal* cells. The most numerous are the septal cells that are responsible for the formation, repair, and maintenance of the connective tissue of the lung. They often are irregular in shape, lying as they do among the elastic and reticular fibers of the interstitium.

Much of the thickness of interalveolar septa is occupied by capillaries, lined by endothelial cells and supported by some pericytes. Capillaries also are limited by basal lamina. Endothelial cells lining the capillaries show dark flattened nuclei and attenuated cytoplasm and resemble surface epithelial (type I) cells, from which they can be distinguished by their relation to capillary blood spaces, which, of course, contain all blood cell types—erythrocytes, granulocytes, lymphocytes, and monocytes. Several of these cells are migratory and may lie outside capillaries in the interstitium or even pass through epithelium into alveolar spaces.

### ALVEOLAR MACROPHAGES

Alveolar macrophages (alveolar phagocytes, or "dust cells") are found not only in the interstitium of interalveolar septa but also on the alveolar surface and in the process of passing through the alveolar wall into the alveolar spaces (Fig. 12–30). The cells are quite large, 15 to 40 μm, often of irregular shape and with an irregular nucleus and a nucleolus. Cytoplasm may appear granular or vacuolated ("foamy"). In addition to the usual organelles, including a prominent Golgi appara-

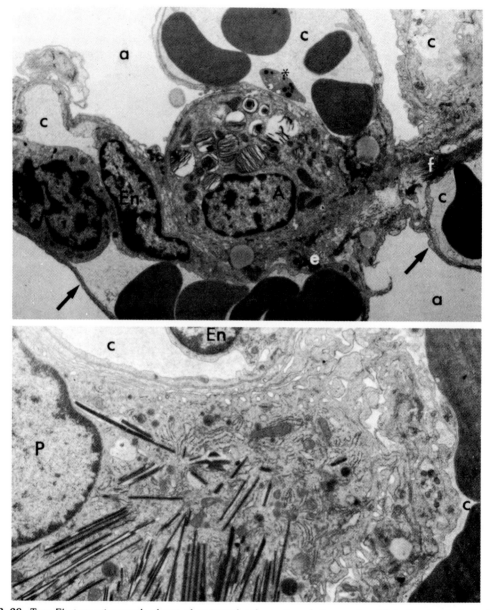

**Figure 12–28.** Top: *Electron micrograph of part of an interalveolar septum, between alveoli (a), showing both thick portions, containing a few collagen microfibrils (f) and small clumps of elastin (e), and thin portions where the blood-air barrier is thin with fusion of the basal laminae of endothelium and alveolar epithelium (arrows). In the septum are capillaries (c) containing erythrocytes and a platelet (asterisk). Also seen are an endothelial nucleus (En) and a type II alveolar cell (A) with its lamellated bodies.* × 5000. Bottom: *Part of an alveolar macrophage, or phagocyte (P), occupies most of the field, with numerous rod-like bodies in its cytoplasm. These probably are asbestos fibers.* × 8500.

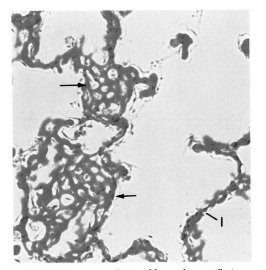

**Figure 12–29.** *Lung capillaries. Here, the capillaries were injected with red-colored gelatin via the pulmonary artery and this thick section demonstrates the rich vascularity in an interalveolar septum (I) and the close meshwork of the capillary net seen particularly well where two alveoli have been sectioned tangentially (arrows). Low power.*

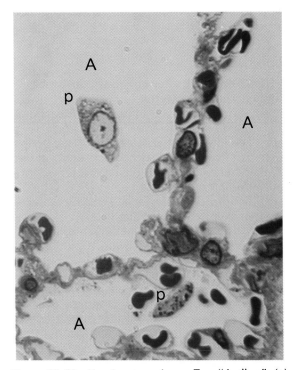

**Figure 12–30.** *Alveolar macrophages. Two "dust" cells (p) are seen, lying free in alveolar spaces (A). Each contains phagocytosed carbon particles. In addition to these alveolar macrophages, interalveolar septa contain numerous capillaries with erythrocytes (blue-black) in their lumina. Toluidine blue. High power.*

tus, the cytoplasm contains a wide variety of membrane-bound bodies that includes primary lysosomes, about 0.5 μm in diameter. These contain a wide range of hydrolytic enzymes. Some macrophages appear vacuolated owing to cytoplasmic lipid (which may be cholesterol), and others contain phagocytosed carbon. One type, the "siderophage" or "heart failure cell," is common when there is stasis of pulmonary blood flow and erythrocytes pass into the interstitium and alveoli (diapedesis). In such a situation, erythrocytes are phagocytosed by the macrophages, and thus, they contain hemosiderin. The macrophages also ingest and destroy bacteria.

Alveolar macrophages originate from stem cells in the bone marrow, being then transported as monocytes in the vascular system and later migrating to the interstitium. Some that lie in the connective tissue of interalveolar septa, in the pleura, and around the vessels and bronchial tubes are relatively static, but most migrate rapidly into alveolar spaces and thence to bronchioles and from there by ciliary action to the pharynx, being eventually eliminated in the saliva by swallowing or expectoration. The turnover rate is very

rapid, and large numbers of macrophages are cleared each hour.

## ALVEOLAR PORES

Even by light microscopy, and confirmed by electron microscopy, small deficiencies, or pores (of Kohn), are seen in interalveolar septa. They vary in size from 6 to 10 μm or more in diameter, lying in spaces between capillaries of the interalveolar septa, and there may be more than one in each septum between adjacent alveoli. Presumably, their function is to equalize pressure between alveoli, particularly those of different bronchioles, to permit collateral ventilation when one bronchiole is obstructed. Thus, even if a bronchiole is obstructed, the alveoli supplied by that bronchiole would not collapse (*atelectasis*), receiving air from adjacent alveoli through alveolar pores.

### BLOOD-AIR BARRIER

The blood-air barrier comprises the structures through which gaseous exchange occurs between air in alveoli and blood in pulmonary capillaries (Fig. 12–31). These are

1. The attenuated pulmonary surface epithelium with its surface fluid film containing *surfactant*, and underlain by its basal lamina.

2. The interstitial space.

3. The basal lamina of the capillary and its lining attenuated endothelium.

*Surfactant*, present in the thin film of fluid that lies over the alveolar epithelium, is produced by the type II alveolar cells (Fig. 12–32). It is a detergent material primarily composed of phosphatidylcholine, mainly dipalmitoyl lecithin. It mixes with water molecules to reduce their cohesiveness, thus diminishing the surface tension of alveolar fluid. In turn, this reduces the force necessary to inflate alveoli and facilitates breathing. Surfactant thus acts as an anticollapse factor and is especially important in the neonate. In lung development, maturation of type II cells occurs at about 24 weeks' gestation. If the amount of surfactant is insufficient, the infant (particularly a premature one) may suffer from the respiratory distress syndrome (hyaline membrane disease), with failure of alveoli to expand on inspiration and collapse of alveoli on expiration. There is a constant turnover of surfactant, new material being released and older material passing from the surface through squamous (type I) alveolar cells and eventually to lymphatics located around alveolar ducts and bronchioles. Some surfactant also is removed by macrophages.

As already indicated, the blood-air barrier varies in thickness. Indeed, in some regions (the *thin portions*), the alveolar wall is specialized for gaseous exchange; in others (the *thick portions*), the function is control of interstitial (tissue) fluid. In the thin regions, the basal laminae of alveolar epithelium and capillary endothelium fuse, and here the interstitium is absent. This arrangement, with a very thin blood-air barrier, obviously facilitates gaseous exchange. In thick regions, where the two basal laminae are separated by an interstitium containing some cells and fibers, there is space for the accumulation of tissue fluid. While fluid does not readily leave pulmonary capillaries, the osmotic pressure of blood usually exceeding a relatively low hydrostatic pressure, some fluid does accumulate in the interstitial space. This can

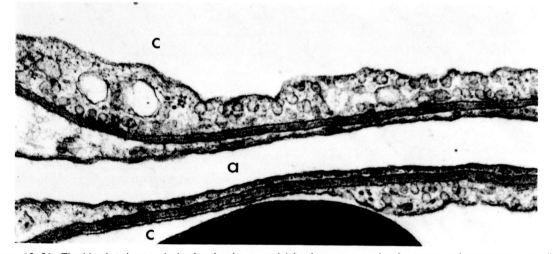

*Figure 12–31.* The blood-air barrier. A slender alveolar space (a) lies between two alveolar septa, each containing a capillary (c). In each case, a single fused basal lamina separates epithelium (type 1 cells) from endothelium, both greatly attenuated. These areas thus are "thin" portions of the blood-air barrier. Endothelial cytoplasm shows micropinocytotic vesicles. × 45,000.

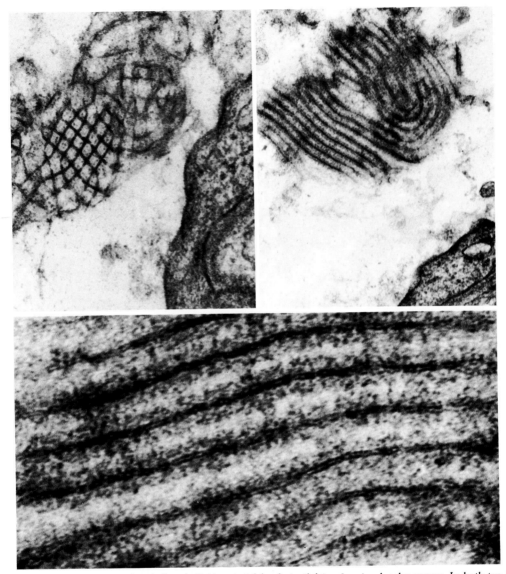

**Figure 12–32.** *Electron micrographs of phospholipid material (surfactant) lying free in alveolar spaces. In both top figures, a small part of a pulmonary surface epithelial cell appears at lower right. Top left and top right, × 42,000; bottom, × 114,000.*

become a problem in pulmonary edema, in which excess fluid accumulates and eventually enters alveolar spaces, thus restricting breathing capacity. This fluid is drained by the lymphatic system, although lymphatics are not present in interalveolar septa, commencing in the walls of alveolar ducts. Thus, in thick regions of the septum, certain quantities of fluid can accumulate (and eventually be drained via the lymphatic system) before entering alveolar spaces, with consequent restriction of gaseous exchange and respiratory distress of the patient.

### The Lung Lobule

The lung lobule, the structural unit of the lung, is pyramidal in shape, with a bronchiole entering at the apex that, usually, is directed toward the hilum (Fig. 12–33). Accompanying the bronchiole is a branch of the pulmonary artery carrying venous blood. Lobules are delineated poorly and incompletely by connective tissue and often are irregular in shape. Generally, they have a base and height both of 1 to 2 cm. Between lobules

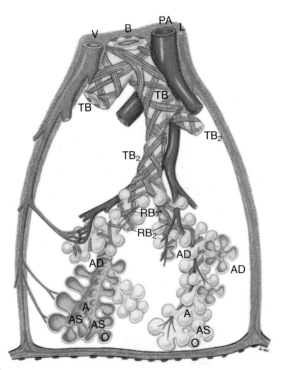

**Figure 12–33.** *Diagram of a lung lobule. It is pyramidal with the base (below) adjacent to visceral pleura (P) and the apex (above) with the bronchiole (B) and branch of the pulmonary artery (PA), the artery containing deoxygenated blood (blue). At the apex, they are joined by lymphatic capillaries (L, green) and the tributary of the pulmonary vein (V), carrying oxygenated blood (red). Pulmonary veins lie in sparse connective tissue of interlobular septa (gray), as do lymphatic vessels connecting pleural lymphatics with those running with the bronchial tree. The lobular bronchiole divides into two terminal bronchioles (TB), each further dividing (TB₂). In turn, these branch to become respiratory bronchioles (RB), which divide again (RB₂) before terminating in alveolar ducts (AD). The alveolar ducts branch before ending in atria (A), from which alveolar sacs (AS) and alveoli (O) arise. One alveolar duct is opened longitudinally to show its dependent alveoli (left), as also are others in transverse section (right).*

in poorly developed interlobular septa are pulmonary veins that, at the apex of the lobule, join the bronchiole and branch of the pulmonary artery. Lymphatic vessels run with pulmonary veins and communicate both with vessels in the pleura and with others around major vessels at the hilum. This relationship is important in the spread of carcinoma of the lung, in which cancerous cells may break through from lymphatics to adjoining pulmonary veins in interlobular septa, this infiltration to the systemic circulation then resulting in widespread metastases, for example, to bone.

Other units of structure in the lung have been described. A *lung acinus* is the tissue supplied by a terminal bronchiole, for example. It is a useful concept in that dichotomous branching is regular, relatively, as far down the bronchial tree as the terminal bronchiole, past which point it becomes less regular and less equal.

### Blood Vessels

The lung has a double blood supply, although the major arterial supply is via the *pulmonary arteries*. These vessels carry deoxygenated blood from the right ventricle and are elastic arteries of large caliber. Their branches accompany those of the bronchial tree as far as respiratory bronchioles, where terminal arterioles break up into a rich capillary plexus situated between alveoli in interalveolar septa. Other vessels leave branches of the pulmonary arteries to traverse lung tissue and terminate in the same capillary plexuses at the lung periphery. Venules from the plexuses, carrying oxygenated blood, join with others draining the pleura and travel in interlobular septa to join the companion arterioles at the apices of lobules.

In addition to this system of pulmonary arteries and veins, there also are *bronchial arteries* and *veins*. The arteries arise from the aorta and supply oxygenated blood to the tissues of bronchi and the connective tissue of the lung and pleura. There are communications between the two systems in that terminal branches of the bronchial arteries join pulmonary arteries via the capillary plexus, and most of the blood in the bronchial arteries returns in pulmonary veins. However, some blood is drained into bronchial veins, which are tributaries of the azygos system.

## Lymphatic Vessels

Two sets of lymphatic vessels are found in the lung, with infrequent interconnections. The *superficial*, or *pleural*, set lies in the pleura, with relatively large lymphatics demarcating lung lobules at the surface of the lung and smaller vessels within this meshwork. They often are blackened by inhaled carbon, particularly in city dwellers, and thus are visible to the naked eye. This set drains around the periphery of the lung to the hilum. The *deep*, or *pulmonary*, set runs with the bronchus, pulmonary artery, and vein. Those with the pulmonary vein commence in interlobular septa; those with the pulmonary artery and bronchi extend peripherally only to the alveolar ducts. All drain centrally to the hilum, where they communicate with efferent channels of the superficial set. Lymphatic nodules are prominent at the hilum and around the bifurcation of the trachea.

## Nerve Supply

Small nerve fibers can be found throughout the lung, particularly in the region of the hilum and related to major bronchi and large vessels. Those associated with the bronchial tree are from the pulmonary plexus, formed by branches of the vagus (parasympathetic, bronchoconstriction) and sympathetic (second to fourth thoracic ganglia, bronchodilation). Both sensory and motor nerves extend as far as terminal bronchioles, and recent studies suggest that nerve endings are found in alveolar ducts and interalveolar septa. These endings mostly are sensory, but some contain dense-cored vesicles and appear to terminate in relation to type II alveolar cells. The latter may account for the reported response of surfactant secretion following nervous stimulation.

Also present in lung are *neuroepithelial bodies*. They are found in the lining epithelium from bronchi to terminal bronchioles, usually at a bifurcation. The bodies are formed by supporting cells that resemble modified Clara cells and neurosecretory cells with small, dense granules situated in basal cytoplasm. Capillaries related to these bodies are lined by type II fenestrated endothelium. The granules of these cells contain serotonin and are released by exocytosis in response to hypoxia (deficiency of oxygen) or hypercapnia (excess of carbon dioxide), presumably into the capillaries, with consequent increase in alveolar capillary circulation and inspiratory effort. These chemoreceptors appear to have both afferent and efferent nerve fibers, and thus, they may be controlled or modified in their activities by the central nervous system.

## The Pleura

The *parietal* pleura lines the wall of the thoracic cavity, and the *visceral* pleura covers the surface of the lung, the two being continuous at the hilum. The pleura is formed by a thin layer of fibroconnective tissue with collagenous and elastic fibers and few cells (principally fibroblasts and macrophages), covered by a layer of mesothelium (Fig. 12–34). Within the connective tissue are numerous lymph and blood capillaries, and some small nerve fibers. The pleura is responsible for the secretion of a small amount of pleural (serous) fluid that permits friction-free movement between parietal and visceral layers.

## DEVELOPMENTAL ORIGIN

The respiratory system originates in the embryo as a ventral outgrowth from the floor of the primitive pharynx, the anterior part of the foregut. This outgrowth passes inferiorly and divides into right and left bronchial buds, each of which later undergoes repeated dichotomous branchings. The primary outgrowth becomes the trachea, with the larynx developing around its origin from the foregut. Each bronchial bud becomes a main (primary) bronchus, and the further orders of branchings the smaller bronchi, bronchioles, and terminal alveoli. Thus, the entire system has a lining that is of endodermal origin, being derived from the foregut lining. Mesoderm forms the accessory coats of the system (e.g., connective tissue, cartilage, and muscle). Initially, respiratory tissue of the lung has a gland-like appearance of epithelium-lined alveoli embedded in mesoderm, and expansion of alveoli does not occur until birth (Figs. 12–35 and 12–36).

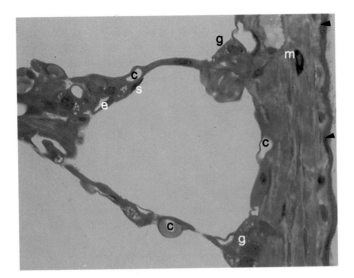

*Figure 12–34.* Pleura. Flattened, dark-staining nuclei (arrowheads) of mesothelial cells of the visceral pleura (right) are supported by fibroelastic connective tissue, in which a mast cell (m) is seen. Two interalveolar septa show capillaries (c) containing erythrocytes, type II alveolar cells (g) with vacuolated cytoplasm, a type I squamous alveolar cell (s), and an endothelial nucleus (e) of a cell lining a capillary. Methylene blue, azure A, basic fuchsin. High power.

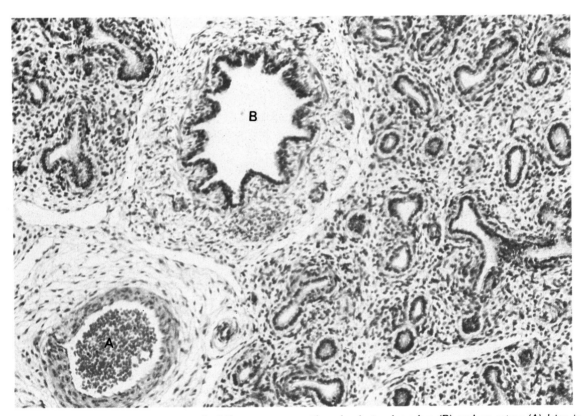

*Figure 12–35.* Fetal lung. This shows a gland-like appearance with a developing bronchus (B) and an artery (A) lying in mesenchyme with numerous endoderm-lined terminal branches that eventually will form alveoli. Hematoxylin, phloxine, safranin. Low power.

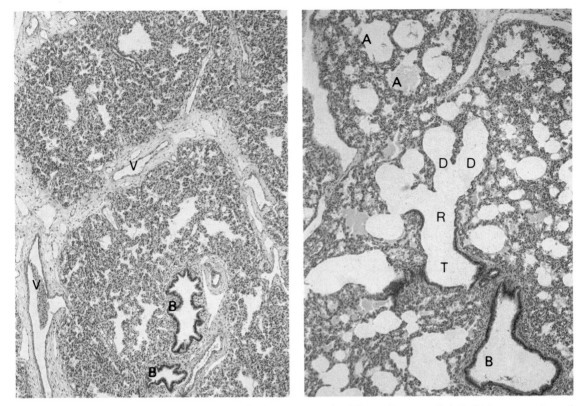

**Figure 12–36.** The lung at birth. Left: Until birth, the lung remains gland-like and unexpanded. At birth, as seen here, the respiratory tissue occupies much of the field and is unexpanded. The lobular nature of the lung at this stage is well seen, with connective tissue "septa" containing tributaries of the portal vein (V) surrounding a lobule that contains two large bronchioles (B) lined by cuboidal epithelium. Right: With inspiration at birth, dilation of respiratory passages occurs. Seen here are a large bronchiole (B), a terminal bronchiole (T), respiratory bronchiole (R), alveolar ducts (D), and alveoli (A), all expanded by respiration, although dilation is not yet complete. H and E. Low power.

## FUNCTION OF THE RESPIRATORY SYSTEM

As stated previously, the main function of the respiratory system is to provide for gaseous exchange. Oxygen in dissolved form diffuses from alveoli through the blood-air barrier to the blood, and carbon dioxide passes in the reverse direction. Essential to the process, however, is the function of the conducting portion of the system in filtering, washing, humidifying, and warming or cooling the inspired air. Additionally, the process involves a loss of water in the expired air that can be regarded as an excretory function. The olfactory mucosa, as the olfactory organ, and the larynx, for phonation, are also accessory parts of the system.

## Summary Table 12–1. The Respiratory System

| Portion | Organ | Lining | Cartilage | Muscle | Glands | Goblet Cells | Special | Additional Function |
|---|---|---|---|---|---|---|---|---|
| CONDUCTING | Nose, vestibule | Skin with hairs | + | Striated (external) | Sebaceous; sweat | No | Hairs stiff | Coarse filter |
| | Nasal cavity, respiratory portion | Pseudostratified ciliated columnar ("respiratory") | +, and bone | No | + | + | Mucoperiosteum, erectile tissue, conchae | |
| | Nasal cavity, olfactory portion | Olfactory | Bone | No | Bowman's | No | Sensory (bipolar) cells | Smell |
| | Nasopharynx | "Respiratory" or stratified squamous | No | Striated | + | + | Lymphatic tissue | |
| | Larynx | Respiratory | + | Striated | + | + | Vocal cords, taste buds | Phonation |
| | Trachea | Respiratory | C shape | Smooth (posteriorly) | + | + | Lymphatic tissue | |
| | Extrapulmonary bronchi | Respiratory | C shape | Smooth (posteriorly) | + | + | Like trachea | |
| | Intrapulmonary bronchi | Respiratory | Irregular, circular | Smooth (internal) | + | + | Ciliated columnar in smaller bronchi | |
| | Large bronchiole | Ciliated columnar | No | Smooth (prominent) | No | Few | Clara cells, 1 mm or less | |
| | Small bronchiole | Ciliated columnar | No | Smooth (prominent) | No | No | Clara cells, 0.3 mm or less | |
| | Terminal bronchiole | Cuboidal | No | Smooth ++ | No | No | Patches of cilia only, Clara cells | |
| RESPIRATORY | Respiratory bronchiole | Cuboidal or squamous | No | ++ | No | No | 0.2 mm or less, Clara cells | Surfactant |
| | Alveolar ducts | Squamous (with pores) | No | At orifices | No | No | Wall is sieve-like | Surfactant |
| | Alveolar sacs and alveoli | Squamous (with pores) | No | At orifices | No | No | "Share" wall as interalveolar septum | Surfactant |

# The Urinary System

## INTRODUCTION

The urinary system consists of the two *kidneys* and their *ureters*, the *urinary bladder*, and the *urethra*. The kidneys are essential for life, functioning in excretion to produce *urine*, which passes down the ureters to the bladder for temporary storage and, eventually, periodic evacuation via the urethra. Urine contains metabolic waste products resulting from food breakdown by the body, particularly nitrogenous compounds such as urea, creatinine, and uric acid, and other foreign substances eliminated through the kidneys. The kidneys also regulate water and electrolyte balance, being the mechanism for excretion of excess water and electrolytes, and, in so doing, maintain the acid-base balance, a process of osmoregulation. Excretion and urine formation involve an ultrafiltration of blood plasma to form a filtrate, which later is modified by selective reabsorption of most of the filtered water and other small molecules and by secretion. The main function of the excretory passages of the ureters, bladder, and urethra is to convey the urine to the exterior, although the male urethra also serves as the pathway for seminal discharge.

The kidneys, in addition to their excretory function, also produce *renin*, a hormone that functions in the regulation of blood pressure, and *erythropoietin*, which is concerned in the regulation of red blood cell formation.

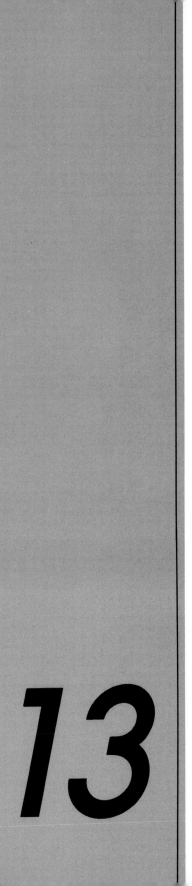

*13*

The kidney can be considered as a compound tubular gland that secretes urine. Each kidney contains a large number of *uriniferous tubules,* each consisting of two parts. The *nephron,* which is some 30 to 40 mm long and is the functional unit, and the *collecting tubule,* about 20 mm long, together form a continuous tubule, although they have different developmental origins. The kidney has an extremely rich blood supply.

## THE KIDNEY

The human kidneys are bean-shaped, about 10 to 12 cm in length, 5 cm wide, and 4 to 5 cm thick, lying behind peritoneum in the posterior region of the upper abdomen, one on each side of the upper lumbar vertebrae (Fig. 13–1). Each is enclosed in a thin fibroconnective tissue capsule that may be stripped easily from the underlying parenchyma, an indication that no septa are present within the kidney.

On the medial aspect is a depression, the *hilum,* from which a space called the *renal sinus* extends into the substance of the kidney. All blood vessels to and from the kidney enter and leave through the hilus, and the excretory duct, the ureter, leaves from the hilus. Within the hilus and the sinus, the upper part of the ureter is expanded as the *pelvis,* subdivided into large and small cups, the *major* and *minor calyces.* Although the pelvis and the calyces together with blood vessels lie within the hilum and sinus, they do not fully occupy the space, and this is filled with areolar-adipose connective tissue.

Usually, there are two major and eight to twelve minor calyces, each minor calyx enveloping a conical protrusion of renal substance called a *papilla.* The apex of each papilla is perforated by the openings of 10 to 25 *collecting ducts,* this being called the *area cribrosa.* The collecting ducts are the terminal segments of the uriniferous tubules, passing urine from the kidney into minor calyces of the renal pelvis. Vertical hemisection of the kidney demonstrates that each papilla is the tip of a pyramidal area of kidney substance that extends from the hilum toward the capsule and that, in the fresh kidney, is pale and radially striated. This area is a *medullary pyramid,* and its striated appearance is due to the presence of straight tubules and parallel blood vessels. The base, or peripheral part, of each pyramid does not show a clear demarcation from the dark, brownish, granular *cortex* of the kidney, since pale, striated, medullary substance extends from the base of the pyramid into the cortex as thin, radially oriented rays, the *medullary rays* (Fig. 13–2). These rays contain bundles of tubules that extend from the pyramid into the cortex. Between adjacent medullary pyramids, cortical material extends centrally as the *renal columns* (of Bertin). The granular appearance of cortical material is accounted for by the presence of spherical bodies, the *renal corpuscles,* and convoluted uriniferous tubules; in any plane of section, the convoluted tubules show ovoid or circular profiles.

In summary, while the bases of the medullary pyramids indicate a line of demarcation between the outer cortex and the inner medulla, it must be appreciated that cortical substance as the renal columns extends centrally into the medulla, and medullary rays extend peripherally into the cortex and are considered part of it. Each pyramid with its associated overlying cortex is regarded as a *lobe;* hence the terms *multipyramidal* or *multilobar* kidney. Some of the lower mammals (e.g., the rat and rabbit) have a unilobar or unipyramidal kidney (Fig. 13–3). In the adult human, the kidney surface is smooth, and the lobes are not demarcated, but in the fetus and the newborn, the kidney surface is irregular with grooves between lobes and is described as *lobated.* Later in development, the grooves disappear, leaving a continuous smooth contour. A *lobule* of the kidney is a smaller, functional unit comprising a medullary ray (in the cortex); the kidney units, or *nephrons,* associated with and draining into it;

*Figure 13–1.* Top: *Diagram of the human kidney, sectioned vertically, with a single nephron (right) showing its component parts and blood supply.* Bottom: *Diagram shows zones of the kidney in relation to segments of outer cortical (A) and juxtamedullary (B) nephrons.* Note: *The outer cortical nephron has a loop of Henle barely penetrating the inner stripe of the medulla with a short, thin segment (black) in the descending limb, whereas the juxtamedullary nephron penetrates deeply into the inner zone and has an extensive thin segment in both descending and ascending arms of the loop. PCT, proximal convoluted tubule; DCT, distal convoluted tubule; CD, collecting duct.*

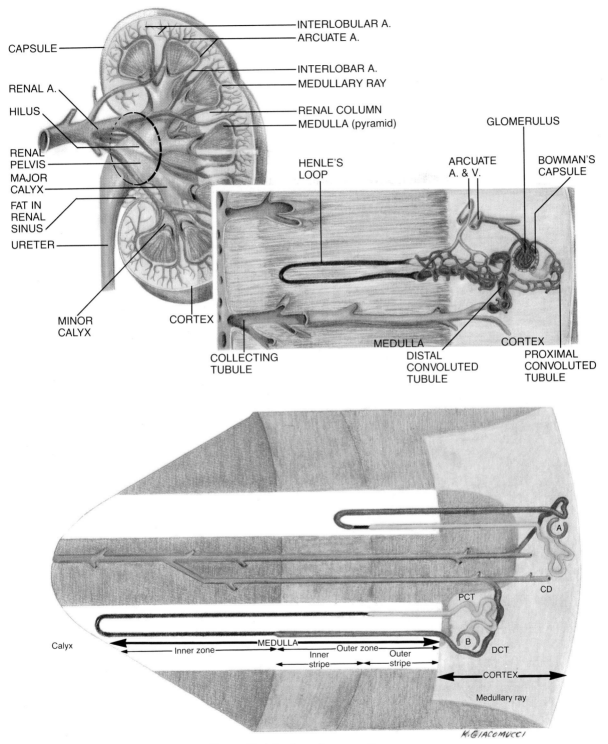

CAPSULE

INTERLOBULAR A.
ARCUATE A.

INTERLOBAR A.
MEDULLARY RAY

RENAL A.
HILUS

RENAL COLUMN
MEDULLA (pyramid)

GLOMERULUS

ARCUATE
A. & V.

BOWMAN'S
CAPSULE

RENAL
PELVIS

HENLE'S
LOOP

MAJOR
CALYX

FAT IN
RENAL
SINUS

URETER

MINOR
CALYX

CORTEX

COLLECTING
TUBULE

MEDULLA
DISTAL
CONVOLUTED
TUBULE

CORTEX

PROXIMAL
CONVOLUTED
TUBULE

A

CD

PCT

Calyx

MEDULLA
Inner zone

Outer zone
Inner
stripe

Outer
stripe

B

DCT

CORTEX

Medullary ray

K. GIACOMUCCI

*Figure 13–1* See legend on opposite page

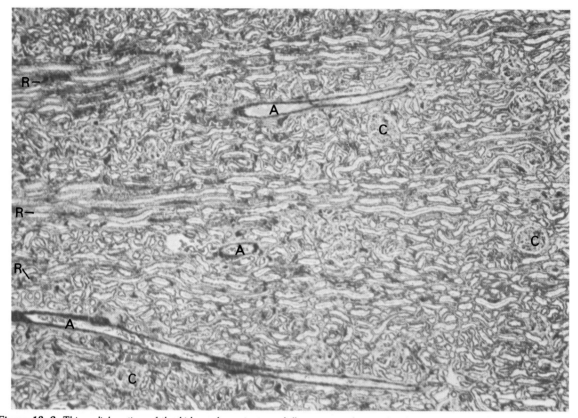

*Figure 13–2.* This radial section of the kidney shows juxtamedullary cortex, that is, the deeper portion of the cortex, with the medulla lying to the left but out of the picture. Passing from the medulla into the cortex are three medullary rays (R), formed by radially oriented collecting tubules, here cut nearly longitudinally. These medullary rays lie at the centers of renal lobules, with lobules demarcated by interlobular arteries (A) also cut mainly longitudinally (top and bottom). In each lobule, the cortex is formed by many nephrons, with their renal corpuscles (C) appearing as larger spherical profiles and their coiled tubules cut in all planes of section, mainly transverse and oblique. Thus, a lobule has a medullary ray formed by collecting tubules at its center, with several interlobular arteries at its periphery, and is composed of the nephrons that drain into the collecting tubules at its center. Mallory. Low power.

and the continuation of the ray in a medullary pyramid. In the cortex, lobules are outlined, but not demarcated, by radially oriented *interlobular* (cortical) blood vessels, while the ray lies at the center, or axis, of the lobule. However, there is no delineation in the medulla. In the medulla, the many specialized segments of the renal (uniferous) tubules are located at specific levels, and this is reflected in distinguishable zones that differ slightly in color, density, and pattern. Thus, there are *inner* and *outer zones* of the medulla, with the outer zone further subdivided into a darker and thicker *inner band*, or *stripe*, and a lighter and thinner *outer band*.

These patterns seen on the cut surface of a normal kidney will be understood better after knowledge of the uniferous tubules is acquired, but essential to that knowledge is an understanding of the blood supply of the kidney.

## Blood Supply of the Kidney

In that the kidneys clean the blood of metabolic waste products, they have a rich blood supply (Fig. 13–4). Each kidney receives a direct branch of the abdominal aorta, the *renal artery*, which enters the hilus, where it usually divides into three

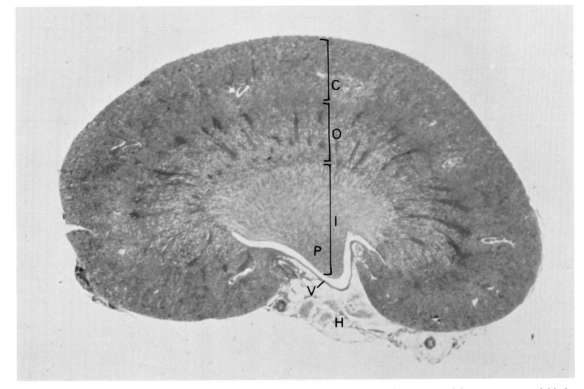

***Figure 13–3.*** *This section is of rabbit kidney, which differs from that of humans in that it is a unilobar or unipyramidal kidney. The hilum (H) lies below with the lining of the pelvis (V), and protruding into it is the renal papilla of the single medullary pyramid (P). The medulla is pale-staining, appears to be radially striated, and is divided into outer (O) and inner (I) zones. The cortex (C) is darker-staining and appears granular. The thin renal capsule is not apparent. H and E. Low power.*

main branches. Two of these pass anterior and one passes posterior to the renal pelvis, with each branch sometimes dividing further. There is little or no anastomosis between these main branches, each supplying three or four medullary pyramids and their associated cortical substance. This area of supply is termed a *renule,* and this arrangement permits surgical removal of one or more renules with preservation of the remainder of the kidney, an operation termed heminephrectomy.

In the adipose tissue of the renal sinus, around the hilum, each major branch divides into smaller *interlobar* arteries that ascend in a column of Bertin between adjacent medullary pyramids, usually eccentrically placed to one side. Interlobar arteries also are found between superior and inferior pyramids and the kidney surface, at upper and lower poles of the kidney. On reaching the base of the medullary pyramids, the interlobar arteries break up into several branches that leave the parent vessel, almost at right angles, to arch over the bases of the pyramids, between cortex and medulla and running parallel to the surface of the kidney. These are the *arcuate arteries,* and from them branch small *interlobular* arteries, passing radially to the surface and located between lobules. Their peripheral terminations reach and supply the capillary bed of the renal capsule.

As they course toward the surface, interlobular arteries give off numerous side branches, the *afferent arterioles,* to supply glomeruli of the renal corpuscles, one arteriole passing to each glomerulus (Fig. 13–5). A single afferent arteriole may branch directly from an interlobular artery, or several may originate from a short common stem, this stem being termed an *intralobular artery.* In

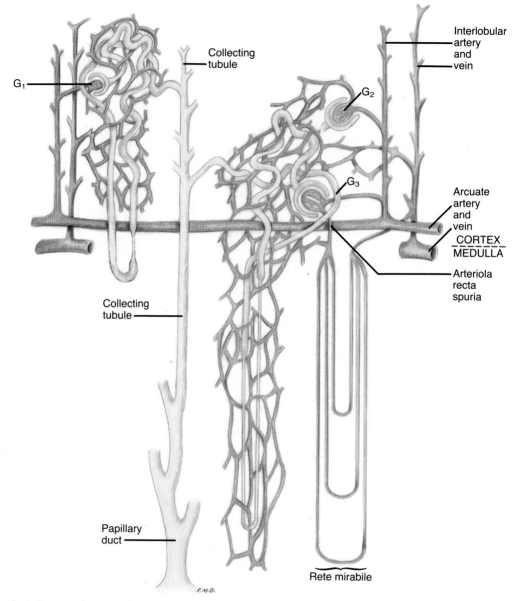

**Figure 13–4.** *Diagram illustrating the blood supply to the kidney. Three glomeruli (G) are shown, of which a cortical (G₁) and a juxtamedullary (G₃) are illustrated with their entire nephrons, a midcortical (G₂) with only the renal corpuscle. Efferent arterioles of cortical glomeruli break up into the cortical, peritubular plexus of capillaries, and eventually this plexus drains to interlobular veins. The efferent arteriole of the juxtamedullary glomerulus (G₃) passes into the medulla as an arteriola recta spuria that branches to form a bundle of vasa recta with recurrent venules, the whole being the rete mirabile, which functions in countercurrent exchange.*

glomeruli, afferent arterioles break up into a tuft of glomerular capillaries that drain not into a venule but into an *efferent arteriole*. Thus, in general, blood passes through glomeruli first before supplying the remainder of the kidney, the glomeruli being the site of filtration of blood plasma. The efferent glomerular arterioles pass from glomeruli to supply the majority of the other portions of the same nephrons, but the arrangement differs between the efferent arterioles leav-

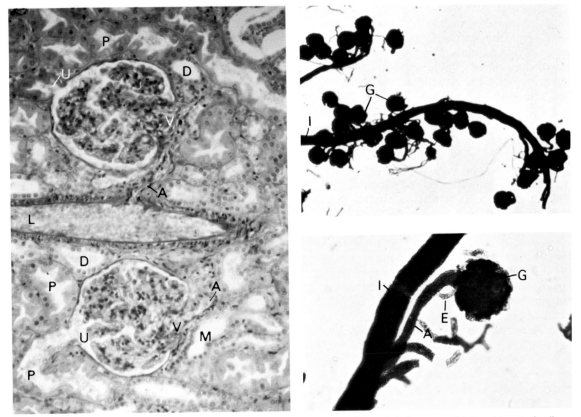

**Figure 13–5.** *Kidney, renal corpuscles, and glomeruli. Left: A portion of an interlobular artery (L) is cut longitudinally, and branching from it on each side is an afferent arteriole (A). Each afferent arteriole passes to the vascular pole (V) of a renal corpuscle to form a glomerulus. Each corpuscle also shows a urinary pole (U) where the thin squamous parietal epithelium of Bowman's capsule changes abruptly to the simple high cuboidal or low columnar epithelium lining the proximal convoluted tubule. The remainder of the field is occupied by profiles of proximal (P) and distal (D) convoluted tubules, and one distal tubule reaches the vascular pole of a corpuscle at a macula densa (M). Masson. Medium power. Right: In these preparations, the renal artery was injected with colored colloidin, and a whole mount prepared. At low power (top), an interlobular artery (I) shows many branches, the afferent arterioles, passing to glomeruli (G), and at medium power (below) an afferent arteriole (A) branches from an interlobular artery (I) to form a glomerulus (G), with an efferent arteriole (E) leaving the glomerulus.*

ing cortical nephrons and those leaving (deeper) juxtamedullary nephrons. Those from cortical nephrons are of relatively small diameter and break up into *peritubular capillary networks* surrounding and supplying their own local uriniferous tubules. Efferent arterioles from juxtamedullary nephrons are of large diameter, and they pass into the medulla as *arteriolae rectae spuriae* (false, straight arterioles). (Arteriolae rectae verae, or true straight arterioles, is a term used to describe direct branches of arcuate and interlobular arteries that bypass glomerular capillaries and pass directly into the medulla. Their presence in the normal kidney is questioned, and probably they are so few as to be of no functional significance.) These arteriolae rectae spuriae, in the medulla, break up into bundles of thin-walled vessels called *vasa recta*. These are slightly larger than capillaries, and, together with the efferent arterioles of the juxtamedullary nephrons, they supply branches to the intertubular capillary network in the medulla.

In the medulla, the vasa recta lie in bundles, parallel to the loops of Henle; at various levels, they take hairpin loops (as do the loops of Henle) and run back toward the corticomedullary junction, with the arterial descending and venous ascending limbs closely approximated and parallel. As descending vessels successively loop and turn back toward the cortex, the bundle becomes smaller, and the whole is termed a *vascular bundle*, or *rete mirabile*. Not only are the arterial limbs of the rete of slightly smaller caliber than the venous limbs, but also the arterial limbs show a continuous lining endothelium (type I), compared with the endothelium of the venous limbs, which is fenestrated (type II). Their structure and close proximity permits rapid interchange of diffusible substances between the descending and ascending limbs. The vasa recta, then, function as an efficient countercurrent exchange system.

Venous drainage is similar to arterial supply, except, of course, that there is no venous component in the glomerulus and its arterioles. In the outer cortex, capillaries collect into small *stellate veins* that join in a star-like pattern to form *interlobular veins*. These pass toward the medulla, lying adjacent to interlobular arteries and receiving tributaries from all levels of the cortex, and drain to *arcuate veins*. The arcuate veins also receive tributaries ascending from the medullary pyramids, and they pass to *interlobar veins* that, in the hilus, unite to form the *renal veins*. Renal veins drain to the inferior vena cava.

Physiologically, blood flow to the cortex is much greater than that to the medulla but may be diminished greatly by sympathetic nerve stimulation. Under stress conditions, blood flow to the cortex virtually ceases, and it becomes pale and ischemic, blood flow being diverted through juxtamedullary nephrons and thence to vasa recta and back to the renal veins by interlobular and arcuate veins.

### The Nephron

The nephron is the functional, tubular unit of the kidney. There are one to two million nephrons in each kidney. Each is simply a long, epithelium-lined tube that starts blindly and terminates by joining an excretory duct, but the nephrons are so tortuous and so intermingled that histological sections of the kidney give no clear idea of their form. This can be achieved by reconstructions from serial sections or by teasing out individual nephrons from kidneys after maceration. Each nephron consists of several segments of different

structure and different function, with each segment located in a definite position in the cortex or medulla.

The first part of the nephron, located in the cortex, is the *renal corpuscle* (of Malpighi), and it consists of two parts. The proximal end of the nephron is blind and dilated into a thin-walled, cup-like expansion called *Bowman's capsule*, which is invaginated by a globular tuft of capillaries called the *glomerulus*. It is here that an ultrafiltrate of plasma leaves the blood and then passes down the uriniferous tubule, where it is altered to form urine both by secretions from tubule cells and by reabsorption of many of its filtered products. Each renal corpuscle has a *vascular pole*, where afferent and efferent arterioles enter and leave the glomerulus, and a *urinary pole*, where the slit-like cavity of Bowman's capsule continues into the lumen of the next segment of the nephron, the *proximal tubule* (Fig. 13–6). This segment has, first, a long, convoluted part followed by a shorter straight part that, in turn, continues into a *thin segment* that passes into straight and convoluted parts of the *distal tubule*. The convoluted part of the proximal tubule (the *proximal convoluted tubule*) and the convoluted part of the distal tubule (the *distal convoluted tubule*) both lie adjacent to their renal corpuscle in the cortex (Fig. 13–7). The remainder of the nephron between them (i.e., the straight part of the proximal tubule, the thin segment, and the straight part of the distal tubule) forms a *loop of Henle* that lies in a medullary ray and extends for a varying distance into the medulla. The loop has radially oriented descending and ascending limbs that are parallel to each other and are connected by a sharp bend.

The length of the loop of Henle and the lengths of the various segments that form it vary with the position of the renal corpuscle in the cortex. Based on the length of the loop of Henle, two types of nephrons are recognized.

1. *Short (cortical) nephrons* are those whose renal corpuscles lie in the outer (subcapsular) part of the cortex. They have short loops of Henle with short thin segments in the descending limbs, the loops extending for only a small distance into the outer zone of the medulla.

2. *Long (juxtamedullary) nephrons* with renal corpuscles in the deep region of the cortex have

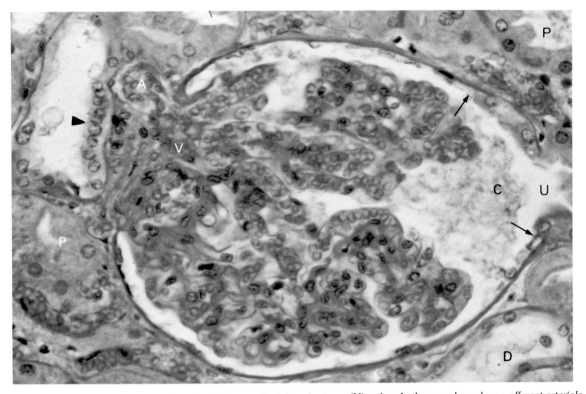

**Figure 13–6.** *This renal corpuscle shows both the vascular (V) and urinary (U) poles. At the vascular pole, an afferent arteriole (A) breaks up into glomerular capillaries filled with erythrocytes (orange), and adjacent to the afferent arteriole is a macula densa (arrowhead) of the distal tubule. In the glomerulus, nuclei are of endothelial cells and of visceral epithelial cells or podocytes, with thin squamous (parietal) epithelium of Bowman's capsule changing abruptly at the arrows to the cuboidal epithelium of the proximal convoluted tubule. The capsular space (C) between visceral and parietal epithelia clearly is continuous with the lumen of the proximal convoluted tubule at the urinary pole. Also seen are proximal (P) and distal (D) convoluted tubules and intertubular capillaries filled with erythrocytes. Masson. High power.*

long loops of Henle with long descending and ascending limbs. Extensive thin segments lie in both descending and ascending limbs, and the loops penetrate deeply into the inner zone of the medulla.

The short type outnumbers the long type. Midcortical nephrons show features intermediate between the long and the short types. As described already, the efferent glomerular arterioles differ significantly in their arrangement in the two types of nephrons. This variation in nephrons accounts for the zonation in the medulla, as illustrated in Figure 13–1 (bottom).

The distal convoluted tubules, the terminal parts of the nephrons, are joined to the collecting duct system. A short connecting segment (the arched collecting tubule) passes to a straight collecting tubule (which lies in a medullary ray), and this passes radially to terminate in a papillary duct (of Bellini) that finally opens into a minor calyx through an area cribrosa.

**RENAL CORPUSCLE**

Bowman's capsule acquires a cup shape that has a double wall by invagination of the glomerular tuft of capillaries into what, originally, was a blind terminal expansion of the nephron. Thus, there is a *parietal* layer of epithelium that, at the vascular pole, is continuous with a *visceral* epithelium, which lies closely applied to the glomerular capillaries. Between the two layers is a slender

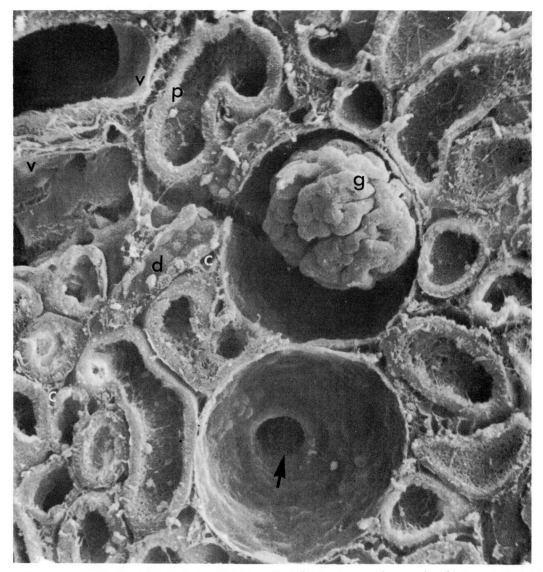

**Figure 13–7.** *Scanning electron micrograph of renal cortex of rat showing two renal corpuscles, the top one containing a glomerulus (g), the lower showing parietal epithelium of Bowman's capsule with a urinary pole (arrow) opening to a proximal convoluted tubule. Proximal (p) and distal (d) convoluted tubules, intertubular capillaries (c), and major blood vessels (v) are seen also. × 750. (Courtesy of Dr. P. M. Andrews.)*

space, the *capsular space*, that at the urinary pole is continuous with the lumen of the proximal convoluted tubule. Here, the parietal layer of Bowman's capsule is continuous with the epithelium of the proximal convoluted tubule.

Renal corpuscles are roughly spherical and vary from 150 to 250 μm in diameter, the juxtamed-

ullary corpuscles being much larger than the cortical ones. The larger, juxtamedullary corpuscles are the first to differentiate during development.

The *parietal layer* of Bowman's capsule is a simple squamous epithelium with nuclei that protrude slightly into the capsular space. These cells show few organelles. At the urinary pole, cell height increases over four or five cells from squamous to low columnar, to become continuous with the lining epithelium of the proximal convoluted tubule.

The *visceral layer* closely invests glomerular capillaries, with nuclei on the capsular side of the basal laminae of the capillaries, but the cells are greatly modified and do not form a complete sheet. The cells are called *podocytes* and are basically stellate in form, with their cell bodies rarely in contact with the basal lamina but separated by a space of 1 to 2 μm (Fig. 13–8). From the cell body, several radiating *major, or primary, processes* extend like the tentacles of an octopus or the limbs of a starfish toward one or more capillary loops, and from these arise numerous *secondary processes, or pedicels,* that attach to the outer, capsular surface of capillary basal laminae. Pedicels of adjacent podocytes and podocytic processes interdigitate in a complex manner, often with the major processes of one podocyte overlying primary processes and pedicels of a neighboring podocyte. Between pedicels is an extensive system of clefts, or intercellular spaces, called *filtration slits* or *slit pores*. This arrangement, whereby much of the capsular surface of glomerular capillaries is covered by interdigitating pedicels between which are filtration slits, provides a large area for filtration, as all slits eventually drain to the capsular space and thus into the lumen of the proximal convoluted tubule. The complexity of the arrangement is demonstrated well by scanning electron microscopy (Figs. 13–9 and 13–10).

Electron microscopy demonstrates that podocyte nuclei often are irregular in outline with deep infoldings and that in the cytoplasm adjacent to the nucleus is a well-formed Golgi apparatus, cisternae of granular endoplasmic reticulum, and some free ribosomes. Cytoplasmic filaments and microtubules are numerous, not only in the perikaryon but also extending into primary and secondary processes. As pedicels extend to the basal lamina of a capillary, they are separated by the filtration slits, about 25 nm wide. However, ad-

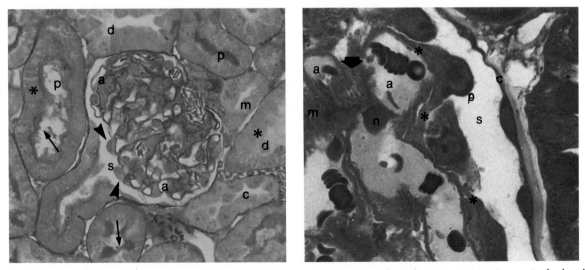

*Figure 13–8.* Renal corpuscle. Left: *This stain colors polysaccharides magenta-pink, and positive staining is seen in the basal laminae of the glomerular capillaries (a) (some of which contain green-stained erythrocytes), in basal laminae around tubules, and in the brush border of proximal convoluted tubules (the glycocalyx, arrows). In the renal corpuscle, nuclei of podocytes (arrowheads) lie external to capillary basal laminae adjacent to the capsular space (s), which is continuous with the lumen of the proximal convoluted tubule. Both proximal (p) and distal (d) convoluted tubules show a faint basal striation (asterisk), and the macula densa (m) and a collecting tubule (c) also are seen. PAS, light green. High power. Right: The parietal (capsular) epithelium (c) of the corpuscle is separated by the capsular space (s) from podocytes (p) of the visceral epithelium. Major processes of podocytes (asterisks) are seen and interdigitate (arrow) between glomerular capillaries (a) containing erythrocytes. A nucleus (n) of an endothelial cell is seen: A possible mesangial cell nucleus (m) also is present. Methylene blue, basic fuchsin. Oil immersion.*

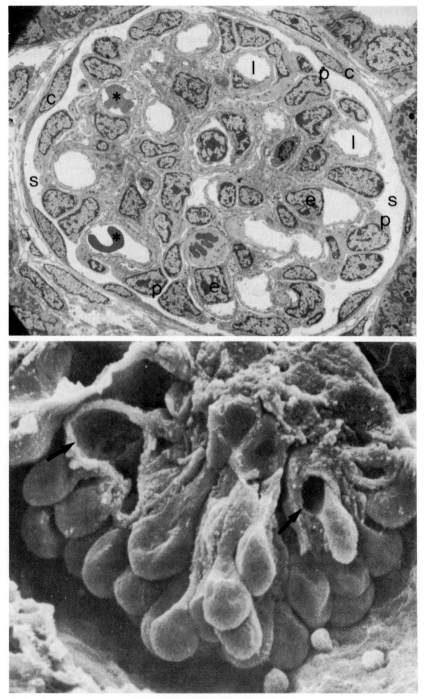

***Figure 13–9.*** *Renal glomerulus. Top: This electron micrograph shows a renal corpuscle with its parietal (capsular) squamous epithelium (c), the capsular space (s), and glomerular capillary lumina (l), some containing erythrocytes (asterisks). Podocytes (p) or visceral epithelium lies external to the capillaries, endothelium (e) lines the capillaries. × c. 2000. Bottom: This SEM shows the glomerulus in three dimensions, with a few capillary loops cut open (arrows). × c. 2500. (Courtesy of Professor M. Miyoshi.)*

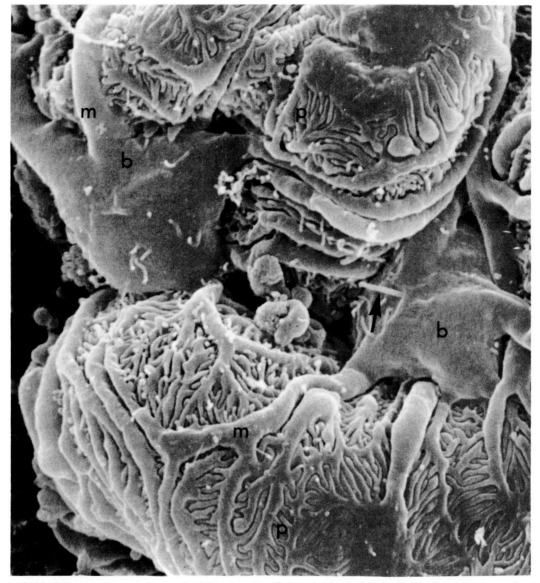

**Figure 13–10.** *Scanning electron micrograph of the visceral epithelium (podocytes) of monkey kidney, showing podocyte cell bodies (b), one with a single cilium (arrow), major processes (m), and pedicels (p). × 7000. (Courtesy of Dr. P. M. Andrews.)*

jacent to the basal lamina, the outer leaflets of the plasma membranes of adjacent pedicels are connected by thin membranes, the *slit membranes*, only 5 to 6 nm thick. These membranes are considered to be similar to the diaphragms closing pores in fenestrated (type II) endothelium. The plasmalemma of pedicels has a prominent glycocalyx containing sialic acid.

The *basal lamina* is about 0.15 to 0.3 μm thick, lying between podocytes and their processes externally and endothelium internally. It shows three zones of varying electron density. Centrally is the electron-dense *lamina densa*, about 0.1 μm thick, with, on each side, the more electron-lucent *lamina rara externa* and *lamina rara interna*. The lamina densa contains type IV collagen, which

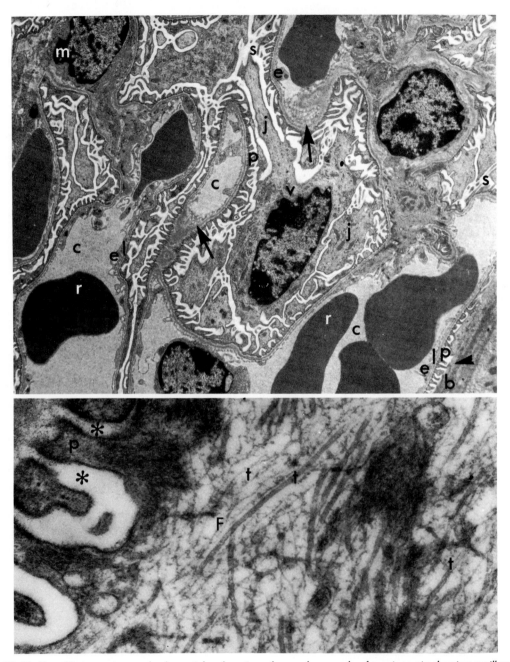

**Figure 13–11.** Top: *Electron micrograph of a peripheral portion of a renal corpuscle of a guinea pig showing capillary lumina (c) containing erythrocytes (r), endothelium (e) showing pores or fenestrae where cut tangentially (arrows), basal laminae ("lamina densa," l), podocytes (v) and their major processes (j) and pedicels (p), a mesangial cell (m), and capsular (urinary) space (s). Parietal epithelium (arrowhead) and the basal lamina (b) of Bowman's capsule are seen at lower right.* × 7000. Bottom: *Part of a major process of podocyte showing microtubules (t) and cytoplasmic filaments (F), with pedicels (p) at left and filtration slits (asterisks) between them.* × 50,000.

acts as a physical filter, and glycosaminoglycans rich in heparan sulfate. The basal lamina is strongly anionic and probably is formed mainly by podocytes with perhaps a contribution from endothelium.

Internal to the basal lamina, the *endothelium* of the glomerular capillaries is greatly attenuated, with numerous pores or fenestrae about 80 nm in diameter (Fig. 13–11). These pores are enclosed by diaphragms similar to those found elsewhere in the body in type II endothelium. The afferent arteriole running to the glomerulus is of greater diameter than the efferent arteriole that leaves it, and consequently, the glomerulus is a relatively high pressure system, aiding in the formation of tissue fluid or filtrate. As it enters the renal corpuscle, the afferent arteriole splits into three to five main branches, from which capillaries arise and, in turn, drain to primary branches or tributaries of the efferent arteriole. Thus, each group of capillaries can be termed a *lobule of the glomerulus*, and anastomoses do occur between capillaries of a lobule and also between capillaries of adjacent lobules (Fig. 13–12). Visceral epithelium (i.e., podocytes) surrounds capillaries, and near afferent and efferent arterioles there are intercapillary spaces where adjacent capillary basal laminae are not lined by endothelium. Such spaces are occupied by *mesangium*, consisting of *mesangial cells* lying in an extracellular matrix of basal lamina–like material. These are stellate cells and resemble pericytes elsewhere, with cytoplasmic processes that sometimes extend between endothelium and the basal lamina, but mesangial cells are phagocytic. They are believed to maintain the basal lamina by removing any filtration residues and probably participate in the removal of old material from its internal surface, while new material is added to the external surface by podocytes. They also provide support for the capillaries and proliferate in some kidney diseases. It has also been suggested that they can contract when stimulated by angiotensin, with a resulting decrease in blood flow through the glomerulus. Mesangial cells extend into the vascular pole, outside the renal corpuscle itself, and are continuous with similar cells that form part of the juxtaglomerular apparatus.

### JUXTAGLOMERULAR APPARATUS

As the afferent arteriole approaches the glomerulus, the smooth muscle cells of its media become "epithelioid" in type. The nuclei become spherical and not elongated, and the cytoplasm contains granules. The granules are not visible in ordinary H and E preparations but are demonstrated by methods such as the PAS reaction and methylene blue, basic fuchsin. These *juxtaglomerular (JG) cells* have a well-developed granular endoplasmic reticulum, a prominent Golgi apparatus, and secretory granules about 10 to 40 nm in diameter, variable in shape, and with a crystalline content that later becomes homogeneous (Figs. 13–13 and 13–14).

JG cells show important functional relationships. In that they are highly modified smooth muscle cells of the media of the afferent arteriole, they are in close contact with the intima and lumen of the arteriole on one side. Indeed, in this location, the internal elastic lamina is thin or even absent. On the other side, the JG cells are related closely to epithelial cells of the *macula densa*. The

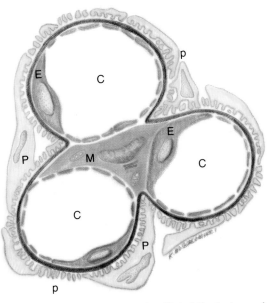

**Figure 13–12.** *This diagram of a "lobule" of glomerular capillaries illustrates the relationship of a mesangial cell (M, green) to endothelial cells (E, red) of capillaries (C), basal laminae (black), and podocytes (P, yellow) and their processes (p).*

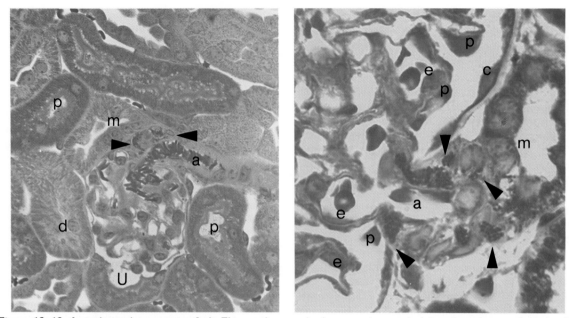

**Figure 13–13.** *Juxtaglomerular apparatus. Left: This renal corpuscle shows a urinary pole (u) and, at the vascular pole, the afferent arteriole (a), packed with erythrocytes, with modified smooth muscle cells in its wall (epithelioid) cells. These are the juxtaglomerular (JG) cells, containing purple-staining granules (arrowheads). Adjacent to them is the macula densa (m) of the distal tubule. Also present are proximal (p) and distal (d) convoluted tubules. Methylene blue, basic fuchsin. Medium power. Right: This vascular pole of a renal corpuscle shows the afferent arteriole (a) with JG cells containing purple-staining granules (arrowheads) in its wall, adjacent to the macula densa (m). In the corpuscle, nuclei of endothelial cells (e), podocytes (p), and parietal or capsular (c) epithelium can be recognized. PAS, hematoxylin. Oil immersion.*

macula densa is a specialized region at the commencement of the distal convoluted tubule as it lies between afferent and efferent arterioles. Here, the cells are taller, and the basal lamina of the tubule is lacking. Also, associated closely with the granular JG cells are some lightly staining, nongranular, extraglomerular mesangial cells (also called *lacis cells*, or polkissen cells) located between afferent and efferent arterioles. Together, the JG cells, macula densa, and lacis cells form the juxtaglomerular apparatus, or complex. Their interrelationships are not understood fully.

Experimental studies have shown that the juxtaglomerular cells produce *renin*. This is an enzyme that, in the blood, acts on *angiotensinogen*, a plasma globulin, to form *angiotensin I*. Angiotensin I itself is inactive but is converted by a converting enzyme in blood plasma (and probably originating in the lung) to *angiotensin* II, the most powerful vasoconstrictor known. The relation of the JG cells to the macula densa is very close topographically, which suggests that some inter-

change occurs between the two. Functionally, changes in blood volume appear to be sensed by the afferent arteriole, and the macula densa detects changes in sodium concentration. The JG cells then release renin, and, in turn, angiotensin II in the blood stimulates the adrenal cortex to release *aldosterone*. Aldosterone then acts upon the collecting ducts and distal tubules of the kidney to increase the reabsorption of sodium and chloride, and thus water, expanding plasma and interstitial fluid volume. This renin-angiotensin system also may function at the level of the individual nephron in the regulation of blood flow through the glomerulus and, thus, of glomerular filtration rate.

### FILTRATION BARRIER

Control of plasma volume and extracellular fluid volume, blood pressure, and cardiac output all are influenced by glomerular filtration. The filtration barrier is the term applied to the struc-

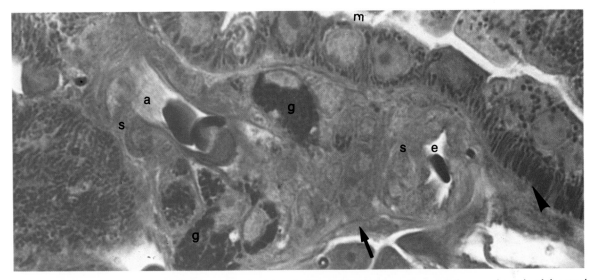

*Figure 13–14.* *Juxtaglomerular complex. Both afferent (a) and efferent (e) arterioles are seen at the vascular pole of the renal corpuscle with smooth muscle (s) in their walls. In the afferent arteriole, the smooth muscle is modified as juxtaglomerular granulated cells (g), closely associated on one side (above) with cells of the macula densa of the distal tubule (m) and on the other with extraglomerular or Lacis cells (arrow), the whole forming the juxtaglomerular apparatus or complex. In the distal convoluted tubule itself (right), cells show characteristic elongated basal mitochondria (arrowhead), while mitochondria of the macula are small, ovoid, and pink-staining. At lower right is a portion of the glomerulus with a proximal convoluted tubule cut obliquely at left. Methylene blue, basic fuchsin. Oil immersion.*

tures that separate blood in glomerular capillaries from filtrate in the capsular space of the renal corpuscle. The barrier comprises (Fig. 13–15):

1. The fenestrated, attenuated endothelium.
2. The basal lamina.
3. The pedicels of podocytes with the filtration slits between them "closed" by slit membranes.

Of these, only the basal lamina is a continuous layer. It is regarded as the main filter preventing passage of large molecules, although the slit membranes also may be significant. Experimentally, large particulate tracers pass through endothelial pores and are held up by the basal lamina; smaller particles such as horseradish peroxidase pass through into capsular space. Additionally, passage of molecules depends not only on size but also on charge, and cationic molecules are held in the basal lamina by binding with anionic sites. As explained earlier, mesangial cells remove such particulate matter by phagocytosis, thus unclogging the basal lamina.

The glomerulus is a relatively high pressure system, and ultrafiltration through the barrier is dependent upon hydrostatic pressure of the blood, usually about 75 mm Hg. Pressure in the glomerulus can be regulated by contraction of the relatively thick smooth muscle media of the efferent arteriole. Physiologically, fluid leaves the blood along the entire extent of the glomerular capillary bed, the total glomerular filtrate being 170 to 200 liters (L) in 24 hours. Of this, some 99 per cent will be resorbed by the uriniferous tubule (the tubular part of the nephron and the collecting duct), so that only 1.5 to 2 L of urine is excreted per day.

### PROXIMAL TUBULE

This segment, commencing at the urinary pole of a renal corpuscle, is about 14 mm long, with an outside diameter of 50 to 60 μm. Each comprises a *convoluted part* (the *proximal convoluted tubule*, or pars convoluta) and a *straight portion* (the pars recta). As the name suggests, the proximal convoluted tubule follows a tortuous course with many small loops and always one large loop toward the capsular surface of the kidney. It eventually returns, to approach its corpuscle of origin before passing into the nearest medullary ray, where it becomes the pars recta, which is the first part of the loop of Henle. As the longest and widest part of the nephron, the proximal convo-

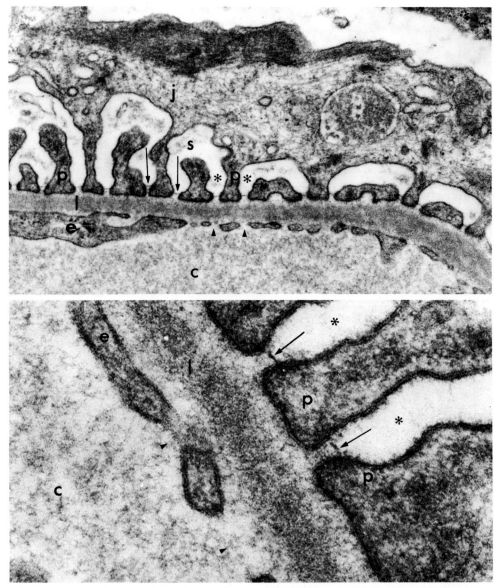

**Figure 13–15.** Electron micrographs showing the "filtration barrier": capillary lumen (c) containing plasma, endothelium (e) with pores (arrowheads), lamina densa (l), pedicels (p) with filtration slits (asterisks) between them, closed by slit membranes (arrows), urinary (capsular) space (s), and major process of a podocyte (j). Top × 32,000; bottom, × 90,000.

luted tubule constitutes the bulk of the cortex, appearing in sections as oblique and transverse profiles.

At its commencement, there is a short *neck* region, where there is a rapid transition from the squamous parietal epithelium of Bowman's capsule to the simple low columnar epithelium of the proximal tubule (Fig. 13–16). The epithelial cells of the proximal tubule are eosinophilic, with a brush border and a basal striation, and the lumen

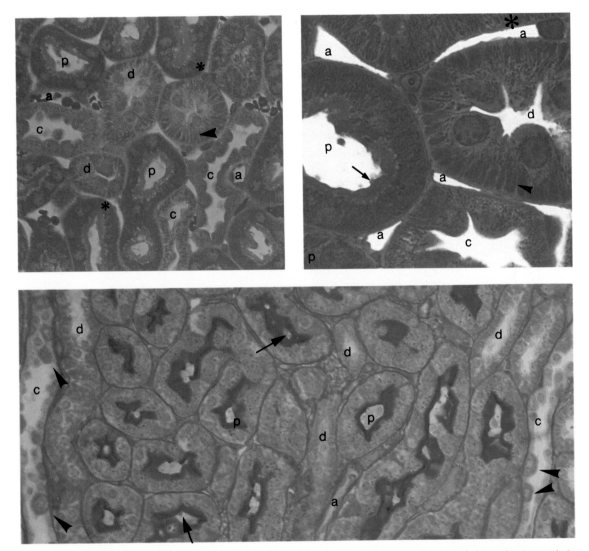

**Figure 13–16.** Kidney, cortical tubules. Top left: Proximal convoluted tubules (p) are lined by a simple low columnar epithelium with a brush or striated border; nuclei are spheroidal and basal, with prominent nucleoli; and cytoplasm stains more darkly than that of distant tubules and has a basal striation (asterisk). Distal convoluted tubules (d) have no brush border, nuclei are spheroidal and sited toward the lumen, and cytoplasm shows a clear basal striation (arrowhead) with elongated (orange-red) mitochondria. In collecting tubules (c), cells are small and cuboidal, with small, ovoid (red) mitochondria. Also seen are intertubular capillaries (a). Methylene blue, basic fuschsin. Medium power. Top right: A higher magnification, showing identical features. In both proximal (p) and distal (d) convoluted tubules, cell interfaces are not clear owing to complex interdigitation of adjacent plasmalemmae. Note the profusion of intertubular capillaries (a). Oil immersion. Bottom: This section shows part of the deep, juxtamedullary cortex in radial section with collecting tubules (c) in medullary rays on each side and cut longitudinally as they pass into the medulla (below, not seen in the section). The magenta stain (PAS technique) stains basal laminae of all tubules and the brush border (arrows), and cytoplasmic lysosome-protein bodies (small granules) of the endocytic process in the proximal convoluted tubules (p). Straight portions (pars rectae) of distal tubules (d) or ascending limbs of the loop of Henle are present, passing from medulla into cortex. In the collecting tubules (c), dark or intercalated cells (arrowheads) are scattered among the principal, light cells (low cuboidal). Centrally in the field is an interlobular artery (a): Thus, the adjacent halves of two lobules are seen. (See also Figure 13–2.) PAS, light green. High power.

usually is widely patent (Fig. 13–17). Lateral cell interfaces are defined poorly owing to a complex interdigitation of plasma membranes of adjacent cells, and basally, a similar interdigitation of basal infoldings is seen, with elongated mitochondria in the compartments so formed, this being responsible for the basal striation (Fig. 13–18). The nucleus is large and spherical and is located centrally, often with a prominent nucleolus, and a Golgi apparatus lies in a supranuclear position. In general, 6 to 12 cells lie around the circumference of a proximal tubule, although rarely are more than four or five nuclei seen because the cells are large compared to section thickness.

The brush border is composed of long, closely packed microvilli with an associated extracellular glycocalyx. This greatly increases the surface available for absorption of, for example, glucose, amino acids, and small peptides. Some protein passes the glomerular filter and is resorbed by an endocytic apparatus. The protein passes into small tubular pits or apical canaliculi that extend downward into cytoplasm between the bases of the microvilli. From these pits, small vesicles bud off, carrying the protein, and pass more deeply, where they coalesce into larger vacuoles. The vacuoles later fuse with lysosomes where the protein is broken down by lysosomal action to amino acids, which then pass to peritubular capillaries. Residual bodies resulting from the process are discharged

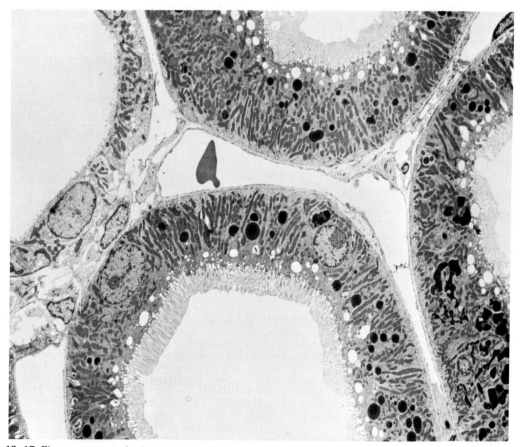

**Figure 13–17.** Electron micrograph of renal cortex showing portions of three proximal convoluted tubules in transverse section, with part of one distal convoluted tubule (top left). The proximal tubules show apical microvilli of the brush border, elongated mitochondria, dense endocytic bodies, and spherical nuclei with prominent nucleoli. The distal tubule here is lined by low cuboidal epithelium with a few scattered, apical microvilli. Intertubular capilaries are extensive. × 3300. (Courtesy of Dr. A. B. Maunsbach.)

into the lumen. Proximal tubule cells also contain peroxisomes, often associated with agranular reticulum, which are involved in the metabolism of hydrogen peroxide. They also may act in gluconeogenesis, utilizing fatty acids.

The basilateral surface of the cells, as indicated, is highly complex, with deep interdigitations. At the base particularly, what appear to be basal infoldings of the plasmalemma in fact are slender basal processes from adjacent cells. Beneath the basal plasma membrane is a continuous basal lamina that separates the epithelial cells from surrounding capillaries that are lined by fenestrated epithelium. The basilateral extracellular space is isolated from the tubular lumen by the presence of junctional complexes between adjacent cells that are located apically, and they prevent the direct passage of sodium and water between cells from the lumen to the peritubular capillaries. Having entered cells by diffusion through the apical plasma membrane, sodium is pumped actively across the basilar plasma mem-

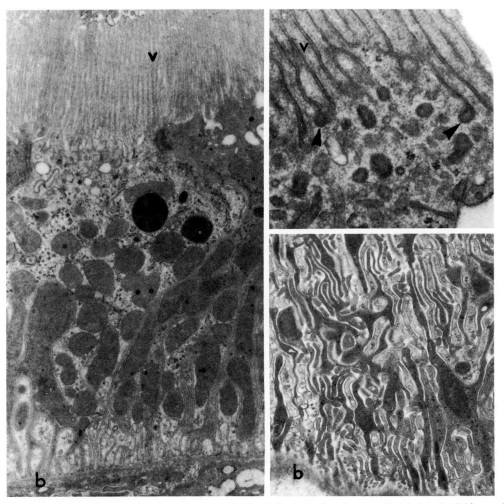

*Figure 13–18.* Electron micrographs of proximal convoluted tubule. Left: Apical microvilli (v), basal infoldings of plasma membrane, and basal interlocking of cytoplasmic processes of adjacent cells (b is the basal lamina) and numerous mitochondria. × 18,000. Top right: Apical canaliculi or tubular pits (arrowheads) between microvilli. × 45,000. Bottom right: Oblique section through the base of a tubule showing the complex interlocking of cytoplasmic processes. × 24,000.

brane to the extracellular space, and water follows passively. From here, water and solutes pass to peritubular capillaries.

The straight portion is continuous with the convoluted portion in a medullary ray, and it then penetrates into the medulla to a varying depth but basically to the inner extremity of the outer stripe, where it passes into the thin segment. Cells in the pars recta are similar to those of the pars convoluta but are lower in height, with fewer mitochondria and less basal interdigitation.

Functionally, the proximal tubule reduces the volume of the glomerular filtrate by 80 to 85 per cent, actively pumping sodium to the extracellular space utilizing the large, numerous mitochondria as the energy source. Chloride ions and water follow passively. Glucose, amino acids, peptides, and proteins as well as bicarbonate are resorbed, as are some essential vitamins. Normally, all glucose is resorbed. However, if the blood level is excessively high (e.g., in diabetes), the capacity for resorption is exceeded, and glucose appears in the urine. In addition, some materials pass to the urine by a process of secretion, for example, organic materials (including penicillin) and dye substances such as iodopyracet (Diodrast) and

phenol red, which are used clinically to assess tubular function.

### THE THIN SEGMENT

As already mentioned, short (cortical) nephrons have a short thin segment continuous with the straight portion of the proximal tubule, the two forming the descending limb of the loop of Henle. At the flexure of the loop, the descending thin limb is continuous with the ascending straight portion of the distal tubule. Thus, there is no ascending thin limb in short nephrons, and the descending thin limb is located in the inner stripe of the outer zone of the medulla (Figs. 13–19 and 13–20; see Fig. 13–1). In long (juxtamedullary) nephrons, the thin segment passes as the deeper part of the descending limb into the inner zone of the medulla, forms the loop, and passes back as the deeper part of the ascending limb to the outer zone, where it continues as the straight portion of the distal tubule. The long nephrons constitute only 15 per cent of the total.

In the outer zone of the medulla, the descending (straight) portion of the proximal tubule abruptly changes to the thin segment, with the

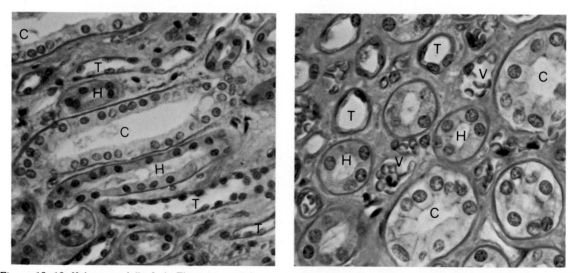

*Figure 13–19.* Kidney, medulla. Left: This section of the inner stripe, outer zone of the medulla shows collecting tubules (c), thick ascending limbs of the loop of Henle (straight portions of distal tubules, H), and thin segments (T), in mainly longitudinal section. The connective tissue of the interstitium stains green and contains a few, elongated, fibroblast-like cells. Right: The same region cut in transverse section, with thick (H) and thin (T) segments and collecting tubules (C) with numerous vasa recta (V) containing erythrocytes (yellow). High power. Masson.

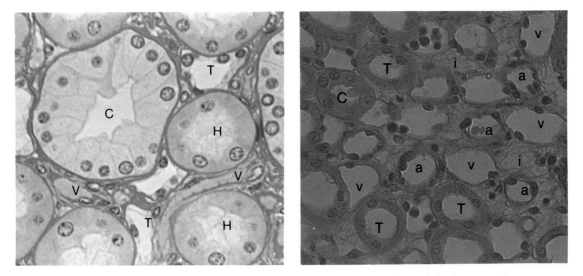

*Figure 13–20.* Kidney, medulla. Left: This section of the inner stripe, outer zone of the medulla shows, in transverse section, collecting tubules (C), thick segments of Henle (H, the straight portions of distal tubules), thin segments (T), and vasa recta (V). Basal laminae of the tubules stain dark pink. H and E. High power. Right: This transverse section of the inner zone of the medulla shows thin (T) segments of the loop of Henle and one small collecting tubule (C) with, centrally, a bundle of vasa recta (the rete mirabile). The descending (arterial) vasa (a) show a thick (nonfenestrated) endothelium, while the ascending (venous) vasa (v) generally have a greater lumen diameter, are lined by thin (fenestrated) endothelium, and are of less regular outline. All vasa lie in the loose interstitium (i) of the medulla. H and E. Medium power.

epithelium changing from cuboidal or low columnar to squamous over a few cells, and the outside diameter from about 60 μm to 12 to 15 μm. The squamous epithelium of the thin segment has a height of only 1 to 2 μm, so the lumen diameter is comparatively large. Nuclei protrude into the lumen, and although the epithelium generally is thicker than the endothelium, thin segments resemble blood capillaries and must be distinguished from them. At the junction, the brush border ceases, although there are a few short microvilli on the luminal surface of thin segment cells. In the thin segment, there are basically two types of epithelium. In type I, there is a simple flat epithelium with little or no interdigitation between adjacent cells, and there are relatively extensive zonulae occludentes between cells near their apices. In type II, the epithelium is a little taller, usually with more apical microvilli, and zonulae occludentes are less extensive. Characteristically, in type II epithelium, there is extensive interdigitation of cell processes, so that in a cross section, up to 20 or more portions of cells may be present, only a few of which contain a nucleus. In short loop nephrons, type I epithelium is seen.

In long loop nephrons, type II epithelium forms both descending and ascending limbs, with type I epithelium forming the loop.

While the functional significance of these differences is not clear, the thin segment concentrates urine by a countercurrent exchange system, to be described later. A loop of Henle is essential for the production of urine that is hypertonic to blood plasma.

### DISTAL TUBULE

The transition between the thin segment and the straight (ascending) part of the distal tubule is abrupt, the cells changing from squamous to cuboidal, this transition occurring at the junction between inner and outer stripes of the medulla in long nephrons. In short nephrons, the change occurs in the descending limb, with the thick segment (straight part of the distal tubule) forming the loop.

The distal tubule is shorter and thinner than the proximal tubule. Three portions are described:

1. A straight portion (pars recta), forming the ascending thick limb of the loop of Henle.

2. The macula densa (pars maculata).

3. The convoluted portion (pars convoluta).

Cells of the *straight* and *convoluted* portions are similar, being cuboidal, lacking a brush border, and with a lumen wider than that of the proximal tubule (Fig. 13–21). Nuclei tend to lie away from the basal lamina and bulge into the lumen. The cells are highly irregular in shape and show a basal striation resulting from extensive infoldings of the basal membrane that form compartments, in which lie long, elongated mitochondria with prominent cristae. As in the proximal tubule, some of the compartments, in fact, are basal processes from adjacent cells. There also is extensive interdigitation of lateral plasma membranes with junctional complexes between cells near their apices. These, however, are not extensive (i.e., not deep) and may permit some intercellular passage of water and solutes.

The straight portion of the distal tubule passes from medulla into cortex and then reaches its renal corpuscle of origin to lie adjacent to afferent and efferent arterioles as the macula densa ("dense spot"), thus completing the loop of Henle.

**Macula Densa.** This specialized region of the distal tubule, which is part of the juxtaglomerular complex, is the short section of the distal tubule immediately adjacent to the afferent and efferent arterioles of the glomerulus, the JG cells, and the extraglomerular mesangium or lacis cells. On the side of the tubule adjacent to the afferent arteriole, the distal tubule cells are packed in a palisade manner, with nuclei close together forming a darkly staining disc. The macula cells differ from those of the straight and convoluted portions of the distal tubule in that

1. They have widely distributed, small, ovoid mitochondria.

2. They show apical vacuolation.

3. They have only shallow folds of the basal plasmalemma.

4. The Golgi apparatus is infranuclear in position.

5. They generally are taller than surrounding cells.

The functional significance of the macula densa remains unclarified, but it is believed that the cells act as a sensor of the osmolarity of the fluid in the distal tubule. If, for example, sodium ion concentration is low, perhaps following decreased glomerular filtration because of low blood pressure, the macula cells may transmit this information to the JG cells with release of renin. In turn, angiotensin II in the blood would cause an increase in blood pressure by vasoconstriction and a release of aldosterone from the adrenal cortex with increased reabsorption of sodium and chloride, and thus water, with expansion of blood volume. The straight portion of the distal tubule actively resorbs sodium, as does the convoluted portion, where the rate of sodium transport is controlled by aldosterone. This is discussed later.

**Distal Convoluted Tubule.** From the macula densa, the nephron continues as the distal convoluted tubule (convoluted part of the distal tubule) that has a short, tortuous course in the renal cortex and terminates near a medullary ray by continuing into a collecting duct (Fig. 13–21). It is much shorter than the proximal convoluted tubule and, thus, in a section appears in smaller numbers. The cells are cuboidal, stain less intensely, have no brush border, and are smaller, with six to eight nuclei seen in a cross section.

The nephron terminates with the distal convoluted tubule, and developmentally, nephrons and collecting tubules or ducts have different origins.

## Collecting Tubules

Junctions between distal convoluted tubules and collecting tubules occur in the cortex of the kidney adjacent to medullary rays, where distal tubules pass into *arched collecting tubules*. Those arched tubules that join juxtamedullary nephrons are longer because they ascend in the cortex before joining with others to form *straight collect-*

---

**Figure 13–21.** Top: *Electron micrograph of distal convoluted tubules from the kidney of a spider monkey. Note the complex infoldings and interdigitation of the basal plasmalemma.* × *4000. (Courtesy of Dr. Ruth Bulger.) Bottom: Electron micrograph of the basal portion of a distal convoluted tubule showing basal infoldings and interdigitation of the basal plasmalemma with elongated mitochondria in the cytoplasmic compartments. Note the peritubular capillary (c) with fenestrated endothelium (pores indicated by arrowheads) and basal lamina (b) of the tubule.* × *24,000.*

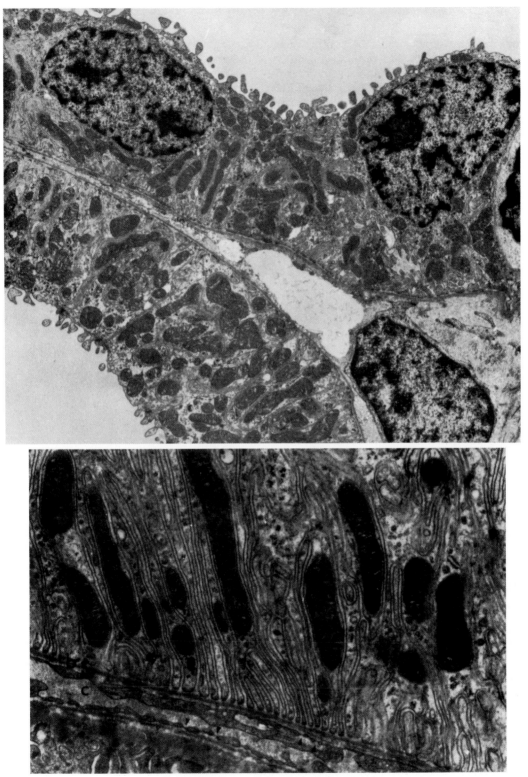

*Figure 13–21* See legend on opposite page

*ing tubules*. These straight collecting tubules pass down in a medullary ray and through the outer zone of the medullary pyramid and then converge and join at acute angles to form the large *ducts of Bellini*. These ducts have an overall diameter of up to 200 μm and pass through the inner zone of the medulla to open on the area cribrosa at the apex of each papilla (Figs. 13–22 through 13–24).

The epithelial cells lining these collecting ducts are pale-staining, with distinct cell boundaries, dark spherical nuclei, and few organelles. Apically are a few microvilli and a single cilium, and the cells increase in height from cuboidal in the arched and straight tubules in the cortex to columnar in

the main ducts of the medulla. Two cell types are present. The *principal, light cells* are as described earlier and are found in tubules from start to termination. Also present are *dark*, or *intercalated, cells* located in arched and straight tubules. Relatively few in number, they contain numerous mitochondria, apical vesicles, and basally located interdigitations between adjacent cells, and on their apical surfaces are many short folds or microplicae.

Collecting tubules conduct urine from the nephrons to the ureteric pelvis and also play a role in the concentration of urine by water absorption, this being controlled by antidiuretic hormone (ADH).

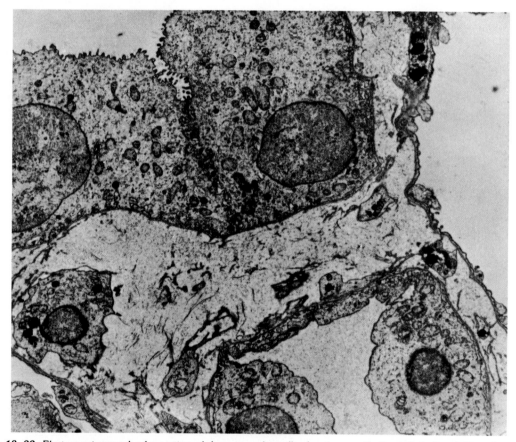

**Figure 13–22.** *Electron micrograph of a section of the rat renal papilla showing a collecting tubule (top left), a thin segment (bottom right), blood capillaries (vasa recta, top right and lower left corner), and, in the interstitium, a small fibroblast-like cell containing several lipid droplets (black). × 4500. (Courtesy of Dr. Ruth Bulger.)*

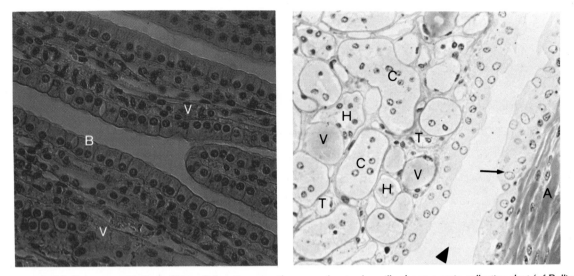

***Figure 13–23.*** *Kidney, papilla. Left: This radial section near the apex of a renal papilla shows a main collecting duct (of Bellini) (B), formed by the union of (two) smaller ducts, lined by columnar, pale-staining epithelium with clear cell interfaces. The ducts open at the area cribrosa, the sieve-like surface of the papilla. Between collecting ducts are parallel vasa recta (V), lined by endothelium. H and E. Medium power. Right: This section shows the periphery of a renal papilla (left) and the surrounding calyx. In the papilla are profiles of collecting tubules (c), thick ascending loops of Henle (H), and thin segments (T), with vasa recta (V), all cut in transverse section. The papilla is covered by transitional epithelium, only two or three cells thick, with similar epithelium lining the outer, pelvic aspect of the minor calyx (arrow) supported by connective tissue (A). The lumen of the calyx (arrowhead) appears between these layers of transitional epithelium. H and E. High power.*

## Renal Interstitium

Connective tissue in the renal cortex is sparse, with thin collagen bundles being more prominent around blood vessels. Fibroblast-like cells are present and are irregular in shape, with long processes that often appear to contact those of adjacent cells. These cells occasionally contain lipid droplets. Also present are a few mononuclear cells that appear to be phagocytic. Presumably, the fibroblast-like cells are responsible for producing and maintaining the collagen fibrils and glycosaminoglycans of the cortical interstitium.

In the medulla, the interstitium is more extensive. It includes fibroblast-like cells similar to those of the cortex with processes that lie around thin limbs and capillaries and that meet at gap junctions. These cells contain lipid droplets and their function is uncertain, although it has been suggested that they secrete a hormone that is involved in the regulation of blood pressure. Also present are pericytes associated with the vasa recta and some mononuclear cells.

## Lymphatic Vessels

Lymphatic vessels are not seen clearly in the kidney, although they are present as two networks located in the capsule and in association with the renal vessels, the two groups interconnected by a few anastomotic channels. In the renal parenchyma, fine channels are present and drain to lymphatics running with interlobular vessels and from there to the kidney hilus. In the outer cortex, some vessels drain to the plexus located in the capsule.

## Nerves

Nerves from the sympathetic plexus enter the kidney with the arteries, with both afferent fibers to the adventitia of the vessels and motor endings to the muscular coat (media). They appear to extend as far as renal corpuscles, but a nerve supply to uriniferous tubules has not been demonstrated conclusively to date. As already men-

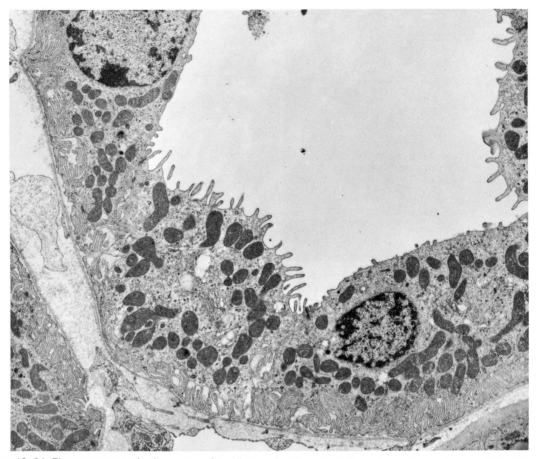

**Figure 13–24.** Electron micrograph of a portion of a collecting duct from the kidney of a spider monkey. × 4500. (Courtesy of Dr. Ruth Bulger.)

tioned, sympathetic stimulation causes blanching of the kidney cortex, with the majority of the blood supply diverted to the medulla.

### Concentration and Dilution of Urine

As already stated, of the 170 to 200 L of filtrate produced each day in the glomeruli, some 99 per cent eventually is resorbed. In the proximal tubule, about 85 per cent of the water and sodium chloride is resorbed, the cells actively transporting sodium, with water and chloride following passively to maintain osmotic equilibrium. Here, also, glucose, amino acids, peptides, proteins, bicarbonate, and vitamins (e.g., ascorbic acid) are conserved by reabsorption, but waste products of metabolism such as urea, creatinine, and uric acid are not totally resorbed and, thus, in part, are eliminated in the urine. Additionally, a loop of Henle is essential for the production of hypertonic urine—the loop, the collecting tubules, and the vasa recta functioning as a countercurrent multiplier and exchange system.

Filtrate leaving proximal tubules, although reduced greatly in volume, has an unchanged osmolarity. Unlike the cortex, interstitial fluid of the medulla has an increased osmolarity. From the corticomedullary junction to the papilla, there is an increase in osmolarity dependent upon the arrangement of the blood vessels and the loop of Henle and the permeability of its various segments. The thick ascending limb (distal tubule) is impermeable to salt and water but actively transports salt from the filtrate to the interstitial fluid, increasing hypertonicity in the outer medulla and inner cortex. At the same time, the fluid in the thick ascending limb becomes more hypotonic owing to loss of salt. The thin descending limb is highly permeable to water but not to salt or urea. Therefore, as it passes into the medulla, where interstitial tonicity is high, water diffuses from it, thus increasing its intratubular concentration of solutes, mainly salt. The ascending thin limb is impermeable to water but permeable to salt, so that after rounding the bend, salt diffuses from the thin ascending segment, with resulting dilution of its fluid content. This thin ascending limb, then, passively helps to maintain the high osmolarity of the inner medulla. Thus, in the ascending limb, fluid becomes more hypotonic, first, by passive loss of sodium in the thin part and, then, by active transport of salt in the thick part.

The remainder of the distal tubule and cortical and outer medullary parts of the collecting tubule are permeable to water but impermeable to salt and urea, and so, passage through this segment results in loss of water and consequent increase in the concentration of urea. In the inner medulla, collecting tubules are permeable to water and urea, which leave the tubule to achieve the final concentration of the urine. Urea in the interstitial fluid of the inner medulla contributes to its high osmolarity.

Involved in this process is the *antidiuretic hormone* (ADH) of the hypophysis. Its action on collecting tubule cells makes them permeable to water, and thus, water leaves the tubules, rendering the urine hypertonic. In the absence of ADH, the tubules are relatively impermeable, water is retained, and the urine remains hypotonic and in excess amount, a condition called *diabetes insipidus*. Aldosterone also is involved in urinary excretion in that it acts upon renal tubules to increase the rate of sodium transport to the interstitium.

The arrangement of the vasa recta in the renal medulla is of parallel descending and ascending vessels with a sharp bend, so that blood runs in opposite directions in the two limbs. The capillaries of both limbs are permeable to sodium chloride and urea, which enter descending vasa recta and leave ascending vessels, the overall result

being that equilibration occurs and that the osmotic pressure and solute content of the interstitium are unchanged. Additionally, water resorbed from collecting tubules and descending limbs of Henle is passed from the interstitium to the ascending vasa recta and is removed, preserving the hyperosmolarity of the medullary interstitium.

## Embryology

The kidney is formed in intermediate mesoderm situated in the posterior abdominal wall. Primitive nephrons develop as cords (strands) of mesenchymal cells that later develop a lumen to become tubular. The blind dilated end of the nephron (the future Bowman's capsule) is then invaginated by the glomerular tuft of capillaries. The ureteric bud, a diverticulum of the mesonephric, or Wolffian, duct, grows upward from the future pelvis and into the mass of developing kidney, or *metanephros*. Later, the mesonephric duct becomes associated with the genital system, and, by differential growth, the ureteric bud that originated from it is taken up into the developing urinary bladder.

Once the growing end of the ureteric bud reaches the metanephros, it undergoes a series of divisions, the major branches becoming the major and minor calyces of the renal pelvis, with the ureteric bud itself becoming the ureter. Each terminal branch of the ureteric bud becomes a collecting tubule, continuous with a developing nephron. The first nephrons to develop are those in the deeper layers of the cortex (juxtamedullary), while the outer cortical nephrons develop later, after birth (Fig. 13–25). At birth, the kidney shows an irregular outline (fetal lobation), with the outer cortical region consisting of undifferentiated mesenchyme, from which additional nephrons will develop. With completion of development after some months, the kidney outline becomes smooth, with no external indication of lobation.

Developmental abnormalities of the kidney and excretory passages are relatively common. Early branching of a ureteric bud before it reaches the metanephros can result in a bifid (or double) ureter or a double kidney. A terminal division of the ureteric bud may fail to connect to, and establish continuity with, an individual nephron,

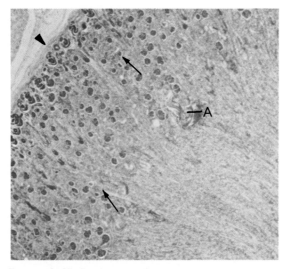

**Figure 13–25.** *Fetal kidney. This radial section of an eight-month fetal kidney shows a clear distinction between cortex and medulla, with a section of an arcuate artery (A) at the junction. The medulla is pale and radially striated owing to tubules cut in longitudinal section, with medullary rays (arrows) extending into the cortex. The cortex is thin and incompletely developed with dark, spherical profiles of renal corpuscles. The juxtamedullary ones are larger and more mature. A connective tissue capsule (arrowhead) covers the surface. The kidney is incompletely developed at birth, the juxtamedullary nephrons developing first. H and E. Low power.*

resulting in a cyst as the nephron dilates. Usually, this abnormality is multiple, with the condition termed multicystic kidney disease.

## EXCRETORY PASSAGES

The excretory passages convey urine from the kidney to the exterior and consist of minor and major calyces, the renal pelvis, the ureter, the urinary bladder, and the urethra. All essentially are simple ducts, the bladder providing temporary storage for urine, but they do add some mucus to the urine and may function to a limited extent to absorb a small amount of fluid. With the exception of the urethra, all show the same general structure of an adventitia (with a serosa in some regions), a muscularis, and a mucosa, the muscularis of smooth muscle being well developed to move urine onward in the tract.

### Pelvis and Ureter

The upper portion of the ureter, the pelvis, is expanded within the hilum of the kidney, where it splits into major and minor calyces. Each minor calyx fits like a cup around a medullary papilla. The wall increases in thickness, with that of the pelvis being thinner than that of the ureter itself. The ureter, 10 to 12 inches (25 to 30 cm) long, lies in the posterior abdominal wall behind the peritoneum and terminates by passing obliquely through the wall of the urinary bladder.

**Mucosa.** In both pelvis and ureter, the lining mucosa consists of transitional epithelium supported by a lamina propria, the epithelium being only two to three cells thick in the pelvis and four to five cells in the ureter (Fig. 13–26). As explained in Chapter 2, the surface cells present a convex border to the lumen, may be binucleate, and show specializations. They vary in shape from cuboidal to squamous (when the organ is distended) and have an irregular, scalloped surface with indentations and, in apical cytoplasm, fusiform vesicles limited by a membrane of a thickness identical to that of the plasma membrane. It is believed that these vesicles form a membrane reserve that is utilized to add to the surface membrane during distention. Apical cytoplasm also contains fine filament bundles. The luminal plasmalemma is unusual in that it is thicker (12 nm) than the usual 7 nm, with the outer lamina thicker than the inner, and it shows a highly ordered substructure of hexagonal units. Together with extensive occluding junctions between surface cells, this special membrane is believed to be a barrier to movement of water (from blood, through the epithelium, to the urine, the urine being hypertonic).

The epithelium rests upon a thin basal lamina, and the lamina propria is a relatively dense, but still areolar, connective tissue in which elastic fibers are prominent. Some loose lymphatic tissue is present, and the outer portion is less dense and is regarded by some as a submucosa. It contains no glands, and, in transverse section, the lumen of the nondistended ureter is stellate in outline owing to longitudinal folds of the mucosa. These folds are "ironed out" when the ureter is distended.

**Muscularis.** This is thick and consists of bundles of smooth muscle cells separated by strands

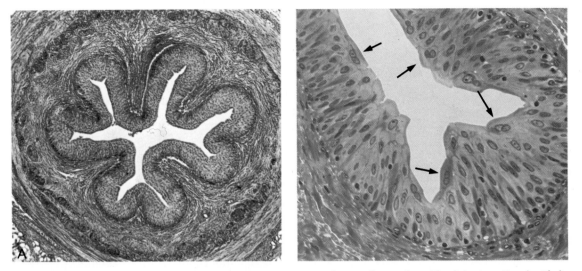

*Figure 13–26. Ureter.* Left: *The lumen of the ureter in transverse section has a stellate outline with a lining transitional epithelium, about five cells thick, supported by a relatively dense fibroconnective tissue lamina propria (green). No submucosa is present, and the muscularis is thick with inner longitudinal (cut transversely) and outer circular layers. Externally is the adventitia with some adipose tissue (A) and peritoneum on the anterior surface of the ureter. Masson. Medium power.* Right: *The transitional epithelium lining the ureter is about five cells thick, with surface cells showing a convex border, being stained more intensely and with some of the cells binucleate (arrows). The supporting lamina propria is relatively dense. H and E. High power.*

of connective tissue. While the muscularis is arranged as inner longitudinal and outer circular coats (the opposite orientation to that in the intestine), the layers are not clearly distinct, and a third, outer longitudinal layer is present in the lower end of the ureter. In the pelvis, associated with minor calyces, only circular muscle is present, and here it is believed to have a squeezing, or "milking," function, aiding the passage of urine from papillary ducts into the calyces. In the lower end of the ureter, as it passes obliquely through the wall of the bladder, there are no circular strands of muscle, and the longitudinal muscle by contracting opens the lumen of the ureter and permits passage of urine into the bladder. Reflux of urine from the bladder is prevented by a flap of bladder mucosa that acts as a valve and by internal distention pressure in the bladder. Urine does not flow continuously down the ureter; rather, waves of peristaltic contraction pass down the ureter, with contraction of the lower longitudinal fibers to open the lumen, resulting in urine entering the bladder in spurts.

**Adventitia.** A coat of fibroelastic connective tissue lies external to the ureter. Above, it blends with the capsule of the kidney at the pelvis and is continuous with the surrounding connective tissue of the posterior abdominal wall along the length of the ureter. The anterior surface of the pelvis and ureter is covered loosely by peritoneum.

There are extensive vascular and lymphatic plexuses in the muscularis and lamina propria of the ureter, which receives arterial supply from several adjacent vessels. Nerves, with some ganglion cells, are present and supply motor autonomic fibers to the muscularis. Sensory fibers extend through the muscularis to penetrate between cells of the epithelium.

### Bladder

The basic structure of the bladder is similar to that of the ureter. However, the lining epithelium is thicker, with six to eight layers of cells (Fig. 13–27). Beneath the epithelium is a discontinuous muscularis mucosae with small, irregularly arranged groups of muscle fibers, richly supplied by nerve fibers. In the lamina propria are a few small mucus-secreting glands with simple or branched ducts, more numerous around ureteric and ure-

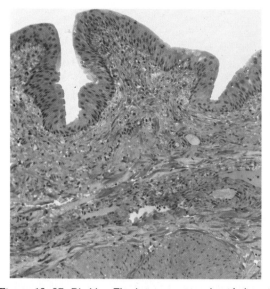

*Figure 13–27. Bladder. The lining transitional epithelium is six to eight cells thick with a thick, dense lamina propria, the external part looser in texture and sometimes called the submucosa. A thick muscularis shows inner and outer longitudinal layers with a thicker middle circular layer, but with intermingling of muscle bundles (the full thickness is not seen here). An adventitia lies externally, with peritoneum on the superior surface only. The mucosa is thrown into folds in the contracted bladder, as seen here. H and E. Low power.*

thral orifices. As in the ureter, the outer layer of the lamina propria is formed by looser tissue, sometimes called the submucosa, which permits folding of the mucous membrane in the contracted bladder. The muscularis is thick and strong, with strands of muscle arranged in three layers, although considerable intermingling of bundles occurs. The outer longitudinal layer is thick on anterior and posterior surfaces, while the inner longitudinal layer is relatively thin and forms an incomplete coat. The thickest, central layer is of circular muscle, highly developed around the internal urethral orifice as the internal sphincter of the bladder and, to a lesser extent, around the ureteric orifices. The adventitia is formed by fibroelastic tissue with peritoneum covering the superior surface of the bladder, where it is attached loosely. There is a rich nerve supply to the bladder, with branches from the sacral nerves (parasympathetic) and hypogastric plexus (sympathetic).

## Urethra

The urethra, the terminal excretory passage between the bladder and the exterior, differs in the sexes.

**The Male Urethra.** This is 15 to 20 cm in length and is divided into three regions (Fig. 13–28):

1. *Pars prostatica.* This short, first part of the urethra passes from the internal urethral orifice of the bladder to traverse the prostate gland. Opening into it are the two ejaculatory ducts and numerous openings of the ducts of the prostate gland.

2. *Pars membranacea.* Only about 2 cm in length, this segment passes between striated muscle of the urogenital diaphragm (which serves as the external sphincter of the urethra) to perforate the perineal membrane and terminate in the bulb of the corpus cavernosum urethrae (corpus spongiosum).

3. *Pars cavernosa (pars spongiosa).* The terminal urethra, or penile urethra, some 15 cm in length, traverses the length of the corpus spongiosum to open at the glans penis.

In the prostatic urethra, the lining epithelium is transitional, similar to that of the bladder. In the remainder of the urethra, it changes to a stratified or pseudostratified columnar epithelium with patches of stratified squamous epithelium, particularly in the penile urethra. At the terminal dilation of the penile urethra, in the fossa navicularis, the epithelium is stratified squamous in type. A few mucous goblet cells may be found. Underlying the epithelium is a loose, fibroelastic, connective tissue lamina propria in which a few slender bundles of smooth muscle are present. The entire urethral mucosa is irregular, with small depressions, or pits, extending deeply as the branching, tubular *glands of Littre*. These are more numerous on the dorsal surface of the penile urethra and are oriented obliquely with blind ends directed toward the root of the penis. These glands are lined by an epithelium similar to that lining the urethra and are mucus secreting.

**The Female Urethra.** This is much shorter than in the male, being only 3 to 4 cm long. The mucosa lies in longitudinal folds and has a lining epithelium that is stratified squamous in type, with patches of pseudostratified or stratified columnar

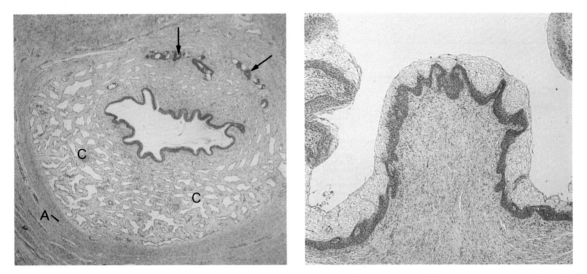

**Figure 13–28.** Male urethra. Left: *The penile urethra is lined by stratified columnar epithelium, continuous with branching tubular glands (of Littre), mainly on the dorsal surface (arrows). The urethra lies in (traverses) the erectile (cavernous) tissue (c) of the corpus spongiosum, surrounded by the dense connective tissue of the tunica albuginea (A). H and E. Low power.* Right: *In the fossa navicularis or terminal urethra at the tip of the penis, the lining is stratified squamous epithelium supported by a lamina propria of relatively cellular fibroelastic connective tissue. H and E. Medium power.*

epithelium (Fig. 13–29). Glandular outpocketings, similar to the glands of Littre of the male, are present. The lamina propria is a loose fibroconnective tissue characterized by the presence of numerous venous plexuses similar to cavernous tissue of the male. Externally, the muscularis is formed by smooth muscle in inner longitudinal and outer circular layers, reinforced by a sphincter of striated muscle around the orifice.

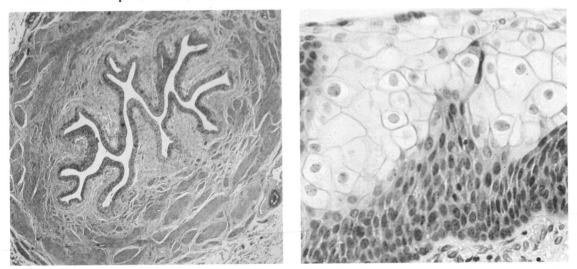

**Figure 13–29.** Female urethra. Left: *A transverse section just distal to the bladder shows a lining transitional epithelium with its lamina propria, a thick muscularis with irregularly arranged muscle fiber bundles, and loose connective tissue externally. The irregular lumen in the contracted state implies a capacity for distention during voiding. Hematoxylin, phloxine, safranin. Low power.* Right: *The distal portion of the female urethra is lined by a stratified squamous epithelium. H and E. High power.*

## Summary Table 13–1. The Nephron

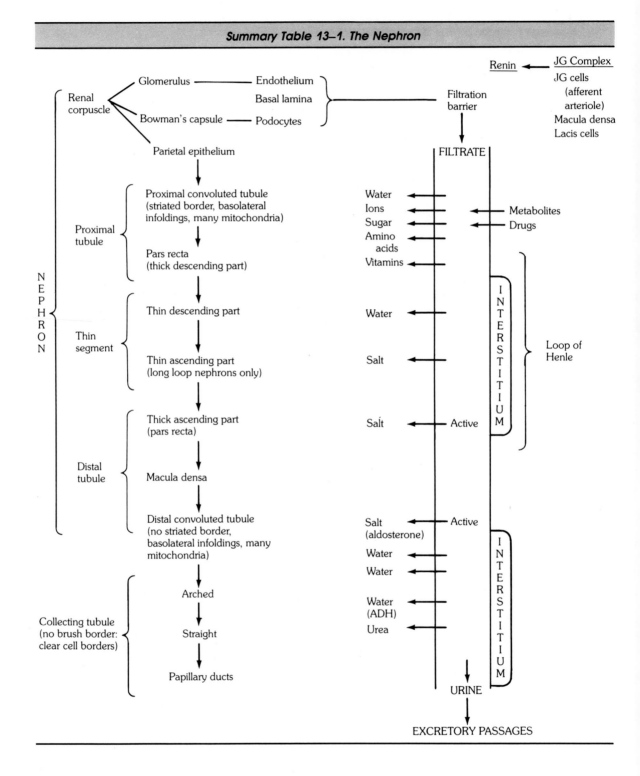

# The Endocrine System

## INTRODUCTION

The endocrine system is composed mainly of duct-less glands whose secretions (*hormones*) are passed directly into the blood or lymph circulation. The endocrine components of the body occur in three forms:

1. As separate entities, which are purely endocrine in function. This group includes the hypophysis (pituitary gland) and thyroid, parathyroid, and suprarenal glands.

2. As scattered masses of endocrine tissue within exocrine glands or other organs. This group includes the pancreatic islets, interstitial (Leydig's) cells of the testis, corpora lutea of the ovary, and juxtaglomerular cells of the kidney. These combined organs are called *mixed glands*. The liver also is a mixed gland, but here each hepatic cell exhibits both exocrine and endocrine functions, secreting bile into the duct system and internal secretions directly into the blood vessels.

3. As isolated endocrine cells, present principally within the lining epithelium of the gastrointestinal and respiratory tracts.

14

The cells are APUD (amine precursor uptake and decarboxylation) cells.

The endocrine glands vary in their embryological derivation; as a group, they are derived from all three germ layers in the embryo:

1. The hypophysis, suprarenal medulla, and chromaffin bodies are of *ectodermal* origin.

2. The suprarenal cortex, testes, and ovaries are derived from *mesoderm*.

3. Parenchymal cells of the thyroid, parathyroid, and islets of Langerhans arise from *endoderm*.

Each endocrine gland secretes one or more specific substances called hormones. Hormones are discharged from cells of endocrine glands into the blood or lymph circulation and eventually are distributed to the tissue fluids everywhere. A hormone has an effect upon a particular tissue or organ or upon the body as a whole. Some hormones affect certain tissues or organs specifically: The organs affected are termed *target organs,* or *receptors.* Only a minute quantity of hormone is required to produce an effect, usually an arousal or activation but occasionally an inhibitory response. Many hormones do not enter target cells but bind to receptors on the cell membrane and activate an enzyme, adenylate cyclase. This membrane enzyme increases intracellular concentrations of *cyclic adenosine monophosphate* (cAMP), which acts as a "second messenger" to initiate the physiological response for which the particular cell is programmed.

The endocrine cells interact to regulate themselves in numerous, complex ways. Additionally, many hormones produce an effect upon the nervous system, and some endocrine cells are regulated by neural mechanisms. This overlapping regulatory control, which involves both endocrine and nervous components, is regarded by many in the field as a single system termed the *neuroendocrine system.*

Hormones differ greatly in their chemical composition. They can be divided into three classes:

1. The *steroid hormones,* for example, the adrenocortical hormones, testosterone, and the estrogens and progesterone. Glands that secrete these hormones include the suprarenal cortex, the ovary, and the testis.

2. The *protein hormones,* for example, prolactin and insulin, secreted by the hypophysis, pancreas, thyroid, and parathyroid.

3. The *amino acid analogues and derivatives,* for example, thyroxine and norepinephrine, secreted by the thyroid and suprarenal medulla.

The major endocrine glands, as a group, have a simple microscopic structure; they consist of either cords, plates, or clumps of cells supported by delicate connective tissue. These glands are highly vascularized by fenestrated capillaries or sinusoids. In some endocrine glands, secretion accumulates within the cells of origin (e.g., pancreatic islets). In others, the secretory product is stored in a central mass surrounded by secretory cells, thus forming a follicle (e.g., the thyroid). In the suprarenal cortex, however, secretion is released almost as rapidly as it is formed.

This chapter discusses the endocrine glands that are separate organs. Other endocrine tissues, which are contained within organs of a wholly different type such as the pancreas and the gonads or which occur as isolated cells, are described in the relevant chapters.

## THE HYPOPHYSIS (PITUITARY GLAND)

The hypophysis (pituitary gland) is the most complex of the endocrine glands. It is composed of two major parts. The *adenohypophysis* (glandular portion) is derived from oral ectoderm that migrates dorsally as *Rathke's pouch* to surround partially the *neurohypophysis* (nervous portion), a ventral evagination from the floor of the diencephalon (forebrain) (Fig. 14–1). The hypophysis is buried in the sella turcica, a bony fossa of the sphenoid bone, and is covered by an extension of the dura mater, the diaphragma sellae. There is a small aperture in the diaphragm, through which passes the hypophyseal stalk.

The hypophysis is about the size of a small, flattened grape. It is approximately 1 cm in length, 1 to 1.3 cm in width, and 0.5 cm in height. It weighs about 0.5 to 0.6 gm in adults. The hypophysis undergoes some enlargement during pregnancy and may weigh 1 gm or more in women who have borne children.

The adenohypophysis, which is pinkish in color in the fresh condition, is divided by the *residual lumen* of Rathke's pouch into two unequal por-

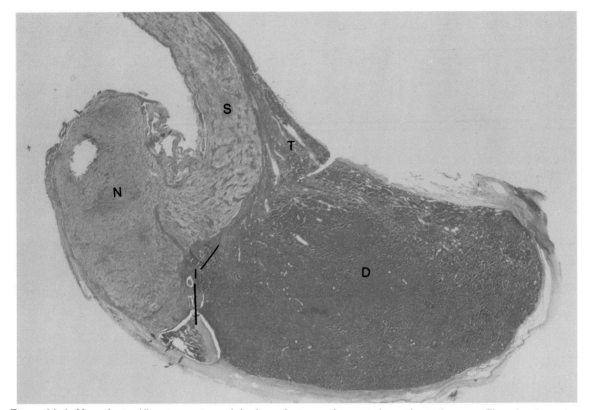

**Figure 14–1.** *Hypophysis. All major portions of the hypophysis are shown in this midsagittal section. The adenohypophysis, which develops from Rathke's pouch and lies to the right, has three parts. The pars distalis (D) is the largest part of the gland, and an extension from it, the pars tuberalis (T), passes superiorly, anterior to the neural stalk. The third part, the pars intermedia (I), is a thin cellular partition in which there are some small cyst-like spaces. Normally, it is separated from the pars distalis by the residual lumen of Rathke's pouch (not apparent on this section). The neurohypophysis also consists of three parts. The major portion is the pars nervosa (N), which superiorly continues into the neural stalk, the lower part of which is the infundibular stem (S). The upper part of the neural stalk, the median eminence of the tuber cinereum, is not present here. The infundibular stem and the pars tuberalis together constitute the hypophyseal stalk. H and E. Low power.*

tions. Anterior to the cleft is the *pars distalis,* an extension of which, the *pars tuberalis,* surrounds the neural stalk (Fig. 14–2). The third component of the adenohypophysis is the *pars intermedia,* which forms a thin cellular partition behind the cleft. The neurohypophysis, which appears white and fibrous in the fresh condition, consists of three parts. The major portion is the *pars nervosa (infundibular process),* which lies immediately posterior to the pars intermedia. Above, the pars nervosa is continuous with the *infundibular stem* and the *median eminence* of the tuber cinereum. The latter two together constitute the *infundibular (neural) stalk.* The *hypophyseal stalk* is composed of the pars tuberalis and the infundibular stalk.

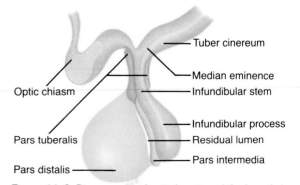

**Figure 14–2.** *Diagram of midsagittal section of the hypothalamus and the hypophysis showing the various divisions.*

**TABLE 14–1. Terminology of the Hypophysis (Pituitary Gland)**

| Adenohypophysis (glandular lobe) | Pars distalis | Anterior lobe |
| | Pars tuberalis | |
| | Pars intermedia | Posterior lobe |
| Neurohypophysis | Pars nervosa | |
| | Infundibular stem | |
| | Median eminence | |

The terms *anterior lobe* and *posterior lobe* are well established in the clinical and endocrinological literature. The anterior lobe refers to the portion of the hypophysis anterior to the residual lumen (i.e., pars distalis and pars tuberalis). The posterior lobe includes the parts posterior to the lumen, pars intermedia and pars nervosa (Table 14–1).

### The Pars Distalis

The pars distalis constitutes about 75 per cent of the hypophysis and is enclosed almost completely in a dense fibrous capsule. The parenchyma is in the form of anastomosing cords and clusters of epithelial cells supported by a network

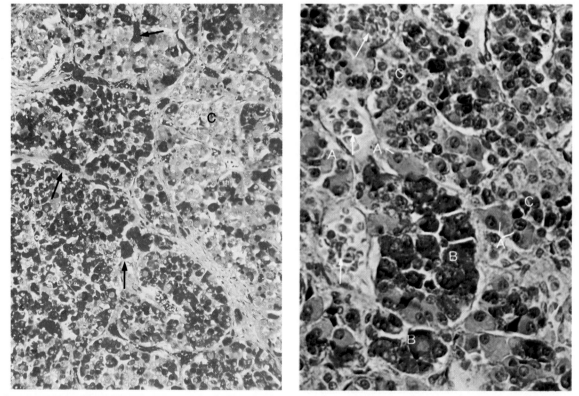

**Figure 14–3.** Hypophysis, pars distalis. Left: The parenchyma of the pars distalis is in the form of anastomosing cords and clumps of epithelial cells supported by a network of reticular fibers (not stained specifically). Large sinusoidal capillaries (arrows) occur between the parenchymal cells, which are of two main types, chromophobes and chromophils. Chromophobes (C), which have little affinity for dyes, are small cells that often appear in large groups. Chromophils are larger cells that are subdivided into acidophils and basophils on the basis of the staining reactions of their cytoplasmic granules. Masson. Low power. Right: Large sinusoids, containing red blood cells (arrows), are present within the delicate connective tissue between cords and clumps of parenchymal cells. The small chromophobes (C) possess little cytoplasm, which usually contains no specific granules. Acidophils, or alpha cells (A), are larger than chromophobes, and their cell boundaries are distinct. The cytoplasm is crowded with small specific granules (deep pink). Basophils, or beta cells (B), tend to be a little larger than acidophils, and their cytoplasm contains small granules that stain deeply basophil. H and E. Medium power.

of delicate reticular fibers continuous at the periphery with component fibers of the capsule. Between the parenchymal cells are sinusoidal capillaries (Fig. 14–3).

The parenchyma is composed of two main categories of cells, *chromophobes* and *chromophils*, distinguished by whether or not their secretory granules take up stain (Fig. 14–4). Chromophils are further subdivided into *acidophils* (*alpha cells*) and *basophils* (*beta cells*) on the basis of the staining reactions of their cytoplasmic granules. Chromophobes, which have little affinity for dyes, sometimes are referred to as *chief*, or *C, cells*. The relative proportions of the cells vary markedly in humans. Chromophobes constitute approximately 50 per cent of cells, acidophils 35 per cent, and basophils 15 per cent. The proportions may be altered considerably by castration, thyroidectomy, or other experimental procedures. Additional cell types may be demonstrated within the alpha and beta groups by special staining techniques and histochemical methods. The cells

also may be identified by immunocytochemical staining, using antibodies prepared against any one of the purified hypophyseal hormones. In this way, it is possible to classify the cell types within the pars distalis on the basis of the one or more hormones they contain (Figs. 14–5 and 14–6).

In the chromophils, it is believed that the granules are actual precursors of the secretion. The cells are thought to secrete cyclically rather than continuously. It appears that some chromophobes represent reserve, or inactive, cells that give rise to chromophils. As the chromophobes become active, granules form within their cytoplasm, and the granules are specific for the different chromophil types. Engorged cells then secrete, and the cells revert to an inactive state.

### CHROMOPHOBES (C Cells)

In the past, these faintly staining cells were known as *reserve cells*. They are small rounded or polygonal cells with relatively little cytoplasm. The boundaries of the cells are not easily visible in ordinary preparations, and generally on light microscopy the cytoplasm lacks specific granules. On electron microscopy, however, many cells exhibit small secretory granules. It appears that most chromophobes are partially degranulated chromophils and, therefore, are capable of differentiating into only one of the chromophil types. Only a small percentage of them may be considered reserve, or nonsecretory, cells. The chromophobes often appear in groups in the center of the parenchymal cords.

### CHROMOPHILS

**Acidophils (Alpha Cells).** The acidophils stain readily and are identified easily in ordinary preparations. They are larger than chromophobes, and their cell boundaries are distinct. The cytoplasm is crowded with small specific granules that are stained by numerous dyes, such as eosin, acid fuchsin, orange G, and azocarmine. Two types of acidophils are distinguished by selective staining methods and by immunocytochemistry.

*Somatotropes.* These acidophils, which often appear in groups, secrete growth hormone (STH, or *somatotropin*) and thus are termed *somato-*

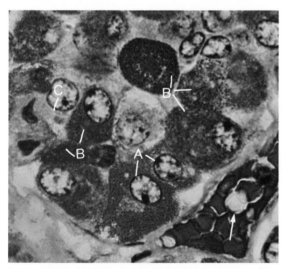

**Figure 14–4.** *Hypophysis, pars distalis. A portion of one clump of parenchymal cells is shown. Acidophils (A) are large cells whose cytoplasm is filled with acidophil granules. Two types of acidophils, somatotropes and mammotropes, are distinguished by selective staining methods and by immunocytochemistry. Basophils (B) tend to be larger than acidophils and less heavily granulated. The granules stain deeply basophil. Thyrotropes, gonadotropes, and corticotropes constitute the three types of basophils. Chromophobes (C) are small cells that are faintly staining. A large sinusoidal capillary (arrow) is closely related to the parenchymal cells. Masson. High power.*

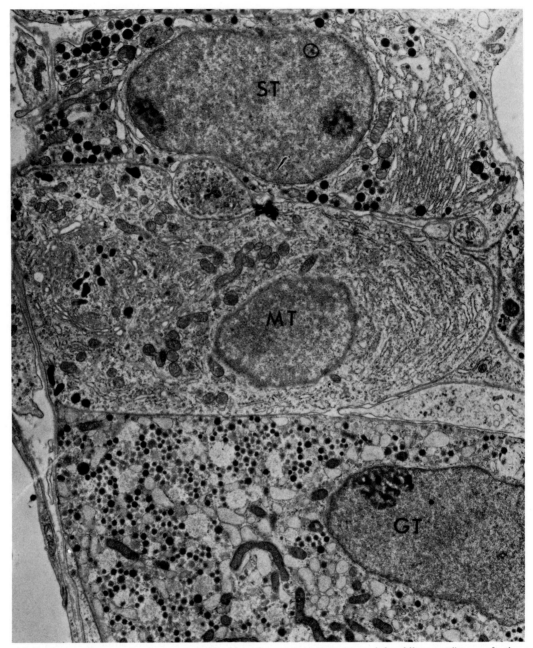

**Figure 14–5.** Electron micrograph of rat pars distalis. Note the varying appearance of the different cell types. In the anterior lobe of the pituitary, there are five morphologically distinct functional cell types: somatotropes (ST), mammotropes (MT), gonadotropes (GT), thyrotropes (not shown), and corticotropes (not shown), so named to denote their association with the production of growth, lactogenic, gonadotropic, thyrotropic, and adrenocorticotropic hormones, respectively. With the light microscope, cell types are distinguished by differences in staining affinities of their secretory granules, somatotropes and mammotropes being acidophil, and gonadotropes, thyrotropes, and corticotropes basophil. With the electron microscope, secretory granule size is the most useful criterion for identification of cell types. × 7000. (Courtesy of M. G. Farquhar.)

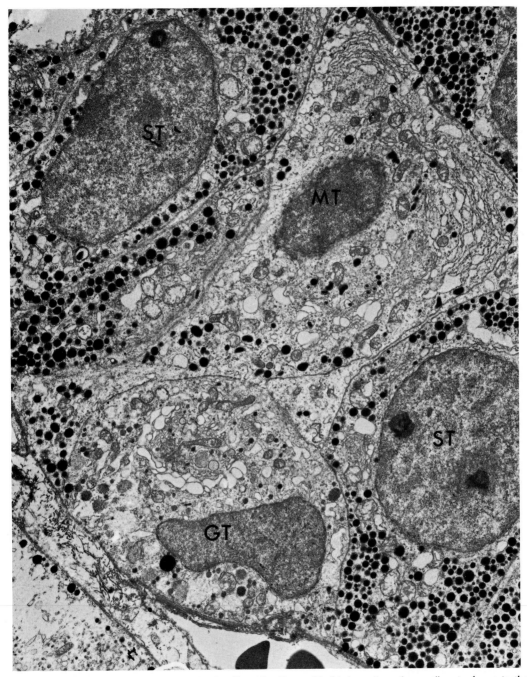

**Figure 14–6.** Electron micrograph of rat pars distalis. (See also Figure 14–5.) A portion of a capillary is shown in the lower center. × 7000. (Courtesy of M. G. Farquhar.)

*tropes*. On electron microscopy, the cells show an extensive development of granular endoplasmic reticulum and contain numerous electron-dense granules, which range from 300 to 350 nm in diameter. Somatotropin stimulates general body growth, particularly growth at the epiphyses of bones. Hypophysectomy causes a cessation of growth, which can be restored to normal by administration of the hormone. Undersecretion leads to *dwarfism* in certain animals. Oversecretion, as in certain tumors of the anterior lobe, causes *gigantism* in children. If oversecretion occurs after closure of epiphyseal discs, a condition known as *acromegaly*, in which the bones become thicker and the hands and feet broaden, results.

**Mammotropes.** Mammotropes are acidophils that tend to be scattered within the parenchymal cords. They are concentrated in the posterolateral regions of the pars distalis and are greatly increased in number during and after pregnancy. Their cytoplasm contains irregular granules that measure 550 to 600 nm in diameter, much larger than granules within somatotropes. Mammotropes secrete a *lactogenic hormone* (*prolactin, luteotropic hormone,* or LTH), which initiates and maintains the secretion of milk after pregnancy and stimulates the corpus luteum of the ovary to secrete progesterone.

**Basophils (Beta Cells).** The basophils tend to be appreciably larger than the acidophils. The granules are less numerous than in acidophils and are smaller (about 150 to 200 nm) in diameter. They stain poorly with hematoxylin but are stained deeply with methylene blue. Basophils are best identified by the periodic acid–Schiff (PAS) technique, for which they are strongly positive (deep pink) owing to the concentration of glycoproteins in their secretory granules. There are three distinct types of basophils.

**Thyrotropes (Beta Basophils).** The cells secrete *thyrotropic hormone* (*thyroid-stimulating hormone,* TSH), a glycoprotein that stimulates both synthesis and release of thyroid hormones. The cells are relatively large and are arranged deeply within the cell cords, usually at some distance from the sinusoidal capillaries. They contain numerous small granules that range in size from 100 to 150 nm or more. Hypophysectomy results in atrophy of the thyroid, which may be restored to activity by administration of hormone extracts. Injections of TSH into normal animals produce all the symptoms and signs of hyperthyroidism. Thyroidectomy results in an increase in the percentage of basophils within the pars distalis.

**Gonadotropes (Delta Basophils).** These basophils usually lie adjacent to sinusoids. They are spherical cells that possess numerous secretory granules, varying in diameter from 200 to 300 nm or more. They possess a prominent Golgi apparatus and a well-developed granular endoplasmic reticulum. The cells produce two hormones, *follicle-stimulating hormone* (FSH) and *luteinizing hormone* (LH). Some workers claim that there are two types of gonadotropes, one secreting FSH and the other LH. Although gonadotropes do exhibit considerable cytological variation, it remains unclear whether both hormones are present in the same granule or occur in different populations of granules.

FSH promotes growth of ovarian follicles in the female and, in the male, stimulates the synthesis of androgen-binding protein by Sertoli's cells of the seminiferous epithelium, thereby promoting spermatogenesis. In the female, FSH acts usually in association with LH, which ensures final maturation of the follicle, ovulation, and subsequent formation of the corpus luteum. In the male, LH (also termed *interstitial cell–stimulating hormone,* or ICSH) stimulates the production of testosterone by the interstitial cells of the testes. Testosterone is essential for sperm maturation and for development and maintenance of the accessory reproductive organs and the secondary sex characteristics. The effect is augmented by the administration of FSH. After castration, the rat hypophysis contains increased amounts of FSH and LH, and the basophils become enlarged and vacuolated (*castration cells*).

**Corticotropes.** The corticotropes are large basophils that contain scattered granules about 200 nm in diameter; an eccentric, indented nucleus; an extensive Golgi apparatus; and a sparse endoplasmic reticulum. They occur throughout the anteromedial portion of the pars distalis and secrete both *adrenocorticotropic hormone* (ACTH) and *lipotropic hormone* (LPH). The corticotropes synthesize a glycoprotein prohormone, containing the amino acid sequences of ACTH and LPH, that undergoes cleavage to yield the two hormones. ACTH promotes growth of the suprarenal cortex and stimulates secretion of glucocorticoids by the zona fasciculata and the zona reticularis of the cortex. The specific functions of LPH in humans are yet to be determined.

### The Pars Intermedia

In humans, the pars intermedia is less well developed than in many other animals and usually is poorly defined. It forms only about 2 per cent of the hypophysis. It is composed of a thin layer of cells and of vesicles that contain colloid (Fig. 14–7). It lies in close relation to the residual lumen, which virtually is obliterated in most adults. Some component cells, polyhedral in shape, are small and pale-staining and resemble chromophobes. Others are somewhat larger and possess numerous secretory granules, 200 to 300 nm in diameter. These cells, which are basophil and resemble corticotropes of the pars distalis, frequently extend as cords for a short distance into the pars nervosa. The cells lining the colloid-containing vesicles commonly are ciliated.

In certain species (e.g., amphibians and fish), the pars intermedia is well developed and produces *intermedin* or the *melanocyte-stimulating hormone* (MSH), which is a polypeptide that influences the production of melanin. In humans, MSH appears not to be a distinct hormone, and it may arise as a result of cleavage of the glycoprotein prohormone found within corticotropes. Thus, many authors feel that the cells responsible for the synthesis of MSH in humans are basophils within the pars distalis.

### The Pars Tuberalis

The pars tuberalis forms a collar of cells around the infundibular stalk. The cells, in close association with numerous blood vessels, are arranged

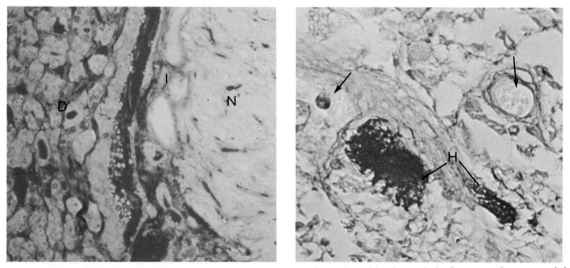

*Figure 14–7.* Hypophysis. Left: Pars intermedia and pars nervosa. Some large blood vessels (red) occupy the center of the field. To the left, there is a small segment of the pars distalis (D). The pars intermedia (I) is represented by a row of small irregular vesicles. The cells lining the vesicles are small and pale-staining and resemble chromophobes. The vesicles in life contain colloid. The pars nervosa (N) contains a few small blood vessels, and like the infundibular stem, it contains numerous unmyelinated nerve fibers and pituicytes (not apparent on this section). Mallory. Medium power. Right: Pars nervosa. Two Herring bodies (H) are present. They stain deeply with hematoxylin and represent accumulations of neurosecretory material. The material is elaborated in the supraoptic and paraventricular nuclei of the hypothalamus and passes along unmyelinated nerve fibers to the pars nervosa, where it is stored within the nerve terminals. Two small blood vessels (arrows) also are present. Gomori's chrome-alum hematoxylin. Medium power.

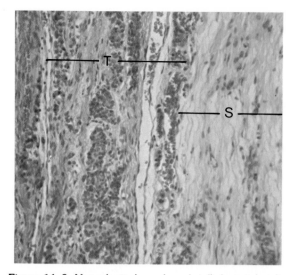

*Figure 14–8. Hypophysis, hypophyseal stalk (pars tuberalis and infundibular stalk). The pars tuberalis (T) contains groups or cords of cells, longitudinally oriented. The cells are small, possess little cytoplasm, and generally are chromophobe-like. They are in association with numerous blood vessels that pass down the length of the stalk, here sectioned longitudinally. The blood vessels are components of the hypophyseal portal system. The infundibular stalk (S) contains numerous unmyelinated nerve fibers (pale pink), whose cell bodies lie within the supraoptic and paraventricular nuclei of the hypothalamus. Only the nuclei (blue-red) of the component cells, or pituicytes, are seen. These cells resemble neuroglial cells found elsewhere within the central nervous system. H and E. Medium power.*

in groups or short cords longitudinally oriented (Fig. 14–8). They include acidophils, basophils, and undifferentiated chromophobe-like cells. The latter appear cuboidal, and the cytoplasm contains fine granules and large accumulations of glycogen. Small islands of squamous cells also may be present.

The function of the pars tuberalis, if any, is unknown.

### The Neurohypophysis

The neurohypophysis includes the median eminence of the tuber cinereum, the infundibular stem, and the infundibular process (pars nervosa). All three portions have the same characteristic cells and the same nerve and blood supply and contain the same active hormonal principle. Some 100,000 unmyelinated nerve fibers, constituting the *hypothalamo-hypophyseal tract*, pass through the infundibular stem to end in the pars nervosa. Their cell bodies lie principally within the supraoptic and paraventricular nuclei of the hypothalamus.

The cells of the neurohypophysis, *pituicytes*, resemble neuroglial cells elsewhere in the central nervous system. Pituicytes are small cells with short branching processes that end in relation either to blood vessels or to delicate connective tissue septa. Within the cytoplasm are fatty droplets, granules, and pigment. Pituicytes, although present throughout the neurohypophysis, are especially abundant in the pars nervosa. They have no known secretory activity, and it is believed that they function like the supporting neuroglia of the central nervous system.

The nerve cells of the supraoptic and paraventricular nuclei are neurosecretory and elaborate material that passes along the unmyelinated nerve fibers of the hypothalamo-hypophyseal tract to terminations of the fibers in the pars nervosa (see Fig. 14–7). Here the secretion is stored in the nerve terminals, which lie in close proximity to the extensive capillary network. With the electron microscope, the nerve terminals are seen to contain membrane-bound granules that have a diameter of 100 to 200 nm. Large groups of these neurosecretory granules, which stain deeply with chrome alum hematoxylin, may be visible on light microscopy as *Herring's bodies.* The neurosecretory material is released from the axon terminals into the perivascular space by exocytosis, in response to impulses that pass down the axons in which it is stored. After release, the hormonal material traverses the thin, fenestrated endothelium of the capillaries and is drained by hypophyseal veins into the systemic circulation.

The two hormones secreted by the neurohypophysis are *oxytocin* and *vasopressin (antidiuretic hormone,* ADH). Although oxytocin is synthesized primarily by nerve cell bodies of the paraventricular nucleus, and vasopressin by cell bodies of the supraoptic nucleus, recent evidence indicates that the two hormones may be synthesized in both nuclei. The nerve cells also synthesize proteins (*neurophysins*) to which these hormones are bound. There is one neurophysin for binding oxytocin and another for vasopressin. The neurophysin-hormone complexes constitute the major portions of the Herring's bodies. The hormones are released at separate nerve terminals in the pars nervosa.

Oxytocin stimulates contraction of the smooth muscle of the uterus during the final stages of pregnancy. It also induces contraction of the myoepithelial cells of the alveoli and ducts of the mammary gland, ejecting milk into the ducts. This phenomenon is initiated during suckling and is known as "milk letdown." Vasopressin causes contraction of vascular smooth muscle, thereby increasing peripheral resistance and elevating the blood pressure. Vasopressin also is known as *antidiuretic hormone* (ADH) because it influences the kidney to produce concentrated urine, thereby conserving water. It accomplishes this by increasing permeability of the distal tubules and collecting ducts of the kidney. Thus, water leaves the tubules and ducts, and a concentration of urine results. In the absence of vasopressin, large volumes of water are lost in the urine, a condition known as *diabetes insipidus*.

### Blood Vessels and Nerves of the Hypophysis

The blood supply of the hypophysis has unusual features and plays an important role in the secretory activity of the gland (Fig. 14–9).

The hypophysis is supplied primarily by two sets of blood vessels, a pair of *inferior hypophyseal arteries* and several *superior hypophyseal arteries*. The inferior hypophyseal arteries, branches of the internal carotid arteries, supply primarily the posterior lobe and send a few small branches to the sinusoidal capillaries of the anterior lobe. The several superior hypophyseal arteries, which arise from the internal carotids and from the posterior communicating artery of the circle of Willis, anastomose freely within the region of the median eminence of the hypothalamus and the base of the hypophyseal stalk and pass into the capillary network within the median eminence. The capillaries of this network drain into small veins that run downward around the hypophyseal stalk to supply the sinusoidal capillaries of the anterior lobe. This system of venous connections between the capillaries of the median eminence and the sinusoidal capillaries of the adenohypophysis constitutes the *hypophyseal portal system*. It must be appreciated, therefore, that the anterior lobe has little, if any, direct arterial supply. The hypophyseal portal system represents a connection by which neurohumeral substances ("hormone-releasing factors") from the median eminence are passed in the blood to the adenohypophysis. It is an important pathway in the regulation of adenohypophyseal function.

Efferent veins from anterior and posterior lobes drain into the cavernous sinuses.

The capillaries of the posterior lobe are smaller than the sinusoidal capillaries of the anterior lobe. Electron micrographs show an attenuated type of endothelium, in both the capillaries and the sinusoids. The deficiencies within the endothelial lining presumably facilitate passage of secretory material into the vessels.

The principal innervation of the neurohypophysis is the hypothalamo-hypophyseal tract, which originates mainly from the supraoptic and paraventricular nuclei (see Fig. 14–9). The unmyelinated nerve fibers of the tract course down the infundibular stalk to the infundibular process, where they end in close relation to the fenestrated capillaries. It is questionable if any nerve fibers extend into the anterior lobe, and there is no evidence to suggest neural control of secretion within the pars distalis.

### THE THYROID GLAND

The thyroid gland consists of two *lateral lobes* connected by a narrow *isthmus*. The isthmus lies over the second to the fourth tracheal cartilages, and the lateral lobes lie in relation to the superior part of the trachea and to the inferior part of the larynx. Frequently, a median *pyramidal lobe*, which extends upward anterior to the larynx, is present in addition. The gland develops as a median downgrowth of the base of the tongue. The thyroglossal duct, which connects the developing gland with the base of the tongue, usually becomes obliterated. Remnants of the duct may give rise to cysts or to the pyramidal lobe, a cranial extension of the isthmus.

The gland is enveloped externally by a connective tissue capsule that is continuous with the deep cervical fascia. Under this, there is an inner, true capsule that is thin and adheres closely to

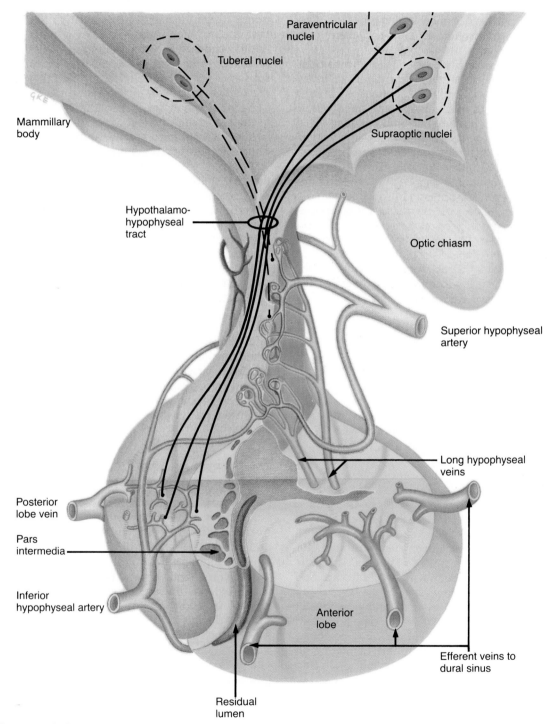

**Figure 14–9.** *Diagram of the principal vascular and nervous relations of the hypophysis. The hypophyseal portal (long hypophyseal) veins commence in the capillary beds of the median eminence and infundibular stem and pass downward to terminate in the sinusoidal capillaries of the anterior lobe.*

the gland. Delicate continuations of the inner capsule extend as septa into the gland, dividing it into indefinite *lobes* and *lobules*.

*Follicles,* the structural units of the gland, compose the lobules (Figs. 14–10 and 14–11). They vary greatly in size, depending upon the degree of distention by secretion. They also vary in shape but usually are irregularly spheroidal. The follicles are embedded within a delicate meshwork of reticular fibers that also supports a close net of fenestrated capillaries.

A follicle consists of a layer of simple epithelium enclosing a cavity that usually is filled with a stiff jelly called *colloid.* The follicular epithelial cells are of two types: *principal,* or *follicular, cells* (which constitute the majority of cells) and *parafollicular cells* (*C, clear,* or *light cells*).

**Principal Cells.** The shape of the principal cells varies but commonly is cuboidal. The cells are low when the gland is hypoactive, high when the gland is hyperactive. Cell height in any one follicle is uniform, and the arrangement is regular. The bases of the cells rest upon a delicate basal lamina, which usually is not resolved with the light microscope. The large, vesicular nuclei of the principal cells lie centrally or toward the base. The cytoplasm is finely granular and basophil and contains numerous mitochondria, abundant granular endoplasmic reticulum, and lysosomes (Fig. 14–12). The Golgi apparatus and centrioles are located above the nucleus. Lipid droplets and other inclusions, principally *colloid droplets,* are found in the cytoplasm of some cells. Junctional complexes are a feature of the interface between cells, and the free border is provided with small microvilli, visible only with the electron microscope. A few, scattered cells possess true cilia.

Colloid fills the follicular lumen. Fresh colloid is homogeneous, clear, and viscous. However, it undergoes shrinkage during the procedures employed in the preparation of microscopic sections and may show irregularities. Spaces often are present between the colloid and the epithelium, and vacuoles may occur within the colloid. The irregularities are indications of the state of the colloid and are most common in activated glands. Colloid stains basophil in active follicles, whereas it stains weakly basophil or acidophil in inactive follicles.

Colloid, which represents a reserve of secretion, is rich in nucleoproteins (hence its basophilia) and contains *thyroglobulin* and enzymes. Thyroglobulin is a glycoprotein containing several iodinated amino acids, the proportions of which vary from

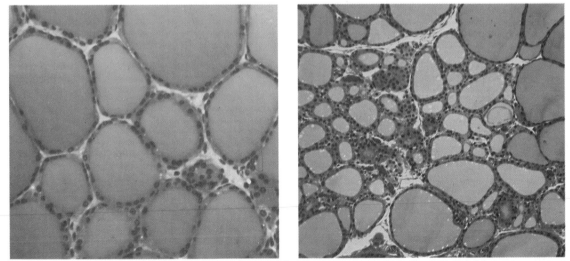

**Figure 14–10.** *Thyroid gland. Follicles, the structural units of the gland, are crowded together with little intervening connective tissue. Each follicle consists of a layer of simple epithelium enclosing a cavity that is filled with colloid. The follicles vary greatly in size, depending upon the degree of distention with colloid. The follicular epithelial cells are of two types, principal cells and parafollicular cells (not visible at this magnification). The principal cells generally appear cuboidal. Plastic sections. H and E. Low power.*

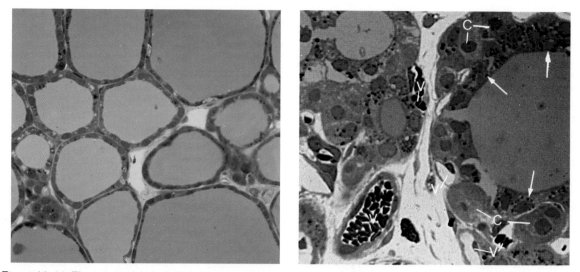

**Figure 14–11.** *Thyroid gland. Left: Follicles are closely packed and are separated by only a delicate, vascular connective tissue. They are lined by a cuboidal epithelium and contain colloid, which appears homogeneous. Plastic section. Toluidine blue. Medium power. Right: The principal cells of the follicular epithelium are irregularly cuboidal and have centrally located, vesicular nuclei. Many cells (arrows) possess discrete colloid droplets (darkly stained) within their cytoplasm. In addition to principal cells, the follicular epithelium contains some paler cells, the parafollicular, or C, cells (C), characteristically located at the periphery of the follicles. These cells, which are larger than principal cells, elaborate thyrocalcitonin. Numerous capillaries (V) lie within the delicate connective tissue of the gland, many in intimate relationship to follicular cells. Plastic section. Toluidine blue. High power.*

follicle to follicle. Thyroglobulin stains deeply with the PAS reaction.

The secretory process is complex and difficult to follow. It involves synthesis of the thyroid hormone, temporary storage, and release into the perifollicular fenestrated capillaries. The thyroid is unique among endocrine glands in that its secretory product is stored extracellularly in the lumen of the follicles. The process involves the following steps:

1. Synthesis of thyroglobulin. Amino acids are synthesized into polypeptides in the granular endoplasmic reticulum and are carried in small transport vesicles to the Golgi complex, where the protein is conjugated into the carbohydrate moiety.

2. Release of noniodinated thyroglobulin into the follicular lumen. From the Golgi complex, the glycoprotein is transported to the apical surface and discharged by exocytosis into the follicular lumen.

3. Iodination of the thyroglobulin. Principal cells take up iodide from the blood stream and concentrate it. Iodide is oxidized to iodine by intracellular thyroperoxidase and then is released into the follicular lumen. Iodination of the tyrosine groups in thyroglobulin occurs rapidly in the follicular lumen immediately adjacent to the microvillous border.

4. Storage of the iodinated thyroglobulin within the follicular lumen until needed.

5. Endocytosis of iodinated thyroglobulin by the principal cells, in response to a secretory stimulus.

6. Hydrolysis of the thyroglobulin. Lysosomes produced by the Golgi complex fuse with the endocytic vesicles, and the contained proteases hydrolyze thyroglobulin, breaking it down into its constituent amino acids, carbohydrates, and the thyroid hormones *triiodothyronine* ($T_3$) and *tetraiodothyronine* ($T_4$, thyroxine).

7. Release of $T_3$ and $T_4$. The thyroxine and triiodothyronine molecules are released through the basal cell membrane and enter the surrounding blood and lymphatic capillaries.

As the hormones enter the capillaries, most of the molecules are bound immediately to a protein called *binding protein*. Triiodothyronine is not as

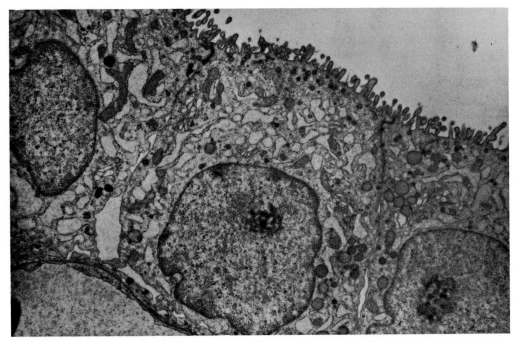

**Figure 14–12.** Electron micrograph of thyroid principal cells. The cytoplasm contains dilated profiles of endoplasmic reticulum and scattered elements of the Golgi apparatus. The apical border is provided with short microvilli that project into the colloid of the follicle. A perifollicular capillary is present in the lower left corner of the figure. × 7200. (Courtesy of S. L. Wissig.)

firmly bound to protein as is thyroxine and is the more potent of the two hormones.

**Parafollicular Cells.** The thyroid contains, in addition to the principal cells of the follicles, a small population of parafollicular cells. Embryologically, these cells arise from the last pair of pharyngeal pouches. In lower vertebrates, they occur as discrete epithelial cell masses, the *ultimobranchial bodies,* but in mammals they are incorporated into the thyroid.

The parafollicular cells, which lie adjacent to the follicles but within the basal lamina, do not abut on the follicular lumen. They are separated from the lumen by processes of neighboring principal cells. Generally, they are larger than principal cells, and their nuclei are placed eccentrically. They are characterized by the presence of numerous membrane-bound granules throughout the cytoplasm. The granules measure 10 to 50 nm in diameter. Immunofluorescent studies have shown that these cells are the site of production of *thyrocalcitonin (calcitonin).*

### Functions of the Thyroid Gland

The most striking effect of the thyroid secretion is its regulation of the metabolic rate. Thyroxine increases cell metabolism and, thus, is concerned with development, differentiation, and growth. In addition to many other effects, it increases the rate of carbohydrate utilization and influences the rate of intestinal absorption, heart rate, and body growth. *Hypothyroidism* in the infant leads to *cretinism;* hypofunction in the adult causes *myxedema.* Symptoms in both conditions are due to a reduction in the metabolic rate and may be removed by the administration of dried thyroid gland. *Hyperthyroidism* leads to overactivity and sometimes is complicated by the development of *exophthalmic goiter.* In hyperthyroidism, the follicles become enlarged, and principal cells increase in height. Colloid is diminished or absent. Surgical removal of a part of the thyroid or the administration of antithyroid drugs or radioiodine reduces the metabolic rate.

The thyroid gland elaborates, in addition to the thyroid hormones, thyrocalcitonin, a product of the parafollicular cells. This hormone is a polypeptide that actively lowers the concentration of calcium in the plasma by a direct action on bone, inhibiting bone resorption by the osteocytes and osteoclasts and the release of calcium. Hypercalcemia is the stimulus for secretion of the hormone, and hypocalcemia inhibits secretion. Therefore, it appears that secretion is controlled by a feedback mechanism operating through the plasma calcium level in a manner similar to that of control of the secretion of the parathyroid hormone, but in the reverse direction.

The thyroid gland has certain interrelationships with the anterior pituitary gland. Thyrotropic hormone (thyroid-stimulating hormone, or TSH) stimulates release of thyroxine. This, in turn, is controlled by thyrotropin-releasing factor (TRF) of the hypothalamus. Low levels of thyroxine in the blood initiate the release of TRF from the hypothalamus, and, in turn, TRF stimulates thyrotropes to secrete TSH. Thyroidectomy results in hypertrophy of the anterior lobe and the appearance of beta cells that morphologically exhibit certain alterations (so-called *thyroidectomy cells*). Secretion of thyrocalcitonin by parafollicular cells is dependent upon blood calcium levels and is not related to pituitary, thyroid, and parathyroid functions.

### Blood Vessels and Nerves of the Thyroid Gland

The thyroid gland receives its blood supply from the superior and inferior thyroid arteries. The blood capillaries form intimate plexuses around the thyroid follicles. They are of the fenestrated type, an arrangement that is thought to aid in the passage of the hormones into the capillary lumen. Arteriovenous anastomoses are common. The architecture of the blood vessels indicates that there are fluctuations in the amount of blood supplied to different regions of the gland. Extensive lymphatic capillary plexuses also surround the follicles and provide an additional route for conveying the hormones from the gland.

Numerous unmyelinated nerve fibers are present in the walls of the thyroid arteries. Most of these fibers are postganglionic sympathetic fibers and are vasomotor in function. Some sympathetic fibers terminate near the basal laminae of the follicles. This finding indicates the possibility that neural stimuli may influence thyroid function through a direct effect upon the follicular cells. However, the major regulator of thyroid activity undoubtedly is thyrotropic hormone secreted by the anterior pituitary.

### THE PARATHYROID GLANDS

There are usually two pairs of parathyroid glands in humans, but accessory glands occur frequently. The glands are small, brownish oval bodies that lie in close relation to the thyroid gland. They measure 3 to 8 mm in length, 2 to 5 mm in width, and 1 to 2 mm in thickness. The upper parathyroids lie on the posterior surface of the thyroid, about midway between the upper and lower poles of the lobes, whereas the lower ones are in relation to the lower poles of the thyroid lobes (Fig. 14–13). The parathyroid glands develop from the endoderm of the pharyngeal pouches, the superior parathyroids from the fourth pouch, and the inferior parathyroids from the third pouch. In their development, the inferior parathyroids are closely associated with the developing thymus and are drawn down with it during its caudal migration. Normally, they migrate only as far as the lower poles of the thyroid gland, but in 5 to 10 per cent of individuals, the lower parathyroids retain their association with the thymus.

Each parathyroid gland is covered by a thin capsule that separates it from the thyroid. Delicate septa, which pass inward from the capsule, carry blood vessels, lymphatics, and a few nerve fibers into the gland. The connective tissue of the capsule and of the septa contains fat cells, which increase in number with age. A network of reticular fibers supports the parenchyma, which is composed of masses and cords of epithelial cells. The epithelial cells are of two types, *chief*, or *principal, cells* and *oxyphil cells*.

**Principal Cells (Chief Cells).** Principal cells measure 7 to 10 μm in diameter and are more abundant than oxyphil cells (Fig. 14–14). They have large vesicular nuclei, centrally placed, and a clear, pale-staining cytoplasm. The cytoplasm

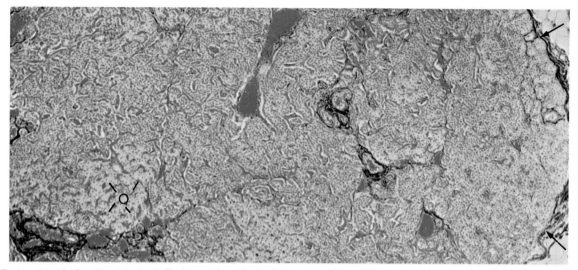

**Figure 14–13.** Parathyroid gland. Each parathyroid gland is covered by a thin capsule of connective tissue (arrows) that separates it from the thyroid gland and from the surrounding cervical fascia. Delicate branching and anastomosing septa (blue) pass inward from the capsule and carry with them numerous small blood vessels (red). The parenchyma of the gland is composed of masses and irregular cords of epithelial cells of two types, principal and oxyphil. Principal, or chief, cells are the most abundant. One group of oxyphil cells (O) is present. These cells are larger than principal cells and have a pale cytoplasm. Mallory-Azan. Low power.

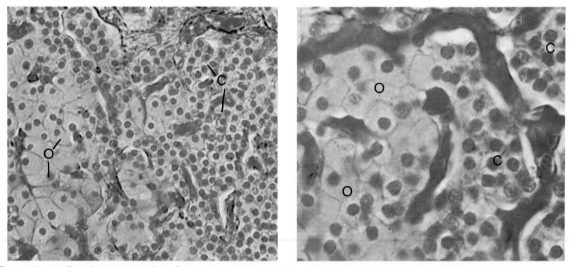

**Figure 14–14.** Parathyroid gland. Left: Principal, or chief, cells (C) occur mainly in anastomosing cords. Individual cell boundaries are difficult to discern. Oxyphil cells (O), present principally in clumps, are larger than principal cells and have distinct cell boundaries. Numerous capillaries (red) occur within the delicate connective tissue between parenchymal cells. Mallory-Azan. Medium power. Right: Principal, or chief, cells (C) form small cords and clumps. Most possess vesicular nuclei, but a few have smaller, more densely staining nuclei. Oxyphil cells (O) are much larger than principal cells and exhibit distinct cell boundaries. They possess small spherical nuclei and a considerable amount of pale-staining, finely granular cytoplasm. The parenchymal cells are embedded in delicate connective tissue (blue) that contains a close network of capillaries (red). Mallory-Azan. High power.

contains, in addition to the usual organelles, lipofuscin granules, large accumulations of glycogen, lipid droplets, and small dense granules limited by a membrane. The latter have been interpreted by some investigators as secretory granules. Some principal cells possess very few dense granules and appear less active than the cells previously described.

**Oxyphil Cells.** Oxyphil cells represent only a minor portion of the cell population and characteristically occur singly or in small groups. They are larger than the principal cells. They have small, darkly staining nuclei that often appear pyknotic. The cytoplasm is strongly acidophil, owing to the presence within the cytoplasm of large numbers of mitochondria, each with closely packed cristae. Small accumulations of glycogen occur between the mitochondria. Oxyphil cells are not present in humans until about 5 to 7 years of age, and thereafter they increase in number, especially after puberty.

Cells with features intermediate between those of principal and oxyphil cells also are seen frequently. Such cells possess a fine granular cytoplasm that is faintly acidophil and nuclei that are smaller and stain more darkly than those of the principal cells.

Most investigators feel that the principal cells are the primary parenchymal elements and that oxyphil and intermediate cells represent only a modification or different functional state.

Small colloid follicles are seen occasionally and are more noticeable in old age. The material they contain has no functional relation to the colloid of thyroid follicles.

### Functions of the Parathyroid Glands

The parathyroid glands elaborate the parathyroid hormone (*parathormone*), a protein consisting of a single polypeptide chain. Although the principal cells are thought to be the primary source of the hormone, there is some evidence to suggest that oxyphil cells also may secrete parathormone, particularly in disease states. The hormone is important in the regulation of calcium metabolism. A lowering of the plasma concentration of calcium is followed by an increased output of the hormone, which, in turn, withdraws calcium from the bones. It is claimed that the action of

the hormone is due to its ability to stimulate the transformation of osteogenic cells into osteoclasts. Parathormone also acts directly on the renal tubules of the kidney to decrease the clearance of calcium and increase the excretion of phosphate, sodium, and potassium. Plasma levels of calcium are prevented from exceeding the optimum by thyrocalcitonin, produced by the parafollicular cells of the thyroid gland.

Atrophy or removal of the parathyroids causes a fall in plasma calcium, which is accompanied by nervous hyperexcitability and muscular spasms, leading to death due to tetany. Administration of calcium or parathyroid extract relieves the symptoms. Hypertrophy of the glands occurs in conditions such as rickets, where there is a calcium deficiency. *Hyperparathyroidism* may result from tumor or hyperplasia and is associated with an elevated blood calcium level and extensive bone resorption.

### Blood Vessels and Nerves of the Parathyroid Glands

The parathyroids have a rich vascular supply from the inferior thyroid arteries or from anastomoses between the superior and inferior thyroid arteries. The larger branches of the blood vessels follow the septa into the interior of each gland. A fine net of fenestrated capillaries lies in relation to the parenchyma.

Unmyelinated nerve fibers, probably vasomotor in function, are scanty.

### THE SUPRARENAL GLANDS

The suprarenal, or adrenal, glands are roughly pyramidal, flattened organs, one at the cranial pole of each kidney (Fig. 14–15). Each measures about 5 by 3 by less than 1 cm and weighs about 5 gm. The hilum is an indentation on the anterior surface. A sectioned, fresh gland shows two regions: (1) an outer cortex, which appears yellow as a result of the presence of lipids, and (2) a thin inner *medulla*, which is reddish brown. These regions are distinct structurally, developmentally, and functionally. The cortex develops from epithelium (mesothelium) lining the primitive body

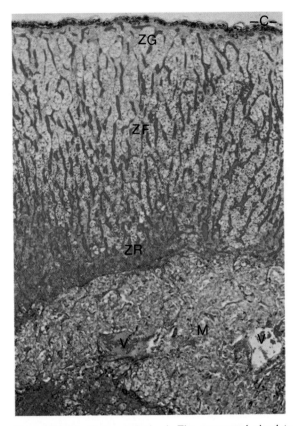

*Figure 14–15. Suprarenal gland. The suprarenal gland is surrounded by a tough fibroelastic capsule (C), from which delicate trabeculae extend radially into the cortex of the gland. The cortex is divided into three ill-defined layers: the zona glomerulosa (ZG), immediately beneath the capsule; the zona fasciculata (ZF), the thickest layer, where cells are arranged in long cords; and the zona reticularis (ZR), the inner zone, where cell cords form an anastomosing network. The medulla (M) is composed of large, ovoid cells that occur mainly in groups or short-anastomosing cords. The gland receives a rich vascular supply. Numerous arterioles pierce the capsule and enter cortical sinusoids (red) that course between the cell cords. Other arterioles pass to the medulla and empty into a capillary plexus. Venous blood both from the cortex and from the medulla drains into venules that join to form large medullary veins (V). Mallory-Azan. Low power.*

cavity (coelom) and overlying the urogenital ridge. The medulla is derived from the neural crest and presumptive autonomic ganglion (*sympatho-chromaffin*) tissue. The cells of this tissue, which are homologues of postganglionic sympathetic neurons that do not develop axons, migrate into the urogenital ridge. In lower vertebrates, the two tissues are not united into a single organ, and in reptiles and birds they may be intermingled in a variety of patterns.

Each gland is surrounded by a tough connective tissue capsule that sends radial trabeculae, consisting principally of reticular fibers, into the cortex. Capillaries penetrate into the gland along the delicate trabeculae. At the corticomedullary junction, the reticular fibers of the trabeculae form a fine meshwork that extends around the groups and cords of medullary cells.

### Cortex

The cortex, the major part of the gland, is divided into three ill-defined layers (Fig. 14–16):

1. A thin, outer zone, the *zona glomerulosa*.
2. A thick, middle zone, the *zona fasciculata*.
3. An inner zone, the *zona reticularis*, directly in relation to the medulla.

In the human, the zona glomerulosa accounts for about 15 per cent of the total cortical volume, the zona fasciculata 78 per cent, and the zona reticularis 7 per cent. The transition from one zone to another is gradual, and boundaries between zones are indistinct.

**Zona Glomerulosa.** This narrow zone, immediately beneath the capsule, consists of pyramidal or columnar cells arranged in ovoid groups or arcades that are continuous with the cell columns of the zona fasciculata. The cells possess deeply staining spherical nuclei, and the cytoplasm, although generally acidophil, contains some basophil material and a few small lipid droplets (Fig. 14–17). On electron microscopy, the most characteristic feature of component cells is the well-developed, smooth-surfaced endoplasmic reticulum, which appears as an anastomosing network of tubules. Numerous mitochondria, with lamellar cristae, are evenly distributed throughout the cytoplasm.

**Zona Fasciculata.** This, the thickest layer of the cortex, is composed of large, irregularly cuboidal or polyhedral cells arranged in long, radial cords usually one or two cells wide (Fig. 14–18). The cords are separated by sinusoidal capillaries. Nuclei of cells of this zone are located centrally and are vesicular. Binucleate cells are seen frequently. The cytoplasm contains basophil masses and is crowded with lipid droplets, composed of cholesterol, fatty acids, and neutral fat. These

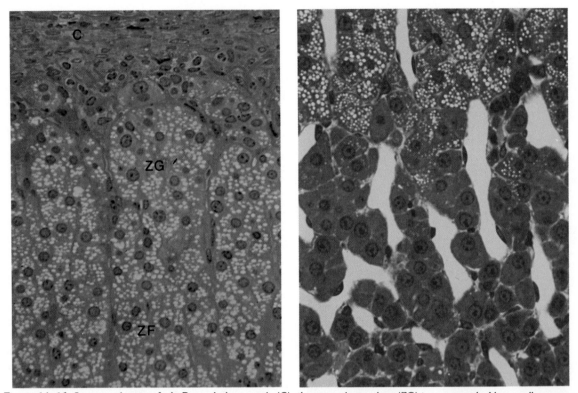

**Figure 14–16.** *Suprarenal cortex. Left: Beneath the capsule (C), the zona glomerulosa (ZG) is composed of large cells arranged in ovoid groups or arcades. The cells appear vacuolated. In the zona fasciculata (ZF), of which only a small portion is shown here, cells are arranged in parallel cords, usually one or two cells wide, and have a spongy appearance: Hence, they are called spongiocytes. The cords are separated by delicate connective tissue trabeculae that contain sinusoidal capillaries. Plastic section. H and E. High power. Right: This section shows the inner portion of the cortex. Note the vacuolated cells (spongiocytes) of the zona fasciculata (above) and the deeply staining cytoplasm of cells of the zona reticularis (below). In the zona reticularis, the cells form an anastomosing network of cords, separated by wide, sinusoidal capillaries. Plastic section. Methylene blue, basic fuchsin. High power.*

substances represent stored precursors of the steroid hormones secreted by the cells. Lipid droplets are most numerous in cells of the outer two thirds of the zone. Since lipids are removed by the usual technical procedures, the cells here appear vacuolated and have a spongy appearance; hence sometimes they are called *spongiocytes.* The inner third of the zone is relatively free of lipid material and is more basophil. The cells contain abundant smooth endoplasmic reticulum and numerous mitochondria with tubular cristae. The plasma membrane is thrown into short, irregular microvilli that extend into the subendothelial space of the sinusoids.

**Zona Reticularis.** The cells of this, the innermost cortical zone, form a network of anastomos-

ing cords that also are separated by sinusoidal capillaries. The parenchymal cells are smaller than those of the zona fasciculata. In general, the cytoplasm contains fewer lipid droplets, the nuclei are more deeply stained, and many cells possess accumulations of lipofuscin pigment granules. Near the zona fasciculata, component cells differ little from those of that zone, but toward the medulla, "light" and "dark" cells can be identified. Nuclei of the light cells are paler staining; those of the dark cells are more intensely stained and shrunken. The significance of these staining differences is unknown. Cells of the zona reticularis possess numerous secondary lysosomes (pigment granules) and, like those of the other zones, abundant smooth endoplasmic reticulum.

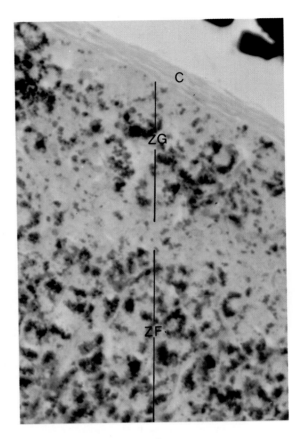

**Figure 14–17.** *Suprarenal cortex, lipid material. This frozen section has been stained specifically to show lipid material. The capsule (C) is unstained, and external to it, there is a small group of fat cells (top right). The outer cells of the zona glomerulosa (ZG) contain some lipid material, which appears as darkly staining droplets, but the inner cells appear almost devoid of lipid droplets. The remainder of the field is occupied by the zona fasciculata (ZF), the component cells of which contain numerous lipid droplets. The inner third of the zona fasciculata and the zona reticularis, not shown here, are relatively free of lipid material. Sudan Black B. Medium power.*

## Medulla

The boundary between cortex and medulla usually is irregular in humans, although in many other animals, the boundary may be sharp. Cells of the medulla are large and ovoid or polyhedral and occur in groups or short anastomosing cords, surrounded by venules and capillaries (Figs. 14–19 and 14–20). Medullary cells have large vesicular nuclei, and their cytoplasm contains fine granules that become brown when treated with potassium bichromate. This is the *chromaffin reaction*, and, therefore, the cells are called *chromaffin* (or *pheochrome*) *cells.* The reaction is due, in large part, to the presence of the catecholamines *epinephrine* and *norepinephrine.* The granules also stain green with ferric chloride and brown with osmium tetroxide.

On electron microscopy, the cells show a well-developed granular endoplasmic reticulum, scattered mitochondria, and an extensive Golgi complex. The cells contain numerous membrane-bound granules that measure 100 to 300 nm in diameter and are of two types. In cells that elaborate norepinephrine, the granules contain very electron-dense cores, whereas cells containing epinephrine possess granules that are homogeneous and less densely staining. The granules, containing either norepinephrine or epinephrine, are released by exocytosis. Each chromaffin cell is said to be oriented with one end abutting on a capillary, the other on a venule.

In addition to chromaffin cells, the medulla contains a few scattered autonomic ganglion cells.

## Functions of the Suprarenal Glands

The cortex and medulla are functionally distinct. The cortex is essential to life. Cortical destruction by tuberculosis (Addison's disease) or removal is fatal unless averted by administration

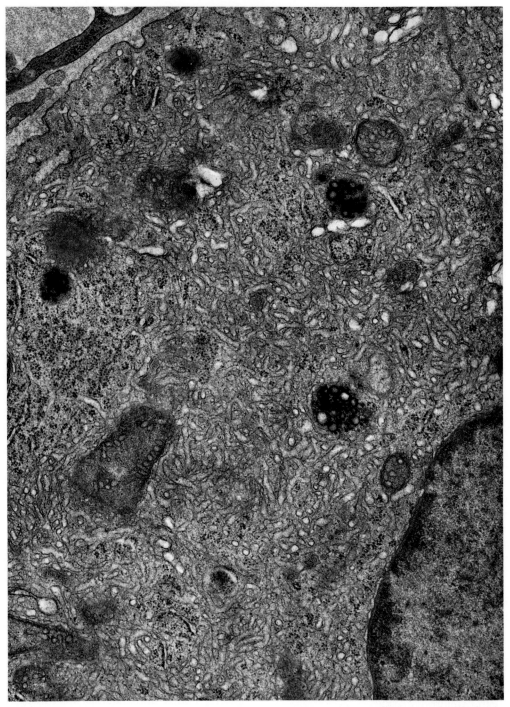

**Figure 14–18.** Electron micrograph of a zona fasciculata cell of human suprarenal cortex. Note the extensive development of smooth-surfaced endoplasmic reticulum (center), which is characteristic of steroid-secreting cells. The dark masses are pigment granules. × 18,600. (Courtesy of J. A. Long.)

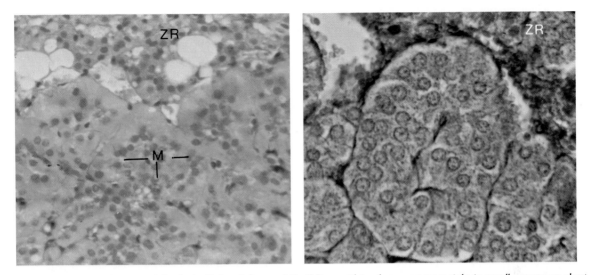

**Figure 14–19.** *Suprarenal medulla. Left: Cells of the medulla (M), ovoid in shape, occur mainly in small groups or short anastomosing cords. Their cytoplasm is finely granular and appears yellow-brown following treatment with potassium bichromate. This is the chromaffin reaction and is due to the presence of catecholamines within cytoplasmic granules. Above, there is a small portion of the zona reticularis (ZR). Chromaffin reaction. Medium power. Right: Cells of the medulla (chromaffin cells) have large vesicular nuclei, and their cytoplasm contains fine granules that stain greenish-gray with zinc chloride. A small portion of the zona reticularis (ZR) is present above the corticomedullary junction (upper right). Zinc chloride. High power.*

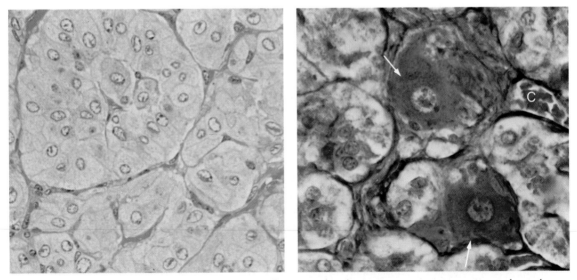

**Figure 14–20.** *Suprarenal medulla. Left: The medullary cells, arranged in discrete groups or anastomosing cords, are large and polyhedral. Nuclei are large and vesicular and generally are centrally placed. The delicate connective tissue that delineates the groups and cords of cells contains numerous capillaries, not visible here. Plastic section. H and E. High power. Right: The medullary (chromaffin) cells here appear pale, with scattered cytoplasmic granules. Also present are two sympathetic ganglion cells (arrows). These cells have large, vesicular nuclei with distinct nucleoli and a densely staining granular cytoplasm. Note also a capillary (C) in the connective tissue between the medullary cell groups and cords. Mallory-Azan. High power.*

of cortical extract. The cortex is necessary to humans in a variety of essential factors. It maintains *water and electrolyte balance* in the body. After ablation of the cortex, there is concentration of the plasma, excessive secretion of sodium, and a shift of water from extracellular spaces to tissue cells. The cortex also maintains *carbohydrate balance.* If control is lost, glycogen stores in liver and muscle are depleted, and *hypoglycemia* results. *Maintenance of the intercellular substances* is an additional function of the cortex.

More than 40 steroid compounds, collectively referred to as *corticosteroids,* have been isolated from the cortex, at least seven of which have been shown to possess physiological activity. In general, the active compounds can be divided into three categories as judged by their type of activity:

1. *Mineralocorticoids (aldosterone* and *deoxycorticosterone),* which control electrolyte and water balance.

2. *Glucocorticoids (cortisol, cortisone,* and *corticosterone),* which influence carbohydrate metabolism.

3. *Gonadocorticoids* (principally *dehydroepiandrosterone*), which normally are of little physiological significance.

**Mineralocorticoids.** Aldosterone and deoxycorticosterone are secreted by cells of the zona glomerulosa. Aldosterone, the most important mineralocorticoid, increases reabsorption of sodium by the distal tubules of the kidney, increases potassium excretion by the kidney, and lowers the concentration of sodium in the secretions of salivary glands, sweat glands, and intestinal mucosa. Aldosterone secretion is controlled by the *renin-angiotensin* system, which is sensitive to changes in blood pressure and to plasma levels of sodium and potassium. Adrenocorticotropic hormone (ACTH) of the adenohypophysis has little or no effect upon secretion of aldosterone.

**Glucocorticoids.** Cortisol, or *hydrocortisone,* is the most important member of the glucocorticoids, which are secreted by the zona fasciculata and zona reticularis. The glucocorticoids increase the formation of glucose in the liver and its storage as glycogen and cause an increase in blood glucose and amino acid levels. These corticosteroids also affect connective tissues to suppress the immune and inflammatory responses. They cause destruction of lymphocytes, inhibit mitoses in lymphoid tissues, and accelerate the sequestration of eosinophils in the spleen and the lungs. The secretory activity of the zona fasciculata and zona reticularis is regulated by the adenohypophysis through secretion of adrenocorticotropic hormone (ACTH). ACTH stimulates steroid synthesis and release, promotes growth of the suprarenal cortex, and increases blood flow in the cortex.

**Gonadocorticoids.** Gonadocorticoids, or *sex steroids,* include both female sex hormones (*estrogen* and *progesterone*) and several *androgenic hormones,* principally dehydroepiandrosterone. These hormones are produced primarily in the zona reticularis, but the amounts produced normally are so small that they are not of physiological significance. However, some tumors that arise in the cortex do produce these steroids in abundance, resulting in a masculinizing or feminizing effect. In the *adrenogenital syndrome,* the inner zones of the cortex become hypertrophic, and increased levels of circulating androgens may cause precocious puberty and increased hirsutism.

Marked changes occur in the human suprarenal cortex after birth. Within two weeks after birth, most of the *inner,* or *boundary, zone* of the cortex (*fetal cortex*) has disappeared, leaving only *subcapsular (permanent) cortex.* The latter consists of zona glomerulosa and zona fasciculata. Zona reticularis does not become established until the end of the third year. The significance of the fetal cortex is poorly understood, but its presence is thought to be dependent upon hormones elaborated by the placenta.

The suprarenal medulla is not essential to life. It produces the catecholamines norepinephrine and epinephrine. Their presence in the cytoplasmic granules can be detected by the chromaffin reaction. The number of chromaffin granules in a cell is an index of its secretory state. Although the two hormones are closely related chemically, there are important qualitative and quantitative differences between them with regard to their physiological effects.

*Epinephrine* has a marked effect upon metabolism, increasing oxygen consumption and mobilizing glucose from liver glycogen stores. It also causes release of ACTH from the hypophysis, which in turn stimulates secretion of glucocorticoids from the suprarenal cortex to offset gluconeogenesis. It increases cardiac output and prepares the body to meet emergency situations.

*Norepinephrine* has little general metabolic action, and its chief function is as the principal transmitter substance or mediator of adrenergic nerve impulses acting upon the heart and blood vessels to elevate and maintain blood pressure. Its effect upon the blood pressure is primarily a consequence of the vasoconstriction it causes in the peripheral segments of the arterial system.

The release of both catecholamines from the parenchymal cells of the medulla is under direct control of the sympathetic nervous system.

### Blood Vessels and Nerves of the Suprarenal Glands

The suprarenal glands receive a rich vascular supply (Fig. 14–21). A variable number of arteries, arising from the inferior phrenic artery, the

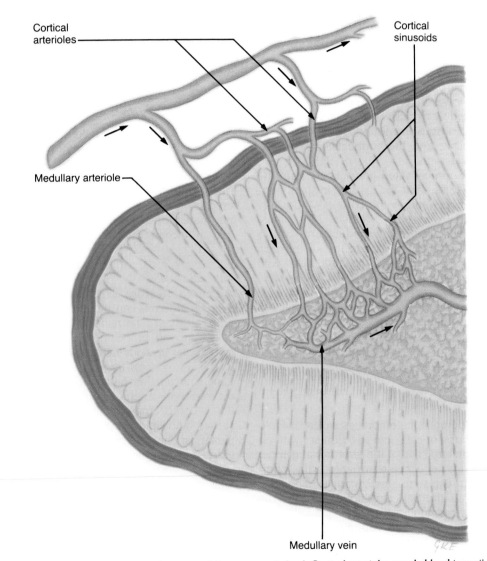

**Figure 14–21.** *Diagram showing the vascularization of the suprarenal gland. Cortical arterioles supply blood to cortical sinusoids, which continue into medullary capillaries. The latter also receive blood directly from medullary arterioles. Blood entering the medullary capillaries from cortical sinusoids is rich in corticosteroids.*

renal artery, and the aorta, supplies each gland. As the arteries reach the gland, they branch into numerous arterioles, which pierce the capsule. *Cortical arterioles* supply blood to the cortical sinusoidal capillaries, which possess a fenestrated endothelium. The cortical capillaries drain into collecting veins at the corticomedullary junction. The collecting veins ultimately join to form a medullary vein. There is no venous system in the cortex. Some arterioles from the capsule pass directly in the connective tissue trabeculae to the medulla as *medullary arterioles*. They provide a direct arterial supply to the rich capillary network surrounding medullary cells. Hence, the medulla has a dual blood supply from cortical sinusoids and from medullary arterioles. The blood reaching the medulla from cortical sinusoids is rich in cortical hormones that may directly influence the activity of medullary cells.

Lymphatic vessels are found only in the capsule, trabeculae, and the connective tissue surrounding large veins.

Numerous unmyelinated nerve fibers from the splanchnic nerves enter the capsule in small bundles. A few fibers end in the cortex, where they are associated with blood vessels. Most fibers follow the trabeculae to the medulla and end as preganglionic fibers in relation to medullary cells. The nerve terminals form typical synapses with the cells, each of which is said to be innervated. Stimulation of the splanchnic nerves causes a heavy discharge of epinephrine, whereas section of the nerves inhibits secretory activity of medullary cells.

## THE PARAGANGLIA (CHROMAFFIN SYSTEM)

The term paraganglia embraces several widely scattered groups of cells that are similar in many ways to medullary cells of the suprarenal glands. The cell groups largely lie retroperitoneally, often in association with sympathetic ganglia. The largest groups are the paired or joined *para-aortic bodies of Zuckerkandl.*

Paraganglia have a thick connective tissue capsule and are highly vascularized. They possess two cell types: *chief cells* and *supporting cells.* Chief cells contain numerous, membrane-bound, electron-dense granules similar to those of supra-

renal medullary cells. The cells exhibit the chromaffin reaction and contain catecholamines, principally norepinephrine. The supporting cells are devoid of secretory granules and partially or completely surround each chief cell. Their function is unknown.

The carotid and aortic bodies, which function as chemoreceptors, are associated with small islands of chromaffin cells.

At present, it is unclear whether paraganglia have an endocrine function, releasing catecholamines into the vascular system, or whether their component cells function as interneurons to inhibit transmission in sympathetic ganglia. They can be important clinically if they release excessive amounts of catecholamines.

## THE PINEAL GLAND

The pineal gland, or *epiphysis cerebri,* is a small, cone-shaped body attached by a stalk to the roof of the third ventricle. It is derived from neuroectoderm of the diencephalon and is covered by pia mater except at its attachment. The pia mater forms a thin capsule that sends septa into the organ, dividing it incompletely into lobules (Fig. 14–22). The lobules are composed of *epithelioid cells,* or *pinealocytes,* and *glial,* or *interstitial, cells.*

Pinealocytes are difficult to define in routine preparations but can be seen well in silver preparations, where they appear as irregularly shaped cells with long, branching processes that terminate in bulbous endings near blood vessels (Fig. 14–23). They possess large, deeply infolded or lobulated nuclei that have prominent nucleoli. The cytoplasm is variable in amount and may contain dense-cored, membrane-bound granules, lysosomes, and lipid droplets. In addition, the cytoplasm is characterized by the presence of an extensive endoplasmic reticulum, mostly smooth-surfaced, and of large numbers of microtubules. Gap junctions, desmosomes, and intermediate types of junctions occur frequently between neighboring pinealocytes.

Glial cells serve as supporting elements and form an interwoven network around and between the cords and clumps of pinealocytes. They are fewer in number than pinealocytes, and their nuclei are elongated and stain more deeply. Cy-

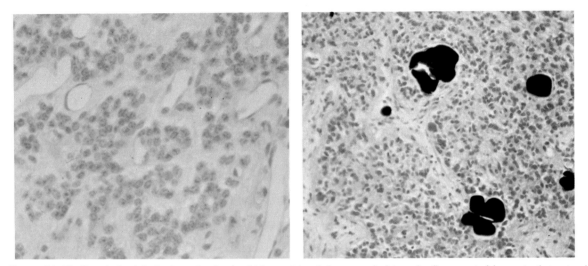

**Figure 14–22.** Pineal gland. Left: Juvenile gland, which consists of clumps and plates of cells separated by septa that extend into the gland from a thin capsule. Two cell types are recognized: The more common epithelioid cells, or pinealocytes, and the glial, or interstitial, cells. The two cell types cannot be distinguished in this H and E preparation. The delicate septa contain numerous small blood vessels. Medium power. Right: Adult gland. The irregular clumps of parenchymal cells, or lobules, are separated by delicate connective tissue septa (pale pink). In the adult, the gland is characterized by the presence of concretions, or acervuli, which are black in this preparation. H and E. Low power.

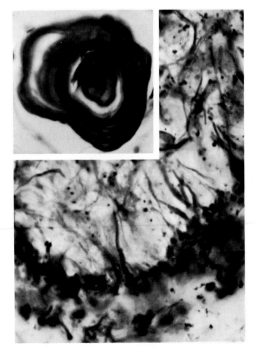

**Figure 14–23.** Human pineal gland in which the pinealocytes have been made visible with silver. Long branching processes of the cells terminate in bulbous endings (below). Del Rio–Hortega silver method. High power. Inset: Acervulus. Acervuli ("brain sand") are lamellated bodies composed primarily of calcium carbonates and phosphates in an organic matrix. Medium power.

toplasmic processes, containing numerous fine filaments 5 to 6 nm in diameter, extend out from the glial cells, giving them the appearance of astrocytes.

The epiphysis attains its maximum development at about seven years of age and thereafter shows retrogressive changes that involve principally the supporting elements. Connective tissue

### Summary Table 14–1. Main Features and Functions of Endocrine Glands

| Gland | Hormone | Source | Functions |
|---|---|---|---|
| Hypophysis<br>Pars distalis | STH (Somatotropin) | Somatotrope (acidophil) | Promotes body growth, particularly growth of long bones |
| | LTH (Prolactin) | Mammotrope (acidophil) | Promotes mammary gland development and lactation |
| | TSH (Thyrotropin) | Thyrotrope (basophil) | Stimulates production of thyroid hormones |
| | FSH | Gonadotrope (basophil) | Stimulates growth of ovarian follicles in female and promotes spermatogenesis in male |
| | LH (ICSH) | Gonadotrope (basophil) | In female: stimulates ovulation and formation of corpus luteum. In male: promotes androgen secretion |
| | ACTH | Corticotrope (basophil) | Stimulates secretion of glucocorticoids by suprarenal cortex |
| | LPH | Corticotrope (basophil) | Unknown in humans |
| Neurohypophysis | Oxytocin | Neurons in paraventricular and supraoptic nuclei | Induces contraction of smooth muscle in uterus and of myoepithelial cells in the mammary glands |
| | ADH (vasopressin) | Neurons in paraventricular and supraoptic nuclei | Promotes water resorption and conservation, and causes contraction of vascular smooth muscle |
| Thyroid | Thyroid hormones (T$_3$ and T$_4$) | Principal cell | Regulates basal metabolic rate and influences body growth and development |
| | Thyrocalcitonin | Parafollicular cell | Lowers blood calcium levels by inhibiting bone resorption |
| Parathyroid | Parathormone | Principal cell (? plus oxyphil) | Raises blood calcium levels by promoting bone resorption and increasing calcium resorption in the kidneys |
| Suprarenal cortex | Mineralocorticoids (principally aldosterone) | Zona glomerulosa cells | Increase reabsorption of sodium by kidney tubules |
| | Glucocorticoids (principally cortisol) | Zona fasciculata and zona reticularis cells | Promote carbohydrate metabolism and suppress inflammatory and immune responses |
| | Gonadocorticoids (sex steroids) | Zona reticularis cells | (Amount too small to produce significant effects) |
| Suprarenal medulla | Epinephrine | Chromaffin cell | Increases oxygen consumption and mobilizes glucose |
| | Norepinephrine | Chromaffin cell | Increases heart rate, blood pressure |
| Paraganglia | Norepinephrine | Chief cell | ? As above |
| Pineal | Melatonin | Pinealocyte | Function unclear but may influence gonadal development |

increases in amount, and the lobules become well delineated. *Acervuli (brain sand, or corpora arenacea)* are concretions that appear mainly in the capsule and in the septa. They are lamellated bodies that vary greatly in size and in number. They are composed primarily of calcium carbonates and phosphates within an organic matrix. Their functional significance, if any, is unknown.

## Blood Vessels and Nerves

A few blood vessels and nerve fibers, both myelinated and unmyelinated, supply the gland. The capillaries within the gland are of the thin, fenestrated type. The nerve fibers, from the sympathetic portion of the autonomic nervous system, arise in the superior cervical ganglia. The nerve terminals end directly in relation to the pinealocytes and are thought to influence their secretory activity.

## Functions of the Pineal Gland

The epiphysis of mammals is a vestige of the photoreceptive pineal system of lower vertebrates. In mammals, the epiphysis appears to have a secretory endocrine function. The pineals of many mammals, including humans, have been shown to secrete various substances, of which *melatonin* is the best understood. In the rat, the gland secretes *serotonin,* a precursor of melatonin, and the amount of the hormone in the gland and in the blood shows diurnal fluctuations. The level is lowest during daylight hours and highest during darkness. It appears that light entering the eye stimulates neurons to transmit impulses via a series of pre- and postganglionic neurons to the pineal gland. Here, they inhibit the secretion of melatonin. In this way, the gland acts as a neuroendocrine transducer, converting a neural input (its sympathetic neurons releasing norepinephrine) into a hormonal output (melatonin) that modifies the functional activity of other endocrine organs and synchronizes endogenous rhythms.

Melatonin, when injected into rats, slows the estrous cycle and causes the ovaries to lose weight. The ability of melatonin to modify gonadal function suggests that its secretion may be concerned with the timing of the estrous and menstrual cycles. In seasonal breeders, as autumn approaches, the shortening of the days leads to increased melatonin secretion and atrophy of the gonads. Whether melatonin acts by suppressing the release of hypophyseal gonadotropins or directly affects the gonads is not clear.

In humans, it has been suggested that the pineal exerts an influence upon gonadal development, particularly in the period prior to sexual maturity. Male infants with brain tumors that destroy the pineal exhibit hypertrophy of the gonads and precocious puberty. On the other hand, pineal tumors in children commonly are associated with delayed puberty as a result of increased pineal activity.

# The Female Reproductive System

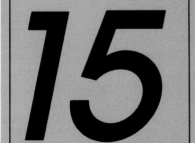

15

## INTRODUCTION

The female reproductive system comprises the ovaries, a system of genital ducts (the uterine tubes, uterus, and vagina) (Fig. 15–1), and the external genitalia. The mammary glands, although not one of the genital organs, are included in this chapter, since they are important glands of the female reproductive system. The principal functions of the system, which are controlled by hormonal and nervous mechanisms, are production of female gametes, the ova, by a process of oogenesis; reception of male gametes, the spermatozoa; provision of a suitable environment for fertilization of ova by spermatozoa and for development of the fetus; a mechanism for expulsion of the developed fetus into the external environment; and nutrition of the newborn.

The development and differentiation of the organs of this system are not completed until the hypophyseal gonadotropic hormones begin to appear at about ten years of age. Under the influence of these hormones during *puberty*, the generative organs increase in size, the mammary glands enlarge, and pubic and axillary hair appears. These changes culminate with the initiation of the menstrual cycles at *menarche*, which occurs at about 13 years of age. Thereafter, throughout the reproductive period, the ovaries, genital ducts, and mammary glands undergo cyclic changes in structure and function associated with the menstrual cycle, which averages about 28 to 30 days in length. At *menopause*, which occurs between the ages of 45 and 55, the menstrual cycles become irregular and eventually cease. The reproductive organs cease to function and undergo atrophy in the postmenopausal period.

## OVARY

The ovaries are classified as double glands, since they produce both exocrine (cytogenic) and endocrine secretions. They are slightly flattened, ovoid bodies, measuring about 4 cm in length, 2 cm in width, and 1 cm in thickness. One lies on each side of the uterus on the lateral wall of the pelvic cavity. Each is attached at one of its margins, the *hilum*, by the *mesovarium*, a fold of peritoneum, to the broad ligament of the uterus. At the hilum, the vascular connective tissue of the mesovarium becomes continuous with the ovarian stroma. The peritoneal covering of the mesovarium at the hilum is continuous with a layer of cuboidal cells, the *germinal epithelium*, that covers the surface of the ovary. The term germinal epithelium is a misnomer, since this layer is not the site of germ cell formation. Beneath the epithelium, there is a poorly delineated layer of

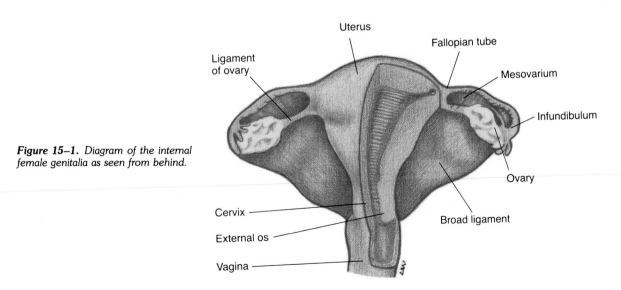

**Figure 15–1.** *Diagram of the internal female genitalia as seen from behind.*

Uterus

Ligament of ovary

Fallopian tube

Mesovarium

Infundibulum

Ovary

Cervix

External os

Vagina

Broad ligament

dense connective tissue, the *tunica albuginea,* which increases in density with advancing age.

In sections of the ovary, two zones may be distinguished: (1) an outer layer, the *cortex,* and (2) an inner portion, the *medulla,* that merges with the vascular connective tissue core of the mesovarium at the hilum (Figs. 15–2 and 15–3). There is no distinct line of demarcation between the two zones. The medulla consists of loose fibroelastic connective tissue containing numerous large blood vessels, lymphatics, and nerves. The stroma contains scattered strands of smooth muscle fibers.

The cortex consists of a compact, cellular stroma that contains the *ovarian follicles* (Figs. 15–4 and 15–5). The stroma is composed of networks of reticular fibers and spindle-shaped cells, arranged in irregular whorls. Elastic tissue is sparse and occurs only in the walls of blood vessels. The follicles may be seen in all stages of development, and the appearance of the ovarian cortex depends upon the age of the individual and the stage of the ovarian cycle (Fig. 15–6). Before puberty, only *primordial,* or *primitive, follicles* are seen (Fig. 15–7). Sexual maturity is characterized by the presence of *growing follicles* and their end products *(corpora lutea, atretic follicles)*. After menopause, follicles disappear, and the cortex eventually becomes a narrow zone of fibrous connective tissue.

## Ovarian Follicles: Growth and Development

### PRIMORDIAL FOLLICLES

In the newborn infant, the follicles are believed to number about 400,000. Their number de-

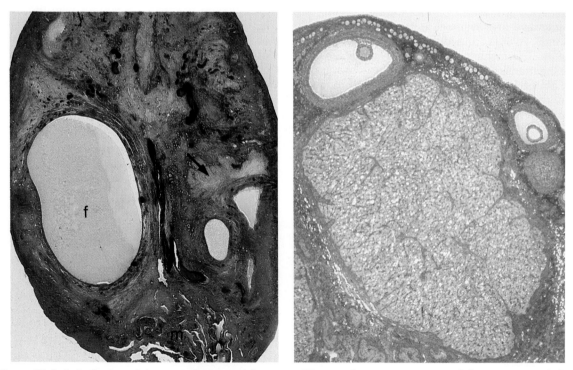

***Figure 15–2.*** Left: *Section of the ovary from an adult woman. The vascular connective tissue of the mesovarium (m) is continuous above with the narrow medulla, in which are large blood vessels. The cortex contains follicles in various stages of differentiation and one large follicle (f) shows an antrum cavity. Also present is a corpus albicans (arrow). Mallory-Azan. Low power.* Right: *Ovary from a pregnant cat. The majority of the field is occupied by a large, pale-staining corpus luteum. Also present is a row of primordial follicles (just below the free surface) and two large follicles. H and E. Low power.*

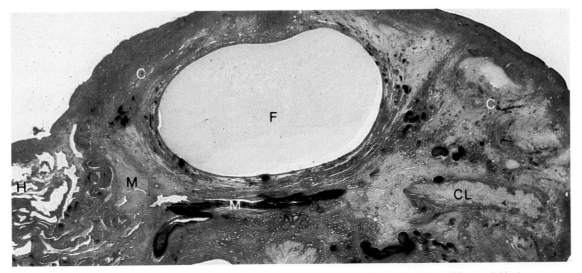

**Figure 15–3.** *Ovary, same preparation as Figure 15–2 (left). The ovary is attached at the hilum (H) to a fold of peritoneum, the mesovarium, that continues to the broad ligament. Two zones may be distinguished within the ovary. The outer zone, the cortex (C), is a compact cellular stroma that contains the ovarian follicles. One large follicle (F) shows an antrum cavity. Also present is a degenerating corpus luteum (CL). The inner zone, the medulla (M), is loose connective tissue that merges into the core of the mesovarium at the hilum. It contains numerous large blood vessels. Mallory-Azan. Low power.*

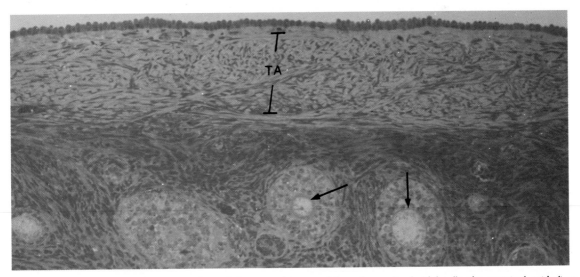

**Figure 15–4.** *Ovary, cortex. The free surface of the ovary is covered by a layer of cuboidal cells, the germinal epithelium. Beneath this, there is a zone of dense connective tissue, the tunica albuginea (TA). The underlying cortex consists of a compact, cellular stroma that contains three primary follicles. The follicular cells form a stratified layer around the immature ovum (seen in two follicles) and are separated from it by the zona pellucida (arrows). Plastic section. Methylene blue, azure A, basic fuchsin. Low power.*

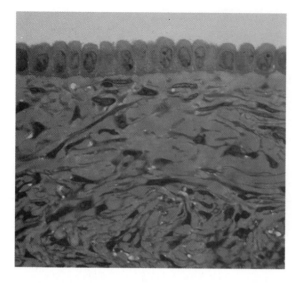

*Figure 15–5. Ovary, germinal epithelium. The germinal epithelium is composed of a single layer of cuboidal cells. At the hilum, this layer is continuous with the mesothelial (peritoneal) covering of the mesovarium. Beneath the epithelium is the dense, irregular connective tissue of the tunica albuginea. Plastic section. Methylene blue, azure A, basic fuchsin. High power.*

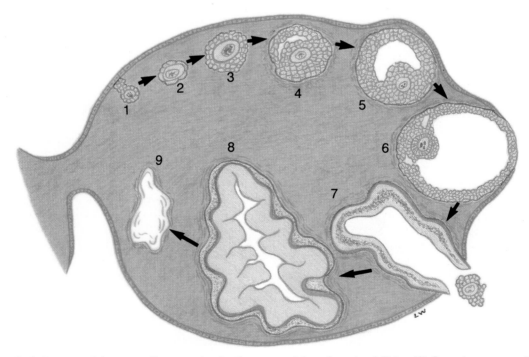

*Figure 15–6. Diagram of the ovary, illustrating the development and fate of ovarian follicles. (1) Oogonium, surrounded by follicular cells. (2) Primordial follicle. (3–5) Growing follicles. (6) Graafian follicle. (7) Ruptured follicle. (8) Corpus luteum. (9) Corpus albicans.*

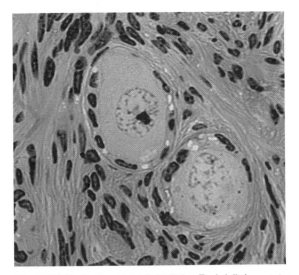

*Figure 15–7.* Ovary, primordial follicles. Each follicle contains an immature ovum (primary oocyte) with a large vesicular nucleus. The nucleus of the upper oocyte also shows a prominent nucleolus. The oocytes are surrounded by a single layer of flattened follicular cells. The follicles lie within the cellular stroma of the cortex. Plastic section. H and E. High power.

creases progressively throughout life until virtually none is left soon after the menopause. Most follicles seen are primordial follicles, which measure about 40 micrometers (μm) in diameter. A primordial follicle consists of an immature ovum, the *primary oocyte*, surrounded by a single layer of flattened epithelial (*follicular*) cells.

The oocyte is a spheroidal cell with a large vesicular nucleus and a prominent nucleolus. The cytoplasm is opaque and finely granular and contains annulate lamellae, a prominent Golgi complex, and numerous mitochondria and small vesicles. The single layer of flattened follicular cells surrounding the oocyte is separated from the ovarian stroma by a thin basal lamina.

### GROWING FOLLICLES

The progressive development of follicles that occurs after puberty is characterized by growth and differentiation of the ovum, proliferation of follicular cells, and organization of surrounding stromal cells into a connective tissue sheath (Fig. 15–8).

The immature ovum increases in size, and a refractile, deeply staining membrane, the *zona pellucida*, is formed around it. The zona pellucida contains glycoproteins, appears homogeneous in the fresh condition, and stains brilliantly with the periodic acid–Schiff (PAS) technique. Although elaborated principally by the surrounding follicular cells, the oocyte also may contribute to its formation.

The flattened follicular cells become first cuboidal and then columnar in shape. They divide actively to produce a stratified layer around the ovum, the *stratum granulosum*, composed of *granulosa cells*. The unilaminar primordial follicle thus is transformed into a multilaminar *primary follicle*.

As the primary follicle increases in size, the adjacent stroma organizes into a capsule, the *theca folliculi*, separated from the stratum granulosum by a basal lamina (the *glassy membrane*). The theca folliculi differentiates into two layers, an inner vascular layer, the *theca interna*, and an outer fibrous layer, the *theca externa*. The theca interna consists of enlarged stromal cells that are secretory and between which are numerous capillaries. The theca externa, composed of closely packed collagenous fibers and fusiform cells, merges peripherally into the surrounding ovarian stroma.

The proliferation of follicular cells continues and occurs more rapidly on one side of the ovum, so that the follicle becomes ovoid in shape, and the ovum eccentric in position. As this occurs, the follicle gradually comes to lie deeper in the cortex. When the stratum granulosum reaches 8 to 12 layers thick, irregular small spaces filled with a clear fluid appear within the follicular mass. The fluid-filled spaces fuse to form a single cavity, the *antrum*, within the follicular layer. The follicle now is identified as a *secondary*, or *antral, follicle* (Fig. 15–9).

The antrum of the secondary follicle contains the *liquor folliculi*, a viscid fluid rich in hyaluronic acid. The ovum, surrounded by a group of granulosa cells, is pressed to one side and forms a definite projection into the antrum cavity. This eccentric mound is known as the *cumulus oophorus*. The granulosa cells of the cumulus oophorus directly in relation to the ovum become radially arranged to form the *corona radiata*, separated from the ovum only by the zona pel-

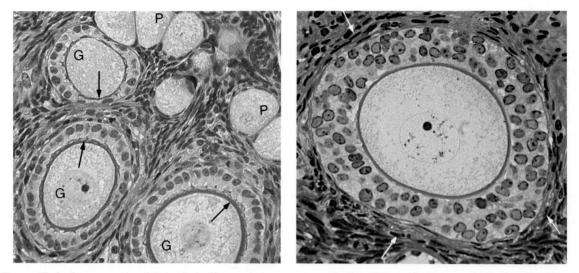

**Figure 15–8.** *Ovary, growing follicles.* Left: *The cortical stroma is markedly cellular and contains spindle-shaped cells with elongated nuclei. Embedded in the stroma are primordial (P) and primary growing (G) follicles. The former consist of an immature ovum surrounded by a single layer of flattened follicular cells. In the primary follicles, the follicular cells assume a cuboidal shape and later produce a stratified layer around the ovum. A refractile, deeply staining membrane—the zona pellucida (arrows)—is interposed between the ovum and the follicular cells. Plastic section. H and E. Medium power.* Right: *Primary follicle. The large immature ovum shows a pale vesicular nucleus with a distinct nucleolus and an opaque and finely granular cytoplasm. It is surrounded by the zona pellucida, which separates it from the stratified layer of cuboidal follicular cells, the stratum granulosum. The surrounding stromal cells are condensing to form a capsule, the theca folliculi (arrows), around the follicle. Plastic section. H and E. High power.*

lucida. Phase and electron microscope studies have shown that processes from the corona radiata cells extend through the zona pellucida to contact the cell membrane of the ovum. Additionally, microvillous processes of the ovum pass into the zona pellucida. Elsewhere, the stratified epithelium, composed of granulosa cells, forms a continuous regular layer around the antrum cavity. Small accumulations of densely staining, extracellular material, the *Call-Exner bodies,* appear among the granulosa cells. These bodies stain positively with the PAS reaction; their origin and significance are unknown.

### MATURE GRAAFIAN FOLLICLES

It is believed that a follicle requires 10 to 14 days to reach maturity. A mature Graafian follicle is 10 mm or more in diameter, occupies the full breadth of the cortex, and indents the medulla. It bulges on the free surface of the ovary. At this point, called the *stigma,* the tunica albuginea and

the theca folliculi become attenuated. The large antrum, distended with fluid, is bounded by the stratum granulosum. The ovum has attained its full size, and it is surrounded by a thick zona pellucida and a conspicuous corona radiata. As follicular maturity is attained, small irregular spaces, filled with fluid, appear between the cells of the corona radiata, thus weakening the connection of the ovum with the stratum granulosum.

The theca folliculi attains its greatest development in the mature follicle. The component cells of the theca interna assume the cytological features of a steroid-secreting endocrine gland and elaborate the precursor of the female sex hormones, *estrogens.* The theca externa, composed of collagenous fibers and fusiform cells, does not appear to have a secretory function.

### OVULATION

As the follicle reaches maturity, there is increased secretion of liquor, more watery than that

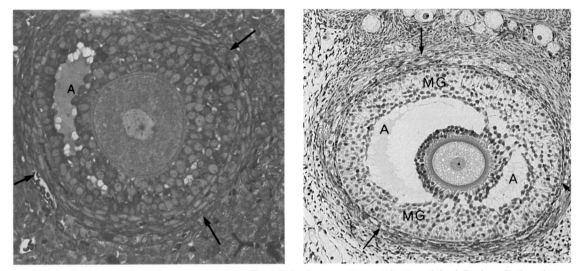

**Figure 15–9.** *Ovary.* Left: Secondary (antral) follicle. This follicle shows greater stratification of the follicular cells than that seen in Figure 15–8 (right) and early development of the antral cavity (A). It is filled with a clear fluid, the liquor folliculi. A capsule of stromal cells, the theca folliculi (arrows), surrounds the follicle. Plastic section. Methylene blue, basic fuchsin. Medium power. Right: Graafian follicle. The cortical stroma contains a row of primordial follicles (top) and an almost mature Graafian follicle. The primary oocyte of the latter, with a vesicular nucleus and a prominent nucleolus, is surrounded by the zona pellucida and by a group of follicular cells, the corona radiata. The whole mound of tissue, the cumulus oophorus, projects into the antral cavity (A). A stratified layer of follicular cells forms a continuous irregular layer, the stratum granulosum or membrana granulosa (MG) around the antral cavity. A well-defined theca folliculi (arrows) surrounds the membrana granulosa. Plastic section. H and E. Medium power.

formed previously, which causes further expansion in diameter of the follicle. This is termed *preovulatory swelling.* The follicle, covered with thinned cortex, ruptures at the stigma, and follicular fluid oozes out into the peritoneal cavity. The ovum, which is surrounded by the zona pellucida and cells of the corona radiata, is torn away from the cumulus and is discharged with the liquor. This process constitutes *ovulation.* The precise mechanisms involved in rupture of the follicle and extrusion of the ovum are poorly understood.

Usually, only one ovum is discharged at one time, but in some cases two or, rarely, more may be released. Drugs may stimulate ovarian activity and cause the simultaneous maturation of several follicles, thus increasing the possibility of multiple birth.

The free ovum usually is directed into the infundibulum of the fallopian tube and retains the capacity to be fertilized only for 24 hours. In the human female, ovulation normally occurs at intervals averaging 28 days.

## Maturation of the Ovum: Oogenesis

The ovum that is released at ovulation is actually a *secondary oocyte* and technically is immature. In preparation for fertilization, the ovum passes through a series of nuclear changes similar to that described for spermatozoa (see Chapter 16). The end result is the same as with spermatogenesis, that is, reduction of the chromosomes to one half the somatic (diploid) number.

*Oogonia,* or primitive ova, which contain the diploid number of chromosomes, divide mitotically to produce *primary oocytes* in the fetal ovary. During follicular development, the primary oocyte grows and then passes through a period of maturation in which it undergoes two maturation divisions, as a result of which the chromosomes are reduced to the haploid number. The first maturation division occurs shortly before ovulation and within the mature follicle. The chromatin is divided equally between the daughter cells, but the division of cytoplasm is extremely unequal. One of the daughter cells, the *secondary oocyte*, receives practically all the cytoplasm of the mother cell; the other becomes the *first polar body,* which soon degenerates. In each, the chromosome assortment is reduced to a single set of 23 chromosomes. At about this time, ovulation occurs, and the secondary oocyte is released from the follicle. At this time, the nucleus of the secondary oocyte commences the second maturation division, which stops in the metaphase and remains in this condition until fertilization. Penetration of the spermatozoon head into the oocyte stimulates it to complete the second maturation division. Again the cytoplasm is divided unequally. The majority of cytoplasm is retained in the mature *ovum*. The other daughter cell is the *second polar body*. Thus, only one daughter cell of a primary oocyte becomes functional.

### Corpus Luteum

After ovulation, there is sometimes a little bleeding into the cavity of the follicle (Fig. 15–10). The wall of the follicle collapses and is thrown into folds. The follicular wall becomes transformed into a temporary glandular structure, the *corpus luteum*. The granulosa cells of the follicle differentiate into large, pale-staining cells with large vesicular nuclei. The cytoplasm acquires an accumulation of fine lipid droplets and lipofuscin pigment granules, which are lysosomal in nature. Dispersed within the cytoplasm are numerous mitochondria with tubular cristae and abundant granular and agranular endoplasmic reticulum. The transformed granulosa cells are called *granulosa lutein* cells, and they form a thick, folded layer about the remains of the follicular cavity (Fig. 15–11).

Cells of the theca interna, which prior to ovulation had increased in size, form *theca lutein cells*. They are smaller in size than granulosa lutein cells and possess compact, dark-staining nuclei. They aggregate peripherally, especially in the recesses between the folds of granulosa lutein cells. The theca externa retains its regular ovoid outline, and component cells do not undergo transformation.

The basal lamina (glassy membrane) that separated the granulosa cells of the follicle from the

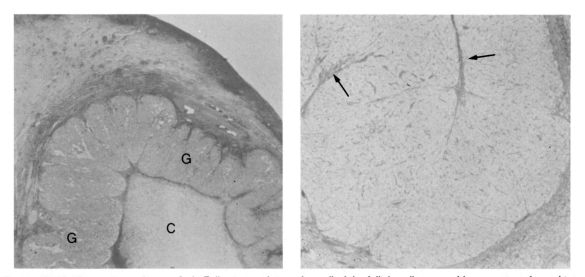

**Figure 15–10.** *Ovary, corpus luteum. Left: Following ovulation, the wall of the follicle collapses and becomes transformed into a temporary glandular structure, the corpus luteum. The central portion of the follicle, initially filled with blood, is replaced by a primitive type of connective tissue (C). The granulosa cells of the follicle differentiate into granulosa-lutein cells that form a thick, folded layer (G) about the remains of the follicular cavity. Right: Late corpus luteum. The corpus appears pale owing to the large size of the component granulosa-lutein cells. Delicate connective tissue septa (arrows), containing blood vessels, pass from the theca (dark red) into the interior of the corpus luteum. Both H and E. Low power.*

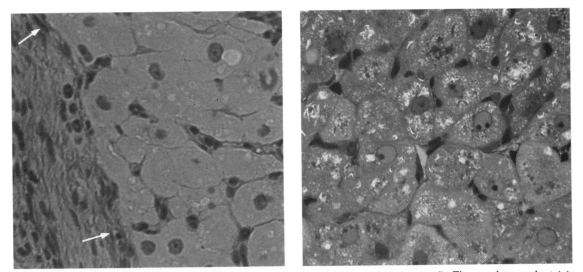

**Figure 15–11.** *Corpus luteum. Left: The majority of the field is occupied by granulosa-lutein cells. They are large, pale-staining cells with vesicular nuclei and abundant cytoplasm that appears vacuolated owing to the removal of lipid material during preparation. Fine connective tissue strands containing capillaries run between the cells. The corpus luteum is bounded by cells of the theca externa (arrows), which retain their fusiform shape. Plastic section. H and E. High power. Right: A group of granulosa-lutein cells is shown. Many cells exhibit nuclei with distinct nucleoli. The extensive cytoplasm is finely granulated and contains numerous vacuoles. The appearance is typical of a steroid-producing gland. Numerous capillaries lie between component cells. Plastic section. Methylene blue, azure A, basic fuchsin. High power.*

theca interna undergoes depolymerization, and numerous capillaries and connective tissue from the theca invade the lutein mass. Fibroblasts organize a delicate reticulum throughout the corpus luteum and form a continuous lining on the inner surface of the lutein cells in relation to the reduced follicular cavity.

If the discharged ovum is not fertilized, the corpus luteum attains its greatest development about nine days after ovulation and then begins to degenerate. This is the *corpus luteum of menstruation*. The former rich vascularization declines, and component cells decrease in size and undergo a fatty degeneration. Connective tissue between lutein cells increases in amount and becomes hyalinized, and gradually the corpus luteum is transformed into a white scar, the *corpus albicans*.

If the ovum is fertilized, the corpus luteum increases in size and becomes the *corpus luteum of pregnancy*. The cells continue to grow in size until the middle months of pregnancy, and thereafter a slow involution occurs. After delivery, involution proceeds rapidly. The resulting corpus albicans is large and usually causes a retraction

of the surface of the ovary, owing to contraction of fibrous tissue formed as a result of involution.

### Atresia of the Follicles

Only about 1000 follicles reach full maturity. Large numbers of follicles undergo *atresia* during fetal life, early postnatal life, and puberty. The period of reproductive activity in the human female is about 30 years. During this time, groups of follicles begin to mature each menstrual cycle, but ordinarily only one ovum is discharged each month. All unsuccessful follicles undergo degeneration, either as primordial follicles or after a varying period of growth (Fig. 15–12).

Atresia appears to occur initially in the ovum. This is followed by degeneration of the follicular cells. In atresia of primordial follicles, the space resulting is filled with stromal tissue. Atresia of growing follicles is a more complicated process. As in primordial follicles, the first degenerative signs occur in the ovum and follicular cells. The zona pellucida swells and may persist for some

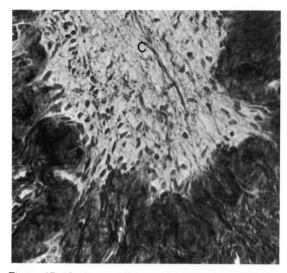

**Figure 15–12.** *Atretic follicle. At any time during development of a follicle, the process may be arrested and the follicle replaced by a mass of connective tissue, the atretic follicle. Here, a portion of an atretic follicle resulting from the degeneration of a Graafian follicle is shown. The center (C) is occupied by connective tissue that has replaced the follicular cells. The thecal margins of the original follicle and the glassy membrane remain as a thick hyalinized band, here stained blue. Ovarian stroma surrounds the atretic follicle. Azan. Medium power.*

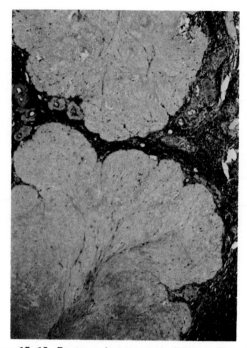

**Figure 15–13.** *Portions of two corpora albicantia. There has been complete replacement of the corpora lutea by connective tissue. Low power.*

time after the disappearance of the ovum and follicular cells. Macrophages invade the atretic follicle and remove degenerating material, including fragments of the zona pellucida. Cells of the theca interna initially develop much like those in a corpus luteum. They increase in size and become arranged in vascularized, radial strands. The glassy membrane also increases in thickness and forms a hyalinized band that is characteristic of follicles in later stages of atresia. After final resorption of follicular cells, the theca cells degenerate and are replaced by connective tissue. The resulting masses of scar tissue are similar in appearance to corpora albicantia but are smaller (corpora atretica) (Fig. 15–13).

### Interstitial Cells

Large epithelioid cells are present in the ovarian stroma of some mammals, particularly rodents. These are the so-called *interstitial cells,* which are

large spheroidal cells containing small lipid droplets. They appear similar to luteal cells and are thought to be derived from the theca interna of follicles undergoing atresia. Thus, they are most abundant when atresia is most marked. In the human, this is in the first year of life. In the adult human ovary, they either are absent or are present as small radiating cords of cells.

In the human, the interstitial cells have been shown to secrete estrogens, whereas in other species, they produce progesterone.

### Hormones of the Ovary: The Ovarian Cycle

The ovaries, in addition to producing sex cells (a cytogenic secretion), secrete the female sex hormones, *estrogens* and *progesterone,* which are steroids. Estrogens (principally estradiol) are produced mainly by the growing follicles, progesterone primarily by the corpus luteum. Estrogens induce growth and development of the female reproductive tract and of the mammary glands. Progesterone causes the uterine glands to secrete and renders the mucosa receptive to a nidating ovum.

Since the sequence of structural changes in the ovary is follicular growth, ovulation, and formation of a corpus luteum, the levels of the two hormones normally exhibit regular cyclic fluctuations. Secretion of estrogens is high during the preovulatory period (*follicular phase*), and progesterone production increases rapidly during luteinization of the ruptured follicle and remains at a high level until the corpus luteum regresses (*luteal phase*). These rhythmic changes in ovarian secretory activity are responsible for the cyclic changes that occur in the structure of the female reproductive tract, notably in the mucosa of the uterus (see Fig. 15–22).

The ovarian cycle in turn is activated and governed by the gonadotropins secreted by the anterior lobe of the hypophysis. The gonadotropins, follicle-stimulating hormone (FSH) and luteinizing hormone (LH), control the maturation of follicles and the formation of corpora lutea. At the beginning of an ovarian cycle, the increased production of FSH by the hypophysis causes many primordial follicles to initiate development. One follicle enlarges more rapidly than the others, which degenerate and become atretic. In conjunction with FSH, LH induces ripening of the mature follicle and ovulation and is responsible for the development and maintenance of the corpus luteum. The rising levels of progesterone produced by the corpus luteum inhibit further release of LH from the hypophysis, and if pregnancy does not occur, the corpus luteum is not maintained. As the corpus luteum declines, the ievels of estrogens decrease. This results in release of FSH by the hypophysis to initiate a new cycle of follicular development.

Recently, it has been shown, principally by immunohistochemical methods, that the corpus luteum of pregnancy secretes *relaxin* in addition to estrogens and progesterone. Relaxin is a polypeptide hormone similar in structure to insulin. Although little is known about the regulation of relaxin secretion, it appears that this hormone may play an essential role in the normal progression of pregnancy and parturition. In lower mammals, the hormone has been shown to cause a "relaxation" of the connective tissue of the symphysis pubis, thus facilitating parturition, and to promote distensibility of the uterine cervix. Additionally, relaxin restrains uterine contractile activity during pregnancy and also may influence mammary gland growth and function.

### Blood Vessels, Lymphatics, and Nerves

Large branches from the ovarian artery anastomose with branches from the uterine artery and pass through the mesovarium to the hilum of the ovary. Here they divide into a number of spiral vessels, the *helicine arteries*, which form a plexus at the boundary zone between cortex and me-

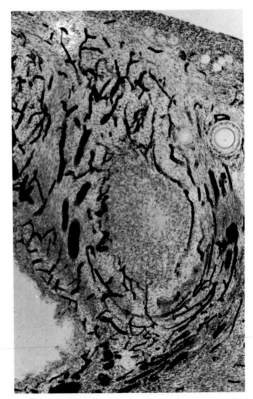

**Figure 15–14.** Section of a portion of an ovary in which the blood vessels have been injected with colored gelatin prior to sectioning. Note the abundant capillary networks in relation to the growing follicles. Low power.

dulla. From this plexus, smaller twigs pass into the cortex to ramify around follicles. Capillary networks are abundant in the theca interna of growing follicles (Fig. 15–14). Veins, which arise from the capillary networks, accompany the arteries and leave the ovary at the hilum.

Lymph capillaries commence in the theca externa of follicles and unite to form larger vessels that pass to the medulla and leave at the hilum. There, they are combined into a smaller number of lymphatic trunks that drain into lumbar (aortic) lymph nodes.

Nerve fibers, mostly unmyelinated, follow the blood vessels and supply their muscular coat. Some fibers penetrate into the cortex and form delicate plexuses around the follicles and beneath the germinal epithelium. Sensory nerve endings are scattered within the ovarian stroma.

## FALLOPIAN TUBES

The *Fallopian (uterine) tubes,* or *oviducts,* are paired structures that extend from the ovaries to the uterus in a fold of peritoneum, the upper free margin of the broad ligament. Each tube is 12 to 15 cm long and about 1 cm in diameter. The end of the tube in relation to the ovary opens into the peritoneal cavity; the other end opens into the uterine cavity. The tube receives the ovum released at ovulation, provides the appropriate environment for its fertilization and initial development, and transports it to the uterine cavity.

The uterine tube shows four regions:

1. The *infundibulum,* which is the funnel-shaped opening into the peritoneal cavity. Its margins are drawn out into numerous fringed folds, the *fimbriae,* which extend toward the ovary.

2. The *ampulla,* the expanded intermediate segment, that comprises two thirds of the length of the tube. It is thin-walled.

3. The *isthmus,* the narrow medial third, adjacent to the uterus.

4. The *intramural (interstitial) portion,* which is the continuation of the canal through the uterine wall.

The wall of the tube thickens progressively toward the uterus, whereas the lumen diminishes in size in this direction.

## Histological Organization

The wall of the fallopian tube consists of the following layers (Fig. 15–15):

1. A mucous membrane.
2. A muscular layer.
3. A serosa.

### MUCOSA

The mucosal lining is thrown into characteristic longitudinal folds, or *plicae.* In the ampulla, the folds branch in a complex manner to divide the lumen into a labyrinth of spaces (Fig. 15–16). In the isthmus, the folds rarely branch; in the intramural portion of the tube, the folds are low (Fig. 15–17).

The epithelium consists of simple columnar cells, some of which are ciliated, whereas others are not (Fig. 15–18). The nonciliated cells are narrow and peg-shaped and appear to be secretory in nature, contributing nutritive material for the ovum. Ciliated cells occur in small groups, alternating with groups of cells that are nonciliated. The proportion of cells with cilia is greatest at the infundibulum and least at the isthmus. Most cilia beat toward the uterus and are thought to play a major role in transportation of the ovum through the ampulla to the ampullo-isthmic junction, the normal site of fertilization. The two types of epithelial cells probably are different functional states of a single cell type.

The epithelium shows cyclic changes associated with the ovarian cycle. The height of the epithelium is greatest during the follicular phase and lowest during the latter part of the luteal phase. In the luteal phase, ciliated cells lose many of their cilia, and "peg" (secretory) cells exhibit augmented secretory activity. The loss of cilia is greatest in the infundibulum and is less marked in the isthmus. The cilia are affected by steroid hormones, estrogens being responsible for the development and maintenance of cilia and progesterone causing an increase in the rate at which they beat.

The lamina propria of the mucosa is composed of an unusually cellular connective tissue containing a network of reticular fibers and numerous fusiform cells, similar to those of the ovarian stroma. It is separated from the epithelium by a thin basal lamina. At the rim of the infundibulum,

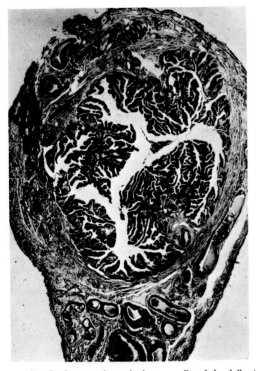

**Figure 15–15.** *Section through the ampulla of the fallopian tube. The lumen appears markedly irregular owing to extensive folding of the mucosa. The thin muscularis is composed mainly of fibers arranged circularly. The surrounding serosa, which constitutes the upper free margin of the broad ligament, contains numerous large blood vessels. Low power.*

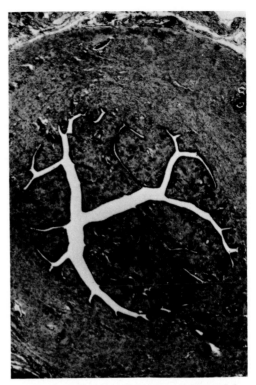

**Figure 15–17.** *Fallopian tube, isthmus. Folding of the mucosa is much less than in the ampullary region, and the folds are low. The muscularis is increased in thickness. Low power.*

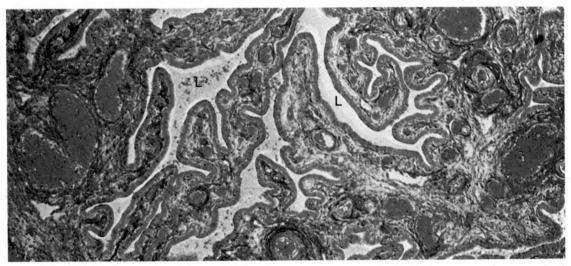

**Figure 15–16.** *Fallopian tube, ampulla. The mucosal lining is thrown into longitudinal folds, here sectioned transversely, that branch to divide the lumen (L) into a labyrinth of spaces. The epithelium is simple columnar and rests upon a markedly cellular lamina propria that contains numerous large blood vessels (red). The surrounding muscularis, not shown here, consists of a broad inner circular layer and a thin, incomplete, outer longitudinal layer. Mallory-Azan. Low power.*

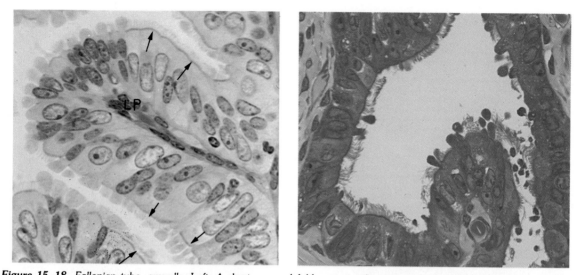

**Figure 15–18.** Fallopian tube, ampulla. Left: A short mucosal fold occupies the majority of the field. The simple columnar epithelium, here sectioned slightly obliquely, contains two cell types, ciliated and nonciliated. The ciliated cells, which occur in groups and become fewer in number as the isthmus is approached, have numerous cilia and show basal bodies that are visible as dense, closely opposed granules in the apical cytoplasm (arrows). The nonciliated cells generally are narrow and peg-shaped, with blebbing of the apical cytoplasm. These cells are thought to be secretory in nature. The core of the mucosal fold consists of a cellular lamina propria (LP), component cells of which are fusiform and similar to those of the ovarian stroma. Plastic section. H and E. High power. Right: Ampulla in pregnancy. The base of a mucosal fold is shown. During pregnancy, the simple columnar epithelium is low (compare with left figure). It still contains two cell types, ciliated and nonciliated. During pregnancy and the luteal phase of the menstrual cycle, there usually is an increase in the number of nonciliated, peg-shaped cells, but it is not apparent here. Plastic section. Methylene blue, azure A, basic fuchsin. High power.

the mucosal lining of the tube becomes continuous with the mesothelium of the serosa.

### MUSCULARIS

The mucosa rests directly upon the muscular coat, with no intervening submucosa. The muscularis consists of a broad inner circular layer and a thin outer layer, but there is no distinct boundary between the two. The outer layer is not continuous and consists of scattered bundles of fibers, oriented longitudinally. Toward the uterus, the muscularis increases in thickness.

Contractions of the muscular coat, occurring in peristaltic waves, aid in the movement of the ovum down the tube to the uterine cavity.

### SEROSA

The uterine tube is invested with a fold of reflected peritoneum, the serosa, consisting of loose connective tissue surfaced with mesothe-

lium. The deeper layers of the connective tissue contain some of the longitudinal bundles of the muscularis.

### Blood Vessels, Lymphatics, and Nerves

Numerous blood vessels and lymphatics are present in the lamina propria and the serosa. Large lymphatic capillaries particularly are abundant in the lamina propria. Nerves form a rich plexus in the serosa, from which nerve fibers pass to supply the muscularis and the serosa.

### UTERUS

The uterus is the thick-walled segment of the tubular female reproductive system that is interposed between the Fallopian tubes and the vagina (Fig. 15–19). It receives the fertilized ovum from

recognized: (1) the expanded upper portion, the *body* (*corpus uteri*), and (2) the lowermost, cylindrical portion, the *neck* (*cervix*), a part of which projects into the vagina as the *portio vaginalis*. The term *fundus* refers to the rounded upper end of the body, from which the Fallopian tubes extend. The *isthmus* is the narrow zone of transition between the body and the cervix. The *cervical canal* passes through the cervix and communicates above with the uterine cavity at the *internal os* and below with the vagina at the *external os*.

### Histological Organization

The wall of the uterus consists of three layers:
1. The outer layer, the serosa (*perimetrium*).
2. The middle layer, the muscularis (*myometrium*).
3. The inner layer, the mucosa (*endometrium*).

#### PERIMETRIUM

The perimetrium is a typical serosa consisting of a single layer of mesothelial cells supported by a thin layer of connective tissue. It is continuous on each side of the organ with the peritoneum of the broad ligament and is deficient over the lower half of the anterior surface, where the urinary bladder abuts. Here, in the absence of peritoneum, the myometrium is covered by connective tissue, or *adventitia*.

#### MYOMETRIUM

The myometrium is a massive coat of smooth muscle, about 12 to 15 mm in thickness. The muscle fibers are arranged in bundles, separated by connective tissue. Individual fibers are large, and their length varies from 40 to 90 μm. During pregnancy the fibers increase greatly in size and may attain a length of 600 μm or more. In spite of the increase in the muscle mass, the myometrium is thinned during pregnancy as the uterus becomes distended.

Three layers of muscle may be distinguished, although they are somewhat ill-defined owing to the presence of interconnecting bundles:

1. An inner muscular layer consisting mostly of longitudinally oriented fibers, the *stratum subvasculare*.

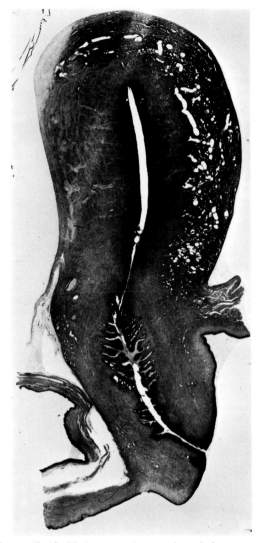

**Figure 15–19.** *Median sagittal section through the uterus and upper portion of the vagina. Note the thickness of the uterine wall (principally myometrium, which contains numerous large blood vessels), the prominent plicae palmatae of the cervix, the portio vaginalis, and a portion of the bladder (anterior) to the left. Low power.*

the Fallopian tube and all subsequent embryonic and fetal development occurs within it.

In the nonpregnant condition, the uterus is a pear-shaped organ, somewhat flattened in a dorsoventral direction, and averages 7 cm in length, 5 cm in width at its broadest part, and 2 to 3 cm in thickness. Two major portions may be

2. A thick middle layer of circular and oblique muscle fibers with numerous blood vessels, the *stratum vasculare.*

3. An outer, thin, longitudinal muscle layer immediately beneath the perimetrium, the *stratum supravasculare.*

The myometrium does undergo intermittent contractions that usually are not of sufficient intensity to be perceived. The contractions may be increased during sexual stimulation or during menstruation, resulting in cramp-like pains. During pregnancy, the contractions are reduced, possibly owing to the presence of the hormone relaxin. At parturition, strong contractions of the myometrium occur to expel the fetus. The contractions are increased by oxytocin, a hormone of the neurohypophysis, and by prostaglandins, which are released from the fetal membranes during parturition.

### ENDOMETRIUM

The endometrium (mucosa), which is firmly adherent to the underlying myometrium, throughout the reproductive period is subject to cyclic changes in response to ovarian secretory activity. These changes culminate in partial destruction of the mucosa, leading to tissue necrosis and hemorrhage, an event known as *menstruation.* Menstruation occurs typically at intervals of about 28 days and lasts for 3 to 5 days. The first day of menstruation is counted as the first day of the menstrual cycle.

The endometrium consists of a surface epithelium, which is invaginated to form numerous tubular *uterine glands,* and of a thick lamina propria, the *endometrial stroma.* The surface epithelium is a simple columnar epithelium that possesses scattered groups of ciliated cells. From the surface epithelium, uterine glands extend through the full thickness of the stroma. They are simple tubules that may branch toward their basal ends. They are separated from each other by the connective tissue of the stroma. Stromal cells, which resemble mesenchymal cells, are irregular, stellate cells that have large, ovoid nuclei. They lie within a framework of reticular fibers that is condensed beneath the epithelium to form a basal lamina. Wandering lymphocytes, granular leukocytes, and macrophages also are present in the stroma.

### Blood Vessels, Lymphatics, and Nerves

A knowledge of the pattern of blood supply within the uterus is essential to an understanding of the mechanism by which cyclic changes occur in the endometrium. Numerous branches from the uterine arteries penetrate to the middle layer of the myometrium (stratum vasculare), where they form *arcuate arteries* that run circumferentially within the myometrium (Fig. 15–20). These arteries give rise to two sets of branches. One set

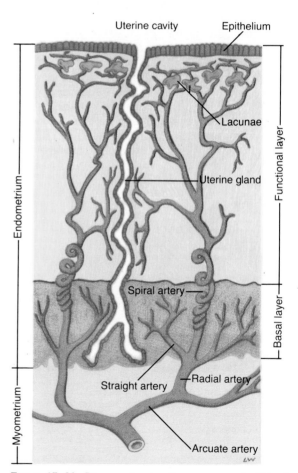

**Figure 15–20.** *Diagram showing the arrangement of blood vessels in the endometrium. Arcuate arteries within the myometrium give rise to radial arteries that pass to the myometrial-endometrial junction. Here, the radial arteries branch into straight (basal) arteries, which supply the basal part of the endometrium, and spiral arteries. The latter supply a rich capillary bed and thin-walled lacunae in the superficial part of the endometrium (functional layer).*

of branches supplies the superficial layers of the myometrium. The second set of branches sends *radial arteries* toward the endometrium. At the myometrial-endometrial junction, these arteries give off *basal* or *straight arteries* to supply the basal part of the endometrium. The radial arteries continue upward into the endometrium and become highly coiled as *spiral arteries*. The latter ramify into arterioles that supply a rich capillary bed in the superficial portion of the endometrium and thin-walled dilated vascular units, the *lacunae*. Thus the endometrium is supplied by a basal and a superficial set of vessels. The basal set, the straight arteries, does not undergo changes during the menstrual cycle, but the coiled, or spiral, arteries show pronounced modifications.

The venous system also forms an irregular network of venules and sinusoidal enlargements in the endometrium. This network drains via a plexus at the myometrial-endometrial junction into large veins present within the myometrium.

Lymph vessels are abundant and form plexuses throughout the layers of the uterus, with the exception of the superficial zone of the endometrium.

Myelinated nerve fibers enter the mucosa and form a plexus beneath the epithelium. Unmyelinated nerve fibers supply blood vessels and muscle bundles.

### Cyclic Changes in the Endometrium

Beginning with puberty and ending at the menopause, the endometrium undergoes periodic changes. Four stages can be recognized in a continuous cycle of events, and each stage passes gradually into the next (Figs. 15–21 through 15–24).

1. The *menstrual stage*, during which there is external menstrual discharge.

2. The *proliferative (follicular) stage,* which is concurrent with follicular growth and secretion of estrogens.

3. The *progestational (luteal) stage,* associated with an active corpus luteum, secreting progesterone.

4. The *ischemic (premenstrual) stage,* when there is interruption of blood flow in the coiled (spiral) arteries.

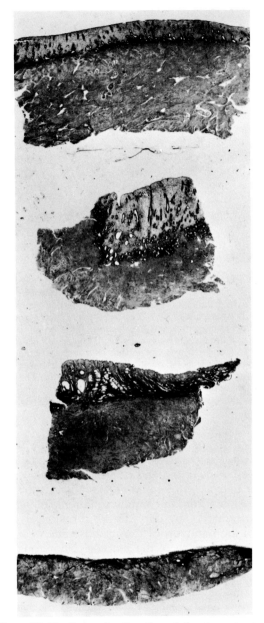

**Figure 15–21.** *Series of sections through the uterus at various stages during the menstrual cycle. From top to bottom, early proliferative (follicular) stage, late proliferative stage, late progestational (luteal) stage, and late menstrual stage. Note the varying heights of the endometrium and the character of the uterine glands. Low power.*

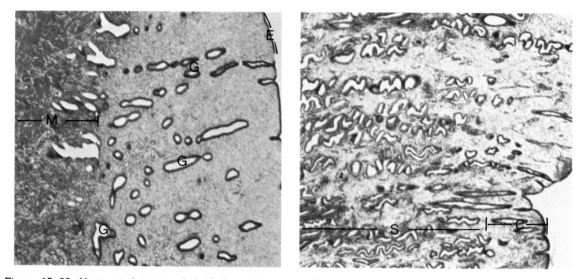

**Figure 15–22.** Uterine endometrium Left: Early proliferative stage. The endometrium, or uterine mucosa, consists of an epithelial lining and an endometrial stroma. The epithelial lining (E) is a simple columnar epithelium from which uterine glands (G) extend through the full thickness of the mucosa. These are simple tubules that may branch toward their basal ends. The glands are separated by a connective tissue stroma (lamina propria) that is highly cellular. Beneath the endometrium, a small portion of myometrium (M) containing large, empty blood vessels is shown. Right: Progestational stage. Only the superficial layers of the endometrium are shown. The endometrium is thick (compare with left figure), and the glands are markedly coiled and lie within a stroma that appears pale because of the presence of edema fluid within it. Once the structural changes associated with the progestational stage become apparent, three endometrial zones can be recognized. The narrow surface zone, or compact layer (C), contains the straight necks of the glands. The tortuous portions of the glands occupy the middle zone, or spongy layer (S). These two layers together constitute the functional layer that is lost at menstruation. The blind ends of the glands lie in the deepest zone, or basal layer, not shown here. (See Figure 15–23, left.) Both H and E. Low power.

**The Proliferative (Follicular) Stage.** This stage begins at the end of a menstrual flow and is characterized by rapid regeneration of the endometrium from the narrow zone remaining after menstruation (see Fig. 15–22). Epithelial cells from the remnants of torn glands glide over the denuded surface of the mucosa. Numerous mitoses occur in cells of the glands and of the endometrial stroma. The mucosa increases in thickness from 1 mm or less to 2 mm or more. This increase coincides with growth of ovarian follicles and secretion of estrogens. The glands proliferate, lengthen rapidly, and become closely packed. Rebuilding of the lamina propria occurs as a result of the mitotic activity of stromal cells and the accumulation of ground substance.

Toward the end of the proliferative phase, the lumina of the glands widen, and they become wavy in outline. Glycogen accumulates in the basal region of the glandular cells, but only a thin mucoid secretion is released at this stage. Coiled arteries grow into the regenerating tissue, but they are only moderately coiled and are not found in the superficial third of the endometrium, which possesses only capillaries, lacunae, and venules.

The proliferative phase continues for about a day after ovulation, and thus it extends until about the middle of the cycle (day 14 of a 28-day cycle).

**The Progestational (Secretory, or Luteal) Stage.** This stage occurs in response to the formation of the corpus luteum (after ovulation), which secretes progesterone (see Figs. 15–22 through 15–24). The endometrium increases in thickness to 4 mm or more in depth. The increase is due largely to hypertrophy of gland cells and to an increase of edema fluid. The glands swell and secrete profusely. Secretory material at first is localized in the basal portions of the cells. During the latter half of this stage, the secretion moves to the apical zone of the cells and then

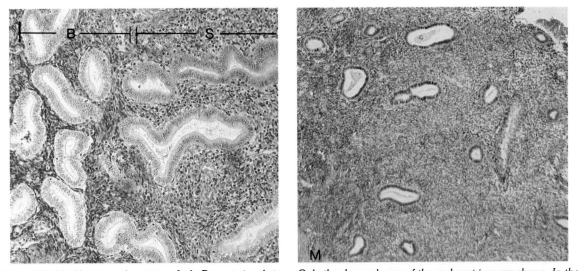

**Figure 15–23.** Uterine endometrium. Left: Progestational stage. Only the deeper layers of the endometrium are shown. In the spongy layer (S), the glands are tortuous and lie within a stroma that is markedly cellular, containing stromal cells and wandering lymphoid cells and granular leukocytes. The basal layer (B) contains the blind ends of the uterine glands, which participate little in the cyclic changes and are not lost at menstruation. Mallory-Azan. Medium power. Right: Early menstrual stage. The surface layers of the endometrium (right) have been lost, and the remaining glands lie within a dense, avascular stroma that is heavily infiltrated with leukocytes. The basal layer (lower left) is intact and contains extravasated blood (red) within its stroma. A small portion of the myometrium (M) also is present. Van Gieson. Low power.

into the lumina of the glands. The secretion is thick and mucoid, and rich in glycogen. The glands become serrated, and their lumina become wider. Coiled arteries grow nearly to the surface. Toward the end of this stage, stromal cells enlarge to become *decidual cells*. Their cytoplasm contains numerous free ribosomes, abundant granular endoplasmic reticulum, and scattered glycogen. These cells form aggregations around the coiled arteries and beneath the surface epithelium.

Once the structural changes associated with this stage become apparent, three zones of the endometrium can be distinguished:

1. Nearest the surface is the *compact layer*, which is a relatively narrow zone. It contains the straight necks of the glands and shows little edema.

2. Under this layer is a thick *spongy layer*, in which are the tortuous portions of the glands, separated by a lamina propria that is grossly edematous. The compact and spongy layers together are termed the *functional layer*, which is lost at menstruation and at parturition.

3. Deepest of all is the thin *basal layer*, containing the blind ends of the glands. This layer participates little in the cyclic changes and is not lost at menstruation or at parturition.

**The Ischemic (Premenstrual) Stage.** This stage occurs 13 to 14 days after ovulation, in response to a reduction in progesterone levels, with early involution of the corpus luteum. The coiled (spiral) arteries constrict intermittently. The functional layer becomes pale and shrinks as a result of anemia and anoxia. The stroma increases in density and becomes infiltrated with leukocytes. However, blood continues to flow into the basal layer of the endometrium through the straight arteries.

**The Menstrual Stage.** The functional layer undergoes necrosis and is shed. After a number of hours, the spiral arteries relax, the walls of the vessels near the surface break, and blood is added to the secretion of the glands and the necrotic endometrial tissue. Patches of tissue separate and are lost. Blood oozes from veins exposed by the shedding process. The menstrual discharge thus

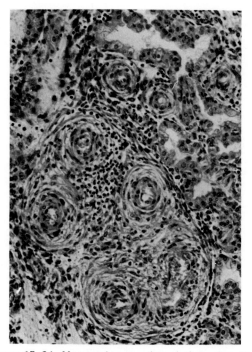

**Figure 15–24.** *Horizontal section through the endometrium during the progestational stage of the cycle. Note the irregular outlines of the glands and the prominent coiled (spiral) arteries within the stroma. Medium power.*

contains arterial and venous blood, disintegrated epithelial and stromal cells, and glandular secretions. Finally, the entire functional layer of the endometrium is lost, leaving a raw surface.

The surviving basal layer remains intact, epithelial cells glide out of the torn ends of glands, and the surface epithelium is quickly restored once the menstrual discharge ceases.

### RELATIONSHIP TO OVARIAN CYCLE

As stated previously, the uterine changes are related closely to the ovarian cyclic changes (Fig. 15–25). The proliferative stage corresponds to the preovulatory period of follicular maturation and the secretion of estrogens. The progestational stage is associated with the formation and activity of the corpus luteum. The time lapse between its commencement and the onset of bleeding is quite uniform, regardless of the length of the menstrual cycle. The onset of bleeding corresponds to the involution of the corpus luteum.

### ANOVULATION

In certain instances, the ovary may not produce a ripe follicle in the course of a cycle. In such an *anovulatory cycle*, the proliferative endometrium develops as usual, but it does not proceed to the progestational stage, since ovulation does not occur and no corpus luteum is formed. Nevertheless, bleeding will occur, but from a proliferative endometrium at the expected time.

## Pregnancy

After fertilization occurs in the ampulla of the Fallopian tube, the ovum completes the second maturation division and extrudes the second polar body. The fertilized ovum undergoes segmentation, a series of mitotic divisions without cell growth, as it moves down the Fallopian tube and enters the uterus. At this time, the ovum consists of a mass of cells, the *morula*, the individual cells of which are called *blastomeres*, surrounded by the zona pellucida.

Soon after this, fluid penetrates the zona pellucida and diffuses between the blastomeres. The fluid increases in amount, the intercellular spaces become confluent, and a single cavity, the *blastocele*, is formed (Fig. 15–26). The zona pellucida disappears, and the morula becomes the *blastocyst*.

The blastocyst remains free within the uterine cavity for about a day and then becomes attached to the endometrium six or seven days after fertilization (Fig. 15–27). At this time, the endometrium is in the progestational phase. It is thick and edematous, and the glands are large and swollen with secretion. The site of attachment may be anywhere on the wall of the uterus but usually is high up toward the fundus.

The blastocyst wall is composed of a single layer of cells, the *trophoblast*, and an *inner cell mass* in the cavity of the blastocyst. The inner cell mass will not be considered further here, since it is from this mass that the embryo is destined to form. As the blastocyst attaches to the endometrium, trophoblast cells proliferate rapidly, and the trophoblast becomes several cells thick. The lining epithelium of the uterus breaks down at the point of attachment, and the blastocyst sinks into the endometrial stroma. The defect in the endome-

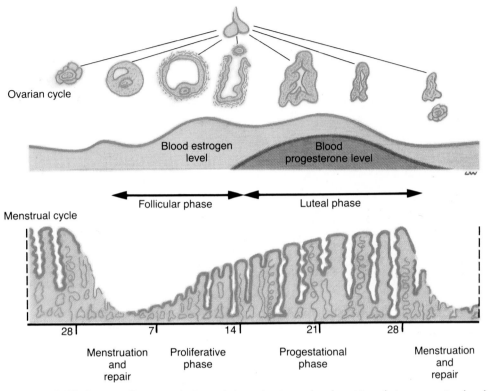

**Figure 15–25.** *Diagram illustrating the interrelations of ovary and endometrium during a menstrual cycle.*

trium is closed temporarily by a plug of fibrin, but later the endometrial epithelium grows over the embedded blastocyst to restore continuity of the uterine lining.

Once the blastocyst becomes embedded within the endometrium, which occurs by about the eleventh day of development, the trophoblast over the entire surface of the blastocyst proliferates. It consists of two layers of cells:

1. The inner layer of cells, the *cytotrophoblast*, is composed of cells with clearly defined cell boundaries.

2. The outer layer is thicker and consists of a multinucleated protoplasmic mass, the *syncytial trophoblast*. The cytotrophoblast exhibits active mitosis and contributes cells to the syncytial trophoblast.

From the surface of the syncytial trophoblast, epithelial cords erode and extend out into the surrounding endometrium. These are the *primary (primitive) villi*. Later, primitive embryonic con-

nective tissue comes into relation with the trophoblast, and the two layers together constitute the *chorion*. Connective tissue, containing fetal blood vessels, then extends into the villi, which now are termed *secondary (chorionic) villi*. With vascularization, the secondary villi become the *tertiary villi*.

Villi on the deeply embedded surface of the blastocyst grow rapidly and form the fetal component of the placenta, the *chorion frondosum*. Villi of the chorion frondosum are attached to a firm, disc-like portion of the chorion, the *chorionic plate*. Villi on the surface of the chorion facing the uterine cavity do not grow as rapidly as on the deeply embedded surface, and they degenerate by the end of the third month of pregnancy. This portion of the chorion is known as the *chorion laeve*.

The endometrium also shows important structural changes during pregnancy. Since all the endometrium, except the deepest layer, is des-

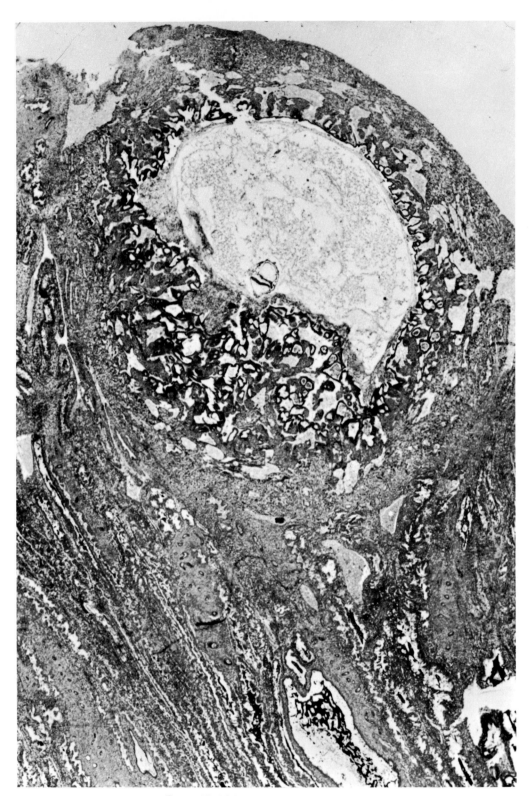

*Figure 15–26* See legend on opposite page

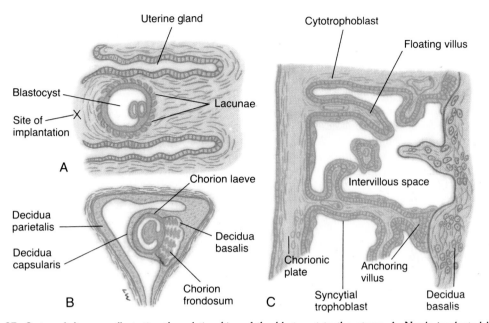

*Figure 15–27.* Series of diagrams illustrating the relationships of the blastocyst to the uterus. A, Newly implanted blastocyst within the endometrium. B, Components of the decidua. C, Small segment of the early placenta, showing fetal and maternal contributions.

tined to be shed at parturition, the endometrium in a pregnant uterus is referred to as *decidua*. Three regions of the decidua are distinguished:

1. Overlying the blastocyst is the *decidua capsularis*.

2. Underlying it is the *decidua basalis*.

3. All the remaining mucosa of the body of the uterus is the *decidua parietalis*. As the embryo increases in size, the decidua capsularis becomes attenuated and eventually contacts the decidua parietalis on the opposite surface of the uterus. At this time, about the end of the third month of pregnancy, the uterine cavity is obliterated.

It is the decidua basalis that becomes the maternal component of the placenta. In the early part of pregnancy, the endometrium increases in thickness. A characteristic feature is the presence of *decidual cells*, which are enlarged stromal cells. The cytoplasm is vesicular or finely granular and contains large amounts of glycogen. The function of these cells is obscure.

As chorionic villi grow into the decidua basalis, they erode and destroy the endometrium, leaving spaces, or *lacunae*. With further expansion of villi, lacunae become interconnected and contain blood liberated by penetration of the maternal vessels by the trophoblast. Diffusion of dissolved substances now can occur between the maternal blood within the lacunae and fetal blood in the capillaries of the villi.

*Figure 15–26.* Section through the implantation site of a 15-day ovum. A differentiating inner cell mass lies within a large trophoblast cavity (blastocele). The trophoblast, which is invading the endometrium, already shows more extensive development toward the decidua basalis (chorion frondosum, below) than toward the decidua capsularis (chorion laeve, above). Low power.

## Placenta

By 16 weeks, the chorion frondosum is well developed, and the placenta is discoid in shape. It continues to increase in size throughout most of the gestational period, owing mainly to growth of the villi. It consists of both a fetal and a maternal component.

**Fetal Component.** The fetal component consists of the chorionic plate and the villi that arise from the plate. The villi lie in lacunae through which maternal blood circulates. Villi usually are classified into two types, *anchoring villi* and *free villi*. Anchoring villi pass from the chorionic plate to the decidua basalis. They give rise to numerous branches that float in the lacunae.

Villi are alike histologically. In the loose connective tissue core of each villus, there is a fetal capillary lined with typical unfenestrated endothelium (Fig. 15–28). Scattered within the connective tissue core are large cells with large spherical nuclei and a vacuolated cytoplasm. These are *Hofbauer's cells*, which are thought to be tissue macrophages. The trophoblast covering each villus consists of two layers until approximately the tenth week of pregnancy, after which time the cytotrophoblast progressively disappears.

The cytotrophoblast, also called *Langerhans's layer*, rests upon a basal lamina and consists of large, discrete, pale cells. The cytoplasm contains vacuoles and some glycogen. Desmosomal contacts occur between adjacent cytotrophoblast cells and between cytotrophoblast and syncytial trophoblast layers. Growth and mitotic activity of the cytotrophoblast are responsible for the development of the syncytial trophoblast. In the second half of pregnancy, proliferation slows while fusion of daughter cells into the syncytial trophoblast continues. This results in a loss of cytotrophoblast cells, and, at parturition, only isolated clumps of its cells remain.

The syncytial trophoblast is a dark layer of variable thickness in which numerous small dark nuclei are present. No intercellular boundaries can be distinguished. The outer, free surface is irregular in outline and possesses numerous mi-

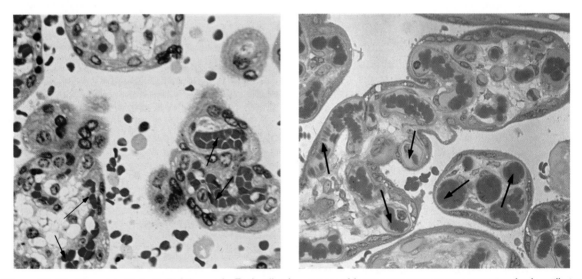

*Figure 15–28.* *Placental villi. Left: Eighth month. Each villus has a core of loose connective tissue containing fetal capillaries (arrows) and a covering of trophoblast. At this stage, the trophoblast consists principally of syncytial trophoblast, which shows dense nuclei and a dense, acidophil cytoplasm. Intercellular boundaries cannot be distinguished. Earlier during pregnancy, a layer of cytotrophoblast is interposed between the syncytial trophoblast and the connective tissue core of the villi, but at this stage, only isolated clumps of cytotrophoblast remain (not seen here). The space between villi is the intervillous space that contains maternal blood. H and E. High power. Right: Ninth month. Each villus is covered by an attenuated layer of syncytial trophoblast. Many of the fetal capillaries, lying within the core of loose connective tissue, are closely opposed to the syncytial trophoblast (arrows). A portion of the chorionic plate is present (above right). Plastic section. Methylene blue, azure A, basic fuchsin. High power.*

crovilli. The cytoplasm is densely basophil and contains abundant granular endoplasmic reticulum, multiple Golgi complexes, and numerous primary and secondary lysosomes. In the latter half of pregnancy, the syncytial trophoblast thins out over the fetal capillaries to form a narrow layer (Fig. 15–29). In other regions, it often becomes aggregated into protuberances called *syncytial knots*, or *sprouts*. On the surface of the villi, irregular masses of an acidophil, homogeneous substance called *fibrinoid* are present. This becomes increasingly abundant in older placentae.

**Maternal Component.** The maternal component of the placenta is the decidua basalis. The enlarged endometrial stromal cells are known as decidual cells. Epithelial cells lining the glands are rich in glycogen and lipid droplets. By the third month, the glands of the decidua basalis become

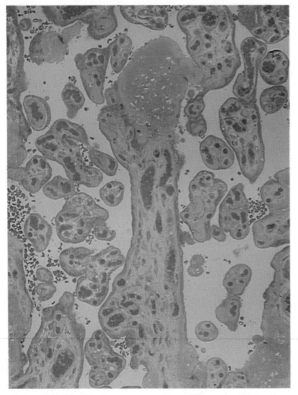

**Figure 15–29.** Placenta at parturition. The syncytial trophoblast covering the villi is thinned out over the fetal capillaries and in many regions forms only a narrow layer. On the surface of the central villus, cut longitudinally, there is an irregular acidophil mass of fibrinoid material (top center). Methylene blue, azure A, basic fuchsin. Medium power.

stretched and appear as horizontal clefts. Passing through the decidua basalis are spiral arteries that open into the intervillous spaces.

The decidua is eroded more deeply opposite the anchoring villi than elsewhere, and this leaves projections of decidual tissue between the main villous trees. Such projections are termed *placental septa*, and they divide the placenta into lobules, or *cotyledons*. There may be a total of 15 to 30 cotyledons. At the margin of the maternal component of the placenta, the decidua basalis becomes continuous with the decidua parietalis. From the fourth month on, the decidua basalis becomes loose in texture owing to the development of a dense venous plexus within it.

### PLACENTAL CIRCULATION AND FUNCTIONS

The placenta transfers from the maternal to the fetal circulation the nutritive and other substances necessary for the growth of the embryo. It also transfers waste products of fetal metabolism to the maternal circulation. Blood poor in oxygen is carried from the fetus to the placenta in a pair of *umbilical arteries*. These arteries divide into numerous radially arranged arteries at the chorionic plate that send branches into the stem villi. These branches ramify in the main villous trees and form extensive capillary networks in the free villi. The oxygen-rich venous blood is collected into a sytem of veins that converge upon a single *umbilical vein* (Fig. 15–30).

On the maternal side, blood from the arcuate arteries is carried by spiral arteries through the basal plate of the placenta into the intervillous spaces. The blood flow is pulsatile and is directed deeply into the spaces. Numerous communications between the spaces and dilated veins in the decidua basalis return the blood to large veins within the myometrium.

Exchange of gases, nutritive substances, and metabolic products ocurs as maternal blood passes over the villi. The maternal circulation is separated from the fetal circulation only by the syncytial trophoblast, the cytotrophoblast (in the first trimester of pregancy only), the basal lamina of the trophoblast, fetal connective tissue, the basal lamina of fetal capillaries, and the fetal endothelium. These structures constitute the so-called *placental barrier*, which is selective against particulate matter, such as microorganisms, and

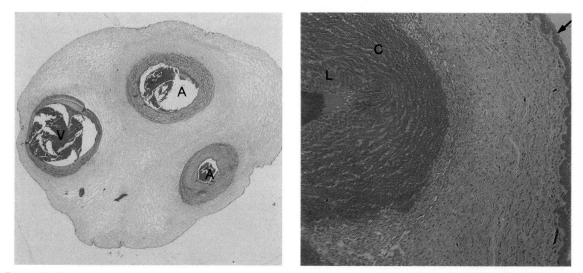

**Figure 15–30.** *Umbilical cord.* Left: *The umbilical cord is covered by a single-layered epithelium of the enveloping chorion and has a core of mucous connective tissue (Wharton's jelly). Within the cord are two umbilical arteries (A) and a single umbilical vein (V). Each artery has a thick muscular coat, or tunica media. The vein, which carries oxygenated blood from the placenta, is unusual in that its wall, unlike that of most veins, consists principally of a tunica media. The tunica adventitia is difficult to define and merges into the surrounding mucous connective tissue. H and E. Low power.* Right: *The umbilical artery (here sectioned transversely), unlike most arteries, possesses a media composed of two thick muscular layers: an inner longitudinal layer (L) and an outer circular layer (C). It also lacks an internal elastic membrane. A portion of the lumen, darkly staining, lies to the left. The artery lies within the delicate, mucous connective tissue, covered externally by the chorion (arrow). Plastic section. Methylene blue, azure A, basic fuchsin. Medium power.*

against chemical substances over a certain molecular size.

The placenta also functions as a major endocrine gland. It elaborates estrogens, progesterone, *chorionic gonadotropin*, and *chorionic somatomammotropin*. All these hormones are thought to be synthesized by the syncytial trophoblast. The cytotrophoblast, previously considered to be active in the synthesis of hormones, functions chiefly in the formation of the syncytial trophoblast.

The placental estrogens contribute to the growth of the uterus and to the development of the mammary glands. Progesterone stimulates development and proliferation of decidual cells and contributes to development of the mammary glands. Enough progesterone is produced by the placenta by the end of the fourth month to maintain pregnancy if the corpus luteum fails to function. Chorionic gonadotropin stimulates secretion of estrogens and progesterone by the corpus luteum during early pregnancy, and chorionic somatomammotropin has a growth-promoting action and stimulates development of the

mammary glands. The latter hormone also influences carbohydrate and fat metabolism of the mother and makes more glucose available for the fetus.

### Cervix

The cervix is the lowest segment of the uterus. The mucous membrane of the cervical canal comprises an epithelium and a lamina propria and forms complex, deep furrows, or clefts, termed *plicae palmatae*, which on section appear as large, branching glands (Fig. 15–31). The epithelium consists of tall, mucus-secreting columnar cells. The oval nuclei lie at the bases of the cells, and the supranuclear cytoplasm is pale. Some of the cells are ciliated, with the cilia beating toward the vagina. Obstruction of the irregular furrows, or clefts, may lead to accumulations of mucus secretion and the appearance of large cysts, the *Nabothian follicles*. The lamina propria is a cellular connective tissue that contains no coiled arteries.

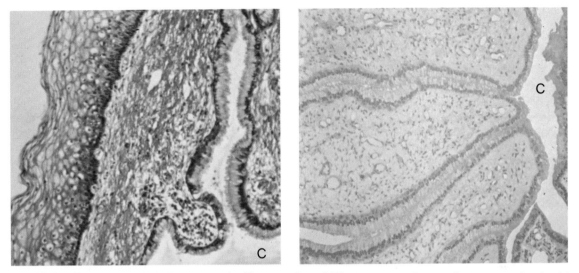

**Figure 15–31.** *Uterine cervix. Left: Portio vaginalis. The cervical canal (C) appears irregular in outline owing to the glandular invagination of the lining epithelium, which is simple tall columnar in nature, to form plicae palmatae. Immediately beneath the epithelium, the lamina propria is cellular, but its deeper layers contain closely packed collagenous fibers (green). The thick epithelium (left), which covers the portion of the cervix that projects into the vagina, is stratified squamous nonkeratinizing. The junction between the two types of epithelia is not shown here, but it would occur just below this section (at the external os). Masson trichrome. Medium power. Right: Cervical canal. The mucous membrane of the cervical canal (C) consists of an epithelium and a lamina propria. The simple columnar epithelium is composed of tall, mucus-secreting cells. The ovoid nuclei lie at the bases of the cells, and the apical cytoplasm is pale, owing to the presence of secretory material. Numerous long, branching clefts, the plicae palmatae, extend from the lining epithelium into the lamina propria, which is a delicate, cellular and vascular connective tissue. Plastic section. H and E. High power.*

The portion of the cervix that projects into the vagina is covered by stratified squamous nonkeratinizing epithelium. The transition between the simple columnar epithelium of the cervical canal and the stratified squamous epithelium of the portio vaginalis is abrupt and occurs usually just inside the external os of the cervical canal. The mucosa of the cervical canal does not desquamate during menstruation, although minor changes in the structure of the plicae palmatae do occur. However, during the menstrual cycle, there are changes in both the quantity and the properties of the cervical mucus, which is a concentrated solution of glycoproteins rich in carbohydrates. Spermatozoa can penetrate midcycle cervical mucus, which is less viscid and more highly hydrated, much more readily than the viscid mucus that is secreted during the progestational stage. During pregnancy, the plicae palmatae secrete large amounts of a more viscous secretion that forms a plug in the cervical canal.

The mucosa rests upon a myometrium that is composed chiefly of dense collagenous connective tissue. Smooth muscle present is arranged mainly in irregular bundles. The thin outer longitudinal layer continues into the vagina. Smooth muscle is absent in the portio vaginalis. Toward the end of pregnancy, changes occur in the fibrous and amorphous components of the myometrium, resulting in softening of the cervix. These changes are brought about by relaxin, the polypeptide hormone secreted by the corpus luteum of pregnancy.

## VAGINA

The vagina is a fibromuscular sheath extending from the cervix to the vestibule. Under ordinary conditions, it is collapsed, and the anterior and posterior walls are in contact. In the virgin, the lower end of the vagina is marked by a fold of mucous membrane, the *hymen*. The wall of the vagina consists of three coats (Fig. 15–32):

1. The mucosa.
2. The muscularis.
3. The adventitia.

### Mucosa

The mucosa exhibits transverse folds, or *rugae*. It is lined with thick stratified squamous epithelium that is nonkeratinizing. Component cells are loaded with glycogen, and thus they appear vacuolated in most histological sections. Like the epidermis, the vaginal epithelium contains Langerhans's cells, which appear as scattered clear cells in the basal and intermediate layers of the epithelium. The epithelium, which lacks glands, is lubricated by mucus that originates from the cervix. Beneath the epithelium, there is a lamina propria that is a dense connective tissue. Numerous elastic fibers are present immediately below the epithelium, and, throughout the lamina propria, there are polymorphonuclear leukocytes, lymphocytes, and occasional lymph nodules. Many lymphocytes and polymorphonuclear leukocytes invade the epithelium, especially around the time of menstruation.

The surface cells of the vaginal epithelium are desquamated continuously and may be studied by the smear method. Glycogen, released into the vagina with desquamated cells, is metabolized by indigenous bacteria to produce an acid fluid that coats the vagina. The glycogen content of the epithelial cells is controlled by secretion of estrogens. The pH of vaginal fluid, which normally is low, thus rises during the luteal phase of the cycle, since less glycogen is formed within the vaginal epithelium. The low pH of the vaginal fluid inhibits the growth of pathogenic bacteria, and the administration of estrogens may aid in the treatment of vaginal infections.

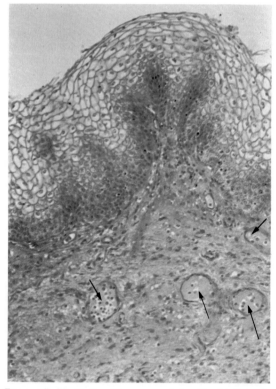

**Figure 15–32.** *Vagina. The mucosa is lined by thick stratified squamous epithelium that is nonkeratinizing. Component cells are loaded with glycogen and thus appear vacuolated in this preparation. The underlying lamina propria is relatively dense connective tissue that contains numerous lymphocytes and polymorphonuclear leukocytes and blood vessels (arrows). The junction between epithelium and lamina propria is irregular because of the presence of connective tissue papillae. The mucosa is surrounded by a muscularis, composed of interlacing bundles of smooth muscle, and a dense connective tissue adventitia (not shown here). H and E. Medium power.*

### Muscularis

The muscularis of the vagina is composed of smooth muscle fibers that are arranged in interlacing bundles. The inner portion, where most muscle bundles are circularly arranged, is thin. The thick outer portion contains longitudinal bundles that are continuous above with the myometrium of the uterus. At the introitus, skeletal muscle fibers of the bulbospongiosus form a kind of sphincter.

### Adventitia

The adventitia is a thin layer of dense connective tissue that blends with that of surrounding organs.

### Blood Vessels, Lymphatics, and Nerves

Blood vessels and lymphatic vessels are abundant in the wall of the vagina. Veins are particularly numerous and give the adventitia the appearance of erectile tissue. There is a rich plexus of venous sinuses in a lamina propria, and engorgement of these veins during sexual excitement probably accounts for the fluid transudate that passes into the vaginal lumen at this time.

The vagina receives both myelinated and unmyelinated nerve fibers. The latter form a ganglionated plexus in the adventitia and supply the muscularis and the walls of blood vessels. Myelinated nerve fibers terminate in special sensory endings in the mucosa.

## EXTERNAL GENITALIA

The female external genitalia, known collectively as the *vulva*, include the clitoris, the labia majora and minora, and certain glands that open into the vestibule.

### Clitoris

The clitoris is homologous to the dorsal part of the penis. It consists of two erectile bodies, the *corpora cavernosa*, which end in a small *glans clitoridis*. It is covered with a thin, stratified squamous epithelium that is associated with numerous, specialized sensory nerve endings.

### Labia Minora

The *labia minora* are folds of mucous membrane that form the lateral walls of the vestibule. They are covered with a stratified squamous epithelium, which contains pigment in its deeper layers, and have a core of richly vascularized connective tissue (Fig. 15–33). Tall papillae of connective tissue penetrate far into the epithelium. Numerous large sebaceous glands occur on both surfaces of the fold, which is devoid of hair follicles.

### Labia Majora

The *labia majora* are folds of skin that cover the labia minora externally. The inner surface is smooth and hairless, and the outer surface is covered by cornified epidermis that contains

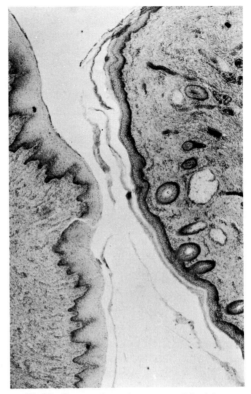

*Figure 15–33.* Section through portions of the labium minus (left) and the labium majus (right). The former is covered with nonkeratinized stratified squamous epithelium and has a core of richly vascularized connective tissue. The latter is a fold of skin, the inner surface of which (shown here) is hairless. Numerous sweat and sebaceous (pale) glands lie beneath the cornified epidermis. Low power.

coarse hairs (see Fig. 15–33). Sebaceous and sweat glands are numerous on both surfaces. The core of each fold contains a considerable amount of adipose tissue and some smooth muscle fibers.

### Vestibule

The *vestibule*, into which the vagina and urethra open, is lined by a typical stratified squamous epithelium and contains numerous small glands, the *minor vestibular glands*. These are located mainly around the urethral opening and near the clitoris. They resemble the urethral glands (of Littre) and contain mucous cells. The *major vestibular glands (glands of Bartholin)*, analogous to the bulbourethral glands in the male, are located in the lateral walls of the vestibule. They are tubuloalveolar glands that secrete a lubricating mucus. Their ducts open near the base of the hymen, and their secretion moistens the inner surfaces of the labia minora.

## MAMMARY GLAND

The mammary glands are modified sweat glands located within the subcutaneous tissue. They are present in both sexes, and they develop only slightly during childhood. At puberty, the glands enlarge rapidly in the female, principally as a result of development of adipose and other connective tissue, but very slowly in the male. The glands remain incompletely developed in the female until pregnancy occurs. After puberty, there is no further development of the glands in the male.

The gland consists of 15 to 20 individual lobes, each of which is an independent gland with a duct opening at the apex of the nipple. A lobe is surrounded by interlobar connective tissue containing many fat cells. The fat and connective tissue also divide each lobe into numerous lobules. The intralobular connective tissue is loose, delicate, and cellular. Intralobular ducts drain into interlobular ducts, which join to form a single excretory duct from each lobe, the *lactiferous duct*. The lactiferous duct courses through the nipple and dilates near its termination at the summit of the nipple into a *lactiferous sinus*.

### Nipple and Areola

The nipple is covered by keratinized stratified squamous epithelium that is pigmented. The underlying dermis is characterized by the presence of unusually long dermal papillae and bundles of smooth muscle fibers. The muscle bundles are arranged circumferentially within the nipple and longitudinally along the lactiferous ducts. Contraction of the muscle in response to certain stimuli hardens and elevates the nipple. The nipple is traversed by lactiferous ducts, each of which opens by a pore on the surface. There are fewer

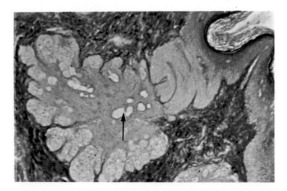

*Figure 15–34. Nipple, areolar gland. This section shows the epidermis (right) and one large areolar gland (left). The epidermis of the areolar skin is relatively thick and exhibits marked cornification (red). The underlying dermis (blue) contains an areolar gland (gland of Montgomery), which is a branched gland intermediate in structure between a sweat gland and a true mammary gland. Large, vacuolated secretory cells lie at the periphery of the gland, and centrally a narrow coiled duct (arrow) extends toward the surface epidermis. Azocarmine. Low power.*

pores than main ducts, owing to terminal fusions. Near their terminations, the ducts are lined by stratified squamous epithelium.

The *areola*, an area of skin that encircles the base of the nipple, is pigmented and contains special *areolar glands (glands of Montgomery)*, which are large, branched glands that produce small elevations on the surface of the areola (Fig. 15–34). These glands are intermediate in structure between sweat glands and true mammary glands. Sweat and sebaceous glands and a number of coarse hairs are present also.

### Parenchyma

The parenchyma of the mammary gland shows extensive structural changes that are dependent upon the functional condition (Fig. 15–35).

#### INACTIVE (RESTING) MAMMARY GLAND

The ducts are the principal epithelial tissue seen. Intralobular ducts are grouped together into lobules. The lining of the ducts changes from a simple cuboidal to a two-layered epithelium from

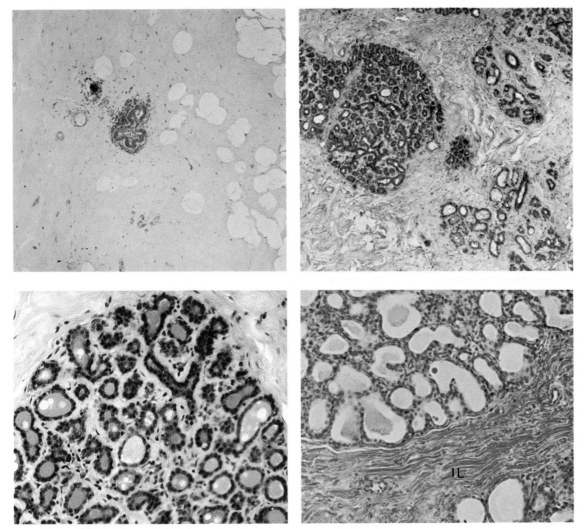

**Figure 15–35.** *Mammary gland, different functional conditions. Top left: Prepubertal (inactive) gland. Prior to puberty, ducts are the principal epithelial elements of the gland. Here, a small intralobular duct, lined by a simple cuboidal epithelium, is surrounded by delicate, cellular intralobular connective tissue. The embedding interlobular connective tissue is dense and contains small amounts of adipose tissue. Top right: Gland in pregnancy. During pregnancy, ducts within the lobules of each lobe proliferate and form buds that enlarge into alveoli. Lobules expand, and interlobular connective tissue and fat decrease in amount. Here, several lobules are shown. They contain groups of alveoli and scattered, wide intralobular ducts and are embedded within a loose, cellular connective tissue. The surrounding interlobular connective tissue is relatively dense and contains a few fat cells. Lower left: Gland in late pregnancy. A portion of one lobule is shown. Alveoli vary in size and are lined by a simple cuboidal epithelium. A layer of myoepithelial cells (not visible here) occurs between the alveolar epithelium and the basal lamina. The lumina of many alveoli contain acidophil secretory material. Intralobular ducts histologically appear similar to alveoli, and functionally they are true secretory ducts that also possess myoepithelial elements. The embedding intralobular connective tissue is cellular, whereas the surrounding interlobular connective tissue is relatively dense. Lower right: Lactation. Portions of two lobules are shown. Alveoli are dilated and may appear as saccules. The lumina of some contain pale-staining, secretory material. The surrounding intralobular connective tissue is condensed and appears markedly cellular owing to infiltration with lymphocytes. The interlobular connective tissue (IL) also is condensed and consists principally of collagenous fibers. All H and E. Top figures, low power; bottom, medium power.*

the small to the main ducts. Near their terminations, the main ducts are lined by stratified squamous epithelium. Alveoli, if present, are small buds of epithelial cells that occur at the blind ends of the intralobular ducts. These cells enlarge during the second half of each menstrual cycle, and the surrounding connective tissue becomes highly vascular. The increase in the size of the mammary gland and the sense of engorgement experienced by some women prior to the onset of menstruation are due to increased blood flow and the accompanying edema of the intralobular connective tissue.

Between the epithelium and the basal lamina, there is an incomplete layer of myoepithelial cells. These highly branched cells possess long, slender processes that embrace the alveoli and ducts. Interlobular connective tissue is dense and abundant and contains varying amounts of adipose tissue. Intralobular connective tissue is loose and more cellular.

### PREGNANCY

The gland exhibits extensive changes in preparation for lactation. During the first half of pregnancy, intralobular ducts undergo rapid proliferation, branch, and form buds that enlarge into alveoli (see Fig. 15–35). Owing to the increase of glandular tissue and the expansion of the lobules, interlobular fat and connective tissue decrease in amount, and the 15 to 20 lobes become distinct entities. Intralobular connective tissue also decreases in amount and becomes infiltrated with lymphocytes, plasma cells, and granular leukocytes.

During the second half of pregnancy, hyperplasia of the glandular tissue slows, but the alveoli enlarge and begin to elaborate some secretory material. At the end of pregnancy, some cloudy watery fluid, *colostrum*, is secreted. This secretion is rich in proteins and lactose but contains practically no lipid. It does contain considerable amounts of antibodies, which provide some degree of passive immunity to the newborn.

During pregnancy, increased deposition of melanin occurs in the skin of the nipple and areola.

### LACTATION

Soon after parturition, the mammary gland begins active secretion of milk, which is rich in fat, sugar, and protein. Many alveoli become dilated and appear as saccules (Fig. 15–36; see Fig. 15–35). They are distended with milk and have a low epithelial wall. Other alveoli are resting; they have a relatively tall epithelial lining and narrow lumina. Individual alveolar cells, which contain an extensive system of granular endoplasmic reticulum and numerous free ribosomes, undergo a cyclic process of secretion.

The secretory process appears to be partly merocrine and partly apocrine. Milk proteins are synthesized within the granular endoplasmic reticulum and are condensed into small vacuoles within the Golgi complex. These membrane-bound granules move to the apical surface, where their contents are released by exocytosis. This

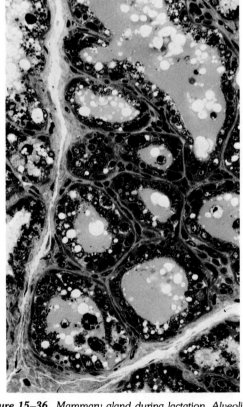

*Figure 15–36. Mammary gland during lactation. Alveoli are distended with milk and are lined by a low epithelium. The cytoplasm of alveolar cells is crowded with dense granules and large lipid globules. Between alveolar cells and the basal lamina are basket (myoepithelial) cells (not visible here), which are contractile. Plastic section. High power.*

THE FEMALE REPRODUCTIVE SYSTEM • **631**

process, which involves no loss of cytoplasm or of cell membrane, is merocrine in type. The fatty components of milk are elaborated and discharged in a different manner. Small fat droplets appear within the cytoplasm and later coalesce to form large fat globules at the cell apex. As these globules are released, they carry with them a portion of the apical cell membrane and a thin coating of cytoplasm. This is an apocrine type of secretion, although the extent of cytoplasmic loss is less marked than in most glands of this type. The secretory cycle then is repeated.

The lumen of each alveolus is filled with these two types of discharged cellular products suspended in a watery fluid. Tight junctions encircle each secretory cell. They provide mechanical adhesion and limit transepithelial permeability. The secretory epithelium rests upon a basal lam-

ina. Between the alveolar cells and the basal lamina are stellate *basket* (myoepithelial) *cells*. These are contractile and aid in the movement of milk from the alveoli into the ducts.

Intralobular ducts histologically appear similar to alveoli. Functionally, they are true secretory ducts that also possess myoepithelial elements.

### REGRESSION

After cessation of lactation, the gland undergoes retrogressive changes and returns to a resting state (Fig. 15–37). Within a few days, milk remaining in the alveoli and ducts is absorbed. Alveoli decrease in size, and some cells degenerate. Connective tissue and fat again become abundant. However, the gland usually does not return to the nulliparous state; many alveoli remain recognizable as such, and remnants of secretory material may be retained within the ducts for a considerable time.

### INVOLUTION

After the menopause, the mammary gland undergoes involution. The secretory epithelium atrophies, and only a few remnants of the duct system persist. Cystic dilation of the remaining ducts occurs frequently. The connective tissue becomes less cellular, increasingly dense, and more homogeneous. It stains only faintly acidophil.

### Hormonal Control

Growth of the duct system, which occurs at puberty, is influenced by *estrogens* and *progesterone* secreted cyclically by the ovaries. While the cyclic response of the mammary gland is minimal, some structural changes can be observed. Further growth of the gland in pregnancy is due to continuous and prolonged production of both estrogens and progesterone by the ovaries and placenta. To obtain full development in late pregnancy, other hormones appear to be necessary. These include *prolactin*, produced by the adenohypophysis, *somatomammotropin*, produced by the placenta, and *suprarenal corticoids*.

At parturition, the levels of circulating estrogens and progesterone fall abruptly, and the increased production of prolactin results in the secretion of

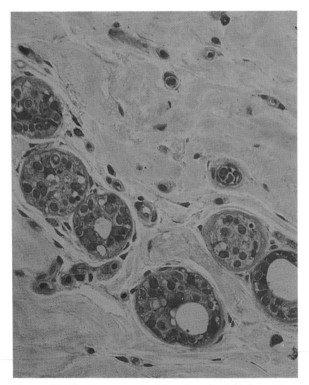

*Figure 15–37.* Mammary gland, inactive, after lactation. After cessation of lactation, the gland undergoes retrogression and returns to a resting state. The lobules, one of which is shown here, are composed principally of ducts, but some alveoli remain. The surrounding connective tissue contains numerous capillaries, which increase in extent during the second half of each menstrual cycle. Plastic section. Methylene blue, azure A, basic fuchsin. High power.

milk. Maintenance of lactation requires continuous secretion of prolactin, which occurs as a result of a neurohumoral reflex initiated by suckling. Frequent breast feeding thus is important to maintain lactation. Regular suckling also causes release of *oxytocin* from the neurohypophysis. The oxytocin stimulates the myoepithelial cells to contract, leading to ejection of milk from alveoli and ducts.

After the menopause, in the absence of stimulation by ovarian hormones, parenchymal cells degenerate and atrophy, and the gland involutes.

### Blood Vessels, Lymphatics, and Nerves

The arteries of the mammary gland arise from the internal thoracic artery, thoracic branches of the axillary artery, and the intercostal arteries. The arteries ramify in the stroma, principally in relation to the large ducts, and terminate in rich capillary plexuses around the intralobular ducts and alveoli. The vascular supply becomes much richer in the active gland. From the capillaries, veins arise, which accompany the arteries and terminate in the axillary and internal thoracic veins.

Lymph vessels are found in the connective tissue around alveoli and intralobular ducts, in the interlobular connective tissue, and in the areola. Collecting lymphatics pass to the axillary and subclavicular nodes. A few lymphatics follow the branches of the internal thoracic artery to terminate in parasternal nodes.

Afferent nerve fibers supply the tactile organs of the nipple. Some nerve fibers follow the interlobular connective tissue and form delicate plexuses around the alveoli.

### EMBRYOLOGY OF THE FEMALE AND MALE REPRODUCTIVE SYSTEMS

The primordia of the gonads arise as thickenings of mesodermal epithelium, the *genital ridges,* on the mesial surface of the mesonephros. The epithelial cells of the ridge proliferate and form a band of tissue composed of two types of cells. Most cells are small, cuboidal elements, and scattered between them are large, spheroidal cells, the *primitive sex cells.* The epithelial cells penetrate the underlying mesenchyme to form *sex cords.*

### Sexual Differentiation

In the male human embryo, the testis becomes recognizable at about seven weeks of gestation. The sex cords become more distinct and elongate to form the seminiferous tubules. Their peripheral ends anastomose and unite with a number of mesonephric tubules to form the rete testis. Prior to the onset of puberty, component cells of the seminiferous tubules differentiate into spermatogonia and Sertoli's cells.

Differentiation of the ovary does not commence until about the eighth week of gestation. The sex cords formed during the indifferent stage gradually disappear. The surface (germinal) epithelium continues to proliferate and produces the primitive cortex of the ovary. This mass of cortical cells is subdivided by strands of mesenchyme into clusters of cells that surround one or more primitive germ cells to form the first follicles. The ovary now has its full complement of germ cells (primary oocytes).

### Genital Ducts

Genital ducts develop in close connection with the embryonic urinary system. They are laid down initially as two paired longitudinal ducts, the *mesonephric (Wolffian)* and the *paramesonephric (Müllerian) ducts,* the latter from mesoderm lining the celomic cavity. In the male, the mesonephric duct is transformed into ductus epididymidis and ductus deferens. Connection of the ductus epididymidis with the rete testis is established by a number of mesonephric tubules that become the ductuli efferentes. The paramesonephric duct involutes, leaving only small rudiments.

In the female, the mesonephric ducts regress, and the paramesonephric ducts transform into the female genital ducts. Caudally, the two paramesonephric ducts fuse to form a single tube that opens into the urogenital sinus (cloaca). The paired upper portions form the Fallopian tubes, and the fused terminal portion becomes the body and cervix of the uterus. The vagina arises from a proliferation on the posterior wall of the urogenital sinus. The proliferating epithelium extends cranially as a solid bar, the *vaginal plate*. This eventually joins with the lower end of the fused paramesonephric ducts and canalizes to form the vagina.

In humans, as in most mammals, the XY and XX sex chromosome complements determine male and female sex, respectively. In the former, the genetic determinant on the Y chromosome is responsible for differentiation of the indifferent gonad into a testis, which otherwise develops as an ovary. The differentiating testis produces substances that suppress paramesonephric duct development and promote mesonephric duct differentiation. In the absence of a testis, paramesonephric ducts differentiate, and mesonephric ducts fail to undergo differentiation.

## Vestigial Structures

Certain vestigial structures occur in relation to the ovary.

The *epoophoron* consists of several blind tubules situated in the broad ligament between the ovary and the Fallopian tube. The tubules fuse into a longitudinal canal, the *duct of Gartner*, which passes along the lateral wall of the uterus.

The *paroophoron*, consisting of a few blind tubules, lies in the connective tissue of the broad ligament close to the hilum of the ovary.

Both epoophoron and paroophoron are remnants of mesonephric tubules. Gartner's duct represents a remnant of the mesonephric duct.

## Mammary Glands

The primordia of the mammary glands develop as two vertical bands of ectoderm, the *mammary ridges*, that extend from the axilla to the inguinal region. In the human, a single pair of glands develops in the pectoral region, and the remainder of the ridges usually disappears. However, additional accessory nipples or glandular masses are not uncommon. As the glands develop, 15 to 20 solid buds of ectoderm invade the underlying mesenchyme. Each bud will form the branching lactiferous duct of one lobe.

## SUMMARY

The ovary is a double gland, producing both exocrine (cytogenic) and endocrine secretions and exhibits two zones, the cortex, covered by germinal epithelium, and the medulla. The cortex consists of a compact, cellular stroma containing ovarian follicles. Prior to puberty, only primordial follicles are present. Each consists of a primary oocyte surrounded by a single layer of flattened follicular cells. After puberty, under the influence of FSH and LH, there is progressive development of follicles. The follicular cells increase in number and in size to become granulosa cells, and the oocyte enlarges and acquires a zona pellucida. As each follicle approaches maturity, an antrum develops, and the oocyte comes to lie within the cumulus oophorus. The surrounding stromal cells organize to form the theca folliculi. Just prior to ovulation, the primary oocyte undergoes the first maturation division (meiosis) to form the haploid secondary oocyte and the first polar body. At ovulation, the secondary oocyte, surrounded by the zona pellucida and cells of the corona radiata, enters the Fallopian tube and the follicular wall becomes transformed into the corpus luteum. If pregnancy does not occur, the corpus luteum commences to degenerate after about nine days and is replaced by a corpus albicans. During the preovulatory period (follicular phase), secretion of estrogens is high, and progesterone production increases and remains at a high level during the luteal phase. These rhythmic changes in ovarian secretory activity are responsible for the cyclic changes that occur in the uterine endometrium.

The epithelium of the Fallopian tube contains both ciliated and nonciliated (secretory) cells and exhibits cyclic changes associated with the ovarian cycle. Fertilization usually occurs within the ampulla and stimulates completion of the second maturation division. The resulting zygote undergoes cleavage as it is transported down the Fallopian tube by peristaltic and ciliary action. It enters the uterus as a blastocyst.

The endometrium of the uterus consists of a simple, surface epithelium, which is invaginated to form uterine glands, and an endometrial stroma. It has two layers, a functional layer (compact and spongy zones), supplied by spiral (coiled) arteries, and a basal layer, supplied by straight arteries. During the menstrual stage of the cycle, the functional layer undergoes necrosis and is shed. Following this, the endometrium enters the proliferative stage, concurrent with follicular growth and secretion of estrogens. Epithelial and stromal cells proliferate and the tubular glands lengthen but remain straight. During the progestational stage that follows, the glands become tortuous and sacculated under the influence of progesterone secreted by the corpus luteum. When the corpus luteum regresses, progesterone levels fall, the spiral arteries undergo intermittent vasoconstriction, and the functional layer suffers anoxia and necrosis.

The blastocyst becomes embedded within the endometrium during the progestational stage. The trophoblast, which consists of syncytial trophoblast and cytotrophoblast, continues to erode into the endometrium, and the blastocyst becomes surrounded by lacunae filled with maternal blood. By 16 weeks, the placenta is discoid in shape and consists of fetal and maternal components. The fetal component, the chorion frondosum, is the chorionic plate and the branching, tertiary villi that arise from the plate. The maternal component is the decidua basalis, and passing through it are spiral arteries that open into the intervillous spaces. Exchange of gases, nutritive substances, and metabolic products occurs across the placental barrier, composed of syncytial trophoblast, cytotrophoblast (in the first trimester of pregnancy only), the trophoblastic basal lamina, fetal connective tissue, and the basal lamina and endothelium of fetal capillaries. The placenta also func-

tions as an endocrine organ, producing estrogens, progesterone, chorionic gonadotropin, and chorionic somatomammotropin. All these hormones are synthesized by the syncytial trophoblast, and the cytotrophoblast functions principally in the formation of syncytial trophoblast. The myometrium, by muscular contractions, is responsible for expulsion of the fetus at parturition.

The mucosa of the uterine cervix, which does not desquamate at menstruation, has a mucus-secreting epithelium that produces a thick, viscid mucus throughout most of the cycle but a thin, less viscid mucus at midcycle. The cervical myometrium is composed chiefly of dense connective tissue that softens at parturition under the influence of relaxin, secreted by the corpus luteum of pregnancy.

The mammary glands are modified sweat glands, and each gland has 15 to 20 individual lobes. The glands enlarge at puberty, principally because of an increase in adipose tissue, following secretion of estrogens and progesterone by the ovary. Further growth in pregnancy, during which the intralobular ducts proliferate and form buds that develop into alveoli, is influenced by continuous production of estrogens and progesterone and, in late pregnancy, by prolactin, somatomammotropin, and suprarenal corticoids. At parturition, secretion of milk results from the increased production of prolactin and is maintained by a neurohumeral reflex initiated by suckling. Regular suckling also causes release of oxytocin, which stimulates contraction of myoepithelial cells, resulting in ejection of milk.

# The Male Reproductive System

## INTRODUCTION

The male reproductive system comprises the testes, the ducts of the testes, the auxiliary glands associated with them, and the penis (Fig. 16–1). The genital duct system includes the tubuli recti, rete testis, ductuli efferentes, ductus epididymidis, ductus deferens, and ejaculatory duct. The auxiliary glands are the seminal vesicles, prostate, and bulbourethral glands. The testes produce the sex cells, spermatozoa, which are conducted to the exterior by the genital duct system and the penis. The auxiliary glands produce secretions that, together with the spermatozoa, constitute the seminal fluid.

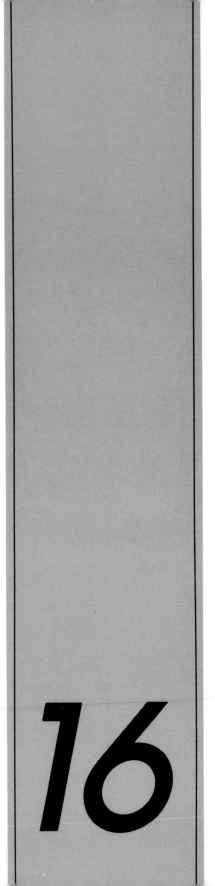

**16**

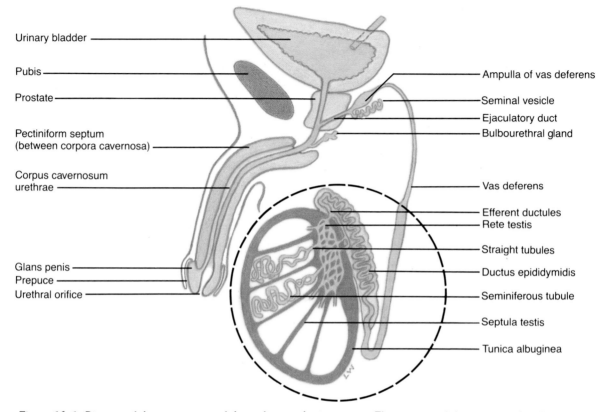

**Figure 16–1.** *Diagram of the components of the male reproductive system. The portions of the system within the circle are represented as more highly magnified than the other components of the system.*

## TESTIS

The testis, like the ovary, is a double gland, since functionally it is both exocrine and endocrine (Figs. 16–2 and 16–3). The exocrine product is chiefly the sex cells, and thus the testis may be referred to as a cytogenic gland. The endocrine product is an internal secretion elaborated by certain specialized cells.

### Testicular Capsule

The testis is suspended within the scrotum and is immediately surrounded by the *testicular capsule*, which is composed of three layers:

1. The outer layer, or *tunica vaginalis.*
2. The middle layer, or *tunica albuginea.*
3. The innermost layer, or *tunica vasculosa.*

The *tunica vaginalis* is a single layer of attenuated mesothelial cells that frequently are destroyed during histological preparation. This visceral layer is part of a closed serous sac, derived from peritoneum, that surrounds the anterior and lateral surfaces of the testis. On the posterior aspect of the testis, this mesothelium is reflected onto the scrotal sac, which it lines to form the parietal layer of the tunica vaginalis. The serous cavity between visceral and parietal layers allows the testis to move freely within it.

The visceral layer of the tunica vaginalis rests upon a basal lamina that separates it from the middle and most prominent layer, the *tunica*

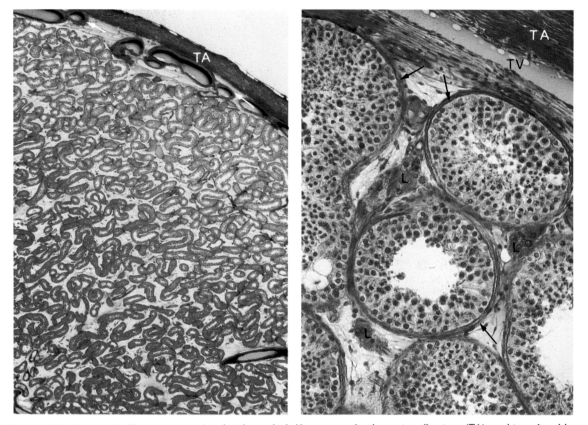

**Figure 16–2.** *Testis.* Left: *The testis is enclosed within a thick fibrous capsule, the tunica albuginea (TA), and is surfaced by a single layer of mesothelial cells, the tunica vaginalis (not shown here). On the inner aspect of the tunica albuginea, dense connective tissue is replaced by a loose connective tissue containing numerous blood vessels, the tunica vasculosa (arrows). Connective tissue septa that extend between the capsule and the mediastinum testis to divide the testis into pyramidal compartments, the lobuli testis, are not apparent on this section. The seminiferous tubules, since they are convoluted, are cut in various planes. Iron hematoxylin, aniline blue. Low power.* Right: *Portions of the tunica albuginea (TA) and of the tunica vasculosa (TV) are present above. Beneath the capsule, sectioned seminiferous tubules, separated by interstitial connective tissue, generally show wide lumina, some containing spermatozoa. The seminiferous epithelium, composed principally of spermatogenic cells, is stratified and is surrounded by the boundary (peritubular) tissue (arrows). The latter contains connective tissue fibers and cells and some myoid cells. The interstitial tissue is a loose, vascular connective tissue containing epithelioid cells, the interstitial cells of Leydig (L). Iron hematoxylin, aniline blue. Medium power.*

*albuginea.* The tunica albuginea is a thick layer of dense fibroelastic connective tissue that contains some smooth muscle cells. In the human, although the smooth muscle elements are widely scattered, they are concentrated predominantly on the posterior aspect of the testis adjacent to the epididymis. The innermost layer of the testicular capsule, the *tunica vasculosa,* consists of a network of blood vessels embedded within a delicate areolar connective tissue.

The testicular capsule is not, as previously thought, an inert covering to the testis but acts as a dynamic membrane capable of periodic contractions. The contractions probably serve to maintain an appropriate pressure within the testis, regulating movement of fluid out of, and back into, the capillaries, and to massage the duct system and thus aid in the movement of spermatozoa in an outward direction. Additionally, the capsule appears to possess the characteristics of a semipermeable membrane and to be involved in several aspects of testicular physiology.

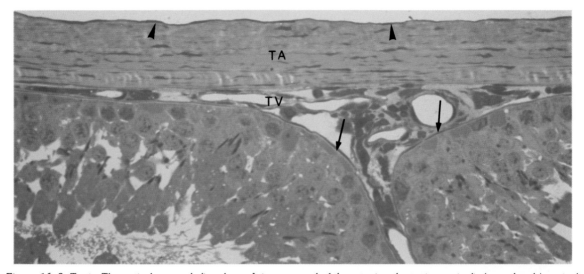

*Figure 16–3.* Testis. The testicular capsule lies above. It is composed of three tunics: the tunica vaginalis (arrowheads), a single layer of attenuated mesothelial cells; the tunica albuginea (TA), a thick layer of fibroelastic connective tissue that also contains smooth muscle cells (not apparent here); and the tunica vasculosa (TV), containing numerous blood vessels. In relation to the latter are groups of interstitial cells of Leydig (darkly staining). Portions of two seminiferous tubules, surrounded by boundary tissue (arrows), underlie the testicular capsule. Plastic section. Methylene blue, azure A, basic fuchsin. Medium power.

The tunica albuginea is thickened along the posterior surface of the testis where it projects into the gland as the *mediastinum testis.* Thin, fibrous partitions radiate from the mediastinum testis to the capsule and divide the interior of the testis into about 250 pyramidal compartments, the *lobuli testis,* with their apices directed toward the mediastinum. The septa show numerous deficiencies and the lobules thus intercommunicate freely. Each lobule contains one to four highly convoluted *seminiferous tubules,* which are embedded within a loose connective tissue stroma containing vessels, nerves, and several types of cells, principally the *interstitial cells* (of Leydig). These are large cells, commonly occurring in groups, and they are important because of their endocrine role.

### Seminiferous Tubules

Each seminiferous tubule is highly convoluted and is about 0.2 mm in diameter and 30 to 70 cm long (Fig. 16–4). The tubules commence as free blind ends or as anastomosing loops either with neighboring tubules of the lobule or, less frequently, with tubules of adjoining lobules. At the apex of a lobule, each tubule loses its convolutions and becomes a *straight tubule.*

The seminiferous tubule is lined by a complex *germinal,* or *seminiferous, epithelium,* which is a highly modified stratified cuboidal epithelium (Figs. 16–5 and 16–6). The epithelium rests upon a thin basal lamina and is covered externally by a specialized zone of fibrous tissue, the *boundary* or *peritubular tissue,* which contains numerous connective tissue fibers, flattened fibroblasts, and some cells with the characteristics of smooth muscle cells. These *myoid cells* exhibit junctional complexes between neighboring cells that retard, but do not entirely prevent, the passage of macromolecules from the interstitial space to the seminiferous epithelium.

The organization of myoid cells shows considerable species variation. In most rodents, myoid cells form a single layer, but in humans, other primates, and several lower species, the peritubular tissue contains three or five layers of myoid cells. It is thought that the myoid cells, by their rhythmic contractions, may alter the diameter of the seminiferous tubule and aid in the movement

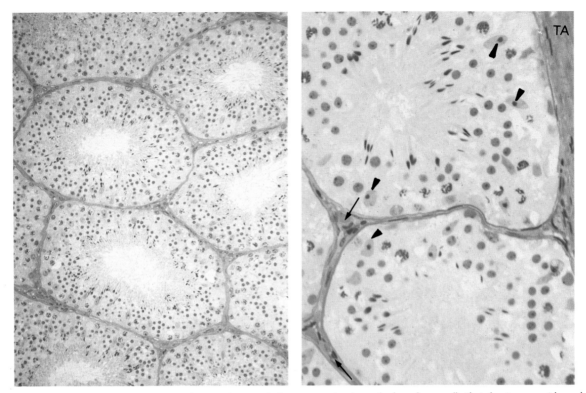

**Figure 16–4.** Testis. Left: In this material, seminiferous tubules appear closely packed, and generally their lumina are wide and empty. The boundary tissue around each tubule is acidophil (pink), and there is little intervening interstitial tissue between the tubules. Plastic section. H and E. Medium power. Right: A portion of the tunica albuginea (TA) lies to the right. The seminiferous tubules are surrounded by the boundary tissue and separated by a narrow interstitial space (arrows) containing blood vessels. The seminiferous epithelium contains two distinct categories of cells—supporting cells and germ, or spermatogenic cells, and nuclear characteristics distinguish supporting cells, or sustentacular cells of Sertoli, from spermatogenic elements. Nuclei of Sertoli's cells (arrowheads) are pale and ovoid, with the long axis of each generally directed radially, and each possesses a distinct nucleolus. Spermatogenic cells differentiate progressively from the basal region to the lumen. The densely staining heads of spermatozoa are present close to the lumen. Plastic section. H and E. High power.

of spermatozoa along the length of the tubule. The thickness of this zone varies with age and shows a great increase in extent in many clinical conditions, particularly those associated with some chromosomal abnormalities (such as Klinefelter's syndrome). An extensive system of lymphatic capillaries lies external to the boundary tissue.

The seminiferous epithelium contains two distinct categories of cells, *Sertoli's cells,* which are nutrient and supporting elements, and the germ, or *spermatogenic, cells.* The latter form the vast bulk of the epithelium and, by proliferation and complex differentiation, give rise to the spermatozoa.

## SERTOLI'S CELLS

The supporting cells, or *sustentacular cells* of Sertoli, are relatively few in number and are spaced along the tubule at fairly regular intervals, crowded between the germ cells (Fig. 16–7). They are tall, pillar-like cells, with their bases resting upon the basal lamina of the tubule. The cell outline is irregular, indistinct, and very complex, since the heads of maturing spermatozoa lie within deep recesses of the cytoplasm. The nucleus is located some distance above the base of the cell and is pale and ovoid, with its long axis directed radially. The definite nucleolus of these cells readily distinguishes them from the sperma-

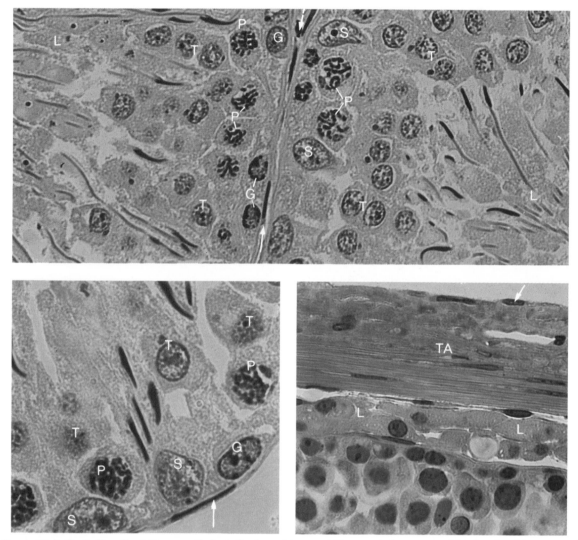

**Figure 16–5.** Testis. Top: Seminiferous epithelium. Portions of two seminiferous tubules, separated by their basal laminae and boundary tissue (arrows), are shown. Sertoli's cells (S), with their characteristic nuclei, lie close to the basal lamina of each tubule. Spermatogonia (G) are located directly above the basal lamina and show spherical or ovoid nuclei. Primary spermatocytes (P) lie in the next layer, immediately above the spermatogonia, and are the largest germ cells. Sperm heads are densely staining, and tails project into the lumen. Plastic section. H and E. High power. Bottom left: A portion of one seminiferous tubule, surrounded by boundary tissue (arrow), is shown. Sertoli's cells (S) show indefinite cell boundaries. The apical cytoplasm of one of them is closely associated with sperm heads. A spermatogonium (G) lies immediately in relation to the basal lamina. The next layer contains primary spermatocytes (P), above which are spermatids (T). Secondary spermatocytes are not present; they are seen rarely, since they rapidly divide to produce spermatids. Plastic section. H and E. Oil immersion. Bottom right: Leydig's cells. The tunica albuginea (TA), covered by the mesothelium of the visceral layer of the tunica vaginalis (arrow), lies above, and below is a portion of a seminiferous tubule. Between the two, there is a group of interstitial cells of Leydig (L). They are large, epithelioid cells that show spherical nuclei with distinct nucleoli and a finely granular cytoplasm. Plastic section. H and E. High power.

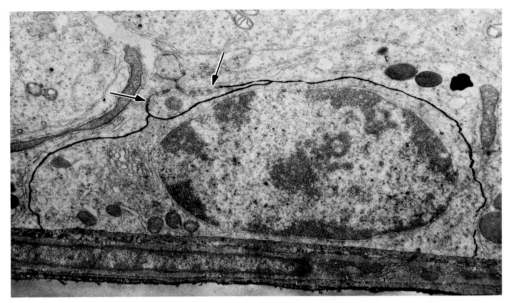

**Figure 16–6.** Electron micrograph of the basal region of the seminiferous epithelium. Lanthanum nitrate, an electron-opaque tracer, was perfused into the testis with the fixative, and it surrounds a spermatogonium. The junctional complexes between Sertoli's cells (arrows) prevent the tracer from penetrating into the adluminal compartment. × 15,000. (Courtesy of Dr. L. D. Russell.)

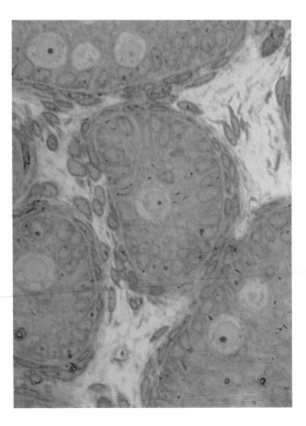

**Figure 16–7.** Early prepubertal testis. The seminiferous tubules exhibit no lumina, and the epithelium is composed principally of Sertoli's cells. The only germ cells present are spermatogonia, which appear pale. The boundary tissue of the tubules and the surrounding interstitium is more cellular than in the adult. Plastic section. Methylene blue. Medium power.

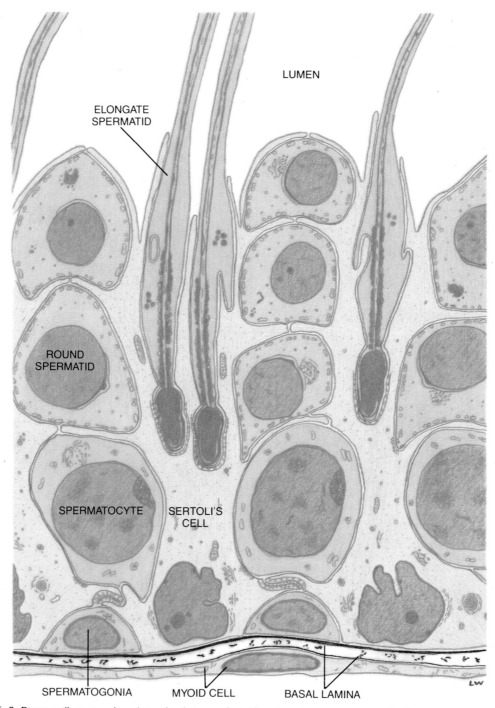

**Figure 16–8.** *Diagram illustrating the relationship between Sertoli's cells and spermatogenic cells. Note the occluding junctions (arrows) situated near the bases of the Sertoli's cells that subdivide the seminiferous epithelium into two compartments: a basal compartment containing the spermatogonia and an adluminal compartment containing the spermatocytes and spermatids. (Courtesy of Dr. L. D. Russell.)*

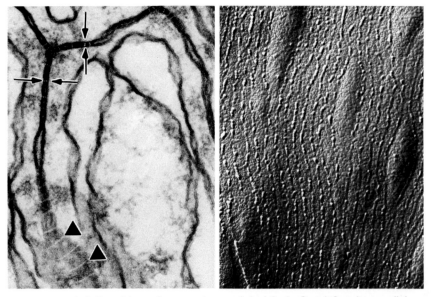

**Figure 16–9.** Electron micrograph (left) and freeze-fracture micrograph (right) of a Sertoli-Sertoli intercellular occluding junction. Note the electron translucencies in the membrane (left), some of which are focal (opposing arrows), and some of which appear linear (arrowheads), in en face sections. These translucencies correspond to the rows of particles seen in freeze-fracture images (right), which are the occluding junctions forming the Sertoli's cell barrier. Left, × 120,000; right, × 90,000. (Courtesy of Dr. L. D. Russell.)

togenic elements within the tubule; it is prominent and of a compound nature, consisting of a central acidophil portion and smaller peripheral concentrations of basophil material.

In fixed preparations, the cytoplasm has a reticular appearance and contains small fibrils, lipid droplets, small discrete granules that stain with iron hematoxylin, and small elongated mitochondria. On electron microscopy, the cytoplasm exhibits profiles of agranular endoplasmic reticulum, scattered free ribosomes, and primary and secondary lysosomes. Occasionally, one can also see a tapering crystalloid body near the nucleus. The chemical nature and the function of this inclusion, the *crystalloid of Charcot-Böttcher,* are unknown.

On light microscopy, the extent and morphology of the cell membrane are poorly defined, but its complexity is clearly demonstrated on electron microscopy. Where two Sertoli's cells border on each other, the contiguous surfaces show complex occluding junctional specializations. There is evidence that these sites of membrane apposition and fusion, together with the peritubular tissue, constitute the morphological basis of the *blood-*

*testis barrier.* The extensive junctions between Sertoli's cells form a continuous barrier that is impermeable to the electron tracer, lanthanum nitrate, and in effect they define two distinct compartments within the seminiferous tubule (Figs. 16–8 and 16–9). The *basal compartment* extends between the junctions and the basal lamina and permits relatively free interchange of nutrients and other materials between the interstitial vasculature and the spermatogenic cells that lie within it. The *adluminal compartment,* which lies between the junctions and the lumen of the seminiferous tubule, is isolated from such a direct interchange, and spermatogenic cells within it, which represent more differentiated stages than those within the basal compartment, must rely upon Sertoli's cells for the availability of nutrients and other substances. Additionally, the barrier prevents proteins from spermatogenic cells within the adluminal compartment from reaching the interstitial vasculature and inducing the formation of antibodies.

During their period of differentiation, spermatids (immature germ cells) attach to the Sertoli's cells and are nourished by them. Sertoli's cells are resistant to various noxious influences that destroy the spermatogenic cells.

### SPERMATOGENIC CELLS

These *germ cells* comprise a stratified layer of epithelium, four to eight cells deep, lining the seminiferous tubule. The spermatogenic cells differentiate progressively from the basal region of the tubule to the lumen. Proliferation pushes the cells toward the lumen, and those nearest the lumen transform into spermatozoa and detach from the epithelium, coming to lie free within the lumen. The sequence of events is referred to as *spermatogenesis*, which involves the two processes of cell multiplication, including reduction from the diploid to the haploid number of chromosomes, and cellular differentiation (*spermiogenesis*).

**Spermatogenesis.** Spermatogenesis, a process that is thought to occupy about 64 days, commences with the *spermatogonia*,* which lie within the basal compartment immediately adjacent to the basal lamina (Fig. 16–10). Each spermatogonium contains a diploid number of chromosomes within its nucleus (44 autosomes and two sex chromosomes, XY).

In the human, three types of spermatogonia are recognized:

1. *Type A dark spermatogonia* possess an ovoid nucleus that stains darkly. They serve as reserve stem cells and divide infrequently to maintain the number of spermatogonia and also to form some type A pale spermatogonia.

2. *Type A pale spermatogonia* possess ovoid nuclei that stain lightly. They divide mitotically to give rise to type B spermatogonia as well as to other type A pale spermatogonia.

3. *Type B spermatogonia* have spherical nuclei that contain densely stained chromatin masses in relation to the nuclear membrane.

The three types of spermatogonia are spherical cells that measure about 12 μm in diameter and possess a pale-staining cytoplasm. They are distinguished by the morphology and staining characteristics of their nuclei.

When type B spermatogonia divide by mitoses, they produce daughter cells that all eventually differentiate to become *primary spermatocytes*.

---

*Greek *sperma*, seed; *goné*, generation.

More complex classifications of spermatogonia have been proposed by some authors; for example, since the number of type B spermatogonial generations in humans is four, they have been designated as types $B_1$, $B_2$, $B_3$, and $B_4$.

*Primary spermatocytes* at first resemble type B spermatogonia and lie within the basal compartment. They increase in size and show a change in the character of the nucleus as it enters the initial stages of division. Following this differentiation, the tight junctions between adjacent Sertoli's cells that lie to the luminal side of the primary spermatocytes disappear, thus permitting the spermatocytes to migrate from the basal to the adluminal compartment. Tight junctions between the Sertoli's cells then re-form at a level between the spermatocytes and the underlying spermatogonia. The spermatocytes now occupy the middle zone of the epithelium and are the largest germ cells seen within the seminiferous epithelium, being 16 μm or more in diameter. Each cell is spherical or ovoid in outline, and the nucleus is usually in some stage of karyokinesis. The cell division that occurs within primary spermatocytes is a reduction division, *meiosis*, in which whole chromosomes (synaptic mates, or the halves of the bivalent chromosomes) move to opposite poles of the spindle, unlike a somatic mitosis in which individual chromosomes split and the half chromosomes separate. As a result of the meiotic division, 23 chromosomes (22 autosomes plus one sex chromosome, either X or Y) pass into each daughter cell, or *secondary spermatocyte*. The meiotic division also is peculiar in that cytokinesis is incomplete, and the two daughter cells (secondary spermatocytes) remain connected by a bridge of cytoplasm. The two conjoined secondary spermatocytes later divide mitotically, and the resultant four cells (*spermatids*) remain in a syncytial cluster, since cytokinesis again is incomplete.

The *secondary spermatocytes* are about half the volume of the primary spermatocytes and lie nearer the lumen. They are seen rarely in sections of seminiferous tubules, since they are short-lived and divide quickly to produce spermatids. The division here, mitosis or the second meiotic division, occurs in the secondary spermatocytes without prior duplication of deoxyribonucleic acid (DNA), or genetic material. Thus, the spermatids are haploid in both chromosome number (23)

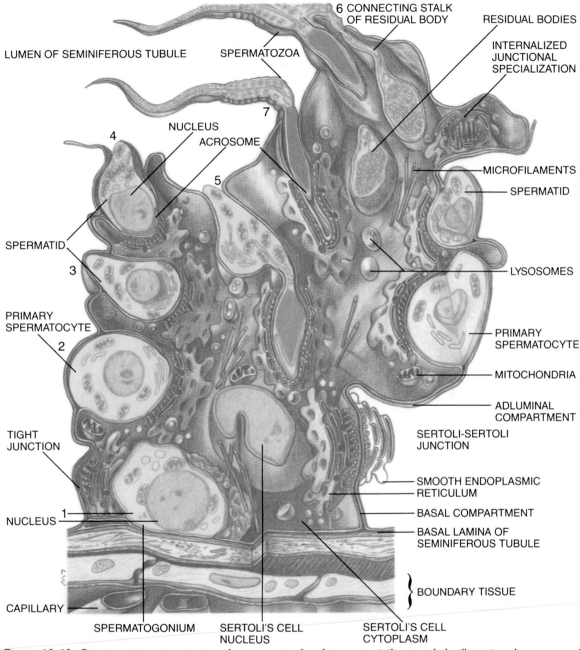

LUMEN OF SEMINIFEROUS TUBULE

SPERMATOZOA

6 CONNECTING STALK
OF RESIDUAL BODY

RESIDUAL BODIES

INTERNALIZED
JUNCTIONAL
SPECIALIZATION

NUCLEUS

ACROSOME

4

7

5

MICROFILAMENTS

SPERMATID

SPERMATID

3

LYSOSOMES

PRIMARY
SPERMATOCYTE

2

PRIMARY
SPERMATOCYTE

MITOCHONDRIA

ADLUMINAL
COMPARTMENT

TIGHT
JUNCTION

SERTOLI-SERTOLI
JUNCTION

SMOOTH ENDOPLASMIC
RETICULUM

NUCLEUS

1

BASAL COMPARTMENT

BASAL LAMINA OF
SEMINIFEROUS TUBULE

BOUNDARY TISSUE

CAPILLARY

SPERMATOGONIUM

SERTOLI'S CELL
NUCLEUS

SERTOLI'S CELL
CYTOPLASM

**Figure 16–10.** *Diagrammatic representation of a segment of a human seminiferous tubule illustrating the process of spermatogenesis. The seminiferous epithelium rests upon a basal lamina and is surrounded by myoid cells of the boundary (peritubular) tissue. The relationship of a Sertoli's cell to the spermatogenic cells is shown. A spermatogonium lies within the basal compartment of the seminiferous epithelium, below the junctional complexes between Sertoli's cells. Primary spermatocytes, spermatids, and spermatozoa are located within the adluminal compartment, above the junctional complexes.*

and DNA content. With the division, there is a further reduction in volume to half that of the secondary spermatocyte.

The *spermatids* lie close to the lumen and are spherical or polygonal cells about 6 μm in diameter. No further division occurs, and each spermatid is transformed by an extensive differentiation (spermiogenesis) into a spermatozoon. The cytoplasmic continuity between clusters of spermatids may constitute a basis for the synchrony of their later differentiation. Soon after their appearance, spermatids become closely applied to the surface of Sertoli's cells, where commonly they lie in deep recesses formed by the irregular surface of the sustentacular cells. In this environment, they undergo metamorphosis into sper-

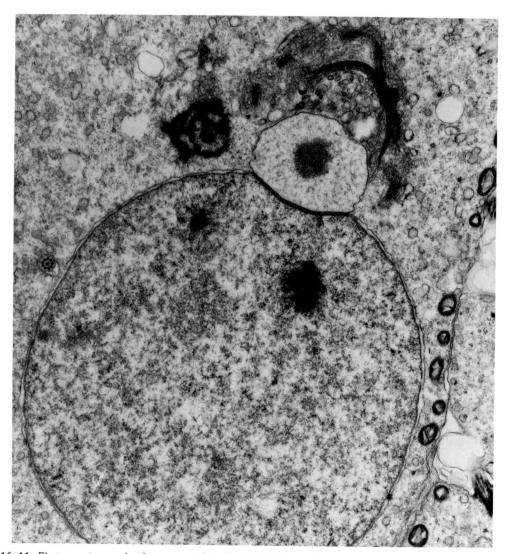

**Figure 16–11.** *Electron micrograph of a spermatid in the Golgi phase of spermiogenesis. The acrosome, comprising the acrosomal granule within the acrosomal vesicle, lies between the main components of the Golgi zone (above) and the nucleus (below), which at this stage is not condensed. Where the acrosomal vesicle exhibits a close relationship with the nuclear envelope, the nuclear envelope is modified. × 15,000. (Courtesy of Dr. L. D. Russell.)*

matozoa. The cytoplasmic continuity between individual spermatozoa finally is broken when they are released from Sertoli's cells into the lumen of the seminiferous tubule.

**Spermiogenesis.** The newly formed spermatid contains a centrally located spherical nucleus with a well-delineated Golgi zone nearby, numerous mitochondria, and a pair of centrioles. Spermiogenesis to produce a spermatozoon involves marked differentiation of all these cellular structures. Initially, during the Golgi phase of differentiation, several small granules appear within the numerous small vesicles of the Golgi zone (Fig. 16–11). They coalesce to form a single large granule, the *acrosome*, which lies within the *acro-somal vesicle* (Fig. 16–12). This complex lies between the main components of the Golgi zone and the nucleus. The membrane bounding the acrosomal vesicle, derived from the Golgi zone, then adheres to the outer layer of the nuclear membrane. The acrosomal vesicle grows over the surface of the nuclear membrane and eventually covers about half of the nuclear surface (Fig. 16–13). Part of the enlargement of the acrosomal vesicle and of the acrosome is contributed to by the Golgi zone, which later migrates from the region of the acrosomal vesicle and comes to lie at the opposite pole of the nucleus. With the migration of the Golgi zone, there appears to be resorption of the fluid content of the acrosomal

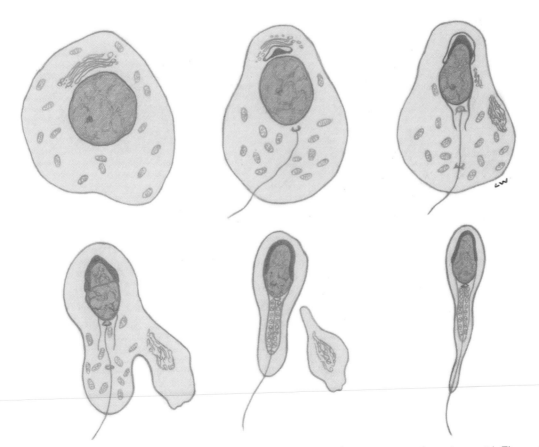

**Figure 16–12.** *Six successive stages in the transformation of the spermatid into the spermatozoon (spermiogenesis). The nucleus condenses to form the sperm head; the acrosome, which appear initially within the Golgi zone, gives rise to the head cap. The flagellum arises in relation to one of the centrioles, and mitochondria migrate around the flagellum to form the sheath of the middle piece.*

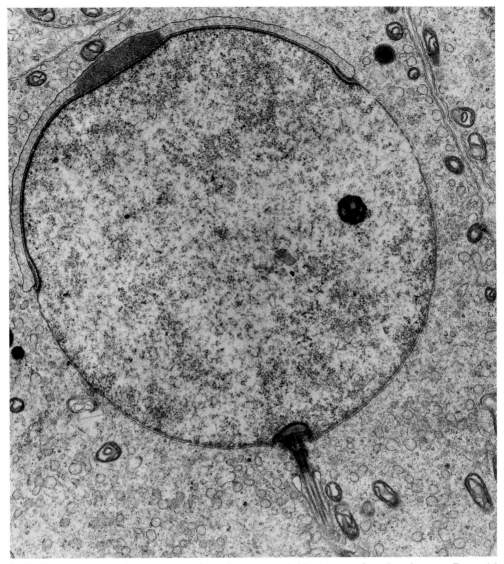

**Figure 16–13.** Electron micrograph of a spermatid in a later stage of differentiation than that shown in Figure 16–11. The acrosomal vesicle (above) has grown over the surface of the nuclear membrane to cover about half of the nuclear surface. At the opposite pole of the nucleus (below), a slender flagellum has grown out from the centriole. Mitochondria still are dispersed throughout the cytoplasm, and the nucleus is not condensed. × 14,000. (Courtesy of Dr. D. Russell.)

vesicle, which collapses onto the acrosome and forms a close-fitting *head-cap* over the nucleus, containing the acrosome between its layers (Fig. 16–14). The acrosome contains hydrolytic enzymes, including hyaluronidase, acid phosphatases, acrosin, and neuraminidase.

As acrosome formation is in progress at one pole of the nucleus, the centrioles become asso-ciated with the nuclear membrane at the opposite pole, and a slender flagellum, the *axoneme,* grows out from one of them. As the axoneme grows, a thin, filamentous sheath, the *caudal tube,* or *manchette*, is laid down around the axial filaments of the flagellum, and the other centriole migrates toward the cell surface and encircles the longitudinal axial filaments as a ring, or *annulus.*

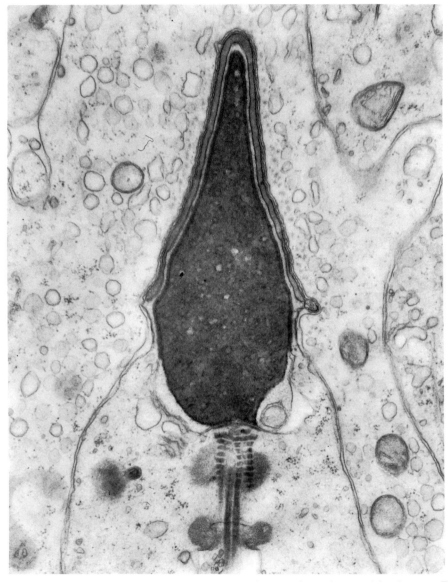

**Figure 16–14.** *Electron micrograph of a section of a human spermatid at an advanced stage of development. The head cap is complete, and the acrosome can no longer be identified as a separate entity. A well-developed flagellum extends from the lower pole of the nucleus.* × *27,500.*

The nucleus becomes condensed, slightly flattened, and elongated and is displaced toward the cell membrane, where it then forms the definitive sperm head. Meanwhile, there is a shift of the bulk of the cytoplasm toward the tail end of the cell. Mitochondria, until now randomly distributed in the cytoplasm, migrate to the region between the basal centriole and the annulus. There they become aligned in a spiral array, or helix, around the proximal portion of the flagellum as the *mitochondrial sheath*, thus delineating the *middle piece* of the future spermatozoon.

As differentiation proceeds, most of the cytoplasm is associated with the middle piece, and only a thin layer of cytoplasm remains as a cover over the nucleus and the tail piece of the spermatozoon. The tail piece is similar in structure to a cilium, containing the same number and arrangement of longitudinal filaments. In the final stages of differentiation, most of the surplus cytoplasm is partitioned off and shed as the *residual body*, and the spermatozoon is released from its intimate contact with the Sertoli's cell (*spermiation*). The residual bodies, which have a high lipid content, are phagocytosed by sustentacular cells. There is some evidence that the lipid is utilized by sustentacular cells in the production of a hormone that might play an important role in regulating spermatogenesis locally.

At the time of their release, spermatozoa appear morphologically mature, but they are immature functionally, in that they are nonmotile and are limited in their ability to effect fertilization of the ovum. The final step in the maturation of spermatozoa, a process known as *capacitation*, is thought to occur after ejaculation into the female. It involves a process of activation that precedes fertilization, but the mechanism is uncertain.

In many lower mammalian orders, spermatogenesis occurs in definite cyclic waves along the length of the seminiferous tubules, but in humans the waves are less distinct. In most species, spermatids at specific stages of spermiogenesis are associated with spermatogonia and spermatocytes also at specific stages of differentiation. On the basis of morphological changes in germ cell nuclei and the development of the acrosome during spermiogenesis, the human spermatogenic cycle may be divided into six characteristic stages. The features of these stages are complex and will not be detailed here. However, the student should recognize that because of the cyclic nature of spermatogenesis, not every stage can be seen at the same time at a given point along the seminiferous tubule. Thus, spermatozoa will be seen in some regions of the seminiferous tubules, and only spermatids in others.

### Mature Spermatozoa

The mature human spermatozoon that lies free within the lumen of a seminiferous tubule consists of a head, middle piece, and tail (Fig. 16–15). The head comprises the condensed nucleus and a head cap, including the dense acrosome at its anterior margin. The head contains the DNA. The acrosome contains hyaluronidase and other hydrolytic enzymes that facilitate the passage of the spermatozoon between the cells that surround the unfertilized ovum, thereby aiding fertilization.

The middle piece, which is separated from the head by a narrow neck, contains a core of longitudinal filaments surrounded by a mitochondrial sheath, and it is thought that it is responsible for control of movements of the tail.

The tail is composed of the *principal piece* and the *end piece*. The principal piece, the longest portion, consists of the axoneme and the nine peripheral double filaments (an arrangement essentially identical to that in a cilium) enclosed by a sheath of circumferential fibers. The end piece consists only of the axoneme ensheathed by a thin layer of cytoplasm.

### Interstitium

The interstitial tissue, within the lobuli testis, lies between the seminiferous tubules. It contains some collagenous fibers, blood and lymphatic vessels, nerves, and several cell types, including fibroblasts, macrophages, mast cells, and some undifferentiated mesenchymal cells. Blood and lymphatic vessels and nerves enter and leave at the mediastinum and form networks around the tubules. The specific *interstitial cells of Leydig* are a marked feature of this tissue (Fig. 16–16). They lie in compact groups, usually in the angular areas created by the packing of seminiferous tubules. They are large polyhedral cells. The nucleus contains coarse chromatin granules and a distinct nucleolus. Binucleate cells are common. The cytoplasm contains numerous lipid droplets that appear as vacuoles in light microscopy preparations. On electron microscopy, the most striking feature of these cells is the extensive development of agranular (smooth-surfaced) endoplasmic reticulum. This appears as a fine meshwork of anastomosing tubules, to the surface of which no ribosomes are attached. Unlike the endoplasmic reticulum associated with ribosomes, which is

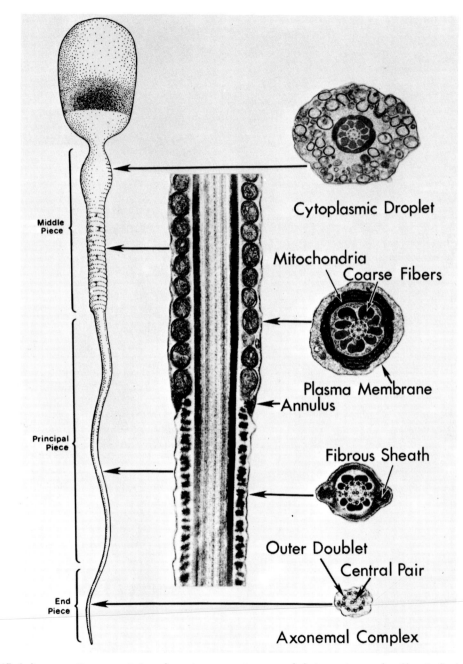

Cytoplasmic Droplet

Mitochondria
Coarse Fibers

Plasma Membrane
Annulus

Fibrous Sheath

Outer Doublet
Central Pair

Axonemal Complex

Middle Piece

Principal Piece

End Piece

***Figure 16–15.*** *A diagrammatic representation of a mature spermatozoon and electron micrographs of longitudinal and transverse sections through the middle piece, principal piece, and end-piece of the flagellum. (Courtesy of Dr. L. D. Russell.)*

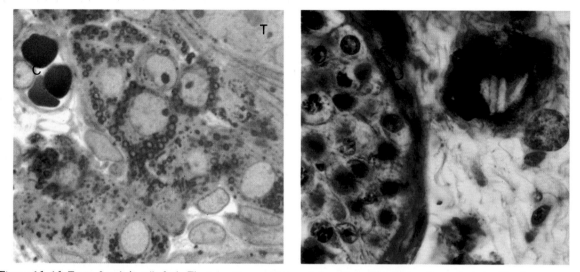

**Figure 16–16.** *Testis, Leydig's cells. Left: The interstitium contains a large group of Leydig's cells, characterized by the presence within their cytoplasm of numerous lipid droplets (dark blue). Nuclei are vesicular and contain distinct nucleoli. Also present within the interstitium are small connective tissue cells, principally fibroblasts, and a capillary (C) containing red blood cells. A portion of a seminiferous tubule (T) lies above right. Plastic section. Toluidine blue. Oil immersion. Right: A portion of a seminiferous tubule, surrounded by boundary tissue, lies to the left. Within the loose connective tissue of the interstitium (right), there is one large Leydig's cell. The cytoplasm is finely granular and deep-staining, and within it pale, rod-shaped crystalloids, the crystals of Reinke, are apparent. Iron hematoxylin, aniline blue. High power.*

concerned with protein synthesis, the agranular reticulum is the site of synthesis of steroid hormones.

A unique feature of human Leydig cells is the presence of peculiar rod-shaped crystalloids, the *crystals of Reinke* (Fig. 16–17). These crystals are not stained with common histological stains and appear as negative images on light microscopy. On electron microscopy, they exhibit a highly ordered structure. Their functional significance is unknown.

### Blood Vessels, Lymphatics, and Nerves

As the testicular artery approaches the testis, it is surrounded by an extensive plexus of veins, the *pampiniform plexus,* which precools the arterial blood by a countercurrent heat exchange mechanism (Fig. 16–18). Within the mediastinum testis, branches from the testicular artery pierce the tunica albuginea and pass to the tunica vasculosa. Smaller arteriolar branches follow the septa to the parenchyma, where they terminate

in networks of capillaries. Venous drainage occurs principally through the mediastinum testis.

Small lymphatic vessels form extensive networks within the interstitial tissue. They drain into larger lymphatic vessels that pass through the mediastinum and along the spermatic cord to para-aortic abdominal lymph nodes.

Nerves accompany the major blood vessels and form fine plexuses around smaller blood vessels and in relation to interstitial cells.

### Functional Considerations of the Testis

The principal endocrine secretion of the testis is testosterone, produced by the interstitial cells, which constitute a peculiar type of endocrine gland in that they develop not from an epithelial surface, as do most endocrine glands, but from the mesenchymal stroma of the testis. In the stroma, abundantly supplied with capillaries, they have easy access for their secretory product into the vascular system. The production of testosterone by the testis depends upon stimulation by

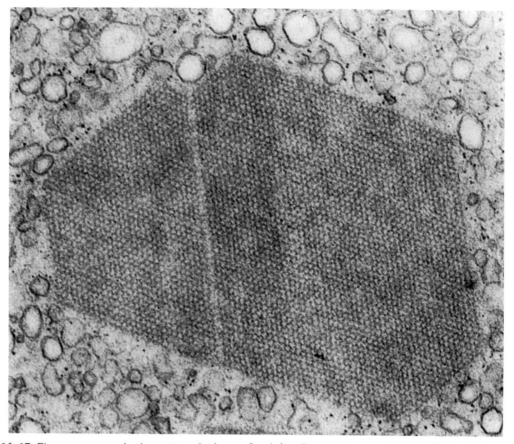

**Figure 16–17.** *Electron micrograph of a portion of a human Leydig's cell containing a crystalloid of Reinke. The surrounding cytoplasm exhibits numerous profiles of agranular endoplasmic reticulum.* × 40,000.

luteinizing hormone (LH) of the anterior lobe of the hypophysis. Since the target organ here is represented by the interstitial cells, luteinizing hormone often is referred to as interstitial cell–stimulating hormone (ICSH) in this context. When testosterone levels are low, cells of the hypothalamus secrete a gonadotropin-releasing factor that causes release of ICSH by the adenohypophysis. In addition to its influence upon spermatogenesis, testosterone controls the appearance of secondary sex characteristics, the sex impulse, and the proper development and maintenance of the genital ducts and auxiliary glands.

The principal exocrine function of the testis, the production of male sex cells, is dependent upon numerous factors. Follicle-stimulating hormone (FSH) of the anterior lobe of the hypophysis stimulates spermatogenesis in mammals, although the effect is not as marked in humans as in lower forms. FSH does act directly upon Sertoli's cells to stimulate the synthesis and release of *androgen-binding protein*, which combines with testosterone and is released into the lumina of seminiferous tubules. The presence of testosterone within the adluminal compartment apparently is necessary to maintain active spermatogenesis. Sertoli's cells also synthesize another testicular hormone, *inhibin*, which passes into the blood stream and inhibits secretion of FSH by the anterior lobe of the hypophysis. Inhibin also is thought to aid in regulating the number of spermatogonia entering spermatogenesis.

A suitable temperature is critical for spermatogenesis. This is furnished principally by the posi-

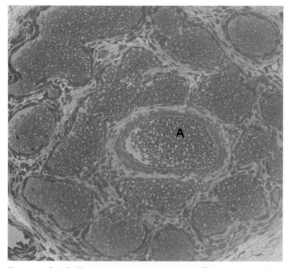

*Figure 16–18. Testis, pampiniform plexus. This section of the external region of the mediastinum testis shows a branch of the testicular artery (A) surrounded by an extensive plexus of small veins, the pampiniform plexus. The plexus precools the arterial blood entering the testis by a countercurrent heat exchange mechanism. Plastic section. H and E. Low power.*

tion of the testis in the scrotum. In cases of *cryptorchidism* (maldescent of the testis), spermatogenesis does not proceed to completion, although Leydig's cells exhibit normal androgenic function.

In humans, spermatogenesis is a continuous process throughout sexual maturity. The sex-determining role of spermatozoa is correlated with the production of spermatozoa of two genetically different types. Half of the secondary spermatocytes contain a female-determining chromosome (X) and the other half a male-determining chromosome (Y), this distinction continuing into daughter spermatids and into spermatozoa.

## MALE GENITAL DUCTS

### Tubuli Recti

At the apex of each testicular lobule, the component seminiferous tubules join to form a straight tubule (*tubulus rectus*). Each straight tubule is short and devoid of convolutions and has a

diameter of about 25 μm. At the point of continuity with the seminiferous tubules, the spermatogenic cells disappear, and only Sertoli's cells remain, forming a simple columnar or cuboidal epithelium. Component cells contain numerous fat droplets. The epithelium rests upon a basal lamina, and the surrounding loose connective tissue is devoid of smooth muscle cells.

### Rete Testis

The tubuli recti course from the apices of the lobules to the dense connective tissue of the mediastinum testis, where they enter a network of anastomosing channels, the *rete testis* (Fig. 16–19). The lining of these irregular spaces is simple cuboidal or squamous epithelium, component cells of which bear a single cilium and a few short microvilli. The epithelium rests upon a delicate basal lamina and is surrounded by the highly vascular connective tissue of the mediastinum.

Passage of spermatozoa through the tubuli recti and the rete testis is thought to occur rapidly, since in sections one rarely sees spermatozoa within the lumina.

### Ductuli Efferentes

In the superior portion of the posterior border of the testis, some 10 to 15 spirally wound, efferent ductules (*ductuli efferentes*) emerge from the rete testis to form *lobules of the epididymis* (Fig. 16–20; see Fig. 16–21). The lobules form the major portion of the head of the epididymis.

Each ductule is about 6 to 8 cm long and about 0.05 mm in diameter. The ductules are bound by connective tissue, and each is surrounded by a thin layer of circularly arranged smooth muscle fibers. The muscle layer becomes progressively thicker as the ductules approach the ductus epididymidis.

The ductuli efferentes are lined by a typical epithelium, mostly simple columnar, which rests upon a thin basal lamina. Externally each ductule has a regular outline, but internally the lumen is irregular in outline, owing to the varying height of the epithelium. Groups of tall columnar cells alternate with groups of much shorter cuboidal cells. The tall cells have a dense acidophil cyto-

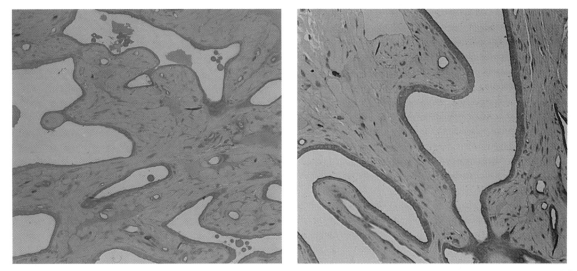

**Figure 16–19.** *Rete testis. The rete testis is a network of anastomosing channels within the dense connective tissue of the mediastinum testis. The irregular channels are lined by a simple epithelium that generally is simple cuboidal. Component cells of the epithelium bear a single cilium (not visible here). The surrounding connective tissue contains a few small blood vessels. Plastic sections. Left: H and E. Low power. Right: Methylene blue, azure A, basic fuchsin. Medium power.*

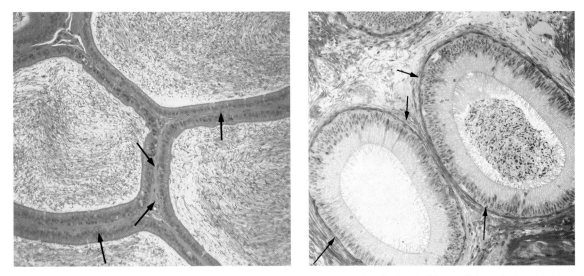

**Figure 16–20.** Left: *Ductuli efferentes. The spirally wound efferent ductules within the head of the epididymis here are sectioned transversely. The ductules are lined by a simple layer of epithelium, mostly simple columnar, which is ciliated. Although the height of the epithelium appears regular in this section, typically it exhibits irregularities at the luminal surface owing to the presence of alternating groups of tall columnar and cuboidal cells. A thin band of circularly arranged smooth muscle cells (nuclei of which are arrowed) surrounds each ductule. The presence of spermatozoa within the lumina is unusual. Plastic section. H and E. Medium power.* Right: *Ductus epididymidis. The ductus epididymidis is highly tortuous and forms part of the head, the body, and the tail of the epididymis. In sections through these regions, the duct is cut numerous times. The epithelium is uniform in height and is pseudostratified, with scattered basal cells and tall columnar, principal cells. The latter possess ovoid nuclei, situated either basally or centrally within the cells. The apical cytoplasm is acidophil and the cells bear stereocilia on the free surface. The lumen may be empty, or it may contain large concentrations of spermatozoa. The duct is surrounded by a basal lamina and by a layer of smooth muscle cells (arrows), which thickens toward the tail of the epididymis. Plastic section. H and E. Medium power.*

plasm containing fat droplets and pigment granules, and many are ciliated. The cilia beat toward the ductus epididymidis and assist in transporting spermatozoa through the ductules. The shorter cells, which contain many lysosomes, mostly are nonciliated. They possess numerous microvilli on their free surface and are absorptive in function. Thus, in addition to acting as a conduit for spermatozoa, the efferent ductules absorb a large proportion of the fluid produced within the seminiferous tubules.

### Ductus Epididymidis

The efferent ductules progressively unite to form a single *ductus epididymidis* (Figs. 16–21 and 16–22; see Fig. 16–20). This duct, which is surrounded by connective tissue, is highly tortuous and forms the remainder of the head, the body, and the tail of the epididymis. It is a long storage duct (5 to 6 m long) through which

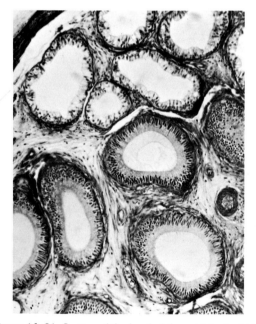

*Figure 16–21.* Section of the head of the epididymis. At the top of the picture are cross sections of efferent ductules and below are sections of the ductus epididymidis. Note the tall, pseudostratified epithelium of the latter and the irregular height of the epithelium of the efferent ductules, owing to the presence of alternating groups of tall columnar and cuboidal cells. Low power.

spermatozoa pass slowly. In their passage, they acquire motility and optimal fertilizability.

The duct has a cylindrical outline both inside and outside, since the epithelium, unlike that of the efferent ductules, is uniform in height. The epithelium is pseudostratified columnar, composed of *basal cells* and tall columnar *principal cells*. Lipid droplets are found in the cytoplasm of both cell types, and the principal cells also contain pigment granules, lysosomes, and secretion droplets. The latter cells also possess a remarkably large supranuclear Golgi complex and, on their free surface, bear a tuft of nonmotile *stereocilia* (long slender cellular processes, which differ from microvilli in the repeated branching near their bases). The secretory product of the epithelium passes into the lumen through this irregular surface. The epithelium also functions in resorption of fluid. Experimental studies have indicated that more than 90 per cent of the fluid leaving the testis is resorbed in the ductuli efferentes and ductus epididymidis.

The basal cells are small, rounded cells located at the base of the epithelium. They are simple in structure, with a pale-staining cytoplasm containing few organelles.

The epithelium is surrounded by a definite basal lamina and by a thin lamina propria, external to which there is a thin layer of circularly arranged smooth muscle fibers. The muscle layer gradually thickens toward the tail of the epididymis and, immediately prior to the union with the ductus deferens, becomes organized into three layers (inner longitudinal, middle circular, and outer longitudinal). These differences in morphological organization of the muscle layer are correlated with differences in muscular activity. In the head and body, the duct exhibits spontaneous peristaltic contractions that aid in transporting spermatozoa along the duct. The peristaltic contractions are reduced in the tail region, which is the principal site of storage of spermatozoa.

### Ductus Deferens

The ductus epididymidis straightens out at its termination and becomes continuous with the *ductus deferens*, which ascends from the scrotum to the inguinal region, traverses the inguinal canal, and courses down the side wall of the pelvis

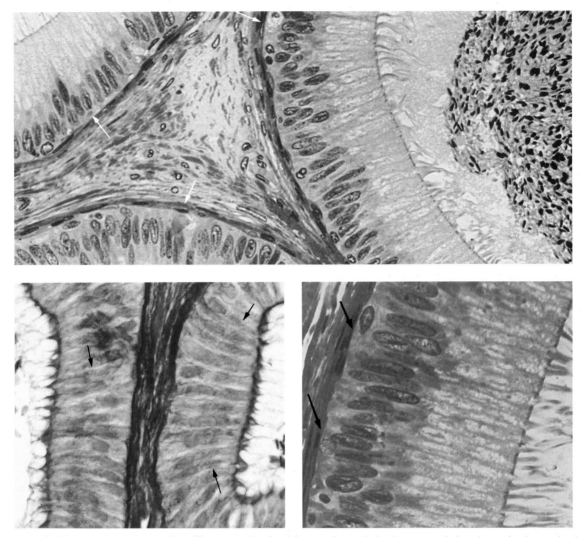

***Figure 16–22.*** *Ductus epididymidis.* Top: *The regular height of the pseudostratified columnar epithelium lining the duct is clearly apparent. Scattered small basal cells, with small spherical nuclei, lie immediately in relation to the basal lamina. The ovoid nuclei of the tall columnar, principal cells lie either basally or more centrally within the cells. The apical cytoplasm is pale and vacuolated, and long stereocilia project into the lumen. A thin layer of circularly arranged smooth muscle cells (arrows) surrounds the duct, which is embedded in a loose, cellular connective tissue. Plastic section. H and E. High power.* Bottom left: *Portions of two segments of the duct are shown. The apical cytoplasm of the principal cells contains secretory droplets (pink, arrows), and the stereocilia exhibit a positive reaction with periodic acid–Schiff (PAS). PAS, light green. Medium power.* Bottom right: *The nuclei of the principal cells are ovoid, and the apical cytoplasm is finely granular and vacuolated. On their luminal surface (right), the cells bear tufts of stereocilia (long, slender branching microvilli that are nonmotile). A layer of circularly arranged smooth muscle cells (arrows) surrounds the duct. Plastic section. H and E. High power.*

retroperitoneally toward the urethra (Figs. 16–23 and 16–24). Relatively, its wall is thick and the lumen narrow. In the scrotum and inguinal canal, the ductus deferens lies within the spermatic cord, where it is easily palpable because of its thick wall. The spermatic cord contains, in addition to the ductus, arteries, veins of the pampiniform plexus, lymph vessels, nerves of the testis and

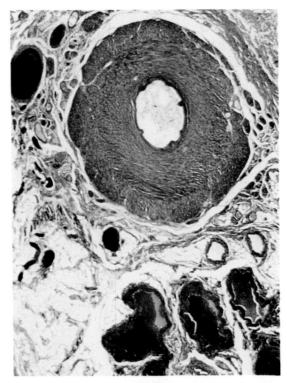

*Figure 16–23.* Spermatic cord. The spermatic cord contains the ductus deferens, arteries, veins, lymphatic vessels, and nerves of the testis and epididymis, and strands of skeletal muscle, the cremaster muscle. The ductus deferens has an extremely thick wall, owing principally to the presence of a large amount of smooth muscle. In the connective tissue immediately surrounding the ductus, there are some small blood vessels that supply the duct. More peripherally, there are numerous large veins, their lumina filled with blood. These are components of the pampiniform plexus. Iron hematoxylin, aniline blue. Low power.

epididymis, and longitudinal strands of skeletal muscle, the *cremaster* muscle. Prior to its termination, the duct dilates into a spindle-shaped enlargement, the *ampulla.*

The epithelium of the ductus deferens is pseudostratified, and many of the tall cells bear stereocilia. A delicate basal lamina intervenes between the epithelium and a thin lamina propria, which is characterized by the presence of numerous elastic fibers. The mucosa rises into longitudinal folds, which are responsible for the stellate outline of the lumen one sees in cross sections. Beneath the lamina propria, there is an ill-defined submucosa, containing numerous blood vessels,

which separates the mucosa from the muscular coat. This coat is thick and is composed of three distinct layers of smooth muscle. The middle, or circular, layer is markedly robust, and beyond this there is another well-developed layer in which the muscle fibers are arranged longitudinally. A fibrous adventitia surrounds the muscular coat and blends with that of adjoining tissues.

Near its termination, the ductus deferens dilates to form the *ampulla.* Here, the lumen is wider, and the mucosa is much more folded than in the main portion of the ductus. Many of the epithelial folds branch and fuse with each other, producing a number of pocket-like recesses. The simple epithelium may show evidence of secretion. The musculature is much less regularly arranged than in the rest of the ductus deferens. Usually, only the external longitudinal layer retains its identity.

The smooth muscle layers of the ductus deferens are associated with an extensive network of autonomic nerve fibers. This accounts for the powerful contractions that occur during ejaculation, transporting spermatozoa rapidly through the ductus deferens.

## Ejaculatory Duct

The *ejaculatory duct* is the short, terminal segment of each genital duct system. It is formed by the union of the ampulla of the ductus deferens and the excretory duct of the seminal vesicle. It is about 1 cm in length and pierces the prostate gland to open into the urethra just to the side of the prostatic utricle.

The ejaculatory duct is lined by a simple columnar or pseudostratified epithelium, probably capable of secretion, which shows some mucosal outpocketings similar to those of the ampulla but less extensive. The supporting wall is fibrous connective tissue that merges into the fibromuscular stroma of the prostate gland.

## AUXILIARY GENITAL GLANDS

The glands associated with the duct system of the testes are the seminal vesicles, the prostate, and the bulbourethral glands. Secretions from them form a substantial part of the seminal fluid.

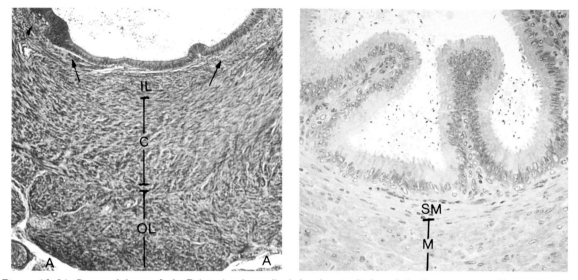

**Figure 16–24.** *Ductus deferens. Left: Relatively, the wall of the duct is thick and the lumen narrow. The epithelium is pseudostratified and is surrounded by a delicate lamina propria. The mucosa rises into short longitudinal folds, here sectioned transversely. Beneath the mucosa, there is a narrow band of submucosa (arrows), composed principally of collagenous fibers. The muscular coat is thick and contains bundles of smooth muscle fibers oriented into three layers: a thin inner layer of longitudinal bundles (IL), a broad middle circular layer (C), and an outer longitudinal layer (OL). A fibrous adventitia (A) surrounds the muscle coat. Iron hematoxylin, aniline blue. Low power. Right: As the ampulla of the duct is approached, the lumen becomes wider and the mucosal folds are more marked. The epithelium is pseudostratified columnar, and the tall cells bear tufts of stereocilia. The mucosal folds contain a core of delicate lamina propria. A narrow zone of submucosal connective tissue (SM) separates the mucosa from the underlying muscle coat (M). Plastic section. H and E. Medium power.*

## Seminal Vesicles

Each *seminal vesicle* is a tortuous, elongated diverticulum off the ductus deferens at the termination of the ampullary portion and is situated posterior to the prostate gland (Fig. 16–25). Since each vesicle is so tortuous, it may be observed in sections in different orientations. The lower portion of the vesicle becomes a narrow straight duct that joins with the ductus deferens to form the ejaculatory duct.

The wall consists of an external connective tissue adventitia containing numerous elastic fibers, a smooth muscle coat thinner than that of the ductus deferens and consisting of inner circular and outer longitudinal layers, and a mucosa that is markedly folded. The high primary folds of the mucosa themselves branch into secondary and tertiary folds that project far into the lumen and merge with one another frequently. As a result, numerous compartments of different sizes are formed. All communicate with the lumen, although in sections many appear to be isolated. The lamina propria of the mucosa is a loose connective tissue that contains many elastic fibers and is richly vascularized.

The epithelium typically shows many variations. It is usually pseudostratified but may be simple columnar. The height of the epithelium varies with the phase of secretion, age, and other influences. Component cells, either columnar or cuboidal, contain secretory granules and a yellow pigment that increases in amount with age. The secretion is a yellowish, viscid liquid that in sections appears as a deeply acidophil coagulum within the lumen. The secretion contains numerous substances, including globulin, ascorbic acid, fructose, and prostaglandins. Fructose is important for the nutrition of spermatozoa, and prostaglandins may assist fertilization by a direct influence upon the female reproductive tract.

The epithelium depends upon hormonal support, testosterone, for its maintenance and activity. Castration is followed by involution and loss

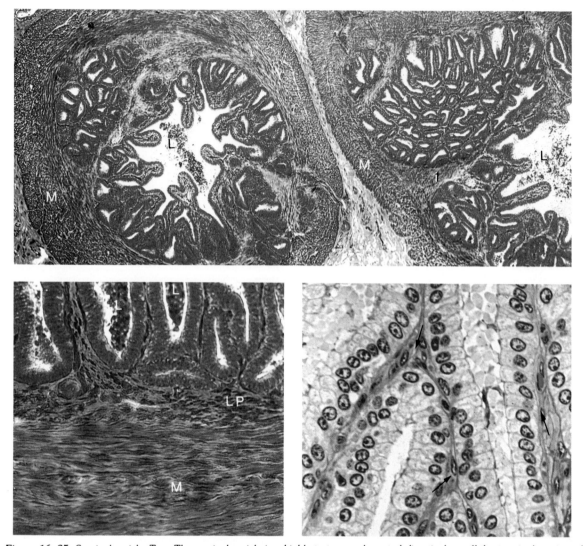

**Figure 16–25.** *Seminal vesicle. Top: The seminal vesicle is a highly tortuous, elongated diverticulum off the terminal portion of the ductus deferens. Two segments of the vesicle are shown here. The mucosa is markedly folded. High primary folds (1) branch into secondary and tertiary folds that project far into the lumen (L) and frequently merge with one another. Thus, the lumen appears to be divided into numerous compartments, although all do communicate freely. The mucosa is surrounded by a thick muscle coat (M) in which most of the bundles of smooth muscle fibers are circularly arranged, although peripheral bundles tend to be more longitudinal in their orientation. The surrounding adventitia contains coarse collagenous fibers (blue). Mallory. Low power. Bottom left: The bases of several mucosal folds that extend into the lumen (L) are shown. The lumen contains some densely staining masses of secretion. The epithelium generally is pseudostratified columnar, and the folds contain a core of delicate connective tissue continuous with that of the underlying lamina propria (LP). Mallory. Medium power. Bottom right: A branching mucosal fold occupies the majority of the field. Although the epithelium of the seminal vesicle typically is pseudostratified, it shows many variations. Here it is simple columnar, with distinct cell boundaries. It rests upon a delicate, cellular connective tissue (arrows) that forms the core of the mucosal folds. Plastic section. H and E. High power.*

of secretory function of the gland, which is promptly restored by the administration of testosterone. The seminal vesicle functions as a gland, secreting and storing the viscid component of the seminal fluid. It is not a site of storage of spermatozoa, although some spermatozoa may be seen within the lumen after death, presumably as the result of back flow.

### Prostate

The *prostate* surrounds the urethra at its origin from the bladder. It is an aggregate of 30 to 50 small compound tubuloalveolar glands that drain into the prostatic urethra by 15 to 30 small excretory ducts (Figs. 16–26 through 16–28). The glandular elements are distributed in three different areas, more or less concentrically ar-

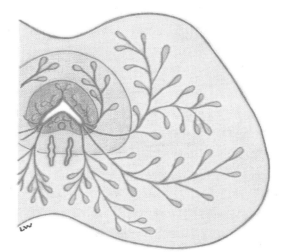

*Figure 16–27. Diagram of a cross section of the human prostate. Note the distribution of the mucous, submucous, and main, or principal, components of the gland. Also depicted are the prostatic urethra, the utriculus prostaticus, and the ejaculatory ducts.*

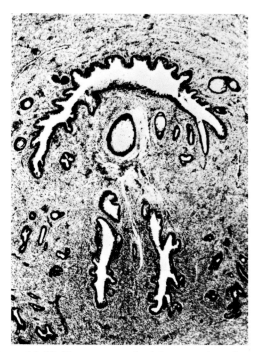

*Figure 16–26. Photomicrograph of the prostatic urethra and surrounding tissue. Immediately below the urethra, which appears crescentic in outline, is the utriculus prostaticus and, below it, portions of both ejaculatory ducts. Each duct is lined by a simple columnar or pseudostratified epithelium and is embedded within fibrous connective tissue that merges into the prostatic stroma. The latter contains portions of some ducts of the prostate gland. Low power.*

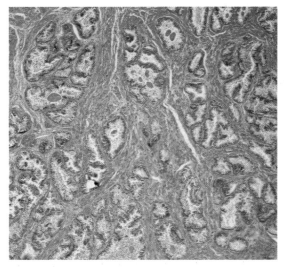

*Figure 16–28. Prostate gland. The prostate gland is an aggregate of numerous small compound tubuloalveolar glands of different sizes. The smallest glands lie within the mucosal layer of the urethra, the next largest within the submucosal layer, and the largest (shown here) within the prostatic stroma. The secretory alveoli and tubules vary in size and are very irregular, and the lining epithelium is folded and pseudostratified or simple cuboidal or columnar in type. The lumina of some alveoli contain prostatic concretions (red). The glands are embedded in the stroma, which is a fibroelastic connective tissue that contains numerous strands of smooth muscle fibers. H and E. Low power.*

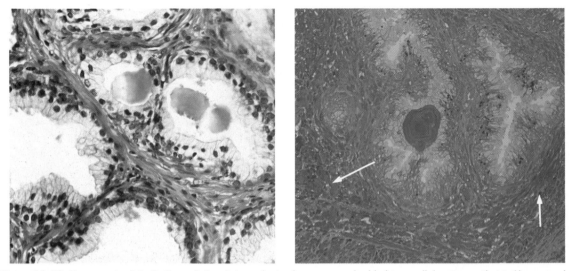

**Figure 16–29.** Prostate gland. Left: Several alveoli, irregular in shape, are embedded in a cellular stroma that is fibromuscular. The alveoli are lined by an epithelium that is simple cuboidal to simple columnar in type. The lumina of several alveoli contain acidophil condensations of secretory material—the prostatic concretions, or corpora amylacea. H and E. Medium power. Right: Two large, irregular alveoli are embedded in a cellular stroma that contains numerous small bundles of smooth muscle fibers (arrows). The lining epithelium of alveoli is simple columnar, and the apical cytoplasm stains palely. A prostatic concretion, exhibiting concentric layering, is present in one alveolus. Plastic section. Methylene blue, azure A, basic fuchsin. High power.

ranged around the urethra. Small glands lie in the mucosa of the urethra, and these are surrounded by submucosal glands. The main, or principal, glandular elements lie peripherally and constitute the bulk of the gland. The whole gland is surrounded by a fibroelastic capsule containing some smooth muscle fibers on its inner aspect and an extensive plexus of veins. The glandular components are embedded in an abundant, dense stroma that is continuous at the periphery with the capsule. This stroma is again fibroelastic and, in addition, contains numerous strands of smooth muscle fibers that, by contraction, aid in the discharge of the prostatic secretion during ejaculation.

The secretory alveoli and tubules are very irregular and vary greatly in size and form (Fig. 16–29). They branch frequently, and both alveoli and tubules have wide lumina. There is no distinct basal lamina, and the epithelium is very folded. It is simple or pseudostratified in type and varies from columnar to low cuboidal, depending upon endocrine status and glandular activity. The cytoplasm of epithelial cells contains numerous secretory granules, lysosomes, and lipid droplets. The

ducts, too, have irregular lumina and resemble smaller secretory tubules. As with the seminal vesicles, the development and functional activity of the prostate gland are dependent upon testosterone.

The secretion of the prostate is a thin, milky fluid that is slightly acidic and is rich in proteolytic enzymes, principally fibrinolysins, which aid in liquefaction of the semen. It also contains large amounts of acid phosphatase. In prostatic carcinoma, there frequently is a pronounced discharge of this enzyme, which may result in high concentrations of it within the blood. In stained sections, the secretion appears as an acidophil granular mass. It frequently contains spherical or ovoid bodies, the *prostatic concretions* (*corpora amylacea*), that are condensations of the secretions, which may become calcified.

### Bulbourethral Glands

The *bulbourethral glands* (or *glands of Cowper*) are paired bodies, each the size of a pea, lying in the connective tissue behind the membranous

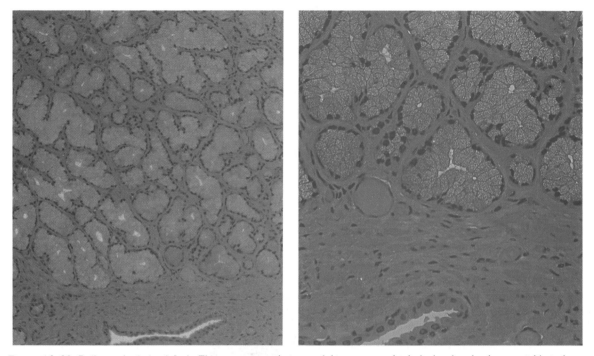

***Figure 16–30.*** *Bulbourethral gland. Left: The secretory end-pieces of this compound tubuloalveolar gland are variable in form, being either alveolar, saccular, or tubular. The lining epithelium is either columnar or cuboidal. Nuclei are basally located, and the apical cytoplasm appears pale. The connective tissue septa, which divide the gland into lobules, contain smooth muscle fibers and isolated skeletal muscle fibers. H and E. Low power. Right: The epithelium lining the irregular secretory end-pieces generally is columnar, and the apical cytoplasm is crowded with mucigen droplets. A secretory duct (bottom center) is lined by a pseudostratified epithelium and lies within a connective tissue septum containing numerous smooth muscle fibers (red). H and E. High power.*

urethra. Each is a compound tubuloalveolar gland whose long duct drains into the proximal part of the penile urethra (Fig. 16–30). The bulbourethral gland is surrounded by a thin connective tissue capsule, external to which are skeletal muscle fibers. Septa pass into the gland to divide it into lobules. The connective tissue septa contain numerous elastic and skeletal and smooth muscle fibers.

The secretory end pieces are variable in form, being alveolar, saccular, or tubular. The epithelium, too, is variable, being either cuboidal or columnar. The cytoplasm contains mucigen droplets and occasional acidophil, spindle-shaped inclusions. Nuclei are spherical and basally located. The secretory ducts are lined by a pseudostratified epithelium resembling that of the urethra and may contain patches of mucous cells.

The secretion is clear, viscid, and mucous and is rich in sialoproteins and amino sugars. It is discharged in response to erotic stimulation and acts as a lubricant for the penile urethra.

## PENIS

The penis serves as the common outlet for urine and seminal fluid and as the copulatory organ (Fig. 16–31). It is formed by three cylinders of erectile tissue: the paired *corpora cavernosa penis* dorsally and the single *corpus cavernosum urethrae* (*corpus spongiosum*) ventrally. The corpus spongiosum encloses the cavernous (penile) portion of the urethra. The paired corpora cavernosa penis are separated from each other prox-

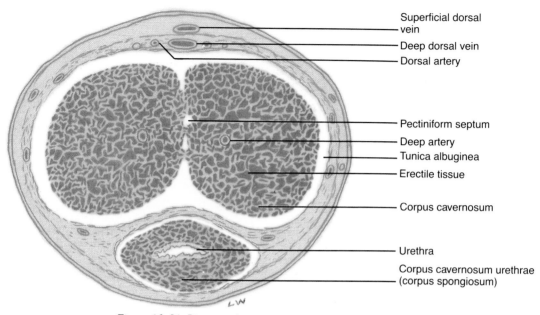

**Figure 16–31.** *Diagram of a cross section of the penis in midshaft.*

imally, where they are attached to the rami of the pubic bone. They join beneath the pubic angle and run forward together, united by a common median partition, the *pectiniform septum*, to the region of the *glans penis* (Fig. 16–32). The deep groove beneath the corpora cavernosa is occupied by the corpus spongiosum. This ends in a cup-shaped enlargement, the glans penis, which forms a cap over the conical ends of the corpora cavernosa penis.

The three cylinders of erectile tissue are surrounded by subcutaneous tissue that is devoid of fat but contains many smooth muscle fibers that proximally are continuous with the dartos tunic of the scrotum. The skin covering the organ is thin and delicate, and terminally it reduplicates over the glans as a fold, the *prepuce*. The inner surface of the prepuce, in relation to the glans, is moist and nonkeratinized. The epithelium over the glans itself is firmly adhered to the fibrous tissue beneath. The skin covering the distal shaft of the penis, unlike that over the root, contains no hair follicles, but it does contain small sweat glands and infrequent sebaceous glands unassociated with hair follicles. On the glans and on the inner surface of the prepuce, there are a number

of modified sebaceous glands, the *glands of Tyson*.

Each cylinder of the corpus cavernosum penis is surrounded by a thick fibrous sheath, the *tunica albuginea*. The collagenous fibers of the sheath are arranged in two layers, the outer longitudinal and the inner circular. The pectiniform septum, common to both cylinders, is pierced by numerous slit-like spaces through which the cavernous spaces of both sides communicate. The erectile tissue consists of numerous *cavernous spaces* created by a network of trabeculae. Trabeculae, continuous with the fibrous sheath, consist of collagenous, elastic, and numerous smooth muscle fibers and form a dense framework within the corpora. The spaces between the framework are lined by a thin squamous endothelium and constitute the cavernous spaces or blood sinuses. The sinuses are continuous with the arteries that supply them and with draining veins. Owing to the arrangement of the trabeculae, the cavernous spaces are largest in the central zone of each cyclinder and gradually diminish in size toward the periphery.

The sheath (tunica albuginea) of the corpus spongiosum is much thinner than that of the

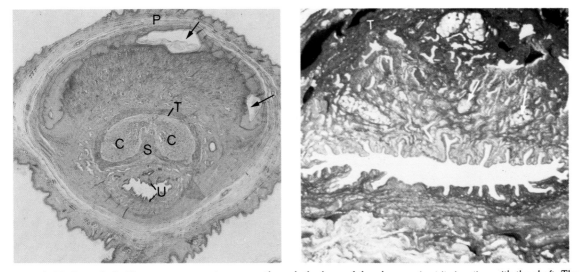

**Figure 16–32.** Penis. Left: *This transverse section passes through the base of the glans penis at its junction with the shaft. The paired corpora cavernosa (C) appear small, since they are sectioned through their conical ends. They are surrounded by a thick fibrous sheath, the tunica albuginea (T), and are separated by a common pectiniform septum (S). The corpus spongiosum (U), which lies in the groove beneath the corpora cavernosa, contains the cavernous (penile) urethra, which exhibits an irregular, crescent-shaped lumen. The mass of erectile tissue above the corpora cavernosa is the base of the glans penis. The subcutaneous tissue surrounding the erectile tissue is delicate and devoid of fat. The skin covering the organ is thin, and terminally it reduplicates over the glans as the prepuce (P). Portions of the space between the prepuce and the glans may be seen in two locations (arrows). Van Gieson. Low power.* Right: *Corpus spongiosum. The urethra is lined by a stratified or pseudostratified columnar epithelium, beneath which there is a loose connective tissue lamina propria (light blue). The entire mucosa appears irregular, and invaginations of epithelium extend deeply to terminate in mucous urethral glands of Littre (arrows). The mucosa is surrounded by erectile tissue of the corpus spongiosum, bounded by a thin sheath of collagenous fibers, the tunica albuginea (T). Iron hematoxylin, aniline blue. Low power.*

corpora cavernosa penis and contains, in addition to collagenous fibers, many elastic and smooth muscle fibers. Trabeculae are thinner and more elastic than those present in the paired corpora. The cavernous spaces are small and almost uniform in size and gradually pass into the small venous spaces surrounding the urethra.

### Blood Vessels and the Mechanism of Erection

The principal arterial branches within the penis are the dorsal arteries, which run in the interval between the corpora cavernosa superiorly on either side of the deep dorsal vein, and the deep arteries traversing each of the corpora. Branches from the dorsal arteries pierce the fibrous capsule along the upper surface to enter the corpora cavernosa, especially near the distal end of the

penis. On entering the erectile tissue, all arteries divide into branches, some of which end in capillary plexuses; others are longitudinal vessels directed distally. In the quiescent state, these vessels, the *helicine arteries*, have a spiral course, their media is thick, and their intima is thrown into longitudinal folds, the *intimal ridges*. These vessels open directly into the sinuses of the erectile tissue. Blood from the cavernous spaces and the capillary plexuses is drained by a plexus of venules within the tunica albuginea. Some emerge from the base of the tunica and converge on the dorsum of the penis to join the deep dorsal vein. Others pass directly out of the upper surface of the corpora cavernosa to enter the same vein. The smooth muscle of the arteries and the trabeculae is supplied both by sympathetic and by parasympathetic fibers.

The structure and organization of the blood vessels within the erectile tissue provide the mech-

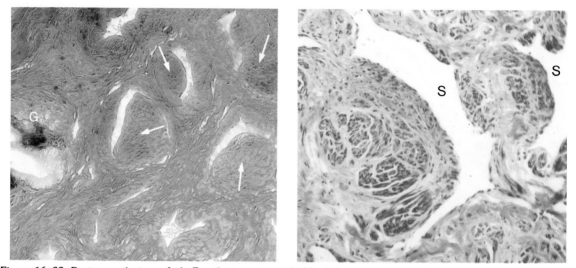

*Figure 16–33.* Penis, erectile tissue. Left: *Erectile tissue is supplied by helicine arteries, which are longitudinal vessels that are directed distally. In the quiescent state, these vessels have a spiral course. Their media is thick, and their intima is thrown into longitudinal folds, the intimal ridges, here sectioned transversely (arrows). Thus, their lumina appear crescentic. These vessels open directly into the cavernous spaces of the erectile tissue, and during erotic stimulation, they straighten out and their lumina dilate. Also present is a mucous urethral gland of Littre (G). Iron hematoxylin, aniline blue. Medium power.* Right: *Erectile tissue is composed of a framework of irregular trabeculae, consisting of collagenous (green), elastic, and smooth muscle (brown) fibers, which are extensions of the tunica albuginea. Within this framework are irregular endothelium-lined spaces, the cavernous spaces or blood sinuses (S). During erotic stimulation, the engorgement of these sinuses with blood results in erection of the penis. Masson. Medium power.*

anism for erection of the penis (Fig. 16–33). Under conditions of erotic stimulation, parasympathetic stimulation produces a relaxation of the smooth muscle, with the helicine arteries straightening out and their lumina dilating. Blood flows freely from them into the cavernous spaces, which become engorged with blood. Thus, there is a rerouting of blood into a greatly enlarged vascular bed. The venous drainage of the periphery of the corpora is said to be diminished as a result of compression of the thin-walled veins under the tunica albuginea by the engorged trabecular spaces. The corpora cavernosa become enlarged and rigid. Since there is less compression of the venous drainage of the corpus spongiosum and a more yielding tunica, there is less rigidity here and the urethra contained within it remains patent to allow for egress of seminal fluid during ejaculation.

At the termination of sexual excitement, the penis returns to a flaccid state through a process of *detumescence*. The arteries regain muscular tone owing to sympathetic stimulation, and the amount of blood supplied to the erectile tissue diminishes. The excess of blood within the corpora cavernosa slowly is pressed out by contraction of the muscle fibers within the trabeculae and by recoil of surrounding elastic fibers, and the normal route of blood flow through the organ is restored.

### SEMINAL FLUID

Seminal fluid (semen) consists of spermatozoa together with the fluid in which they are suspended. The fluid is a product of all the auxiliary genital glands, together with a minor contribution supplied by the system of genital ducts. Semen is a whitish, opaque fluid containing about 100 million spermatozoa per ml, but the number varies greatly. The ejaculate averages about 3 ml and thus contains about 300 million spermatozoa.

The discharge of semen is said to occur in a definite sequence. The bulbourethral glands and the urethral glands of Littre discharge their mucous secretion during erection and lubricate the cavernous urethra. During actual ejaculation, the prostate discharges first. This is followed by the spermatozoa, which are forced out of the distal portion of the ductus epididymidis and the ductus deferens by powerful contractions of the muscular walls. Finally, the thick secretion of the seminal vesicles, which contains fructose and is nutrient to the sperm, is added to the mass.

## SUMMARY

The primary function of the male reproductive system is the production of spermatozoa, which occurs within the germinal epithelium of the seminiferous tubules, for the procreation of the species.

The germinal, or seminiferous, epithelium is composed of a permanent population of supporting cells, Sertoli's cells, and a mobile population of proliferating and differentiating spermatogenic cells. Sertoli's cells possess complex occluding junctional specializations that divide the seminiferous epithelium into basal and adluminal compartments. The tight junctions, together with the peritubular tissue, constitute the morphological basis of the blood-testis barrier.

Spermatogenesis commences with the diploid spermatogonia, which lie in the basal compartment of the seminiferous epithelium. Type A dark spermatogonia are reserve cells that divide infrequently to maintain the numbers of spermatogonia and to produce type A pale spermatogonia. The latter divide frequently to produce other type A pale spermatogonia and type B spermatogonia. Type B spermatogonia divide to produce primary spermatocytes, which increase in size and migrate from the basal to the adluminal compartment. Each primary spermatocyte then undergoes a reduction division, meiosis, to produce two haploid secondary spermatocytes, which remain joined by a bridge of cytoplasm. These cells divide rapidly to produce four conjoined spermatids. No further division occurs, and the spermatids undergo an extensive differentiation, spermiogen-

esis, to transform into spermatozoa. The differentiation occurs in synchrony while the spermatids are associated closely with Sertoli's cells. Spermiogenesis involves development of the acrosome from the Golgi zone, formation of the flagellum in close association with the centrioles, condensation of the nucleus to form the sperm head, and migration and rearrangement of the mitochondria to form the mitochondrial sheath of the middle piece.

The principal endocrine secretion of the testis is testosterone, produced by the interstitial cells of Leydig after stimulation by LH (or ICSH). Testosterone promotes spermatogenesis, the appearance of secondary sex characteristics, and the proper development and maintenance of the genital ducts and of the auxiliary glands. FSH stimulates secretion of androgen-binding protein by Sertoli's cells, which in turn maintains high levels of testosterone within the adluminal compartment of the seminiferous epithelium.

Spermatozoa released into the seminiferous tubules are nonmotile and incapable of fertilization. They are moved into the tubuli recti and rete testis by a flow of testicular fluid (produced by the seminiferous epithelium) and by contractions of myoid elements within the peritubular tissue and testicular capsule. They pass via the ciliated ductuli efferentes into the ductus epididymidis. Most of the testicular fluid is absorbed in the ductuli efferentes and in the proximal portion of the ductus epididymidis. In their slow passage through the ductus epididymidis, the spermatozoa acquire motility and optimal fertilizability. They are stored in the distal ductus epididymidis, and powerful contractions of its muscular wall and that of the ductus deferens transfer spermatozoa to the prostatic urethra.

During ejaculation, the three primary auxiliary genital glands add their secretions to the seminal fluid. The secretions of the bulbourethral glands lubricate the penile urethra. The prostate gland, a complex of compound tubuloalveolar glands, produces an abundant milky secretion rich in acid phosphatase, which is released following contraction of muscle fibers within its stroma. The seminal vesicles produce a viscous secretion that is rich in fructose, which is an important energy source for the spermatozoa.

The penis contains three cylinders of erectile

### *Summary Table 16–1. Histological Features of Male Genital Ducts*

| Duct | Lining Epithelium | Support | Muscle |
|---|---|---|---|
| Tubuli recti | Simple columnar | Loose connective tissue | Absent |
| Rete testis | Simple cuboidal or squamous with single cilium on each cell | Highly vascular connective tissue | Absent |
| Ductuli efferentes | Tall columnar, mostly ciliated, alternating with short cuboidal, mostly nonciliated, with microvillus border | Loose connective tissue | Thin layer of circular smooth muscle |
| Ductus epididymidis | Pseudostratified columnar; tall principal cells with stereocilia; small basal cells | Thin lamina propria | Circular smooth muscle proximally; distally three layers (as in ductus deferens) |
| Ductus deferens | Pseudostratified columnar with stereocilia: in longitudinal folds | Thin lamina propria and indefinite, vascular submucosa | Thick. Three layers: inner longitudinal, middle circular, outer longitudinal smooth muscle |
| Ampulla | Pseudostratified columnar with complex folding | Thin lamina propria, poorly defined | Thin, ill-defined smooth muscle |
| Ejaculatory duct | Simple or pseudostratified columnar, less complex folding | Fibrous connective tissue, merging with prostatic stroma | Absent, except in fibromuscular stroma of prostate |

tissue, the paired corpora cavernosa penis dorsally and the corpus spongiosum ventrally. The latter contains the cavernous portion of the urethra. Following parasympathetic stimulation, dilation of helicine arteries within the erectile tissue causes blood to flow into the cavernous spaces. This, together with accompanying compression of the veins draining the corpora cavernosa, results in an erection. Sympathetic stimulation constricts the arteries and detumescence follows.

### *Summary Table 16–2. Histological Features of Auxiliary Genital Glands*

| Gland | Type | Epithelium | Supporting Tissue |
|---|---|---|---|
| Seminal vesicle | Tortuous diverticulum off ductus deferens | Pseudostratified or simple columnar, with complex folding | Lamina propria, inner circular and outer longitudinal smooth muscle, adventitia |
| Prostate | 30–50 compound tubuloalveolar glands | Variable. Simple or pseudostratified columnar, or cuboidal, with concretions | Dense fibroelastic stroma with smooth muscle |
| Bulbourethral gland | Compound tubuloalveolar gland | Variable. Simple cuboidal or columnar. Ducts lined by pseudostratified columnar | Fibroelastic connective tissue, with skeletal and smooth muscle |

# Organs of Special Sense

## INTRODUCTION

As outlined in Chapter 7, organs of general sensibility are distributed widely in epithelium, connective tissue, muscle, and tendon. Special receptors associated with sensations of smell, taste, sight, hearing, and balance are found in limited areas (receptors for smell and taste already have been described in Chapters 12 and 11, respectively). All receptors, of course, are transducers in the sense that they convert one form of energy into another. They are either nerve endings or cells specialized for this function (Fig. 17–1).

## SENSORY RECEPTORS

Receptors are classified on more than one basis. One classification is based on the source of the stimulus in relation to the body, and thus there are

1. *Exteroceptors*, located in viscera and blood vessels and receiving external stimuli.

2. *Interoceptors*, located in viscera and blood vessels and responding to internal stimuli.

**17**

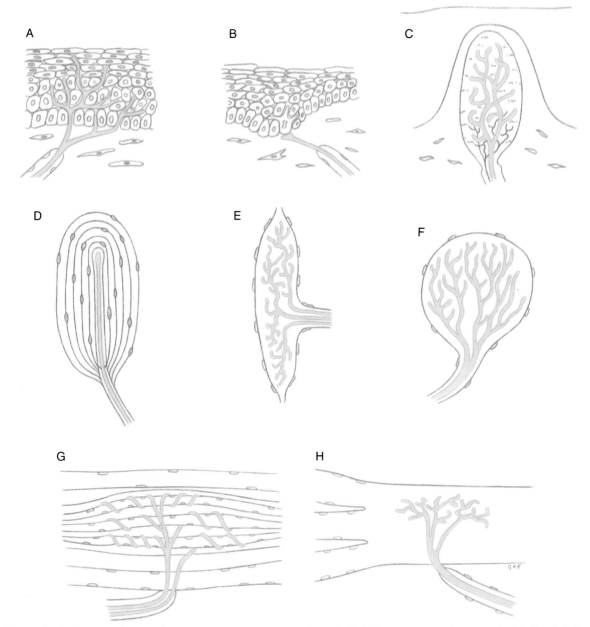

**Figure 17–1.** *Diagram of some of the types of sensory nerve endings. A: Naked nerve endings in cornea (pain). B: Merkel's disc in epidermis (touch). C: Meissner's corpuscle in dermis (touch). D: Lamellated corpuscle (Vater-Pacini) (pressure). E: Ruffini's corpuscle (heat). F: Krause's end bulb (cold). G: Neuromuscular spindle (proprioception). H: Neurotendinous ending (proprioception).*

3. *Proprioceptors*, associated mainly with the musculoskeletal system and responding to movement and change in position.

Another classification depends upon the particular energy type or modality, with

1. *Thermoreceptors*, sensitive to change in temperature.

2. *Mechanoreceptors*, sensitive to touch and pressure.

3. *Chemoreceptors*, sensitive to chemical changes.

4. *Osmoreceptors*, sensitive to change in osmotic pressure.

However, on a *morphological basis*, receptors can be classified as either (Fig. 17–2)

1. Free or naked, unencapsulated endings, or

2. Encapsulated, or corpuscular, endings.

The sensation carried in the nerve of any receptor is specific, and, usually, only a single sensation is appreciated. Not all sensations reach the conscious level, some being concerned with reflex actions.

Where appropriate, some receptors have been described in previous chapters, and only brief accounts follow of the two main morphological types.

### Free Nerve Endings

Free nerve endings of sensory afferent nerve fibers are numerous where sensation is developed highly, for example, in the skin, where they comprise most of the sensory receptors; in cornea; in the oral cavity; and in respiratory mucosa (see Fig. 17–2). In the epidermis, the sensory nerve fibers are unmyelinated or small-diameter myelinated fibers, all losing their investments before terminating, with naked nerve fibers passing between epidermal cells as far as the granular layer. Different fibers probably receive sensations of touch, pain, and temperature. In association with hairs, sets of endings lie around the dermal sheath, with others parallel to the hair shaft and terminating in the outer root sheath. They are stimulated by movement of the hair, with one nerve often branching widely to supply several follicles. These *peritrichial endings* together form an important tactile organ.

Some nerve terminals are associated with specialized epithelial cells. In epidermis, in relation to epithelial cells of hair follicles, and in oral mucosa, nerve terminals form disc-like endings with modified epithelial cells called *Merkel's discs* or *corpuscles* (Fig. 17–3). Merkel's cells are dark-staining, with cytoplasmic processes that extend between adjacent keratinocytes, and the cytoplasm contains 80-nm dense-cored cytoplasmic vesicles with, sometimes, an unusual nuclear inclusion of parallel filaments. It is believed that these are mechanoreceptors, detecting movement between keratinocytes, and some may respond to vibratory stimuli. Other expanded nerve terminals that terminate around single, unmodified basal epidermal cells are believed to be cold receptors.

### Encapsulated Nerve Endings

This type has the terminal nerve fiber ensheathed by a capsule, and they vary greatly in size and shape.

**Lamellated Corpuscles (of Pacini, or Vater-Pacini).** These are distributed widely in subcutaneous tissue, particularly of the palms, soles, and digits and in the nipples, periosteum, mesentery, cornea, pancreas, and loose connective tissue (see Fig. 17–2). They are large (2 to 4 mm by 0.5 to 2 mm), spherical or ovoid, and lightly staining and structurally resemble an onion. Each is supplied by one (or more) large myelinated fibers that lose myelin as they enter the corpuscle; they then pass through the corpuscle to end in an expanded bulb. About 60 closely packed lamellae composed of flattened cells surround the nerve fiber. Externally is a "capsule" of up to 30 concentric lamellae of flattened, endothelium-like cells with basal laminae and a few collagen fibrils between them. These corpuscles respond to pressure and vibration: In relation to joints, they register movement and position.

**Tactile Corpuscles (of Meissner).** These corpuscles are found in dermal papillae (particularly those of digits, lips, nipples, and genitalia) and are cylindrical in shape, 80 μm long, and 40 μm in diameter, with their long axes perpendicular to the skin surface (see Fig. 17–2). A thin connective tissue capsule surrounds a central stack of transversely oriented flattened cells, between which are branches of both myelinated and unmyelinated nerve fibers. These corpuscles are sensitive

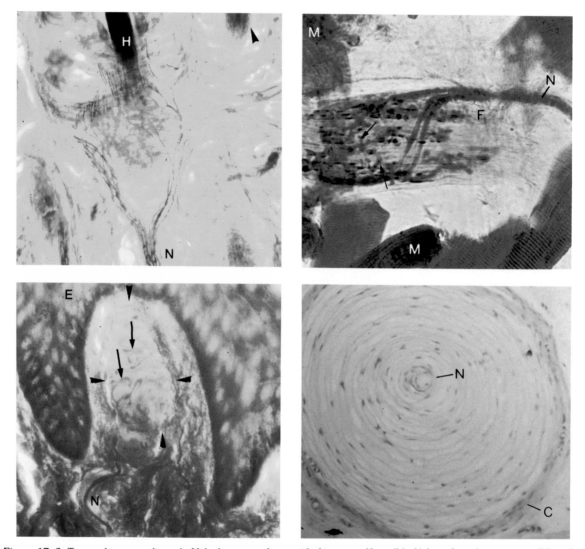

**Figure 17–2.** *Types of nerve endings. A: Naked nerve endings, with thin nerve fibers (black) branching from a nerve (N) in the dermis and passing to a hair follicle (H) to terminate mainly in the glassy membrane of the dermal root sheath. The arrowhead indicates a second hair follicle. These are the peritrichial nerve endings for touch. Golgi. Medium power. B: Neurotendinous (Golgi) organ, with a bundle of tendon fibers (F) in a thin connective tissue capsule and a nerve (N) branching and then terminating in club-shaped endings (arrows). Also present are muscle fibers (M). This is a proprioceptive ending. Gold chloride. High power. C: Meissner's corpuscle (arrowheads), supplied by a nerve (N), lies in a dermal papilla (E is the epidermis) and is sensitive to touch. Golgi. Medium power. D and E: Vater-Pacini lamellated corpuscles. D: The corpuscle is sectioned transversely with a nerve fiber (N) in its core and is surrounded by layers (up to 60) of flattened cells with a sheath of connective tissue (C).*

Illustration continued on opposite page

to touch and permit two-point tactile discrimination (i.e., the ability to distinguish between two closely placed pointed stimuli).

**Bulbous Corpuscles (of Krause).** These spherical corpuscles are about 50 μm in diameter and

are found at mucocutaneous junctions (lip and external genitalia) and in the dermis. There is a thick capsule within which the nerve fiber branches and may become coiled, terminating in club-like endings. These corpuscles decrease in

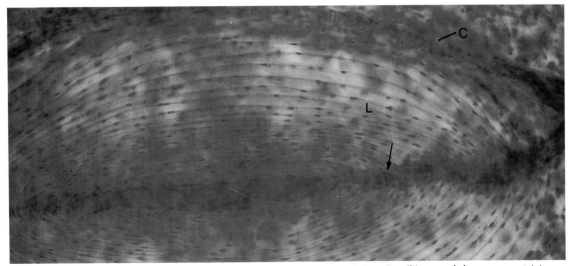

**Figure 17–2** Continued, E: *The corpuscle is seen in longitudinal section with lamellae (L) around the nerve-containing core (arrow). The corpuscles respond to pressure and vibration and, in relation to joints, are proprioceptive. Both H and E, low power.*

number with age, and while they may be mechanoreceptors or cold receptors, they are considered by some to represent a degenerative process in nerve terminals.

**Corpuscles of Ruffini.** These are found in connective tissues, including the dermis and joint capsules, and have a thin capsule containing a spray-like nerve ending with terminal swellings. They are believed to be mechanoreceptors.

**Neurotendinous Endings (of Golgi).** Similar to the corpuscles of Ruffini, these are found in tendons near the muscle junction, consisting of small bundles of tendon fibers (the intrafusal fasciculi) enclosed in a lamellated corpuscle with nonmyelinated nerve endings arborizing around the bundles (see Fig. 17–2). About 500 μm long and 100 μm in diameter, they are proprioceptive and are stimulated by stretching or contraction of the associated muscle.

**Neuromuscular Spindles.** Found in muscle, often near a tendon, they are formed by several small muscle fibers (the intrafusal fibers) with motor and sensory nerve fibers, the whole enveloped in a connective tissue capsule. The spindle is fusiform and up to 2 mm long, and the contained muscle fibers are of two types—"nuclear bag fibers" (numerous central nuclei with few peripheral myofibrils) and "nuclear chain fibers"

(a single central row of nuclei and many small myofibrils). Sensory nerve fibers end as annulospiral endings around nuclear bag fibers and as flower-spray endings on nuclear chain fibers, with small motor fibers ending at modified myoneural junctions on all intrafusal fibers. These sensory endings are mechanoreceptors, responding to stretch.

## THE EYE

The eyeball basically consists of three layers (Figs. 17–4 and 17–5). Internally is the nervous layer, the *retina*, which developmentally and functionally is an isolated part of the central nervous system, to which it remains connected by a tract of nerve fibers, the *optic nerve*. The retina is nourished and protected by two external coats, or tunics, one of vascular and one of fibrous tissue. The outer fibrous coat, corresponding to the dura mater of the CNS, is opaque and white over the posterior five sixths (the *sclera*) and transparent over the anterior one sixth (the *cornea*). Between the retina and the fibrous coat is a vascular, nutrient layer analogous to the pia

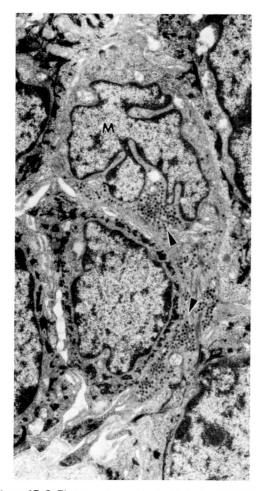

**Figure 17–3.** Electron micrograph of a Merkel's cell (M) from the hard palate of the squirrel monkey. The cell contains concentrations of dense-cored granules (arrowheads) and lies between keratinocytes. × 5200. (Courtesy of Drs. P. R. Garant, J. Feldman, M. I. Cho, and M. R. Cullen.)

the inner surface of the ciliary body and posterior surface of the iris.

There is a potential space, the *perichoroidal space*, between fibrous and vascular tunics except anteriorly at the corneoscleral junction and posteriorly at the exit of the optic nerve; at these sites, the two layers are attached firmly. As the iris reflects inward, the space between fibrous and vascular tunics is expanded as the *anterior chamber*. The *lens* lies immediately posterior to the iris, supported by a *suspensory ligament* or *zonule* that passes from the periphery (equator) of the lens to the ciliary body. The slender space between iris and lens is the *posterior chamber*, and it communicates freely with the anterior chamber through the pupil. The two chambers contain *aqueous humor*, a clear fluid secreted by ciliary epithelium. Posterior to the lens, the cavity of the eyeball is filled with *vitreous humor*, a transparent gel. Thus, to reach the sensory retina that lines the posterior half of the eyeball, light rays must traverse a series of transparent, refractive media consisting of cornea, aqueous humor, lens, and vitreous body.

The eyeball is not truly spherical, being somewhat flattened from above down, and neither does the optic nerve exit at the posterior pole but rather about 3 mm to the nasal side and 1 mm below it. Anterior and posterior *poles* are the central points of corneal and scleral curvatures, the *geometrical axis* being the line joining them. The *fovea*, the area of most distinct vision, lies just to the temporal side of the posterior pole, the *visual axis* being the line between the center of the pupil and the fovea. The *equator* is a circumferential line dividing the eyeball into anterior and posterior hemispheres. Any circle drawn through the poles and crossing the equator at a right angle is termed a *meridian*.

The sclera has a radius of 12 mm, while the cornea is curved more acutely, with a radius of only 8 mm. At the corneoscleral junction, there is a shallow circular sulcus, the external scleral sulcus, and here are attached conjunctiva and bulbar fascia. Arterial suppy to the eyeball is via short posterior ciliary arteries that pierce sclera around the exit of the optic nerve, long posterior ciliary arteries on each side piercing sclera, and anterior ciliary arteries passing just posterior to the corneoscleral junction. Vortex veins drain the

arachnoid. This *uveal* coat consists of the *choroid* posteriorly, the *ciliary body* just behind the corneoscleral junction, and the *iris* anteriorly, the last reflected inward to diverge from the cornea. In the iris is a central, spherical deficiency called the *pupil*, the diameter of which can be varied dependent upon light conditions. The nervous, or sensory, part of the retina lines only the posterior half of the eyeball but continues anteriorly as a non-nervous (i.e., nonphotosensitive) layer to line

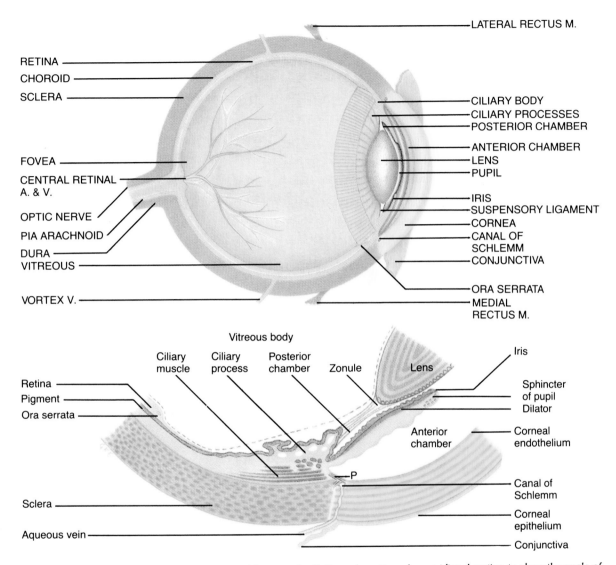

**Figure 17–4.** Top: *Diagram of the eye, sectioned horizontally.* Bottom: *A portion of a meridional section to show the angle of the eye. The letter "P" indicates the pectinate ligament (trabecular meshwork), through which aqueous humor drains from the anterior chamber into the canal of Schlemm.*

choroid, with one leaving each quadrant of the eyeball.

## Fibrous Coat

This, composed of sclera and cornea, provides tough, fibroelastic support for the eye.

### SCLERA

This is dense fibrous tissue, 1 mm thick posteriorly, 0.8 nm thick anteriorly, but only 0.3 mm thick at the equator. It is composed of flat bundles of collagen fibers, mainly running parallel to the surface but intersecting freely, with fine networks of elastic fibers, some ground substance, and a

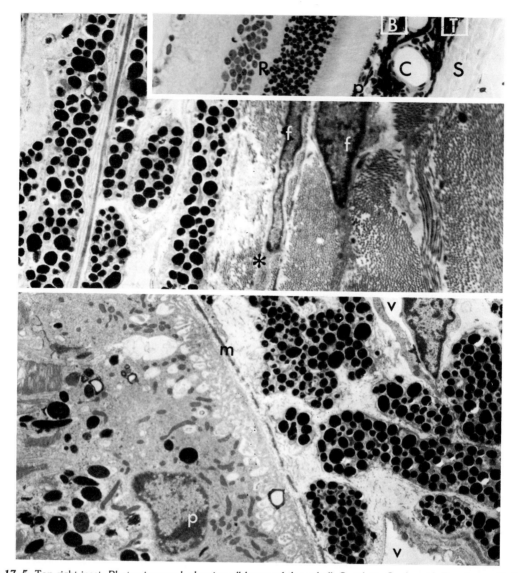

**Figure 17–5.** Top right inset: *Photomicrograph showing all layers of the eyball: S, sclera; C, choroid; R, retina; with "p" the pigment epithelium. The squares roughly indicate regions seen in the top (T) and bottom (B) electron micrographs. In sclera (top right), there are fibroblasts (f) and collagenous bundles, the region of the lamina fusca is marked with an asterisk, and in the choroid there are numerous melanocyte processes (left) containing melanin. Bottom: Deeper choroid is seen (right) with melanocytes and blood vessels (v). Bruch's membrane (m), and pigment epithelium (p). Inset, × 250; top and bottom, × 6000.*

few flattened, branching fibroblasts (see Fig. 17–9). Externally, there is a looser fibroelastic tissue (the episcleral tissue) that is separated from the dense fibrous tissue of Tenon's capsule (the bulbar fascia) by a slender space, traversed by the tendons of the extraocular muscles as they insert onto sclera. This space, and extraocular fat, permits the eyeball to rotate within the orbit. At the inner aspect of the sclera, collagen bundles are smaller, with numerous elastic fibers and melanocytes (the lamina fusca). Posteriorly, the sclera is perforated by the optic nerve at the *lamina cribrosa.*

## CORNEA

The cornea is clear and transparent, and although it has a smooth surface, it is not curved uniformly. The central (optical) zone has a smaller radius of curvature than does the periphery, and the posterior surface is more strongly curved than the anterior. Thus, it is thinner (0.7 to 0.8 mm) centrally than at its margin (1.1 mm). The refractive power of the cornea, a function of its refractive index and its radius of curvature, is greater than that of the lens. Anatomically, the cornea consists of the *cornea proper* and the *limbus*, a transition zone about 1 mm wide at the periphery that contains blood vessels and lymphatics. The cornea proper is avascular.

A cross section of the cornea shows five layers (Fig. 17–6):

1. *Epithelium.* Externally is a stratified squamous nonkeratinizing epithelium, 50 μm thick, with five or six layers of cells—a basal layer of low columnar cells, three or four layers of polyhedral, or "wing," cells, and one or two layers of surface squamous cells (Figs. 17–7 and 17–8). The epithelium is highly sensitive, with numerous free nerve endings, and has excellent regenerative powers, mitoses occurring in the basal layer.

2. *Bowman's Membrane.* This is 8 μm thick, structureless, and acellular; is formed by a feltwork of fine collagen fibrils; and ends abruptly at the limbus.

3. *Substantia Propria.* This, the stroma, forms 90 per cent of the thickness of the cornea and is composed of lamellae of collagen fibrils arranged in many layers, the lamellae at different angles. Interchange of fibrils between adjacent lamellae holds the lamellae together. Ground substance between lamellae contains chondroitin sulfate and keratan sulfate and between the bundles of collagen fibrils are stellate, flattened fibroblasts (keratocytes).

4. *Descemet's Membrane.* This is 5 to 7 μm thick centrally but thickens to 8 to 10 μm peripherally, where it is continuous with material of the *trabecular meshwork* (pectinate ligament) at the *ring of Schwalbe.* While it appears homogeneous

by light microscopy, on electron microscopy it is composed of small fibrils with a 107-nm periodicity arranged in a hexagonal pattern of great regularity.

5. *Endothelium.* This is a single layer of low cuboidal cells lining the internal surface of the cornea, responsible for transporting fluid from the anterior chamber to the stroma. As already stated, the cornea is avascular and for its nutrition (and hydration) depends upon diffusion from blood vessels in the limbus and from aqueous humor, through the endothelium.

The *limbus cornea* is a 1 mm wide transition zone between cornea and sclera. Here, the corneal epithelium thickens to ten or more layers and is continuous with the conjunctiva, Bowman's membrane ends abruptly, Descemet's membrane splits up to become continuous with trabeculae of the pectinate ligament, and the corneal stroma becomes less regular and blends with the sclera. The limbus is well vascularized.

## Uveal (Vascular) Coat

Uvea means "grape-like" and aptly describes the blood vessels and pigment cells of the choroid, ciliary body, and iris.

## CHOROID

This is a spongy, brown membrane with extensive venous plexuses, and while it actually is 0.1 to 0.3 mm thick, it usually collapses after death (Fig. 17–9).

Externally is the *epichoroid*, only 20 to 30 μm thick and consisting of loosely arranged collagen and elastic fibrils that partially bridge the perichoroidal space (between sclera and choroid), with stellate melanocytes between fibrils. The bulk of the choroid is formed by the *vessel layer* formed by a mass of arteries and veins, the larger vessels externally, lying in loose connective tissue that contains many melanocytes (Fig. 17–10). Internal to this is the *choriocapillaris*, a layer of capillaries lined by fenestrated (type II) endothelium. This plexus supplies nutrition to the outer portion of the retina and extends anteriorly only as far as the ora serrata (the junction between nervous and non-nervous portions of the retina). Between

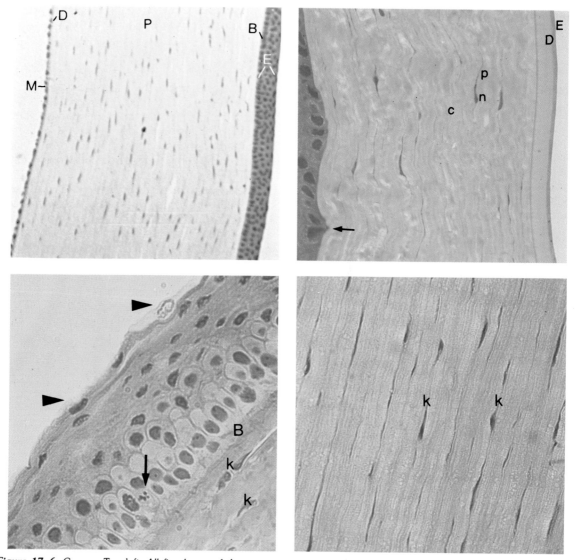

**Figure 17–6.** Cornea. Top left: All five layers of the cornea are seen: epithelium (E), Bowman's membrane (B), substantia propria (P), Descemet's membrane (D), and endothelium (M). To the left would be aqueous humor in the anterior chamber. H and E. Low power. Top right: This shows the deeper layer of the corneal epithelium (left) supported by Bowman's membrane (arrow), nuclei (n) and slender processes (p) of keratocytes with lamellae of collagen fibers (c) forming the substantia propria, the structureless Descemet's membrane (D), and the near-squamous corneal endothelium (E). Methylene blue, azure A, basic fuchsin. Medium power. Lower left: The stratified squamous, nonkeratinizing corneal epithelium is six to eight cells thick, the surface squamous cells being nucleated (arrowheads), the basal layer showing a mitosis (arrow). Beneath is Bowman's membrane (B) and the outer part of the substantia propria with keratocytes (k). H and E. High power. Lower right: The substantia propria shows regular lamellae of collagen fibers (pink) with flattened keratocytes (k) between them. H and E. High power.

choriocapillaris and retina is the *lamina elastica* (Bruch's membrane), a shiny homogeneous membrane only 1 to 4 μm thick, composed of elastic fibers externally and an inner basal lamina.

Anteriorly, it extends into ciliary body, and posteriorly it ends abruptly at the optic disc.

The choroid contains numerous stellate melanocytes lying between the vessels, these involved

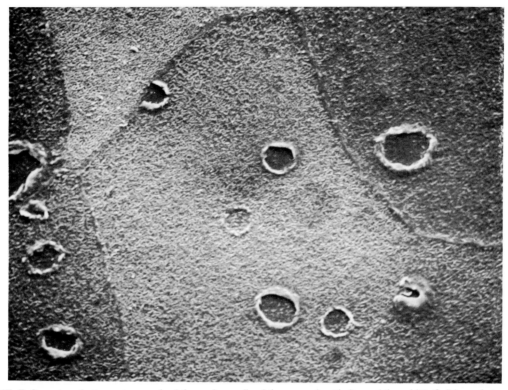

**Figure 17–7.** *Scanning electron micrograph of the surface cells of the corneal epithelium of the rabbit. Cell boundaries are seen clearly, the cell surfaces show microvilli and microplicae (small folds), and the "craters" on the surface may represent secretory vacuoles.* × *6500. (Courtesy of M. J. Hollenberg and B. J. Lewis.)*

in light absorption. Also present are some nerves (sympathetic) and a few ganglion cells associated with these plexuses.

### CILIARY BODY

The ciliary body encircles the eye anterior to the ora serrata and, in meridional section, is triangular, with its base facing the anterior chamber, an outer surface applied to sclera, and an inner surface separated from vitreous by the ciliary (non-nervous) portion of the retina (Figs. 17–11 and 17–12). This inner surface is irregular with shallow grooves, the *ciliary striae*, passing forward from the ora serrata, and deeper ridges and grooves more anteriorly, the *ciliary processes* (Figs. 17–13 and 17–14). Anteriorly, the outer angle attaches to the scleral spur (an inner projection of the anterior extremity of the sclera that projects toward the anterior chamber), and the inner, free angle juts internally just anterior to the equator of the lens.

The ciliary body is the anterior extension of both choroid and retina but does not include any choriocapillaris. Its bulk is formed by smooth muscle fibers arising from the scleral spur and pectinate ligament anteriorly and passing in three layers as meridional, radial, and equatorial bands to function in accommodation (discussed later). Elastic fibers lie between the ciliary muscle fibers, with some melanocytes. Internal to muscle is a vascular layer with capillaries and veins in the cores of the ciliary processes, these vessels probably being the site of formation of aqueous humor. Internally, the ciliary body is covered by the ciliary epithelium, two layers of cells of which the outer is pigmented and continuous with the pigment epithelium of the retina, while the inner is

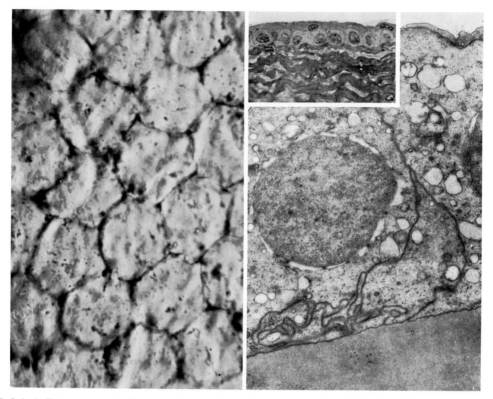

**Figure 17–8.** Left: *Flat preparation of the corneal endothelium, showing the hexagonal cell pattern and penetration of the stain into the interdigitations between cells.* × 950. *(Courtesy of J. Speakman.)* Inset: *Plastic section of corneal endothelium.* × 550. Right: *Electron micrograph of the corneal endothelium with Descemet's membrane beneath.* × 7500.

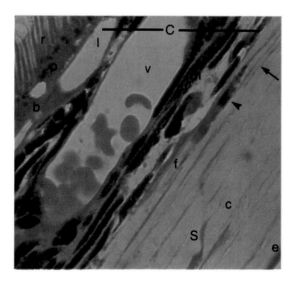

**Figure 17–9.** *Sclera and choroid. The sclera (S) is formed by thick bundles of collagenous fibers (c), less regular than those of the corneal stroma, with scattered branching fibroblasts between the bundles. Looser fibroelastic tissue forms the episcleral tissue (e) externally, and internally is the lamina fusca (f) with smaller collagen bundles (arrow), more elastic tissue, and melanocytes (arrowhead). In the choroid (C), there are large vessels (v), the choriocapillaris (l), and the lamina elastica (Bruch's membrane, b) with numerous melanocytes (m) containing pigment. Above left is the pigment epithelium (p) of the retina and outer segments of rods (r). Methylene blue, basic fuchsin. High power.*

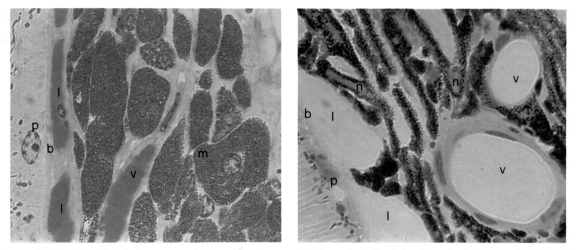

**Figure 17–10.** Choroid. Left: *Larger vessels (v) and melanocytes (m) form the bulk of the choroid, while internally (left) is the choriocapillaris (l), separated from the pigment epithelium of the retina (p) by the lamina elastica (Bruch's membrane, b). H and E. Oil immersion.* Right: *This is similar but shows only the inner portion of the choroid. Melanocytes are stellate, and their nuclei (n) are obscured partially by pigment (melanin) granules. Melanin has a role in the absorption of light rays. Hematoxylin, light green. Oil immersion.*

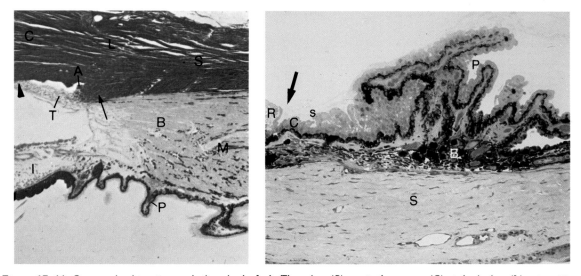

**Figure 17–11.** Corneoscleral junction and ciliary body. Left: *The sclera (S) meets the cornea (C) at the limbus (L), a transition zone. Internally, the sclera terminates at the scleral spur (arrow). The trabecular meshwork (T) passes from the posterior extremity of Descemet's membrane (the ring of Schwalbe, arrowhead) posteriorly to the scleral spur and ciliary body (B). The canal of Schlemm (A) lies external to the meshwork. On the internal surface of the ciliary body is the ciliary epithelium formed by two layers of cells, the outer (external) of pigmented cells continuous with the retinal pigmented epithelium and the inner nonpigmented and representing the forward continuation of the entire thickness of the sensory retina. This surface is deeply ridged and grooved, forming the ciliary processes (P). The ciliary epithelium continues anteriorly to the posterior surface of the iris (I), where both layers become heavily pigmented. Melanocytes (M, black) lie between muscle fibers of the ciliary body. Mallory. Low power.* Right: *Externally (below) is the sclera (S). Internally at the ora serrata (arrow), the nervous portion of the retina (R) is continuous with the non-nervous portion (C), and, between outer and inner layers, the choroid passes into the ciliary body (B), which is somewhat thicker. The internal surface against the vitreous is irregular with shallow grooves or striae (s) posteriorly and with deeper, radial, ridges anteriorly, these called the ciliary processes (P). Methylene blue, azure A, basic fuchsin. Low power.*

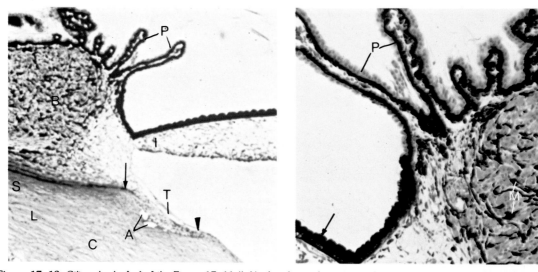

*Figure 17–12.* Ciliary body. Left: Like Figure 17–11 (left), this shows the corneo (C)-scleral (S) junction at the limbus (L), with the canal of Schlemm (A), and the trabecular meshwork (T) extending between the ring of Schwalbe (arrowhead) and the scleral spur (arrow). The ciliary body (B) is formed by ciliary muscle (pink) and melanocytes (black), with ciliary processes (P) internally. The root of the iris (I) shows a posterior pigmented epithelium (above) and an anterior surface (below) that is, in fact, discontinuous and formed by fibroblasts and melanocytes supported by delicate connective tissue. (Compare with Figure 17–19, top.) Right: A higher magnification showing melanocytes (M) and ciliary muscle (pink) of the ciliary body. Ciliary processes (P) are covered by the ciliary epithelium with outer pigmented and inner nonpigmented layers. At the root of the iris, both layers become heavily pigmented (arrow). H and E. Left, low power; right, high power.

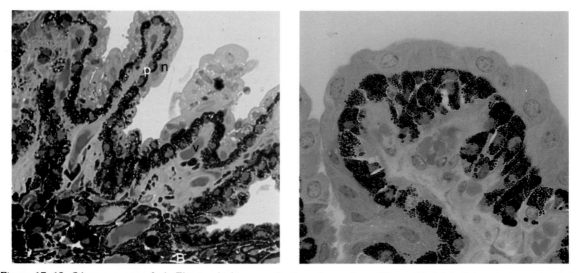

*Figure 17–13.* Ciliary processes. Left: This is a higher magnification of a portion of Figure 17–11 (right), with the ciliary body (below, B) showing numerous blood vessels (the vascular layer) and melanocytes. Internally (above) are the ciliary processes covered by ciliary epithelium, the outer layer pigmented (p), the inner nonpigmented (n). In the cores of the processes is connective tissue with numerous vessels (pink, v), the probable site of formation of aqueous humor. Right: At higher magnification, the two layers of ciliary epithelium are seen clearly, with blood vessels (filled with erythrocytes, pink) in the core of a ciliary process. Methylene blue, azure A, basic fuchsin. Left, high power; right, oil immersion.

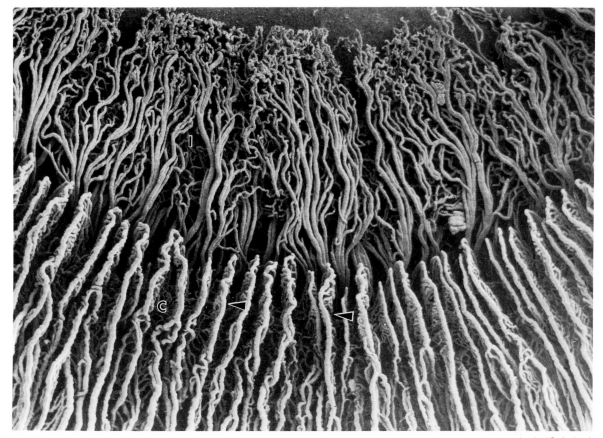

**Figure 17–14.** *Ciliary processes and iris. This scanning electron micrograph is of the blood vessels of the ciliary body (C, below) and iris (I, above) as seen from internally, previously injected with plastic, from the eye of a duckling. The vessels in the cores of the ciliary processes are arranged radially and form ridges (arrowheads) with grooves between. In the iris, the vessels are arranged radially. This SEM indicates the extreme vascularity throughout the uveal coat of the eye. × 76. (SEM courtesy of Dr. F. E. Hossler and Dr. K. R. Olson.)*

nonpigmented and represents the forward prolongation of the neural retina. At the basal (outer) surface of the pigmented layer is a basal lamina continuous with Bruch's membrane, while another, the internal limiting membrane, covers the basal (inner) surface of the nonpigmented layer. (In development from the double-walled optic cup, "basal" surfaces of the two cell layers lie on outer and inner aspects, with the apices of the two cell layers facing each other.) Anteriorly at the root of the iris, the inner layer also becomes pigmented.

## IRIS

The most anterior part of the uvea, the iris (which means "rainbow"), has a central aperture, the pupil (Figs. 17–15 and 17–16; see Fig. 17–14). The iris varies in color among individuals and with age. Peripherally where it attaches to the ciliary body, its root is thin. Its central part is thicker, and then it becomes thin again at the pupillary margin where it rests against the anterior surface of the lens, thus separating the anterior chamber from the posterior. It has the form of a flat, truncated cone, inclining forward from its attachment. Its anterior surface is irregular with crypts and furrows and is divided into a pupillary zone and a wider, peripheral, ciliary zone. Posteriorly, the surface shows shallow furrows and is uniformly black (Fig. 17–17). Developmentally, the anterior layers are part of the uvea (mesodermal), while the posterior ones are ectodermal (pars iridica).

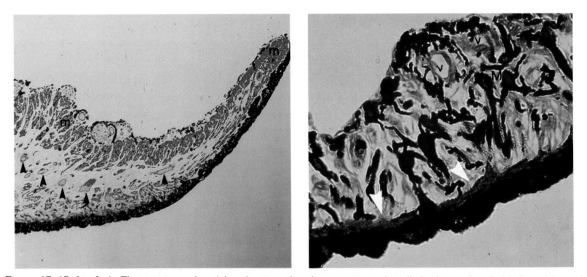

**Figure 17–15.** *Iris. Left: The anterior surface (above) is irregular, the posterior surface (below) is uniformly black and formed by two layers of pigmented cells. In the stroma are smooth muscle cells (m) of the sphincter pupillae muscle, here cut transversely. Only the central area of the iris is seen (pupillary margin to the right). Also present are melanocytes and blood vessels (arrowheads) that are radial in orientation (see Figure 17–14) but spiral, which permits the vessels to accommodate to change in length with change in pupil diameter. Methylene blue, azure A, basic fuchsin. Low power. Right: This section shows the anterior surface (above) without a definite cellular membrane but formed by a discontinuous layer of fibroblasts and melanocytes (black) with delicate connective tissue. In the stroma are blood vessels (v) and stellate melanocytes (M), numerous here in a brown eye, that are responsible for the color of the iris. Posteriorly (below), there are two layers of the pigmented epithelium, the anterior of which are myoepithelial cells, their basal processes (pink, arrowheads) forming the dilator pupillae. This section is of the peripheral, ciliary zone, where the iris is relatively thin. H and E. Medium power.*

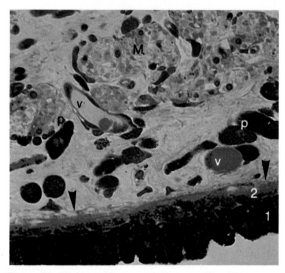

**Figure 17–16.** *Iris, sphincter and dilator pupillae. This section is near the pupillary margin. Smooth muscle (M) of the sphincter pupillae is cut transversely. In the stroma are blood vessels (v) and pigment cells (p) ("clump" cells) that differ slightly from melanocytes that lie more peripherally and anteriorly. Posteriorly (below) is the posterior pigmented epithelium, the posterior layer (1) heavily pigmented, while the anterior, or basal, layer (2) is of myoepithelial cells, their basal processes (pink, arrowheads) forming the dilator pupillae. H and E. High power.*

The anterior surface has no definite cellular membrane and is formed by a discontinuous layer of fibroblasts and melanocytes with, beneath it, a layer of delicate connective tissue with more fibroblasts and melanocytes, the pigmented cells showing elongated processes (Fig. 17–18). Their number determines the color of the iris: Little or no pigment gives a blue color, and increasing amounts impart shades of gray, green, brown, and black. In albinos, in whom pigment is absent or sparse, the iris appears pink owing to its rich vascularity.

Beneath this stroma is a layer of blood vessels running radially. These vessels can accommodate to changes in length (with changes in pupil diameter) and have walls formed by endothelium, pericytes, and a very thick connective tissue adventitia. The posterior surface of the iris is covered by two layers of pigmented cells continuous with ciliary epithelium, the inner nonpigmented layer of the ciliary epithelium becoming heavily pigmented, the numerous melanin granules obscuring all cellular detail. The posterior (inner) surface is covered by a limiting membrane, a typical basal lamina. The cells of the anterior layer of this

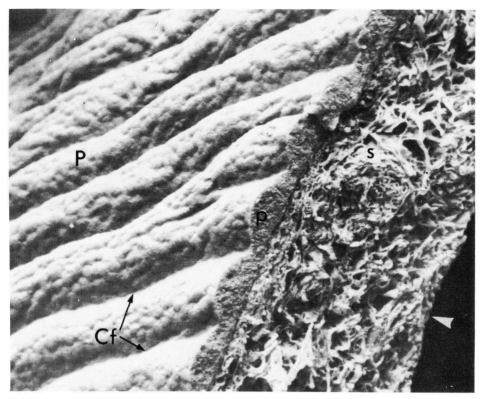

**Figure 17–17.** *This low-power SEM of the iris shows deep circular furrows (Cf) of the posterior pigmented epithelium (P), the cells appearing granular where cut in section (p). The stroma (S) is loose and irregular, with the anterior surface at right (arrowhead).* × 280. *(SEM courtesy of Dr. D. H. Dickson.)*

pigmented epithelium become less pigmented as the *myoepithelium* of the dilator pupillae.

The iris is an adjustable diaphragm and for this has both a *sphincter* and a *dilator pupillae*. The sphincter muscle lies as a ring of smooth muscle at the pupillary margin, supplied by parasympathetic fibers of the third nerve that have synapsed in the ciliary ganglion. The dilator muscle is a thin, radially oriented, indeterminate layer just anterior to the posterior pigmented epithelium. It is not true muscle but is formed by basal processes of the anterior layer of this epithelium, these cells being myoepithelial. It is supplied by sympathetic fibers through the superior cervical ganglion. By variation in the size of the pupil, light entering the eye can be adjusted over a range of brightness. In intense light conditions, the pupil constricts, and this also increases the depth of focus (as in a camera).

## The Chambers of the Eye

**Anterior Chamber.** This is the space bounded anteriorly by the posterior surface (endothelium) of the cornea and posteriorly by the lens, iris, and anterior surface (base) of the ciliary body. Circumferentially, the lateral border of the anterior chamber is occupied by the pectinate ligament (trabecular meshwork), through which aqueous humor is drained into the canal of Schlemm.

**Posterior Chamber.** This is bounded anteriorly by the iris, posteriorly by the lens and zonule, and peripherally by the ciliary processes.

**Aqueous Humor.** This is the thin, watery fluid that fills both anterior and posterior chambers, secreted partially by ciliary epithelium and partially by diffusion from capillaries in ciliary processes. It contains diffusable materials of blood plasma but has a low protein content. It is secreted

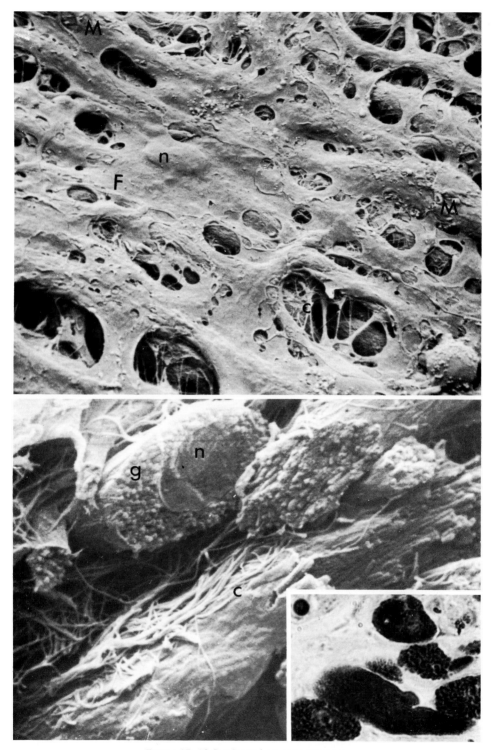

*Figure 17–18* See legend on opposite page

continuously into the posterior chamber, passes through the pupil into the anterior chamber, and is drained through the trabecular tissue into the canal of Schlemm. Usually, the secretion rate is balanced by the drainage rate, and thus intraocular pressure remains constant at about 23 mm of mercury. *Glaucoma* is a relatively common condition in which intraocular pressure is raised and, if uncorrected, can result in blindness. It usually is the result of obstruction to drainage of aqueous humor. In addition to its function in the maintenance of intraocular pressure, necessary for eye function, aqueous humor provides a suitable environment for the functional needs of the cornea, and it also nourishes the lens, which is avascular.

**Canal of Schlemm.** This annular vessel encircles the eye just anterior and external to the scleral spur. Externally is scleral tissue, internally the deeper layer of trabecular tissue. The lumen may be double or even plexiform but usually is single, bounded by a wall of endothelium only 1 μm thick. Its function is to drain aqueous humor, and it has afferent connections through the trabecular spaces and efferent drainage via endothelium-lined tubes. These, about 20 in number, leave the canal around its circumference, pass into sclera, and anastomose to form the deep scleral plexus. A few direct efferent vessels also pass to the episcleral venous plexus that lies external to the limbus (Fig. 17–19). The more anterior channels of this plexus contain only aqueous humor and not blood. These are the "aqueous veins."

**Trabecular Meshwork.** Also known as the pectinate ligament, this sponge-like tissue is interposed between the anterior chamber (and its contained aqueous humor) and the canal of Schlemm (Fig. 17–20). In meridional section, it is triangular, with the apex anteriorly and the base posteriorly, and is formed by trabeculae, or beams, with spaces between them through which aqueous humor drains to the canal of Schlemm. All trabeculae have a core of connective tissue in which there are ordinary collagen fibrils and "long-spacing" collagen with a periodicity of 105 to 124 nm, the core covered by endothelium. A few nerve endings of the supraciliary plexus are present in trabeculae.

All trabeculae arise anteriorly from the ring of Schwalbe, which marks the posterior extremity of Descemet's membrane, and from subjacent corneal lamellae and pass posterolaterally to attach to the root of the iris, the anterior surface (base) of the ciliary body, and the scleral spur. The innermost zone, or uveal meshwork, is formed by thin, delicate trabeculae, while the main, or scleral, meshwork consists of thicker, flattened, perforated bands of tissue. The external part, or endothelial meshwork, consists mainly of perforated sheets of endothelium with little supporting connective tissue, and it forms the inner wall of the canal of Schlemm, the pores within it connecting trabecular spaces with the lumen of the canal of Schlemm.

## The Refractive Media

The refractive media include all transparent structures through which light rays must pass to reach the retina. The cornea and anterior and posterior chambers already have been described, and the remaining components are the lens and the vitreous body.

### LENS

The crystalline lens is biconvex, with the posterior surface more highly curved than the anterior. The *axis* lies between anterior and posterior poles, and the peripheral circumferential border is called the *equator*. The lens inherently tends to become spherical but is flattened by tension in the zonule. The axis (thickness) normally is 3.6 mm, increasing to 4.5 mm in accommodation, with a diameter of about 9 mm.

*Figure 17–18.* Top: *Scanning electron micrograph of anterior surface of the iris showing an incomplete surface layer of fibroblasts (F), much flattened, with a nucleus (n) seen, resting on successive layers of melanocytes (M), and collagen fibrils (c) in the stroma.* × 900. Bottom: *Scanning electron micrograph of a freeze-fracture preparation of the iris stroma showing melanocytes with collagen fibrils (c). One melanocyte is fractured to show clearly the nucleus (n) and melanin granules (g) in its cytoplasm.* × 6700. *(Courtesy of Dr. D. H. Dickson and reproduced by kind permission of the editor, Canadian Journal of Ophthalmology).* Inset, lower right: *Melanocytes within the iris stroma.* × 900.

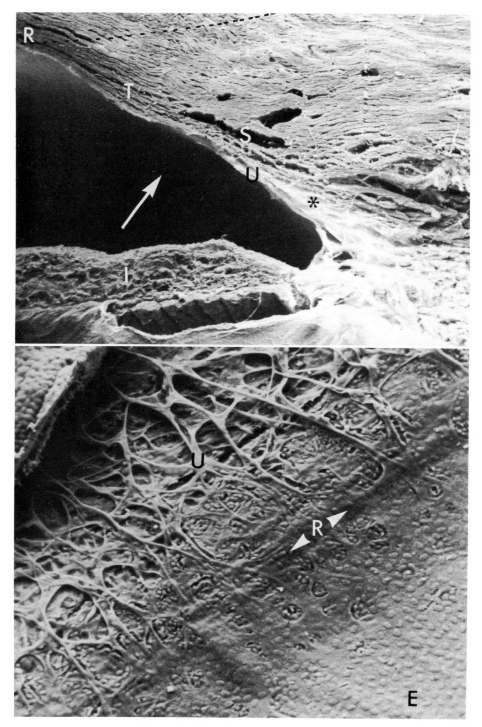

*Figure 17–19* See legend on opposite page

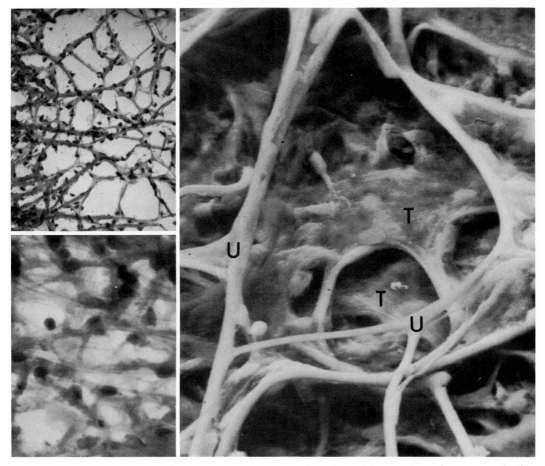

**Figure 17–20.** *Illustrations of the trabecular meshwork. Left: Photomicrographs of flat preparations showing, top, the thin cords of the uveal meshwork with trabeculae covered by endothelium and trabecular spaces between, and bottom, the scleral meshwork with flat, lamella-like trabeculae. Top,* × *225; bottom,* × *350. (Courtesy of J. Speakman.) Right: Scanning electron micrograph of the internal portion of the endothelium-covered trabecular meshwork with rope-like uveal trabeculae (U) and, more deeply, the flattened lamellae of the trabecular (scleral) (T) meshwork.* × *1000. (Courtesy of Drs. D. H. Dickson, N. Carroll, and G. W. Crock.)*

---

**Figure 17–19.** *Top: Low-power scanning electron micrograph of a meridional section through the limbus. (Compare with Figure 17–12, left.) The corneolimbal junction is outlined by the dotted line commencing internally at the ring of Schwalbe (R). The trabecular meshwork, with the rope-like uveal meshwork (U) and the deeper scleral or trabecular meshwork proper (T), separates aqueous humor in the anterior chamber from the canal of Schlemm (S). The scleral spur (asterisk) and the iris (I) are seen also.* × *100. (Courtesy of Dr. D. H. Dickson.) Bottom: Scanning electron micrograph of the internal surface of the limbus as it would appear when viewed in the direction of the arrow in the top figure, with corneal endothelium (E) at lower right, showing nuclei, which become wider apart (i.e., the endothelial cells are larger) at the periphery of the cornea.* × *180. (Courtesy of Drs. D. H. Dickson, N. Carroll, and G. W. Crock.)*

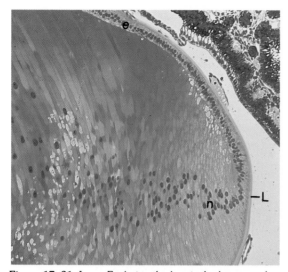

*Figure 17–21. Lens. Enclosing the lens is the lens capsule, a homogeneous and structureless membrane, thicker on the anterior surface (above). Beneath it on the anterior surface only is the subcapsular epithelium (e). This is simple cuboidal, but toward the equator (L), the cells become taller and transform into lens fibers. The lens fibers form the lens substance and are elongated in the shape of a six-sided prism, closely packed and concentrically arranged parallel to the surface. The younger, external fibers retain their nuclei (n), but they are lost from older cells of the inner nucleus. The lens is biconvex, more highly curved on the posterior surface, elastic, and avascular. Ciliary processes are seen at top right. H and E. Low power.*

The *lens* is covered by the *lens capsule*, about 10 μm thick on the anterior surface but only 5 to 6 μm thick on the posterior (Figs. 17–21 and 17–22). It is homogeneous, elastic, and rich in type IV collagen and proteoglycans, and attached to it are the zonular fibers that pass to the ciliary body as the suspensory ligament (Fig. 17–23). Beneath the capsule, on the anterior surface only, is the *subcapsular epithelium*, a single layer of cuboidal cells that have their bases lying externally in relation to the capsule. The cell apices lie internally and form junctional complexes with the lens fibers. Toward the equator, these capsular cells increase in height and transform into lens fibers, permitting growth of the lens by addition of these fibers. The *lens substance* itself is composed of *lens fibers*, each in the form of a hexagonal prism 8 to 10 mm long, 8 to 10 μm wide, and only 2 μm thick (Fig. 17–24). Most are parallel to the lens surface in a concentric arrangement. The younger, external fibers contain nuclei and a few organelles, but the central, older fibers lose their nuclei, the cytoplasm is homogeneous, and adjacent cells show a complex interlocking of cytoplasmic processes with abundant gap junctions and some spot desmosomes.

The lens is avascular, deriving its nutrition from

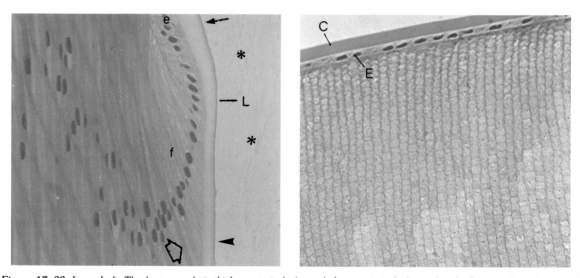

*Figure 17–22. Lens. Left: The lens capsule is thicker anteriorly (arrow) than posteriorly (arrowhead). Zonular fibers (asterisks) of the suspensory ligament appear as fine pink fibrils and attach to the capsule. At the equator (L), subcapsular epithelial cells (e) become taller and transform into lens fibers (f). Individual, elongated lens fibers can be seen (open arrow). Right: Lens fibers show a hexagonal pattern when cut transversely, accounting for the crystalline nature of the lens. No nuclei are seen. Anteriorly (above) is the lens epithelium (E) covered by lens capsule (C). Both, H and E. High power.*

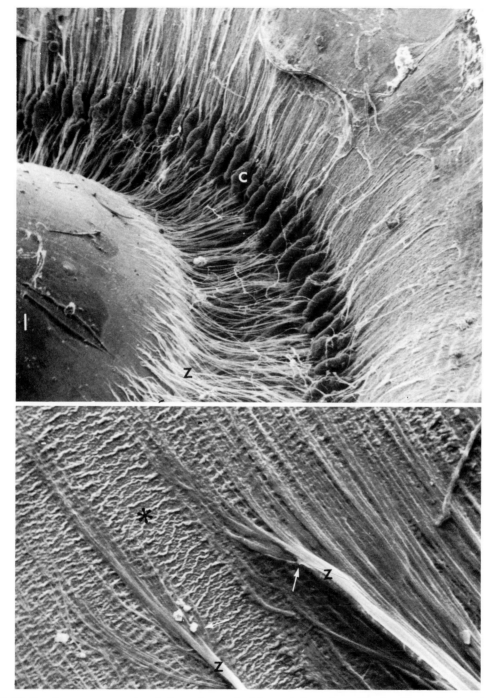

**Figure 17–23.** Top: *Low-power scanning electron micrograph of the posterior surface of the lens (l), zonula (z), and ciliary body (c), with zonular fibers passing from the region of the ora serrata (top right) and ciliary body to the posterior surface of the lens.* × 28. Bottom: *A higher magnification showing that zonular fibers (z), as they approach the lens, splay out (arrow) before contacting the lens capsule, which is crenated (asterisk) by tension of the zonular fibers.* × 660. (*Courtesy of Dr. D H. Dickson.*)

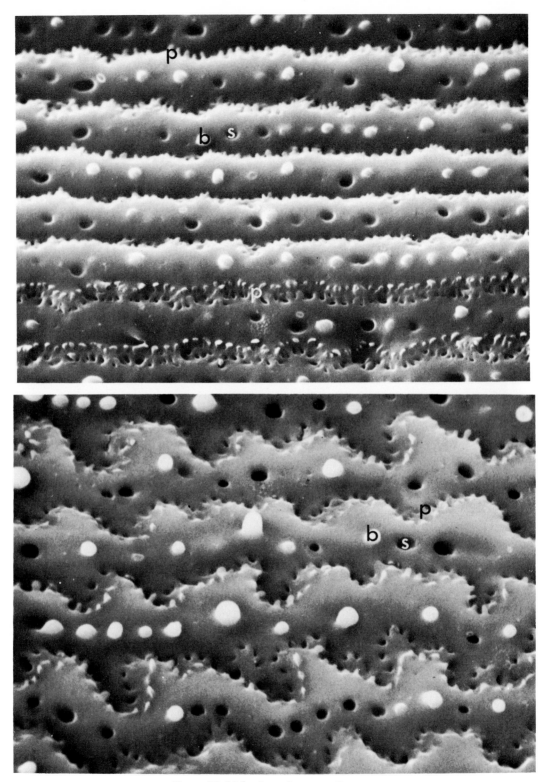

*Figure 17–24* See legend on opposite page

the aqueous humor. It is elastic and transparent. The theory is that transparency depends upon the impermeability of the plasmalemmae of the lens fibers to small ions. A change in permeability results in *cataract* formation, an opacity that results eventually in loss of vision. The lens becomes harder and loses elasticity with age.

The lens is held in place by the *suspensory ligament*, or *zonule*. This consists of zonular fibers or strands formed by bundles of hollow filaments 12 nm in diameter that pass from the ciliary body to the equator of the lens. They split into finer fibers that fuse with the lens capsule on anterior and posterior surfaces. The fine tubular filaments appear to be identical to the microfibrils of elastic tissue.

Light rays entering the eye are focused by the cornea and the lens, eventually to form an inverted, real, reduced image of the object on the photosensitive retina. Focusing is accomplished by alteration in the convexity of the lens. When the eye is at rest, the lens is flattened by elastic tension of the zonule. To focus on a near object, the ciliary muscle contracts, its meridional fibers pulling the choroid and ciliary body forward, the circular fibers narrowing the diameter of the eye at the ciliary body like a sphincter. This reduces tension in the zonule and permits the lens, which is elastic, to become more convex, increasing its refractive power.

### VITREOUS BODY

The vitreous body is a clear, transparent gel filling the space between the retina and the lens and, thus, is spheroidal, with an anterior depression to accommodate the lens. It adheres to the retina, particularly so at the ora serrata and around the optic disc. Nearly 99 per cent of the body is water, and it contains hyaluronic acid and collagen fibrils that lack the usual 64-nm periodicity, arranged in a fine network. These fibers are denser peripherally and around an anteroposterior, fluid-containing, tubular canal (the "hyaloid canal") that originally contained the embryonic hyaloid artery. A few cells are present: "hyalocytes," concerned in the synthesis and maintenance of collagen and hyaluronic acid, and a few macrophages.

The vitreous body maintains the shape and turgidity of the eye and, of course, permits passage of light rays to the retina.

### The Retina

The innermost layer of the eyeball, the retina, comprises an anterior, nonsensitive portion (ciliary and iridial epithelium, already described) and a posterior functional, or optical, portion, the photoreceptor organ. It develops as an evagination of the forebrain, the optic vesicle, that retains its connection to the brain by the optic stalk, the future optic nerve. The optic vesicle later becomes transformed into a bilayered optic cup, the outer layer becoming the pigment epithelium and the inner becoming the neural retina, or retina proper. A potential space remains between the two layers, and while the outer pigment layer is attached firmly to the choroid, the inner layer frequently detaches from the pigment layer during histological preparation. Such a split occurs also in life following trauma ("clinical detachment" of the retina).

The optical (neural) retina lines the choroid, from the papilla of the optic nerve posteriorly to the ora serrata anteriorly. It shows a shallow depression, the *fovea centralis*, about 2.5 mm to the temporal side of the optic papilla. Around the fovea is the *macula lutea* (yellow spot), an area containing a yellow pigment. The fresh retina is almost perfectly transparent when detached from its pigment epithelium, but reddish in color. Large blood vessels lie above and below the central area of the retina (fovea and macula), but only small capillaries are present in the fovea itself,

---

*Figure 17–24. Scanning electron micrographs of lens fibers. Top: The surface of cortical lens fibers (rat) close to the posterior pole of the lens, showing processes (p) of adjacent fibers that are closely interlocked. In addition, upper and lower surfaces of the fibers are held together by interlocking "ball (b) and socket (s)" processes. × 5200. Bottom: Outer surfaces of fibers close to the equator with similar interlocking but with the fibers in a zigzag arrangement. × 6000. (Courtesy of M. J. Hollenberg and B. J. Lewis).*

which increases its transparency. The fovea is the area of sharpest vision. Photoreceptors are absent from the optic papilla, this region being called the "blind spot."

### LAYERS OF THE RETINA

Excluding the fovea, optic papilla, and ora serrata, the retina in transverse section shows ten layers. From external to internal they are (Figs. 17–25 and 17–26):

1. Pigment epithelium
2. Layer of rods and cones
3. External limiting membrane
4. Outer nuclear layer
5. Outer plexiform layer
6. Inner nuclear layer
7. Inner plexiform layer
8. Ganglion cell layer
9. Optic nerve fiber layer
10. Internal limiting membrane

The complexity of this becomes simplified by appreciation of the fact that the retina is only three neurons deep. The first neuron, the photoreceptors (i.e., rods and cones), accounts for the outer layers, with each rod and cone having a sensory end organ (layer 2) lying outermost against pigment epithelium (layer 1), a nucleus

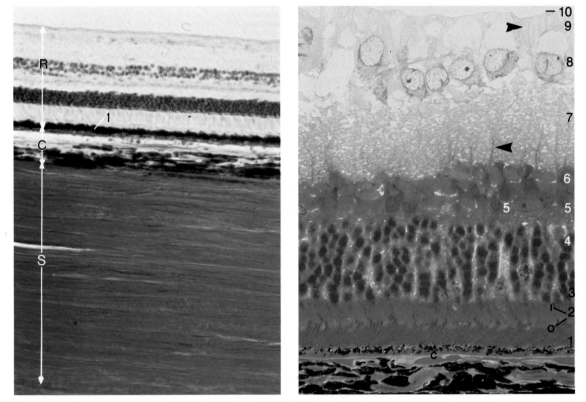

**Figure 17–25.** Left: The full thickness of the eyeball is seen. Externally is the sclera (S) and, internally, the choroid (C) with many blood vessels and melanocytes. This layer appears thinner than it is in life owing to collapse of the blood vessels. The nervous retina (R) shows a regular, layered appearance, with the pigment epithelium (1) most external. Mallory. Low power. Right: Below is the choroid with numerous melanocytes and the choriocapillaris (c) beneath the retina. All layers of the retina are seen: 1, pigment epithelium with melanin granules; 2, photoreceptors with outer (o) and inner (i) segments; 3, external limiting membrane; 4, outer nuclear layer; 5, outer plexiform layer; 6, inner nuclear layer; 7, inner plexiform layer; 8, ganglion cell layer; 9, optic nerve fiber layer; 10, internal limiting membrane. This is peripheral retina where photoreceptors are rods and with comparatively few ganglion cells, with a thin nerve fiber layer. The radially oriented cytoplasmic strands are Müller's supporting cells (arrowheads). Methylene blue, azure A, basic fuchsin. High power.

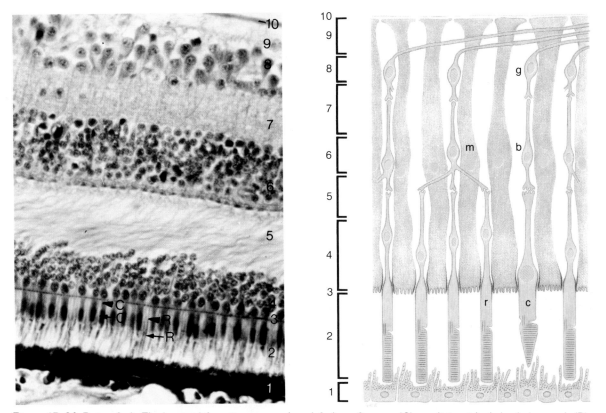

**Figure 17–26.** Retina. Left: *The layers of the retina are numbered. In layer 2, cones (C) are distinguished clearly from rods (R), rods being paler, thinner, and longer with inner (R, arrowhead) and outer (R, arrow) segments, whereas cones are thicker and darker, with inner (C, arrowhead) and outer (C, arrow) segments. Cone nuclei lie just internal to the internal limiting membrane (3), while rod nuclei are in several rows in layer 4. Iron hematoxylin. High power. Right: Diagram illustrating the layers of the retina. Only photoreceptors (rods, r; cone, c), direct conducting neurons (bipolar cells, b; ganglion cells, g) and cells of Müller (m) are illustrated.*

(in layer 4), and an inner terminal fiber passing to the outer plexiform layer (5) (Fig. 17–27). (Layer 3, the external limiting membrane, is formed by processes of supporting [Müller] cells.) The outer plexiform layer (5) is the site of junction (synapse) between the first and second neurons. The intermediate, or second, neurons have nuclei in the inner nuclear layer (6), together with nuclei of other cells (association and supporting), and, in turn, the inner plexiform layer (7) is the site of junction between the second and third neurons. Cell bodies of these third neurons, the ganglion cells, lie in layer 8 together with neuroglia, and their central processes (axons) pass to layer 9 as optic nerve fibers, all of which pass to the optic papilla and thence to the optic nerve. These fibers are unmyelinated but acquire a myelin sheath as

they exit through the cribriform plate at the optic papilla. The internal limiting membrane (layer 10) separates the retina from the vitreous body.

It should be recognized that the retina is gray matter of the central nervous system, while the optic nerve is white matter.

Layer 4, the outer nuclear layer, over most of the retina consists of a single outer row of cone nuclei with four rows of rod nuclei lying more centrally. At the fovea, where only cones are present, layer 4 is formed by several rows of cone nuclei (Fig. 17–28).

**Pigment Epithelium.** This is a single layer of polygonal cells, about 14 μm tall and 14 μm wide, and regular in shape: Cells become more flattened toward the ora serrata. Cell bases show complex interdigitating cell processes, typical of

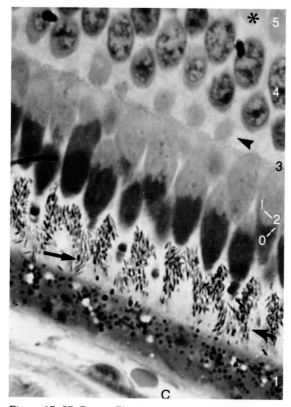

**Figure 17–27.** *Retina. This is squirrel retina, and only cones are present. In layer 2, the cones clearly show outer (dark, O) and inner (light, l) segments. Extending between outer segments are apical processes (arrows) of pigment epithelial cells containing melanin (brown) granules. The nuclei of the cones lie in several rows in layer 4, and also seen are outer cone fibers (arrowhead) and inner cone fibers (asterisk). Beneath the retina (below) are capillaries of the choriocapillaris (C). H and E. Oil immersion.*

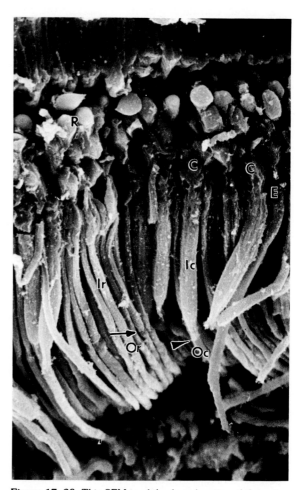

**Figure 17–28.** *This SEM is of the foveal region of the retina with nuclei of cones (C) and rods (R) in the outer nuclear layer (layer 4), with inner and outer segments of cones (Ic and Oc) and of rods (Ir and Or) and neck regions of cones (arrowhead) and rods (arrow). Also seen is the external limiting membrane (E). (SEM courtesy of Dr. Bessie Borwein.)*

actively transporting epithelia, and lateral interfaces show apical junctional complexes. The cell apices show cylindrical outfoldings that surround photoreceptor outer segments, with long microvilli between the photoreceptors. Nuclei are spherical and lie toward cell bases. Numerous mitochondria lie in basal cytoplasm and around nuclei, with a well-developed agranular reticulum, some granular reticulum, a Golgi apparatus, and some lipofuscin granules. Prominent also are numerous melanin granules and premelanosomes, and residual bodies containing lamellar debris resulting from phagocytosis of membrane lamellae of the external tips of the photoreceptor outer segments.

Functionally, the pigment epithelium absorbs light (by the pigment granules) and prevents reflection, is involved in the nutrition of photoreceptors and the turnover of their membrane lamellae, and is essential for the formation of rhodopsin and its movement by storing and releasing vitamin A, a rhodopsin precursor.

## NEURAL RETINA

Several cells are present and fall into four groups:

1. Photoreceptors (rods and cones).

2. Direct conducting neurons (bipolar and ganglion cells).

3. Association and other neurons (horizontal, amacrine, and centrifugal bipolar cells).

4. Supporting elements (Müller's cells and neuroglia).

**Photoreceptors.** Both rods and cones are modified neurons, each with inner and outer segments lying outside the external limiting membrane, an outer conducting fiber (physiologically a dendrite) passing to the cell body in the outer nuclear layer, and an inner conducting fiber (physiologically an axon) extending into the outer plexiform layer (Figs. 17–29 and 17–30). It must be appreciated that light must traverse the thickness of the retina to reach photoreceptors. (Note the inner layers are absent in the fovea, the area of most acute vision.)

*The Rod.* Rods are slender, specialized cells with cylindrical *outer* and *inner segments*, each 1.5 to 2 μm in diameter, the two segments connected by a narrow "neck" (Fig. 17–31). The outer segment is about 28 μm long, with its external tip "embedded" in pigment epithelium and showing transverse striations (Fig. 17–32). The inner segment is 32 μm long and divided into an outer "ellipsoid" containing many mitochondria and an inner "myoid" containing the Golgi apparatus, both granular and agranular reticulum, and glycogen. Microtubules are found in both ellipsoid and myoid.

By electron microscopy, the outer segment is seen to contain numerous (1000 or more) flattened membrane lamellae, or discs, stacked like a pile of pancakes. Each disc is formed by two parallel membranes about 6 nm thick, the two being continuous at the periphery of the disc, thus enclosing a cavity that is only 8 nm deep. These discs are separate from the surrounding plasma membrane and contain rhodopsin. The neck region is eccentrically placed and contains a modified cilium showing nine peripheral doublets (but no central singlets) originating in a basal body found in the ellipsoid of the inner segment.

Outer segments are renewed constantly. Protein is synthesized by ribosomes in the myoid and passes through the neck to the outer segment for incorporation into new membrane discs. As new lamellae are formed and added to the outer segment, the oldest lamellae at the tip are phagocytosed and destroyed by pigment epithelium cells, a cycle of total renewal occupying about ten days.

A rod proper is connected to its perikaryon (in the outer nuclear layer) by a slender *outer rod fiber* that traverses the external limiting membrane. From the perikaryon, an *inner rod fiber* passes into the outer plexiform layer to terminate in a small end knob, or *rod spherule*. This synaptic ending contains synaptic vesicles and a synaptic ribbon that appears as a dense plaque between vesicles. The spherule contacts dendrites of bipolar cells of the inner nuclear layer and is contacted by axons of horizontal cells.

*The Cone.* While similar in structure to rods, cones have a tapering outer segment that swells to a conical inner segment. Some lamellae of the outer segment, particularly the proximal (inner) ones, have membranes continuous with the covering plasma membrane, so their lumina are continuous with the extracellular space. Cone inner segments resemble those of rods, and inner and outer segments also are connected by an eccentric, modified cilium. The cone nucleus is larger than that of the rod, is less dense, and lies just internal to the external limiting membrane; thus, the *outer cone fiber* is short, the *inner cone fiber* is long. It also is thicker than that of the rod and terminates in the outer plexiform layer as a *cone pedicle*, from which short processes emerge (Fig. 17–33).

Cones vary in different regions of the retina. In the fovea, cones are long (75 μm) and slender (1 to 1.5 μm in diameter), but they are only 45 μm long in peripheral retina. In the fovea, nuclei lie in several rows in layer 4, and outer cone fibers are long. In peripheral retina, the cone nuclei lie in a single, outer row in the outer nuclear layer, and outer cone fibers are virtually absent, the myoid blending into the cell body. Turnover of cone discs is not continuous, as it is in rods, with new protein synthesized in the inner segment passing randomly to lamellae of the outer segment. Cones do not contain rhodopsin, but have pigments sensitive to blue, green, and red light. Cones in the fovea connect with a single bipolar cell.

There are estimated to be 130 million rods and 6 to 7 million cones in the human retina.

**Direct Conducting Neurons.** These include bipolar and ganglion cells, the second and third neurons of the three-neuron chain of the retina.

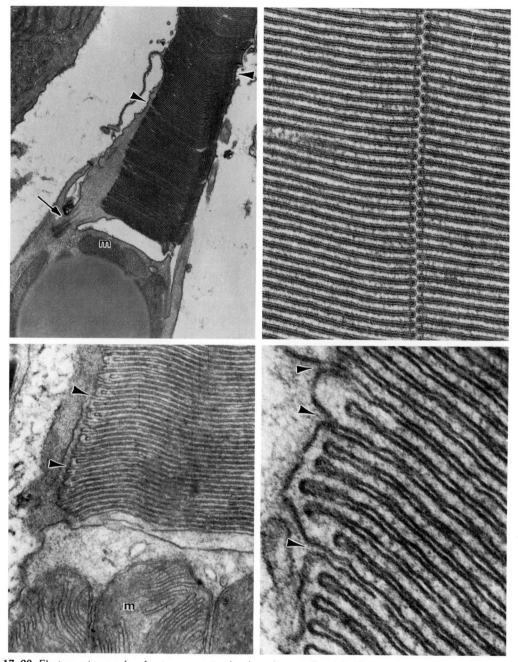

**Figure 17–29.** *Electron micrographs of outer segments of rods and cones.* Top left: *The junction of inner and outer segments of a frog rod with membrane lamellae or discs in the outer segment (above), the discs separate from the enclosing plasma membrane (arrowheads). Below is the inner segment with mitochondria (m), the two segments connected by a modified cilium (arrow).* Top right: *A higher magnification of frog rod outer segment showing the membrane discs. (These micrographs courtesy of Dr. J. Usukura.)* Bottom left: *The junction of inner (below) and outer (above) segments of a squirrel cone, some membrane lamellae appearing as infoldings of (i.e., continuous with) the covering plasmalemma (arrowheads).* Bottom right: *A higher magnification showing continuity of membrane lamellae with the plasmalemma.* Top left, × 18,000; top right, × 85,000, bottom left, × 32,000; bottom right, × 92,000.

**Bipolar Cells.** Perikarya of bipolar cells lie mainly in the central zone of the inner nuclear layer, with two main groups:

1. *Diffuse* bipolars contacting several photoreceptors.

2. *Midget* (monosynaptic) bipolars contacting a single cone.

Dendrites of diffuse bipolars pass to the outer plexiform layer, where they branch and contact several rod spherules or groups of about six cone pedicles. The single axon passes vertically into the inner plexiform layer to contact dendrites of ganglion cells. The midget bipolar synapses with a single cone pedicle, and its axon synapses with a single midget ganglion cell, thus providing a one-to-one pathway from cone to optic nerve fiber.

**Ganglion Cells.** Cell bodies lie in layer 8, with their dendrites in the inner plexiform layer and their axons, which never branch, constituting the optic nerve fibers (layer 9). They are large cells showing prominent Nissl bodies and are of two main types:

1. *Diffuse* cells, their dendrites contacting several bipolar cells.

2. *Midget* (monosynaptic), their dendrites synapsing with a single, midget (cone) bipolar cell.

## Association and Centrifugal Neurons

**Horizontal Cells.** Perikarya of horizontal cells lie in the outer portion of the inner nuclear layer and are somewhat larger than those of bipolar cells. Dendrites terminate in cup-like baskets around cone pedicles, while a single axon branches into an elaborate telodendron to synapse with both rod spherules and cone pedicles, all in the outer plexiform layer. Thus, the horizontal cells laterally connect cones in one area with rods and cones in another area, perhaps affecting the functional threshold between rods and cones and bipolar cells.

**Amacrine Cells.** Perikarya are pear-shaped and lie in the inner portion of the inner nuclear layer. A single process passes inward to the inner plexiform layer and branches extensively to connect with the axonal endings of bipolar cells and the dendritic branches of ganglion cells.

**Supporting Elements.** As in the brain, the retina has an elaborate framework of neuroglia for support, insulation, and nutrition. There is a main network of Müller's fibers with astroglia, perivascular glia, and microglia.

**Müller's Cells.** Also called *retinal gliocytes*, these cells are giant in size, their nuclei located in the inner nuclear layer and with thin cytoplasmic processes extending to both inner and outer limiting membranes (i.e., they extend for nearly the full thickness of the retina) (Fig. 17–34). From these processes, sheet-like extensions wrap around photoreceptors and bipolar and ganglion cells, permitting little in the way of intercellular spaces. At the inner limiting membrane, broad, foot-like processes abut against the membrane, and externally, processes meet rods and cones at zonulae adherentes to form the external limiting membrane.

In addition, there are neuroglial cells, with spongioblasts prominent in the inner nuclear layer and astrocytes in ganglion cell, inner and outer plexiform layers. Astrocytes are numerous in the optic nerve and the region of the disc, and phagocytic microglia are found in all layers.

**Limiting Membranes.** The internal limiting membrane is simply the basal lamina of the Müller's cells, separating retina from the vitreous. The external limiting membrane is not a true membrane but is, in a section, a row of zonulae adherentes between Müller's cell processes and photoreceptors. It is perforate in the sense that photoreceptors traverse it, and, in this region, there are tufts of microvilli extending from the Müller's cell processes between the photoreceptors.

### SPECIALIZED AREAS OF THE RETINA

**Central Area and Fovea.** The distinction between the central area and the remainder of the retina is both structural and functional. The central area has a high concentration of photoreceptors and is specialized for accurate diurnal vision, whereas the peripheral area is of coarser structure and is more suitable for reception of weak stimuli in dim illumination.

Morphologically, there is an accumulation of ganglion cells in more than one row and a density of cones and bipolar cells in the central area. The *macula lutea* is a vague area, characterized by the presence of a yellow pigment in the inner layers, about 3 mm in diameter, that surrounds the fovea.

The *fovea centralis* is pale, lacking pigment and with few blood vessels, and is in the form of a

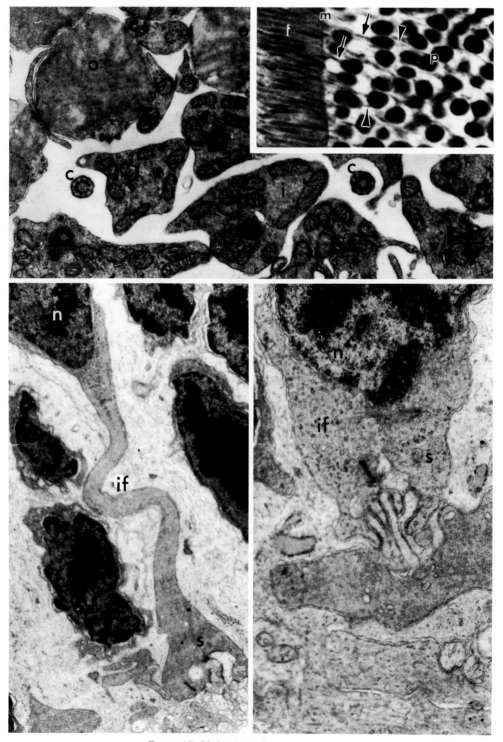

*Figure 17–30* See legend on opposite page

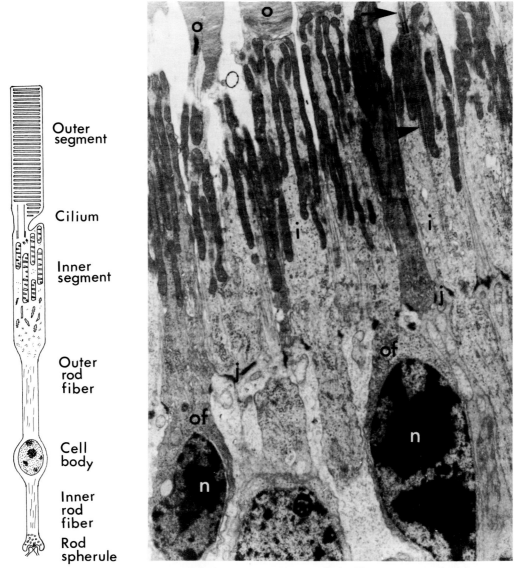

Outer
segment

Cilium

Inner
segment

Outer
rod
fiber

Cell
body

Inner
rod
fiber

Rod
spherule

**Figure 17–31.** Left: *Diagram of a rod as seen with the electron microscope.* Right: *Electron micrograph of the outer portion of rods showing outer segments (o); a connecting cilium in a neck region (arrow); inner segments (i), one showing a striated rootlet of a cilium (arrowhead); the external limiting membrane and its junctional complexes (j); outer rod fibers (of); and rod nuclei (n).* × *4500.*

---

**Figure 17–30.** Top inset: *Photomicrograph showing external limiting membrane (m) with inner segments (i) of rods, outer rod fibers (arrows), rod perikarya (p), and inner rod fibers (arrowheads).* × *900. The electron micrographs illustrate features of rods. Top: A transverse section showing outer segments (o) with membrane lamellae en face, inner segments (i), and neck regions with cilia (c). Bottom left: The central region of a rod showing nucleus (n), inner rod fiber (if), and rod spherule (s) in the outer plexiform layer. Bottom right: A rod nucleus (n) lying centrally in the outer nuclear layer has a short inner fiber (if) passing to a spherule (s). Note the dark, synaptic "ribbons" in spherules.* Top, × *8000; bottom left,* × *4500; bottom right,* × *18,000.*

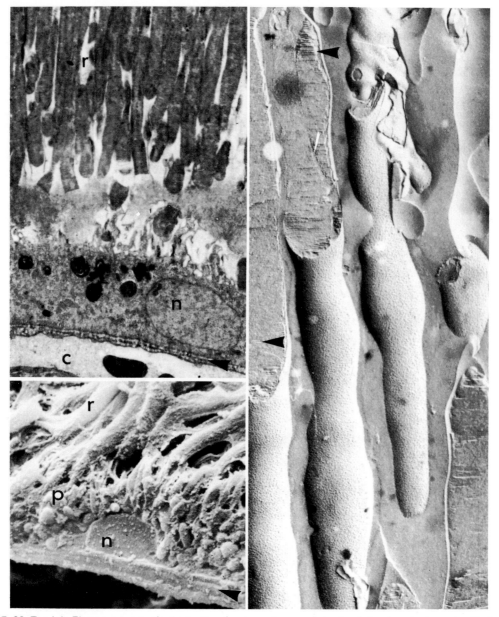

*Figure 17–32.* Top left: *Electron micrograph of rat retina showing outer segments of rods (r, above), pigment epithelium with a nucleus (n), Bruch's membrane (arrowhead) and choriocapillaris (c).* × *3500. Bottom left: A similar area in a freeze-fracture scanning electron micrograph, with pigment granules (p) in the cytoplasm of the pigment epithelial cell.* × *5000. (Courtesy of Dr. D. H. Dickson.) Right: Freeze-etch preparation of rod outer segments showing internal membrane lamellae (arrowheads).* × *12,500.*

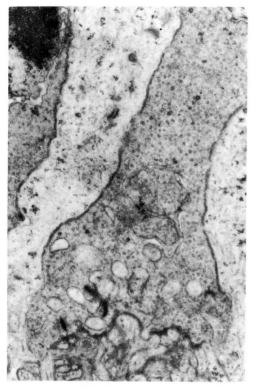

*Figure 17–33.* Electron micrograph of cone pedicle: note the dark, linear bodies (synaptic ribbons) in the pedicle. × 20,000.

shallow rounded pit, 2 to 2.5 mm on the temporal side of the optic disc (i.e., at the visual axis) (Fig. 17–35). The depression results from the absence of the inner layers of the retina in this region and is about 1.5 mm in diameter. Its *fundus*, or floor, is only 550 μm in diameter and contains 30,000 cones that are thinner and longer than elsewhere (i.e., not cone-shaped), and the area lacks rods. These cones synapse with bipolar cells placed obliquely around the margins of the fovea, which has no capillaries. This arrangement permits free passage of light rays to the photoreceptors.

**Optic Disc and Papilla.** The retinal aspect of the optic nerve is called the *optic disc*, which includes the *optic papilla*, this slight protrusion being formed by the heaping up of nerve fibers as they pass from the retina into the optic nerve. The disc is 1.5 mm in diameter and slightly oval and is situated to the nasal side of the posterior pole. With the exception of the optic nerve fibers,

all retinal tissues cease abruptly at the margin of the disc. The absence of photoreceptors accounts for the term "blind spot." As the optic nerve fibers perforate sclera to pass into the optic nerve, they do so through the lamina cribrosa, the dense fibrous plate that is perforated by bundles of optic nerve fibers. At its periphery, the lamina cribrosa is continuous with scleral tissue.

In the optic disc is a small central depression, the "physiological cup," through which the central artery and vein of the retina emerge. In most cases, the central artery is the sole arterial supply to the retina, and its occlusion leads to permanent blindness. In a few individuals, the retina also has a blood supply to the macula from the cilioretinal artery.

**Optic Nerve.** This is not a peripheral nerve but a tract of the central nervous system between retinal ganglion cells and the midbrain (Fig. 17–36). The nerve contains more than a thousand nerve bundles supported by astrocytes (neuroglia, not endoneurium) and passes posteriorly to the optic chiasma. Meninges, with subarachnoid space, pass from the brain as sheaths of the optic nerve. While most fibers in the optic nerve are afferent fibers from retinal photoreceptors, there also are fibers passing to the tectum for pupillary reflexes and to the superior colliculus, a few autonomic fibers, and some efferent fibers of unknown function passing to the retina. The central artery and vein enter the optic nerve at some distance posterior to the eyeball and pass forward to the retina.

### Accessory Organs of the Eye

The eyeball lies in the bony orbit, open anteriorly. The opening can be closed by opposition of the eyelids, which meet at the *palpebral fissure.* The *conjunctiva* is reflected from the corneal perimeter to line the deep surface of the eyelids, the reflections being termed the superior and inferior *fornices.* With the eyelids closed, the conjunctival sac is a closed space anterior to the eyeball and contains a small amount of fluid.

#### EYELIDS

Each eyelid has a core of connective tissue and skeletal muscle covered externally by skin and

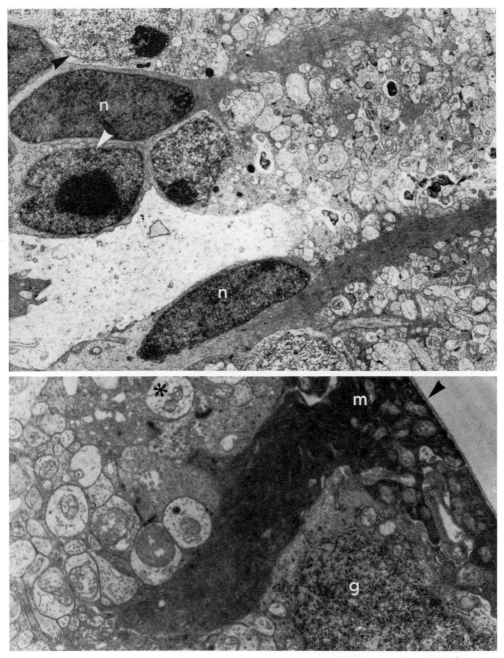

**Figure 17–34.** *Electron micrographs of the deeper portion of the retina showing Müller's cells. Top: Müller's cell nuclei (n) lie in the inner nuclear layer with nuclei of bipolar cells (arrowheads), with processes passing to the right (centrally) in the inner plexiform layer. Bottom: A Müller's cell process (m) abuts against the internal limiting membrane (arrowhead) with the nucleus of a ganglion cell (g) and nerve fibers (asterisk) of the optic nerve fiber layer. Top, × 5000; bottom, × 12,500.*

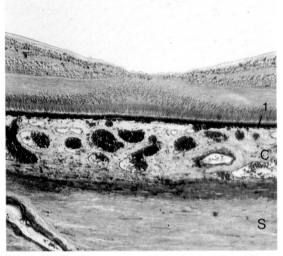

**Figure 17–35.** *Fovea centralis. Below is the sclera (S), traversed by a large blood vessel (left) with the choroid (C) internal (above) to it. Internally is the retina, here specialized as the fovea centralis. In this region, the pigment epithelium (1) is seen associated with very many modified, elongated cones in layer 2, but the inner layers of the retina, from outer plexiform to optic nerve fiber layer, are virtually absent, leaving a shallow surface pit or depression. The elongated cones synapse with bipolar cells located at the margin of the fovea, and thus, their inner core fibers slant out to the margin. The fovea is the area of maximal visual acuity. Iron hematoxylin. Low power.*

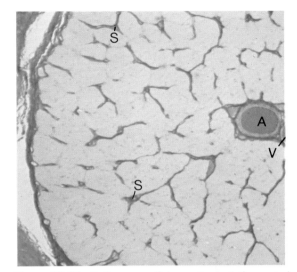

**Figure 17–36.** *Optic nerve. Being a tract of the central nervous system and not a true peripheral nerve, the optic nerve is covered by meninges (blue) that blend with the sclera at the eyeball. Passing into the nerve from the surrounding pia mater are septa carrying blood vessels, the septa (S) dividing the nerve into bundles. Located centrally are profiles of the central artery (A) and vein (V) of the retina. Mallory. Low power.*

internally by a mucous membrane (Fig. 17–37). The skin is thin, with small hairs, sweat and sebaceous glands, and a relatively delicate dermis rich in elastic fibers. At each lid margin, the dermis is more dense and contains three or four rows of long, stiff hairs, the *eyelashes.* Between and behind the eyelashes are large, modified sweat glands (the glands of Moll), characterized by straight and not coiled terminal ducts that open into the hair follicles.

Beneath the skin is a layer of striated muscle, the palpebral part of the orbicularis oculi muscle with, in the upper lid, fibers of insertion of the levator palpebrae superioris muscle. Also present are slips of smooth muscle, the palpebral muscles (of Müller).

Deep to the muscle is a fibrous layer of the septum orbitale, thin peripherally but thickened centrally as the *tarsal plates.* The plates are curved to the convexity of the eyeball, the upper plate being D-shaped and 10 to 12 mm broad, with its lower border coextensive with the lid margin. The lower plate is narrow, only 5 mm broad, and is located in the central region of the lid. In each tarsal plate is a single row of very large sebaceous glands, the *tarsal (Meibomian) glands.* Their ducts open at the lid margin, with many lateral branches from the main duct draining single or multiple secretory alveoli. The deep posterior surface of each tarsal plate blends with conjunctiva.

### CONJUNCTIVA

This mucous membrane is continuous with skin at the margins of the eyelids and with corneal epithelium at the periphery of the cornea, lining the inner surface of the eyelids from which it is reflected onto the anterior surface of the eyeball (Fig. 17–38).

The conjunctival epithelium varies with location. It consists of a basal layer of cuboidal cells, a surface layer of taller cone- or cylinder-shaped cells, and, particularly on the lower lid, one to three intermediate layers of polygonal cells. Mucus-secreting goblet cells are scattered among the epithelial cells. At the corneal margin, the con-

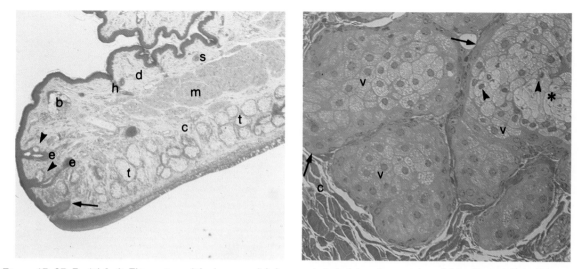

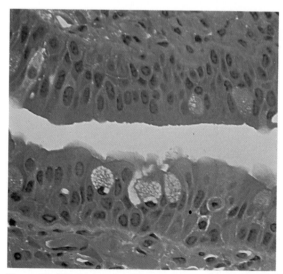

*Figure 17–37.* Eyelid. Left: This section of the lower eyelid shows anteriorly (above) a covering of thin skin with hairs (h), sweat (s) and sebaceous (b) glands, and a dermis (d) of delicate connective tissue. At the lid margin (left), there are two rows of long stiff hairs, the eyelashes (e), with associated sebaceous glands (arrowheads). In the core of the eyelid is striated muscle (m) of the orbicularis oculi and, behind it, dense connective tissue (c) of the septum orbitale, thickened as the tarsal plate (not seen here). In this layer is a single row of tarsal (Meibomian) glands (t), opening by ducts (arrow) at the lid margin. Posteriorly (below), the internal surface is lined by conjunctiva. H and E. Low power. Right: The secretory alveoli or saccules of tarsal glands have a peripheral single row of low cuboidal cells (arrows), in which mitoses occur, and as the cells pass to the center of an aveolus, they accumulate lipid, become vacuolated (v), and increase in size. Eventually, the entire cell breaks down (asterisk) to form the secretory material, a process of holocrine secretion. Nuclei of dying cells are pyknotic (arrowheads). H and E. High power.

*Figure 17–38.* Conjunctiva. The conjunctiva shows a stratified epithelium with a basal layer of cuboidal cells, two or three layers of polygonal cells, and a surface layer of cone- or cylinder-shaped cells. Scattered among the cells are mucus-secreting goblet cells (pale, foamy cytoplasm). The epithelium is supported by a lamina propria, and at the lid margins and corneal margin, the conjunctiva blends into skin and corneal epithelium, respectively. H and E. High power.

junctival epithelium becomes stratified squamous in type, identical to and continuous with the corneal epithelium. Supporting the epithelium is a lamina propria, relatively fine superficially and with numerous lymphocytes, and more dense externally. In the fornices, the lamina propria is attached loosely to intraorbital fat to permit free movement of the eyeball in the conjunctival sac.

### THE LACRIMAL APPARATUS

The conjunctival sac contains fluid, the tears, formed by lacrimal glands whose ducts pass into the sac, with a drainage duct passing from the sac into the nasal cavity.

The main lacrimal gland is located just within the orbital margin at its superolateral corner, just external to the conjunctiva of the superior fornix and in relation to the tendon of levator palpebrae superioris (Fig. 17–39). It is a tubuloacinar serous gland with prominent myoepithelial cells and is almond-sized. Some 10 to 15 excretory ducts drain separate lobes of the gland into the lateral part of the superior fornix. Numerous accessory

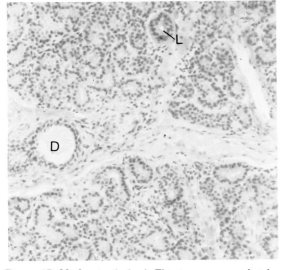

**Figure 17–39.** *Lacrimal gland. This is a compound, tubuloalveolar serous gland. Portions of several lobules are seen here with an interlobular duct (D) located in an interlobular septum and an intralobular duct (L) surrounded by acini. In association with acini, myoepithelial cells are prominent (not seen here). H and E. Medium power.*

lacrimal glands lie in the lamina propria of upper and lower eyelids.

Tears, the sterile secretion of the lacrimal glands, function to keep the conjunctival and corneal epithelia moist and to wash out foreign matter (e.g., dust particles). Blinking of the eyelids spreads fluid over the cornea like windshield wipers, and excessive evaporation is prevented by a film of mucus (from conjunctival goblet cells) and a film of oil (from tarsal glands). Excess tears pass medially to the medial corner of the conjunctival sac, the lacus lacrimalis, and then into the lacrimal canaliculi. These commence at minute orifices, one in each eyelid medially (the lacrimal puncta), and pass to the lacrimal sac located in the medial corner of the eye, whence excess tears pass down the nasolacrimal duct to drain into the inferior meatus of the nose.

### Functions of the Eye

Essentially, the eye is a camera obscura, with the refractive media of cornea, aqueous humor, lens, and vitreous body. Light rays are refracted by the cornea and converge on the lens, where

they are refracted further and focused on the photoreceptors.

In the retina, quanta of light are transduced by the photoreceptors into nerve signals that eventually reach the brain via the optic nerve. The process of transduction involves a photochemical reaction between light and one of the visual pigments located in the lamellae of outer segments, a change in the plasma membrane permeability, and hyperpolarization of the photoreceptor. The pigment of rods is rhodopsin, the rods functioning in dim illumination. Cones are active under diurnal conditions and consist of three types sensitive to red, blue, or green light. Visual pigments are a combination of vitamin A aldehyde and an opsin (protein). With exposure to light, these pigments undergo a change in form that results in depolarization of the receptor cell membranes and the formation of an action potential, which then is conducted by a series of neurons (including bipolar and ganglion cells) to the brain. As indicated, rods are used for dim light perception, containing more photopigment and being more photosensitive than cones. Cones are less photosensitive and are used for color perception and, with fewer interneuronal connections, for fine visual acuity. Hence, only cones are present in the fovea centralis.

### THE EAR

The ear morphologically is divided into the *external ear*, which receives sound waves, the *middle ear*, where sound waves are changed to mechanical vibrations of the small bones contained in the middle ear cavity, and the *internal ear*, where the vibrations stimulate receptor cells (Fig. 17–40). From these receptor cells, nerve impulses are conveyed by the eighth cranial (acoustic) nerve to the brain. Additionally, the inner ear also contains the vestibular organ, which maintains balance and equilibrium.

### The External Ear

The external ear comprises the auricle (the visible appendage), the external auditory meatus

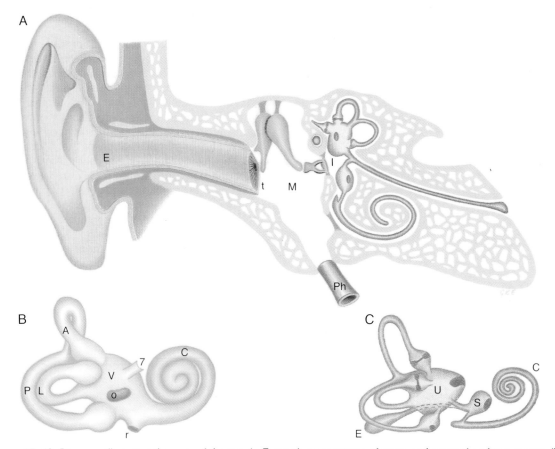

**Figure 17–40.** *Diagrams illustrating the parts of the ear. A: External ear consisting of pinna and external auditory meatus (E); middle ear (M), separated from the external ear by the tympanic membrane (t) and traversed by the three ossicles (malleus, incus, and stapes); and internal ear (i). The pharyngotympanic (eustachian) tube (Ph) extends inferomedially from the middle ear. B: Right osseous, or bony, labyrinth viewed from the lateral side. Anterior (A), posterior (P), and lateral (L) semicircular canals, vestibule (V), and cochlea (C) are shown. The oval (o) and round (r) windows and the canal for the facial nerve (7) also can be seen. C: Membranous labyrinth with semicircular canals, utricle (U), saccule (S), cochlear duct (C), and endolymphatic sac (E) and duct. Neuroepithelial (sensory) areas are indicated in black.*

that passes into the temporal bone, and the tympanic membrane (eardrum).

**Auricle.** The characteristic shape of the auricle is due to a plate of elastic cartilage, 0.5 to 1 mm thick, covered by a perichondrium with a high content of elastic fibers (Fig. 17–41). All surfaces are covered by thin skin in which hairs and sweat glands are present but poorly developed. In the subcutaneous tissue are thin slips of striated muscle, vestigial in humans but more prominent in lower animals that are capable of ear movements.

**External Auditory Meatus.** This canal extends from the auricle to the tympanic membrane. It is oval in section and permanently patent, with a wall of elastic cartilage (continuous with that of the auricle) in the outer third and bone (of the temporal bone) in the inner two thirds. Thin skin with no subcutaneous tissue lines the canal, the dermis blending with perichondrium or periosteum. Numerous hairs associated with sebaceous glands are present in the outer portion, with small hairs and sebaceous glands in the roof only of the inner portion. Also present are *ceruminous glands*, which are large, modified, coiled, tubular sweat glands, their ducts opening directly onto the skin surface or with sebaceous glands into the

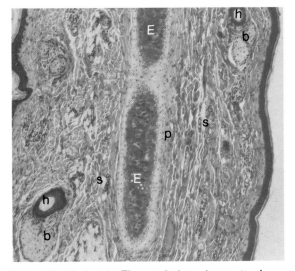

**Figure 17–41.** *Auricle. The auricle (pinna) owes its characteristic shape to a central plate of elastic cartilage (E) here cut near its edge, and with a perichondrium (p) in which elastic fibers are predominant. On external and internal surfaces, it is covered with thin skin, in the dermis of which are hairs (h) and sweat (s) and sebaceous (b) glands. H and E. Low power.*

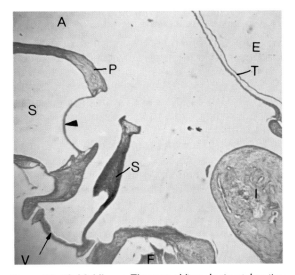

**Figure 17–42.** *Middle ear. This is an oblique horizontal section of the right middle ear cavity, seen from above. At top right is the deepest part of the external auditory meatus (E) extending to the tympanic membrane (T), the tympanic membrane forming the lateral wall of the middle ear cavity. Anteriorly, the cavity is continuous with the pharyngotympanic tube (A). Posteriorly is the head of the incus bone (I) and, medially, the stapes (S) shows a base plate (arrow) occupying the fenestra ovalis. Also in the medial wall is the promontory (P, formed by the basal turn of the cochlea) and the fenestra rotunda, closed by the secondary tympanic membrane (arrowhead). Just posterior to the fenestra ovalis is the canal for the facial (VIIth) nerve (F). In the inner ear (left) are perilymph-filled spaces of the scala tympani (V) and the scala vestibuli (S). H and E. Low power.*

necks of hair follicles. *Cerumen*, found in the external meatus, is a brown waxy material, bitter to the taste and protective in function. It is the combined secretion of ceruminous and sebaceous glands.

**Tympanic Membrane.** This membrane closes the innermost extremity of the external meatus. It is oval and lies obliquely, with a core of connective tissue formed by external radial and internal circular fibers. Externally, it is covered by very thin skin, internally by a cuboidal epithelium of the mucosa of the middle meatus. Attached to its internal surface is the malleus (one of the ossicles), the handle of which extends to the center of the membrane and causes it to bulge into the middle ear cavity. The upper portion of the membrane lacks collagenous fibers and is called the flaccid part (Shrapnell's membrane).

### The Middle Ear

The middle ear is a cleft-like cavity in the temporal bone, the *tympanic cavity,* with a canal or duct, the *auditory (Eustachian) tube,* that connects it with the nasopharynx (Fig. 17–42).

**Tympanic Cavity.** This is a flat, box-like air space, about 1.3 cm high, the same in length, but only 2 to 3 mm transversely. The lateral wall is formed by the tympanic membrane, the medial wall by the inner ear. The bony roof separates it from the middle cranial fossa and temporal lobe of the brain, the floor from the retropharyngeal area. The narrow posterior wall opens into a smaller space, the tympanic antrum, into which open the mastoid air cells, and the anterior wall extends forward as the auditory (pharyngotympanic) tube. The cavity is lined by an epithelium that is simple squamous or low cuboidal with a thin lamina propria blending with periosteum.

The cavity contains the three ossicles, formed of compact bone without a marrow cavity. These form an articulated chain with the *malleus* laterally attached to the tympanic membrane, the footplate of the *stapes* attached by a fibrous joint to the oval window (fenestra ovalis) in the medial wall, and the *incus* lying between them. Both the malleus and the incus are suspended by tiny ligaments from the roof, and between the three ossicles are two synovial joints. The thin periosteum of each ossicle blends with the thin lamina propria beneath the squamous or low cuboidal epithelium lining the cavity.

Two small muscles are associated with the ossicles. Lying in a canal above the auditory tube is the tensor tympani muscle. Its tendon first passes posteriorly and then hooks around a small bony projection to cross the tympanic cavity from medial to lateral walls to insert into the handle of the malleus. The stapedius muscle lies posteriorly, and its tendon passes forward to insert into the neck of the stapes. The two muscles are believed to be "protective," dampening high-frequency vibrations.

The oval window in the medial wall is occupied by the base plate of the stapes, which separates the tympanic cavity from the scala vestibuli of the cochlea, the latter filled with perilymph. The arrangements thus permit vibrations of the tympanic membrane to be transmitted via the chain of ossicles to perilymph of the inner ear. However, the perilymph spaces are closed, and fluid is incompressible, so a "safety valve" is required. This is the fenestra rotunda (round window) lying in the medial wall, below and behind the oval window and closed by an elastic membrane (the secondary tympanic membrane) that separates the tympanic cavity from perilymph in the scala tympani of the cochlea.

**Auditory (Eustachian) Tube.** This connects the tympanic cavity and the nasopharynx. It is about 3.5 cm long, the posterior third having a bony wall and the anterior two thirds a wall of cartilage. The lining epithelium varies from ciliated columnar posteriorly near the tympanic cavity to pseudostratified ciliated columnar with goblet cells near the pharynx, where the lamina propria also contains seromucous glands. Usually, medial and lateral walls are in contact to occlude the lumen, but, by the act of swallowing, the walls are separated, opening the lumen and allowing air to enter or leave the middle ear cavity to equalize pressure on both sides of the tympanic membrane.

## The Inner Ear

Within the petrous part of the temporal bone is a system of cavities and canals called the *osseous labyrinth*, within which is a similar, membrane-bound labyrinth, the *membranous labyrinth*. The osseous labyrinth is filled with *perilymph*, and the membranous labyrinth with *endolymph*, the two fluids separated by the wall of the membranous labyrinth.

### OSSEOUS LABYRINTH

The *vestibule* lies centrally, medial to the tympanic cavity, with the wall between the two perforated by the fenestrae ovalis and rotunda. Opening into the posterior part of the vestibule are three *semicircular canals*, named anterior, posterior, and lateral, each being at right angles to the others (Fig. 17–43). The two lateral canals of right and left ears are in the same plane, and the anterior of one is parallel to the posterior canal of the other side. Each canal has a dilation, or *ampulla*, at one end: Those of the anterior and lateral canals lie adjacent to each other above the fenestra ovalis, that of the posterior canal opens into the posterior part of the vestibule. Although there are three canals, there are only five and not six openings into the vestibule, the nonampullated ends of posterior and anterior canals opening into the medial part of the vestibule by a common opening, the *crus commune*.

Anteriorly, the vestibule is continuous with the bony *cochlea*, a tube that spirals like a snail shell for 2¾ turns. Its total shape is conical, with a base 9 mm in diameter, and a height from base to apex of 5 mm. The axial bony stem, the *modiolus*, is oriented across the long axis of the petrous temporal bone, the base facing the posterior cranial fossa and the apex pointing forward and laterally. A shelf of bone, the *spiral lamina*, projects from the modiolus like the thread of a screw.

The term "osseous labyrinth" may be confusing; it is *not* a separate bone but simply a system of canals and cavities within the temporal bone.

### MEMBRANOUS LABYRINTH

The membranous labyrinth is lined by epithelium, is filled with endolymph, and lies within the

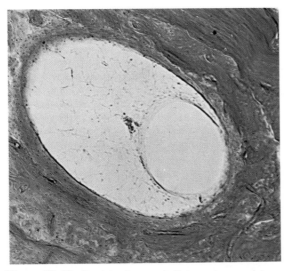

*Figure 17–43. Semicircular canal. Petrous temporal bone contains the three semicircular canals. Within the bony, or osseous, canal is the canal of the membranous labyrinth, placed eccentrically (right), lined by a thin epithelium, and containing endolymph. Thin connective tissue trabeculae traverse the space between bony and membranous labyrinths, the space being filled with perilymph. H and E. Medium power.*

osseous labyrinth. In a few places, the wall of the membranous labyrinth is adherent to periosteum lining the osseous labyrinth but, in general, lies free with perilymph between it and periosteum, although strands of connective tissue containing blood vessels do cross the perilymph space to suspend the membranous labyrinth within the osseous labyrinth.

The general form of the membranous labyrinth is similar to that of the osseous labyrinth with the exception that the vestibule is occupied by two chambers and not one. Posteriorly is the *utricle*, which communicates by five openings with the three membranous semicircular canals, each with a large ampulla. Anteriorly is the *saccule*, nearly spherical and joined to the utricle by a slim Y-shaped tube, the short stems being the utricular and saccular ducts, which join to form the *endolymphatic duct*. This duct passes posteroinferiorly to the posterior surface of the petrous bone to terminate as a blind sac, the *endolymphatic sac*. Anteriorly lies the spiral *cochlear duct*, which communicates with the lower part of the saccule via the short, slender *ductus reuniens*.

Sensory nerve endings lie in the ampullae of the semicircular canals (*the cristae ampullares*) and in the utricle and saccule (*maculae utriculi* and *sacculi*), these subserving static and kinetic senses (Fig. 17–44). The *organ of Corti*, the organ of hearing, lies along the length of the cochlear duct.

The wall of the membranous labyrinth is delicate connective tissue with some fibroblasts and melanocytes, lined by simple squamous epithelium supported by a basal lamina. The sensory areas are specialized.

**Cristae and Maculae.** In the ampulla of each semicircular canal the epithelium is raised into a transverse ridge, the *crista*, covered by sensory epithelium and oriented across the long axis of the duct. In the lateral wall of the utricle and in the medial wall of the saccule are the two *maculae*, each ovoid and 2 to 3 mm in diameter. The two are perpendicular to each other and are formed by three cell types similar to those forming cristae ampullares (Fig. 17–45). These cell types are supporting (sustentacular) cells, and hair cells of two types (Fig. 17–46).

The *type I hair cell* is piriform or flask-shaped, with a nucleus in the globular base and a short neck. The *type II hair cell* is cylindrical, with nuclei at various levels but usually lying in a row placed toward the lumen. In both types, apically there is a sensory hair bundle formed by a single cilium and 30 to 100 hairs or stereocilia. These are constricted at their bases and have a core of fine filaments that extend into apical cytoplasm to become embedded in a prominent, thickened terminal web (cuticular plate). The hairs lie in a regular hexagonal pattern and, at one surface, are only 1 μm long but increase progressively to 100 μm in length on the opposite surface, where the cilium originates from a basal body. This cilium has the regular 9 + 2 pattern of microtubules but is thought to be nonmotile and is called a *kinocilium*. The synaptic contacts with terminal vestibular nerve fibers differ in the two types of hair cells. In type I, the afferent nerve ending shows a cup-like ending with synaptic ribbons in the adjacent cytoplasm of the hair cell, but, in places, pre- and postsynaptic membranes are separated by a space of only 5 nm. In the type II hair cell, there are numerous, separate boutons, believed to be efferent in nature. Similar boutons also contact the nerve terminals of type I cells.

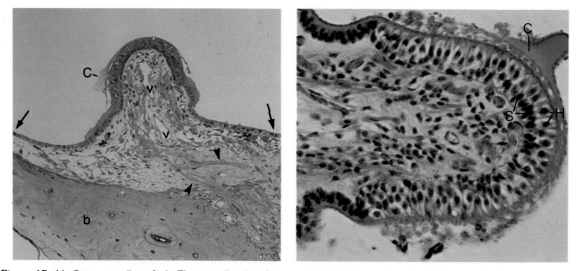

**Figure 17–44.** *Crista ampullaris.* Left: *The ampulla of each semicircular canal contains a crista (crest) lying transversely across the long axis of the canal, here cut transversely. The lining of the membranous semicircular canal itself is of squamous or low cuboidal epithelium (arrows) supported by thin connective tissue. In the crista is a core of connective tissue containing blood vessels (v) and nerves (arrowheads), branches of the vestibular portion of the eighth cranial nerve. At the base of the crista, the lining epithelium changes to a sensory neuroepithelium covered by the gelatinous, homogeneous cupula (C). Below is bone (b) of the surrounding bony labyrinth. Methylene blue, azure A, basic fuchsin. Medium power.* Right: *The complex neuroepithelium of the crista contains sustentacular cells (S), tall and slender with nuclei near the basal lamina, and sensory hair cells (H) with more peripheral nuclei, flask-shaped and with apical hair-like processes extending into the gelatinous cupula (C). In fact, two types of hair cells are present but not distinguishable here. H and E. High power.*

*Sustentacular cells* are tall columnar cells, lying between and around hair cells, and are of irregular shape. Their nuclei are basal in position, and they have a well-developed cytoskeleton of microtu-bules and contain some granules that may be secretory.

In maculae, the hairs are covered by a surface gelatinous layer, the *otolithic membrane*, formed

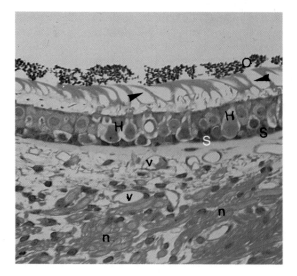

**Figure 17–45.** *Macula. Like cristae, maculae of utricle and saccule show sustentacular and hair cells. The sustentacular cells (S) are tall columnar and darkly staining, with basal nuclei and apical microvilli. Hair (sensory) cells (H) are of two types. Type I is pyriform, type II is cylindrical, the two types poorly distinguished here but both with pale-staining cytoplasm and large, vesicular, spherical nuclei. Apically, both have a sensory hair bundle (arrowheads) formed by a single cilium (kinocilium) and 30 to 100 stereocilia. These hair bundles pass into the overlying otolithic membrane (O), a gelatinous membrane containing numerous crystalline bodies, the otoconia or otoliths, here stained dark purple. In the connective tissue beneath the neuroepithelium are numerous blood vessels (v) and nerve fibers (n) of the vestibular nerve. Methylene blue, azure A, basic fuchsin. Medium power.*

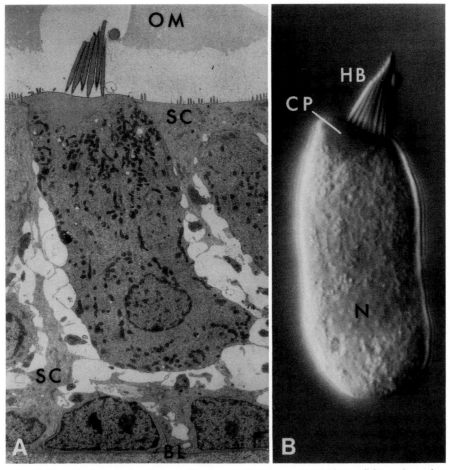

*Figure 17–46.* Hair cell. Left, A: *This section of the bullfrog's sacculus shows a typical hair cell (center) on electron microscopy with adjacent supporting cells (SC) all lying on the basal lamina (BL). From the hair cell, the hair bundle extends to contact the otolithic membrane (OM). Right, B: This light micrograph is of a living hair cell enzymatically isolated from the sacculus. The cell body is cylindrical with a basal nucleus (N) below which there are afferent and efferent synaptic contacts (not seen here). The hair bundle (HB) protrudes from the cuticular plate (CP) at the apex of the cell.* × 2300. *(Courtesy of Dr. A. J. Hudspeth and reproduced by permission from Science, volume 230, 15 November 1985, pp. 745–752. Copyright 1985 by the AAAS.)*

by a jelly-like glycoprotein material in which are suspended minute (3 to 5 μm) crystalline bodies composed of a complex of calcium carbonate and a protein. These bodies are called *otoliths.*

In cristae, hairs are covered by *cupulae,* composed of a gelatinous material similar to the otolithic membrane but lacking otoliths.

Functionally, it is believed that change in position of the head causes changes in pressure or tension in the otolithic membrane with stimulation of the hair cells of the maculae. In cristae ampul-

lares, movement of endolymph follows angular accelerations of the head, causing movement of hairs and their consequent stimulation.

## COCHLEA

The osseous cochlea spirals for 2¾ turns around the modiolus from which projects the spiral lamina (Fig. 17–47). The cavity of the spiral canal is divided into three by two membranes. The *basilar membrane* extends from the spiral

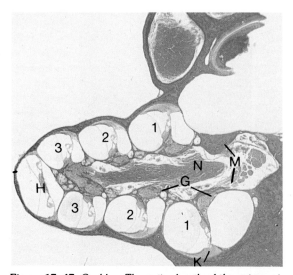

*Figure 17–47. Cochlea. The entire length of the guinea pig cochlea is seen with the apex, or helicotrema (H), to the left. The axial stem, or modiolus (M), contains the auditory (cochlear) nerve (N) with profiles of the spiral ganglion (G) associated with the spiral turns (1, 2, and 3) of the cochlea around the modiolus. The basal turn (1) is of greater diameter. In each turn, the thin basilar membrane extends outward from the region of the spiral ganglion to a thickening of the periosteum (K) called the spiral ligament, with a second thin (vestibular) membrane also crossing the cavity so that each turn is divided into three cavities—the scala vestibuli above the vestibular membrane (to the left), the scala tympani below the basilar membrane (to the right) (these two containing perilymph), and the cochlear duct centrally between the two membranes (and containing endolymph). The organ of Corti lies on the basilar membrane in the cochlear duct. H and E. Low power.*

lamina to the outer wall of the cochlea, where the cochlear periosteum is thickened as the *spiral ligament.* The *vestibular (Reissner's) membrane* passes between the spiral lamina and the outer wall above this. Thus, there are three cavities: the *scala vestibuli* above, the *scala tympani* below, and the *cochlear duct* between the two. The two scalae are filled with perilymph, and their walls consist of connective tissue blending externally with periosteum. The perilymph of the scala vestibuli is continuous with that of the vestibule and reaches the inner surface of the fenestra ovalis, while the scala tympani at its base reaches the fenestra rotunda and the secondary tympanic membrane, which separates it from the tympanic cavity. The two scalae at the apex of the cochlea are in communication by a narrow canal termed the *helicotrema.* Thus, as a sound wave reaches the fenestra ovalis, it ''compresses'' perilymph in

the scala vestibuli, the wave of compression passes to the apex of the cochlea in the scala vestibuli, traverses the helicotrema, and returns down the scala tympani to reach the secondary tympanic membrane at the fenestra rotunda, this acting as the safety valve. The wave of compression also can pass directly between scala vestibuli and scala tympani, crossing the vestibular and basilar membranes and the cochlear duct.

The cochlear duct connects with the saccule via the ductus reuniens but terminates blindly near the helicotrema as the *cecum cupulare.*

The *spiral ganglion* lies incompletely surrounded by bone at the junction of modiolus and osseous spiral lamina (see Fig. 17–50). From its entire length, bundles of nerve fibers perforate bone of the spiral lamina to reach the organ of Corti, situated in the cochlear duct on the basilar membrane. The periosteum of the spiral lamina is thickened as the *limbus spiralis* and bulges into the cochlear duct.

### COCHLEAR DUCT

The epithelium of the cochlear duct varies with location. Over the vestibular membrane it is squamous, higher and irregular over the limbus, and laterally is low columnar with an underlying connective tissue that contains many capillaries. This is termed the *stria vascularis,* believed to be the site of secretion of endolymph. Over the basilar membrane, the epithelium is highly specialized as the organ of Corti.

### ORGAN OF CORTI

As in other sensory areas, the organ of Corti comprises supporting and hair cells (Figs. 17–48 and 17–49).

Most of the supporting cells are tall and columnar, but several groups are described. Extending the full length of the cochlea is a tunnel that is triangular in cross section. Its base is the basilar membrane, and it is bounded medially and laterally by the inner and outer pillar cells. The *inner pillar cell* is a narrow cone shape with a broad base, containing the nucleus and lying on the basilar membrane, and a slender apex that overlies an outer pillar cell. The *outer pillar cell* is longer but of similar shape, with an expanded apex fitting into a depression on the undersurface

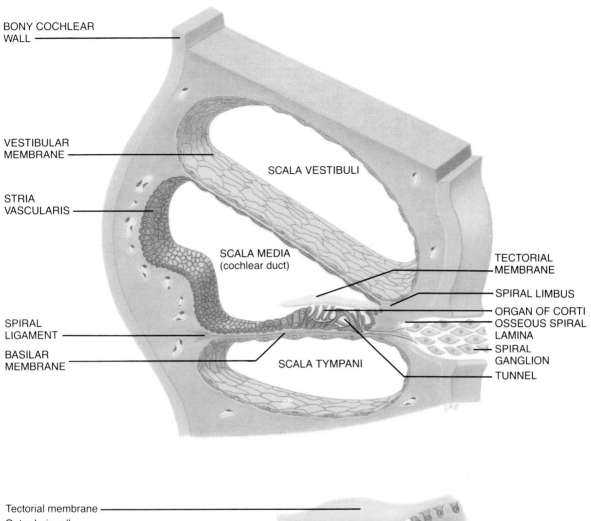

BONY COCHLEAR WALL

VESTIBULAR MEMBRANE

SCALA VESTIBULI

STRIA VASCULARIS

SCALA MEDIA (cochlear duct)

TECTORIAL MEMBRANE

SPIRAL LIMBUS

ORGAN OF CORTI

OSSEOUS SPIRAL LAMINA

SPIRAL LIGAMENT

SPIRAL GANGLION

BASILAR MEMBRANE

SCALA TYMPANI

TUNNEL

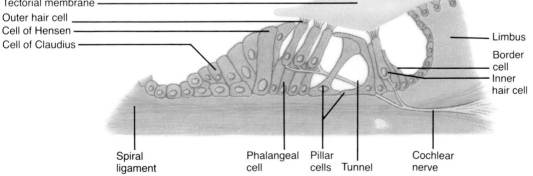

Tectorial membrane
Outer hair cell
Cell of Hensen
Cell of Claudius

Limbus

Border cell

Inner hair cell

Spiral ligament

Phalangeal cell

Pillar cells

Tunnel

Cochlear nerve

*Figure 17–48.* Cochlea, organ of Corti. Top: *This diagram shows one turn of the cochlea with its surrounding bone. The scala vestibuli and the scala tympani are lined by simple squamous epithelium (blue) and filled with perilymph. Centrally, the cochlear duct is limited by the vestibular membrane above and the basilar membrane (dark green), the latter passing from the spiral lamina to the outer wall where cochlear periosteum is thickened as the spiral ligament. The epithelium lining the cochlear duct is thickened laterally with numerous capillaries in the underlying connective tissue. This is the stria vascularis, believed to be the site of formation of endolymph. On the basilar membrane, it is highly specialized as the organ of Corti, covered by the tectorial membrane (pink) extending from a thickening of the spiral lamina called the limbus spiralis (spiral limbus). The spiral ganglion lies medially. Bottom: A diagram illustrating the cell types in the organ of Corti.*

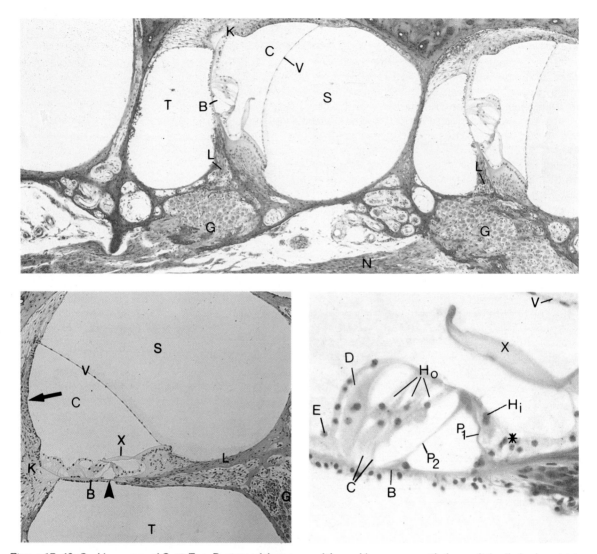

**Figure 17–49.** *Cochlea, organ of Corti. Top: Portions of three turns of the cochlea are seen with the modiolus (below) containing the cochlea nerve (N) and profiles of the spiral ganglia (G). The spiral lamina (L) projects like the thread of a screw from the modiolus, and attached to it is the basilar membrane (B) that passes outward to the spiral ligament (K), a thickening of the periosteum of the outer wall. The thinner vestibular membrane (V) passes from the spiral lamina to the outer wall. The two membranes divide each turn of the cochlea into scala vestibuli (S) and scala tympani (T) (filled with perilymph) and cochlear duct (C) filled with endolymph. The organ of Corti lies upon the basilar membrane. H and E. Low power. Bottom: Two illustrations of the organ of Corti. At left, the cochlear duct lies between the scala vestibuli (S) and scala tympani (T) with vestibular (V) and basilar (B) membranes. Laterally is the spiral ligament (K) and the stria vascularis (arrow). Medially is the spiral lamina (L), with part of the spiral ganglion (G). The organ of Corti shows the central tunnel of triangular outline (arrowhead) with the tectorial membrane (X) above it. High power. With oil immersion (right), part of the cochlear duct lies between vestibular (V) and basilar (B) membranes, and on the latter are inner ($P_1$) and outer ($P_2$) pillar cells surrounding the tunnel with nuclei of a single row of inner ($H_i$) and three rows of outer ($H_o$) hair cells. Other cell types seen are border cells (asterisk), phalangeal cells (C), and cells of Hensen (D) and Claudius (E). The tectorial membrane (X) is artificially raised from the hair cells. H and E. Left, high power; right, oil immersion.*

of the head of an inner pillar cell. The inner pillar cells outnumber the outer pillar cells by a ratio of approximately 3 to 2.

Adjacent to the pillar cells are the inner and outer *phalangeal* cells (of Deiters). The inner cells form a single row that surrounds the inner hair cells. The outer phalangeal cells support the three or four rows of outer hair cells. They are columnar, with their bases on the basilar membrane, but apically they do not reach the surface and leave the upper two thirds of the outer hair cells exposed. Internally, there is a row of border cells that lie on the basilar membrane between the inner phalangeal cells and the limbus, and externally there are elongated, polygonal cells arranged in more than one layer and decreasing in height. These are the cells of Hensen and of Claudius.

The *hair cells* of the organ of Corti lie as a single inner row between the inner pillar cells and inner phalangeal cells, with three rows of outer hair cells between the outer pillar cells and outer phalangeal cells. Inner hair cells are similar to type I hair cells of the vestibular labyrinth. They are short and goblet-shaped, with nuclei lying in expanded bases and with a more slender neck. Apically, they bear 50 to 60 hairs or stereocilia arranged in a U or W. They lack a kinocilium. Outer hair cells are different and, thus, may have a different function. Apical hairs are more numerous, up to 100, and of uneven length. The synaptic contacts of inner hair cells are with the cochlear nerve with pre- and postsynaptic membrane thickenings and synaptic ribbons. The synaptic contacts cover the base of the cell up to the nuclear area, and the cell also receives vesiculated efferent endings. The basal parts of outer hair cells receive both afferent and efferent nerve fibers, the latter being larger.

The surface of the organ of Corti is covered by a ribbon of gelatinous material termed the *tectorial membrane*. It is formed by a protein, and numerous fibrils can be demonstrated within it. Recent evidence suggests that the tips of the hairs are embedded in it, although most preparations show a space between the two that, thus, may be artifactual.

## SPIRAL GANGLION

This ganglion spirals around the modiolus, partially surrounded by bone of the modiolus and

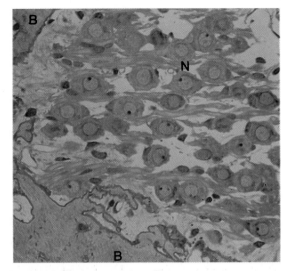

**Figure 17–50.** *Spiral ganglion. The spiral ganglion lies at the junction of the modiolus and the osseous spiral lamina, incompletely surrounded by bone (B). It is formed by bipolar nerve cells (the shape well seen in the cell labeled "N") with their peripheral processes (dendrites) passing to hair cells of the organ of Corti and their central processes (axons) forming the cochlear nerve. Methylene blue, azure A, basic fuchsin. Medium power.*

the spiral lamina (Fig. 17–50). It is formed by bipolar neurons, the central myelinated processes (axons) of which run together to form the acoustic nerve. The peripheral dendrites also are myelinated but lose their sheaths as they perforate bone and pass to the organ of Corti, terminating around hair cells.

In addition to its cochlear division, the eighth (acoustic) cranial nerve also has a vestibular division that supplies the remainder of the labyrinth. Its ganglion lies in the internal auditory meatus, its axons running with the cochlear division. Peripheral dendrites pass to three cristae ampullares and to the maculae of utricle and saccule.

### Functional Summary

Sound waves picked up by the external ear are converted to vibrations at the tympanic membrane, and these vibrations then are transmitted through the chain of middle ear ossicles to the fenestra ovalis, and thence to the perilymph of the vestibule. This sets up pressure waves in the

## Summary Table 17–1. The Eye

| Coat | Part | Structure | Function |
|---|---|---|---|
| Fibrous | Sclera | Dense fibrous tissue | Opaque, provides form and rigidity and attachment for muscles |
| | Cornea | Dense, regular fibrous tissue with anterior epithelium and posterior endothelium. Avascular | Transparent, refracts light |
| Uveal | Choroid | Highly vascular, with melanocytes | Nutrient, absorbs light |
| | Ciliary body | Smooth muscle, melanocytes, vessels, plus non-neural retina | Accommodation. Aqueous humor formation |
| | Iris | Vessels, muscle, pigment cells, plus non-neural retina | Diaphragm, varying pupil diameter, reducing light |
| | Lens | Lens fibers with capsule and epithelium. Avascular | Transparent, focuses image on retina |
| Retina | Pigment epithelium | | Phagocytic, absorbs light, nutrition; stores vitamin A |
| | Rods | First neurons, modified | Low light vision |
| | Cones | First neurons, modified | Diurnal, color vision. Greatest acuity |
| | Bipolar cells | Second neuron | Conducting |
| | Ganglion cells | Third neuron | Form optic nerve |

## Summary Table 17–2. The Ear

| Division | Part | Structure* | Function |
|---|---|---|---|
| External | Auricle | Elastic cartilage covered by skin | Collects sound waves |
| | External auditory meatus | Elastic cartilage (⅓) plus bone (⅔), thin skin with glands and hairs | Conducts sound waves |
| | Tympanic membrane | Modified skin, connective tissue, cuboidal epithelium | Sound waves cause vibrations |
| Middle | Tympanic cavity | Lining of simple cuboidal epithelium. Traversed by malleus, incus, and stapes | Transmits vibrations to internal ear |
| | Auditory tube | Bone (⅓), elastic cartilage (⅔), ciliated (pseudostratified) columnar epithelium | Equalize pressure on tympanum |
| Inner | Osseous labyrinth | Bone with periosteum. Vestibule, three semicircular canals, and cochlea. Filled with perilymph | Houses sense organs |
| | Membranous labyrinth | Filled with endolymph | |
| | | Organ of Corti, in cochlear duct between scalae vestibuli and tympani. | Hearing |
| | | Semicircular canals with cristae. Utricle and saccule with maculae | Vestibular, balance and position |

*All sensory areas—organ of Corti, cristae, and maculae—have hair cells and supporting cells with overlying tectorial membrane (Corti), cupula (cristae), or otolithic membrane (maculae).

perilymph of the scala vestibuli that pass, first, through the vestibular membrane in its floor to endolymph in the cochlear duct, and then across the basilar membrane to perilymph of the scala tympani. The waves finally are dissipated at the round window. The passage of sound waves from scala vestibuli to scala tympani across the cochlear duct causes the basilar membrane to oscillate, different regions oscillating at different frequencies. The oscillation causes shearing forces between the tectorial membrane and the hairs of the hair cells, with depolarization of the cells and resultant afferent impulses in the cochlea nerve, which pass to the auditory cortex.

# INDEX

Note: Numbers in *italics* refer to illustrations; numbers followed by (t) refer to tables.